Tenth Edition

KINESIOLOGY
Scientific Basis of Human Motion

Nancy Hamilton, Ph.D.
Associate Professor, University of Northern Iowa

Kathryn Luttgens, Ph.D.
Professor Emerita, Northeastern University

Boston   Burr Ridge, IL   Dubuque, IA   Madison, WI   New York   San Francisco   St. Louis
Bangkok   Bogotá   Caracas   Kuala Lumpur   Lisbon   London   Madrid   Mexico City
Milan   Montreal   New Delhi   Santiago   Seoul   Singapore   Sydney   Taipei   Toronto

McGraw-Hill Higher Education

A Division of The **McGraw-Hill** Companies

KINESIOLOGY: SCIENTIFIC BASIS OF HUMAN MOTION
TENTH EDITION

Published by McGraw-Hill, a business unit of The McGraw-Hill Companies, Inc., 1221 Avenue of the Americas, New York, NY 10020. Copyright © 2002, 1997, 1992, 1982 by The McGraw-Hill Companies, Inc. All rights reserved. No part of this publication may be reproduced or distributed in any form or by any means, or stored in a database or retrieval system, without the prior written consent of The McGraw-Hill Companies, Inc., including, but not limited to, in any network or other electronic storage or transmission, or broadcast for distance learning.

Some ancillaries, including electronic and print components, may not be available to customers outside the United States.

This book is printed on acid-free paper.

5 6 7 8 9 0 DOC/DOC 0 9 8 7 6 5

ISBN 0-07-232919-X
ISBN 0-07-112243-5 (ISE)

Vice president and editor-in-chief: *Thalia Dorwick*
Executive editor: *Vicki Malinee*
Senior developmental editor: *Michelle Turenne*
Senior marketing manager: *Pamela S. Cooper*
Project manager: *Mary Lee Harms*
Production supervisor: *Enboge Chong*
Coordinator of freelance design: *Rick D. Noel*
Cover designer: *Jamie A. O'Neal*
Cover image: © *Imagedrome, Inc.*
Senior photo research coordinator: *Lori Hancock*
Senior supplement producer: *David A. Welsh*
Media technology producer: *Judi David*
Compositor: *Shepherd, Inc.*
Typeface: *10/12 Times Roman*
Printer: *R. R. Donnelley & Sons Company/Crawfordsville, IN*

Library of Congress Cataloging-in-Publication Data

Hamilton, Nancy (Nancy Patricia), 1946– .
   Kinesiology : scientific basis of human motion / Nancy Hamilton, Kathryn Luttgens. — 10th ed.
    p. cm.
   On the previous ed. Luttgens appears first.
   Includes bibliographical references and index.
   ISBN 0-07-232919-X — ISBN 0-07-112243-5
   1. Kinesiology. I. Luttgens, Kathryn, 1926– . II. Title.

QP303 .L87 2002
612.7'6—dc21   2001030368
                                                  CIP

INTERNATIONAL EDITION ISBN 0-07-112243-5
Copyright © 2002. Exclusive rights by The McGraw-Hill Companies, Inc., for manufacture and export. This book cannot be re-exported from the country to which it is sold by McGraw-Hill. The International Edition is not available in North America.

The Internet addresses listed in the text were accurate at the time of publication. The inclusion of a website does not indicate an endorsement by the authors or McGraw-Hill, and McGraw-Hill does not guarantee the accuracy of the information presented at these sites.

www.mhhe.com

BRIEF CONTENTS

Preface ix

CHAPTER 1

Introduction to the Study of Kinesiology 1

PART I
Anatomical and Physiological
Fundamentals of Human Motion

CHAPTER 2

The Musculoskeletal System: The Skeletal
Framework and Its Movements 21

CHAPTER 3

The Musculoskeletal System:
The Musculature 44

CHAPTER 4

The Neuromuscular Basis
of Human Motion 69

CHAPTER 5

The Upper Extremity:
The Shoulder Region 94

CHAPTER 6

The Upper Extremity: The Elbow,
Forearm, Wrist, and Hand 126

CHAPTER 7

The Lower Extremity: The Hip Region 158

CHAPTER 8

The Lower Extremity: The Knee,
Ankle, and Foot 181

CHAPTER 9

The Spinal Column and Thorax 215

PART II
Fundamentals of Biomechanics

CHAPTER 10

Terminology and Measurement
in Biomechanics 261

CHAPTER   11

The Description of Human Motion 277

CHAPTER   12

The Conditions of Linear Motion 301

CHAPTER   13

The Conditions of Rotary Motion 339

CHAPTER   14

The Center of Gravity and Stability 371

PART III
Motor Skills: Principles
and Applications

CHAPTER   15

The Standing Posture 399

CHAPTER   16

Kinesiology of Fitness and Exercise 412

CHAPTER   17

Moving Objects: Pushing and Pulling 435

CHAPTER   18

Moving Objects: Throwing,
Striking, and Kicking 450

CHAPTER   19

Locomotion: Solid Surface 467

CHAPTER   20

Locomotion: The Aquatic Environment 495

CHAPTER   21

Locomotion: When Suspended
and Free of Support 512

CHAPTER   22

Impact 528

CHAPTER   23

Instrumentation for Motion Analysis 537

Appendices 553

CONTENTS

Preface to the Tenth Edition ix
Preface to the First Edition—1950 (abridged) xiv

CHAPTER 1

Introduction to the Study of Kinesiology 1

The Nature of Kinesiology 2
Components of a Kinesiological Analysis 4
Laboratory Experiences 15

PART I

Anatomical and Physiological
Fundamentals of Human Motion

CHAPTER 2

**The Musculoskeletal System: Skeletal
Framework and Its Movements 21**

The Bones 23
Articulations 25
Orientation of the Body 33
The Fundamental Movements of Major
    Body Segments 38
Analyzing Joint Motions 41
Laboratory Experiences 42

CHAPTER 3

**The Musculoskeletal System:
The Musculature 44**

Skeletal Muscle Structure 45
Skeletal Muscle Function 51
Coordination of the Muscular System 57
Methods of Studying the Actions
    of Muscles 63
Muscular Analysis 66
Laboratory Experiences 66

CHAPTER 4

**The Neuromuscular Basis of Human
Motion 69**

The Nervous System and Basic Nerve
    Structures 70
The Motor Unit 74
Sensory Receptors 75
Reflex Movement 81
Volitional Movement 88
Neuromuscular Analysis 91
Laboratory Experiences 92

CHAPTER 5

The Upper Extremity: The Shoulder Region 94

The Shoulder Girdle (Acromioclavicular
    and Sternoclavicular Articulations) 96

Muscles of the Shoulder Girdle 99
The Shoulder Joint (Glenohumeral
    Articulation) 103
Muscles of the Shoulder Joint 107
Joint and Muscular Analysis of the
    Fundamental Movements of the Arm
    on the Trunk 113
Common Injuries of the Shoulder
    Region 120
Laboratory Experiences 122

CHAPTER 6

**The Upper Extremity: The Elbow, Forearm,
Wrist, and Hand 126**

The Elbow Joint 127
The Radioulnar Joints 130
Muscles of the Elbow and Radioulnar
    Joints 131
Muscular Analysis of the Fundamental
    Movements of the Forearm 135
The Wrist and Hand 136
Muscles of the Wrist and Hand 143
Muscular Analysis of the Fundamental
    Movements of the Wrist, Fingers,
    and Thumb 148
Cooperative Actions Wrist
    and Digits 150
Common Injuries of the Forearm, Elbow,
    Wrist, and Fingers 152
Laboratory Experiences 154

CHAPTER 7

The Lower Extremity: The Hip Region 158

The Pelvic Girdle 159
Relationship of the Pelvis to the Trunk
    and Lower Extremities 163
The Hip Joint 165
Muscles of the Hip Joint 169
Common Injuries of the Thigh, Hip Joint,
    and Pelvis 178
Laboratory Experiences 179

CHAPTER 8

**The Lower Extremity: The Knee, Ankle,
and Foot 181**

The Knee Joint 182
Muscles of the Knee Joint 187
Muscular Analysis of the Fundamental
    Movements of the Leg at the Knee
    Joint 193
The Ankle and the Foot 193
Muscles of the Ankle and Foot 200
Muscular Analysis of the Fundamental
    Movements of the Ankle and Foot (Tarsal
    Joints and Toes) 208
Common Injuries of the Leg, Knee,
    and Ankle 209
Laboratory Experiences 213

CHAPTER 9

The Spinal Column and Thorax 215

Structure and Articulations of the Spinal
    Column 216
Movements of the Spine as a Whole 222
Muscles Operating the Spinal Column 227
Muscular Analysis of the Fundamental
    Movements of the Head and Spine 239
Structure and Articulations of the Thorax 241
Movements of the Thorax 245
Muscles of Respiration 246
Muscular Analysis of Respiration 251
Common Injuries of the Neck, Back,
    and Thorax 252
Laboratory Experiences 253

PART II
Fundamentals of Biomechanics

CHAPTER 10

**Terminology and Measurement
in Biomechanics 261**

Introduction to Terminology 262

Quantities in Biomechanics 263
Vector Analysis 265
Laboratory Experiences 275

CHAPTER 11

The Description of Human Motion 277

Motion 278
Kinematic Description of Motion 284
Laboratory Experiences 299

CHAPTER 12

The Conditions of Linear Motion 301

The Nature of Force 302
Newton's Laws of Motion 311
Forces That Modify Motion 318
Free-Body Diagrams 329
Work, Power, and Energy 331
The Analysis of Linear Motion 335
Laboratory Experiences 336

CHAPTER 13

The Conditions of Rotary Motion 339

Rotary Force 340
The Lever 348
Newton's Laws and Rotational
    Equivalents 358
Centripetal and Centrifugal Forces 365
The Analysis of Rotary Motion 367
Laboratory Experiences 368

CHAPTER 14

The Center of Gravity and Stability 371

Center of Gravity 372
Stability and Equilibrium 374
Finding the Center of Gravity
    in the Human Body 385
Laboratory Experiences 393

P A R T III
**Motor Skills: Principles and
Applications**

CHAPTER 15

The Standing Posture 399

Significance of Posture 400
Support of the Standing Posture 400
Factors Related to the Standing Posture 404
Principles Applied to Posture 406
Postural Adaptations to External Conditions
    and Special Problems 408
Posture Screening 409
Laboratory Experiences 410

CHAPTER 16

Kinesiology of Fitness and Exercise 412

Kinesiology and Exercise Programs 413
Developing Flexibility 413
Exercises for Muscle Strength
    and Endurance 417
Modification of Common Exercises to Fit
    the Progressive Resistance Concept 422
Evaluating Exercises 432
Laboratory Experiences 433

CHAPTER 17

Moving Objects: Pushing and Pulling 435

Pushing and Pulling 436
Principles of Pushing and Pulling
    Motions 437
Push–Pull Applications 439
Analysis of Ergometer Rowing 446
Laboratory Experiences 448

CHAPTER 18

**Moving Objects: Throwing, Striking,
and Kicking 450**

Sequential Movements 451

Principles Relating to Throwing, Striking
and Kicking 456
Examples of Throwing and Striking 460
Laboratory Experiences 465

CHAPTER 19

Locomotion: Solid Surface 467

Locomotion 468
Walking 468
Running 480
Jumping, Hopping, and Leaping 484
Additional Forms of Locomotion 486
Laboratory Experiences 492

CHAPTER 20

Locomotion: The Aquatic Environment 495

Aquatic Locomotion: Swimming 496
Aquatic Locomotion: Rowing, Canoeing,
and Kayaking 506
Laboratory Experiences 510

CHAPTER 21

**Locomotion: When Suspended and Free
of Support 512**

Suspension Activities 513
Nonsupport Activities 521
Laboratory Experiences 527

CHAPTER 22

Impact 528

Meaning of Impact and Its Reception 529
Principles in Receiving Impact 532
Laboratory Experiences 536

CHAPTER 23

Instrumentation for Motion Analysis 537

Instrumentation for Kinematic Analysis 538
Instrumentation for Kinetic Analysis 544
Electromyography 545
Computer Models and Simulation 547
Using Quantitative Analysis 549
Summary 551

APPENDICES

APPENDIX A

Glossary 553

APPENDIX B

**Classification of Joints
and Their Movements 557**

APPENDIX C

Joint Range of Motion 560

APPENDIX D

Muscular Attachments and Nerve Supply 569

APPENDIX E

Mathematics Review 581

APPENDIX F

Table of Trigonometric Functions 586

APPENDIX G

U. S. – Metric Equivalents 588

APPENDIX H

Exercises for Kinesiological Analysis 589

APPENDIX I

Answers to Problems in Part II 608

Index 609

Preface to the Tenth Edition

The tenth edition of *Kinesiology: Scientific Basis of Human Motion,* is dedicated to the memory of Katharine F. Wells, pioneer author and originator of the original version of this text. This edition carries on a proud contribution to the professional literature of human motion study started by Dr. Wells in 1950, and continued with her active participation through the seventh edition. Although much of the content of the current text has changed since that first edition, there remains a significant heritage, which can be traced back to her original work. Through her influence, she helped define and structure the teaching and study of kinesiology for many generations of students. The authors of this tenth edition are honored to be the current stewards for this classic text.

Since the publication of the first edition of this text, courses in kinesiology have undergone many changes in both content and emphasis. Each subsequent edition has reflected these changes, and the tenth edition is no exception. The primary goals of this revision has been to update and expand the material where appropriate and to strengthen the textbook as a pedagogical tool. Several of the chapters have been expanded and updated in light of current research. The resultant content makes this a book ideally suited to help students achieve an understanding of the in-tegrated nature of kinesiology as an area of study that includes both anatomical and biomechanical components.

AUDIENCE

Moving into the twenty-first century, the traditional course often titled kinesiology has been separated into courses in anatomy and biomechanics. This text attempts to integrate the anatomy of human movement with the mechanics of human movement. It is neither an anatomy text nor a biomechanics text, but is an intergrated kinesiology text. The textbook is designed as a basic source to introduce the undergraduate student to the fundamentals of kinesiology. Because the fundamentals are presented without compromise of basic theory, this book may be used as an introductory text. The book presents the subject in a fashion that presupposes some background in anatomy and little in physics. The text does not shy away from presenting material that requires some theoretical foundations in these areas. Whatever background is needed to understand the various applications is supplied, and numerous examples and exercises are provided. There is extensive discussion of both anatomical and biomechanical fundamentals of human motion and the application of these fundamentals to the analysis of a wide variety of motor skills. For these reasons, the text is especially appropriate for use in courses with these objectives:

1. To afford students the opportunity to learn a systematic approach to the analysis of human motion.
2. To provide information that will help students obtain an understanding of the anatomical and biomechanical fundamentals of human motion.
3. To provide the types of experiences that ask students to apply anatomical and biomechanical analysis to the learning and improvement of a broad spectrum of movement activities.

The organization of the text is as follows: Introduction to the Study of Kinesiology

ORGANIZATION

The **Introduction to the Study of Kinesiology** is a single chapter which sets the stage by presenting a kinesiological analysis model. This chapter is intended to lay the foundation for the remainder of the text. It is here that the student will learn to organize the thought process involved in understanding human movement. It is critical that the study of kinesiology begin here—with a systematic approach to learning.

Part I, Anatomical and Physiological Fundamentals of Human Motion, consists of eight chapters, each beginning with a discussion of the anatomical background essential for understanding human movement followed by the presentation of a systematic approach to kinesiological analysis. The emphasis throughout is on the *relation of anatomical structure to function,* not on anatomy as such. It is assumed throughout this section that the student has acquired a basic knowledge of static anatomy as applied to stationary models, skeletons, and cadavers. The emphasis in this text is the dynamic anatomy of the moving body. Applications of the knowledge of structure to the analysis of human motion are introduced in these early chapters so that the stu-

dent can begin to put theory into practice immediately, rather than wait until the knowledge base is more complete. Additional laboratory experiences have been added to assist with this practice.

Major changes in part I include the early presentation of the analysis model, which is then carried through all subsequent chapters. The laboratory experiences for each of the anatomical chapters have been expanded to offer the student the opportunity to participate in a systematic analysis as new knowledge is gained.

Part II, Fundamentals of Biomechanics, presents the fundamentals of biomechanics as they apply to human movement analysis. The first chapter introduces the student to terminology and to the units of measure used when motion and the forces that cause it are studied. This chapter is followed by chapters in which motion and the forces that cause and modify it are described. The section concludes with a chapter on the center of gravity and stability.

Part II provides an elementary approach to the material without oversimplifying to the point where misconceptions could occur. In many instances the student is shown the "proof" of a principle through experimental examples or mathematical derivation. This approach is used in the belief that greater understanding will result. The reward will be greater comprehension of the reasons "why" optimum movement patterns occur as they do. It should be remembered, however, that the emphasis in a first undergraduate course in kinesiology should be on the development of the qualitative method of analysis. The introduction of the quantitative method, if used, should be limited to understanding fundamental concepts and not for extensive application to analysis of movement patterns.

Part III, Motor Skills, utilizes the kinesiological analysis system which has been developed in concert with the anatomical and mechanical concepts that have been presented. This analysis model forms the basis for the organization of the nine chapters in part III. In each of these chapters the basic principles of anatomy and mechanics are identified and applied to specific motor skills. Sample analyses are also included.

PEDAGOGICAL FEATURES

Helpful pedagogical tools in every chapter assist the learning process. These include outlines, objectives, laboratory experiences, and references and selected readings. Internet resources are provided in selected chapters.

There are nine appendices. These are intended to provide material which supplements the basic concepts presented in the text:

A. Glossary
B. Classification of Joints and Their Movements
C. Joint Range of Motion
D. Muscular Attachments and Nerve Supply
E. Mathematics Review
F. Table of Trigonometric Functions
G. U.S.–Metric Equivalents
H. Exercises for Kinesiological Analysis
I. Answers to Problems in Part II

NEW TO THIS EDITION

The analysis model is presented early in part I and is integrated through the remaining chapters. Analysis examples are updated throughout to help better explain anatomical and biomechanical concepts to undergraduates, including a new discussion of ergometer rowing in Chapter 17.

Laboratory experiences for each of the anatomical chapters have been expanded.

Websites have been added at the ends of chapter 1 and the parts to obtain further information to learn about human movement.

An online lab manual accompanies the tenth edition and provides additional labs and applications.

The *Dynamic Human 2.0* CD-ROM is included with each purchase of a new text, and provides an excellent reference that enables students to comprehend the anatomy within the text through the use of its graphics and animation.

Included with each new book purchase of this text, you will find a passcard allowing you to access *PowerWeb,* a new easy-to-use online resource from McGraw-Hill. *PowerWeb* provides current articles, curriculum-based materials, weekly updates with assessments, informative and timely world news, related web links, research tools, student study tools, interactive tools, and much more!

ANCILLARIES

Instructor's Resource Materials
Instructor's Manual and Test Bank

Provides chapter overviews, key points, sample test questions, a sample term project, and Lab Notes to be used in conjunction with the lab experiences in the text.

MICRO TEST III Computerized Test Bank

Available on Hybrid CD for Windows and Macintosh, the latest version of our computerized testing software is available. This allows you to custom design your own tests, use the expanded test bank, and to add your own testing questions.

Internet Resources
Online Learning Center

http://www.mhhe.com/hamilton

This website offers resources to students and instructors. It includes downloadable ancillaries, Web links, student quizzing, additional information on topics of interest, the online lab manual, and more. Resources for the instructor include:

• Downloadable PowerPoint presentation
• Lecture outlines
• Online lab manual
• Concept summaries

Resources for the student include:

• Flashcards
• Online chapter reviews
• Interactive quizzes

Health and Human Performance Discipline Page

http://www.mhhe.com/hhp
McGraw-Hill's Health and Human Performance Discipline Page provides a wide variety of information for instructors and students—including monthly articles about current issues, monthly articles that celebrate our diversity, text ancillaries, a "how to" guide to technology, study tips, and athletic training exam preparation materials. It includes professional organization, convention, and career information, and also includes information on how to become a McGraw-Hill author. Additional features of the Discipline Page include:

- This Just In: This feature provides information on the latest hot topics, the best Web resources, and more—all updated monthly!
- Faculty Support: Access online course supplements such as lecture outlines and PowerPoint presentations, and create your own course website with PageOut!
- Student Success Center: Find online study guides and other resources to improve your academic performance. Explore scholarship opportunities, and learn how to launch your career!
- Author Arena: Interested in writing a textbook or supplement for the college market? Read the McGraw-Hill proposal guidelines and links to the editorial and marketing teams, and meet and converse with our current authors!

Online Lab Manual

This manual takes many of the laboratory experiences from the text and guides the student through the process of using an experiential approach whether it be experimentation, problem solving, observation, or analysis.

PowerWeb

Included with each new book purchase of this text, you will find a passcard allowing you to access *PowerWeb,* a new easy-to-use online resource from McGraw-Hill. *PowerWeb* provides current articles, curriculum-based materials, weekly updates with assessments, informative and timely world news, related Web links, research tools, student study tools, interactive tools, and much more!

Access to *PowerWeb* also gives you:

- Study tips with self-quizzes.
- Links to related sites.
- Weekly updates.
- Current news.
- A daily newsfeed of related topics.
- Web research guide.
- Access to *Northern Light* providing Internet access to articles from 6300 premium sources not available from any other search engine.

PowerWeb is a password-protected website. Ask your McGraw-Hill sales representative how you can create a student package with *Power-Web!*

PageOut: The Course Website Development Center

PageOut enables you to develop a website for your course. The site includes:

- A course home page.
- An instructor home page.
- A syllabus (interactive, customizable, and includes quizzing, instructor notes, and links to the Online Learning Center).
- Web links.
- Discussions (multiple discussion areas per class).
- An online grade book.
- Student Web pages.
- Design templates.

This program is now available to registered adopters of McGraw-Hill textbooks.

Primis Online

www.mhhe.com/primis/online
Create content-rich textbooks, lab manuals, or readers right from our website. Choose the material you would like to include in your own cus-

tomized book. A Primis e-book is a digital version of the text you created (and is sold directly to students as a downloadable file to their computer, or it may be accessed online by a password). And Primis Online customized books are affordable for students. Visit our website for further information.

Interactive CD-ROM
Visual Resource Library

The Visual Resource Library is a bank of images for use in the classroom and in the accompanying PowerPoint presentation. A slide editor tool allows the user to create customized slide shows.

Dynamic Human CD-ROM

With each purchase of a new text, the *Dynamic Human 2.0* CD-ROM is included providing an excellent reference that enables students to comprehend the anatomy within the text through the use of its graphics and animation.

ACKNOWLEDGMENTS

We would like to thank the following individuals who served as reviewers for their helpful comments and suggestions in revising the text:

Joel A. Bloom   *University of Houston*
Michael Delp   *Texas A&M University*
Ro DiBrezzo   *University of Arkansas at Fayetteville*
Inza L. Fort   *University of Arkansas at Fayetteville*
John Green   *Texas A&M University*
Steve Henderson   *California State University at Chico*
Michael J. Higgins   *University of Delaware*
Michelle Molnar   *Newman University (KS)*
Paul A. Smith   *Huntington College (IN)*
Donald H. Sussman   *Old Dominion University*
Thomas E. Temples   *North Georgia College and State University*

Appreciation is also expressed to the authors and publishers who graciously gave permission to quote passages and reproduce illustrations from their publications. The authors also wish to acknowledge their indebtedness to the generations of students whose stimulus has been a vital reason for the existence of this book. Finally, they would like to express their sincere thanks to the editorial and production staffs of McGraw-Hill for their helpfulness throughout the preparation of the edition.

Nancy Hamilton, *Cedar Falls, Iowa*

Kathryn Luttgens, *Wellesley, Massachusetts*

PREFACE TO THE FIRST EDITION— 1950

This book is intended as a kinesiology text both for the teacher and for the student. It is believed that there is enough material to use it as a text for a full year's course yet, at the same time, by judicious selection of the subject matter, by omission of the supplementary material, and by the substitution of classroom demonstrations for some of the laboratory exercises, the book should serve equally well as a text for a one-semester course in kinesiology. It is left to the discretion of the instructor to select the material that meets his particular needs.

In its original form this textbook was an unpublished handbook–laboratory manual. It was used by the author in her kinesiology classes for three years before it was expanded to its present form. The original manual did not serve as an independent textbook. It was intended to be used as a companion book to a kinesiology or anatomy text. Since this limited its usefulness, however, it was decided to expand it to what is intended as a complete and independent textbook. For those who like to use a single textbook for a course it should suffice. To help the student (and the instructor) in collateral reading, most chapters in this text contain a comprehensive bibliography. In many cases there is also a list of readings which are particularly recommended. These bibliographies and reading lists provide a rich source of information for the inquiring student.

In regard to the value of laboratory exercises and projects as a means of learning, James B. Stroud, in his book *Psychology in Education,* points out that "Effectiveness of instruction is not determined so much by what the teacher does, as by what he leads the pupils to do. . . ." Again, "Perhaps one of the most successful procedures for infusing learning with significance has been the [educational method known as] constructive activities. . . . The activity is thus a means of making learning meaningful and of giving it a purpose." In accord with this point of view numerous laboratory exercises are suggested. In conformity to the same principle, only a few complete analyses of skills are presented, for it is the writer's contention that the students will gain far more from making one complete analysis himself or herself than from reading a dozen or more ready-made analyses.

As a further means of enriching the kinesiology course a number of the chapters include supplementary material in the form of brief descriptions of research projects in the field of anatomy and kinesiology. A few of these were carried out by the author, but the majority were conducted by other investigators and reported in professional journals. The purpose of including this material is to broaden the instructor's background and to provide supplementary reading assignments for advanced students.

It has been the intention of the author to write simply and to use nontechnical terminology whenever this conveyed the meaning as clearly and specifically as technical terms. The latter have been used, however, whenever they served to avoid ambiguity. While it is desirable for the kinesiology students to enlarge their scientific vocabulary, a text which confronts him with a staggering list of new and strange words defeats its purpose. Textbooks should stimulate the curiosity of their readers, not frighten them with a forbidding vocabulary.

The author acknowledges her indebtedness to many individuals without whose help it is doubtful if this book could have been written. She wishes to express her grateful appreciation particularly to Professor C. H. McCloy of the State University of Iowa for his continued guidance, encouragement, and criticism, also for his generous permission to use material from his course in The Mechanical Analysis of Motor Skills, and to the students in her kinesiology classes of the last three years who served patiently as "guinea pigs" and who made many constructive suggestions concerning the laboratory exercises.

For the illustrations, which add immeasurably to the usefulness of the text, grateful acknowledgment is made to Miss Mildred Codding, who made the anatomic drawings.

The author is under obligation to a number of individuals for the use of photographs and to several publishers for permission to reproduce copyrighted materials. To all writers and teachers from whom the author, either wittingly or unwittingly, has derived ideas which have provided the necessary background for the writing of this book she humbly acknowledges her indebtedness.

Katharine F. Wells
1950

1

INTRODUCTION TO THE STUDY OF KINESIOLOGY

O U T L I N E

- *The Nature of Kinesiology*
  Reasons for Study
  Methods of Study
- *Components of a Kinesiological Analysis*
  Description of the Motor Skill
  Anatomical Analysis
  Mechanical Analysis
  Prescription for Improvement
    of Performance
- *Laboratory Experiences*

O B J E C T I V E S

At the conclusion of this chapter, the student should be able to:

1. Define kinesiology and explain its importance to the student of human motion.
2. Describe the major components of a kinesiological analysis.
3. Prepare a description of a selected motor skill, breaking it down into component phases and identifying starting and ending points.
4. Determine the simultaneous-sequential nature of a variety of movement skills.
5. Classify motor skills using the classification system presented.
6. State the mechanical purpose of a variety of movement skills.
7. Utilize methods of observation and palpation to identify the joints and basic muscle groups active in a movement skill.

THE NATURE OF KINESIOLOGY

Kinesiology, as it is known in physical education, athletic training, physical therapy, orthopedics, and physical medicine, is the study of human movement from the point of view of the physical sciences. The study of the human body as a machine for the performance of work has its foundations in three major areas of study—namely, mechanics, anatomy, and physiology; more specifically, biomechanics, musculoskeletal anatomy, and neuromuscular physiology. The accumulated knowledge of these three fields forms the foundation for the study of human movement.

Some authorities refer to kinesiology as a science in its own right; others claim that it should be called a study rather than a true science because the principles on which it is based are derived from basic sciences such as anatomy, physiology, and physics. In any event, its unique contribution is that it selects from many sciences those principles that are pertinent to human motion and systematizes their application. However it may be categorized, to the inquiring student it is a door opening into a whole new world of discovery and appreciation. Human motion, which most of us have taken for granted all our lives, is seen through new eyes. One who gives it any thought whatever cannot help being impressed not only by the beauty of human motion but also by its apparently infinite possibilities, its meaningfulness, its orderliness, its adaptability to the surrounding environment. Nothing is haphazard; nothing is left to chance. Every structure that participates in the movements of the body does so according to physical and physiological principles. The student of kinesiology, like the student of anatomy, physiology, psychology, genetics, and other biological sciences, can only look with wonder at the intricate mechanism of the body.

Reasons for Study

Kinesiology is not studied merely to incite our interest in a fascinating and mysterious subject. It has a useful purpose. We study kinesiology to improve performance by learning how to analyze the movements of the human body and to discover their underlying principles. The study of kinesiology is an essential part of the educational experience of students of physical education, dance, sport, and physical medicine. Knowledge of kinesiology has a threefold purpose for practitioners in any of these fields. It should enable them to help their students or clients perform with optimum *safety, effectiveness,* and *efficiency.* Safety is becoming a greater concern of all movement professionals. It is imperative to structure the movements that students or clients do in such a way as to avoid doing harm to the body. At the same time, both the educator and the therapist set goals for effective performance. We judge the effectiveness of a performance by success or failure in meeting those goals. And in producing an effective performance, the movement specialist also strives with the student or client to achieve the movement goal with the least amount of effort, as efficiently as possible. *Safety, effectiveness,* and *efficiency,* then, are the underlying aims in all of our uses of kinesiology for the analysis and modification of human movement.

In the early days of physical education, when few activities were taught other than gymnastics and dance, the content of a course in kinesiology was confined chiefly to functional anatomy. Gradually, as sports and dance assumed a more important place in the curriculum, the concept of kinesiology was broadened to include the study of the mechanical principles that apply to the techniques used in sport, dance, and leisure activities. The principles were applied not only to the movements of the body itself but also to the movements of the implements, balls, and other equipment. In like manner, the development of the kinesiology course in schools of physical therapy and occupational therapy has kept pace with the development of their expanded curricula. Having started as "muscle reeducation," kinesiology has come to include the application of mechanical principles to postural adjustments, to the gait, to the use of tools and household implements, and to the wide variety of technological workstations that are commonplace in today's computerized world. Kinesiology is also frequently used by therapists in the modification of vocational and homemaking activities necessitated by limitations in neuromuscular capacity and skeletal structure.

Kinesiology helps prepare physical educators, coaches, and fitness professionals to teach effective performance in both fundamental and specialized motor skills. Furthermore, it enables them to evaluate exercises and activities from the point of view of their effect on the human structure. The human body improves with use (within limits), *provided it is used in accordance with the principles of efficient human motion.* The function of kinesiology in physical education, therefore, is to contribute not only to *successful participation* in various physical activities but also to the *improvement of* the human structure through the intelligent selection of activities and the efficient use of the body.

The physical or occupational therapist and the athletic trainer are primarily concerned with the effect that exercises and other techniques of physical medicine have on the body. He or she is concerned particularly with the restoration of impaired function and with methods of compensating for lost function. Although effective performance remains a primary goal, to the therapist "effective performance" refers not so much to *skillful* performance in athletic activities as to *adequate* performance in the activities associated with daily living. Whereas the educator applies knowledge of kinesiology chiefly to the movements of the normal body, the therapist is concerned with the movements of a body that has suffered an impairment in function.

Methods of Study

Once the study of kinesiology is begun, one of the most satisfactory ways of proceeding is by supplementing book study with laboratory experimentation. It is a truism that we learn best by doing. Laboratory experiences should include two types of activity. The first type consists of experiments performed under controlled conditions. Activities in this category are selected to help the student gain insight into and understand the nature and complexity of human motion. Although the emphasis is primarily on qualitative analysis in beginning study, some quantification of data is appropriate, as is the use of "laboratory-type" instruments. Especially helpful is the videotape recorder, whose use enables the careful and prolonged study of a very small moment in the performance of a technique and permits the observation of detail unavailable to the naked eye. In more advanced study, the use of advanced measurement methodology and more advanced electronic equipment such as electromyography, force sensing instruments, and computer simulation are common. As these technologies become more sophisticated so does the ability to use them increase the depth of our knowledge and understanding of human motion.

The second type of laboratory experience should consist of practice in analysis under the conditions that exist every day in the gymnasium or clinic. Only through practice under these conditions will the student learn how to apply a knowledge of kinesiology and develop the qualitative skills necessary for accurate observation, diagnosis, and treatment of faulty motor performance.

Whatever method of teaching or study is employed, it is well for the student to keep in mind the aims of kinesiology study and the intended applications for what will be learned. The analysis of motion is not an end in itself but rather a means to the learning of new movement patterns and improving the safety, effectiveness, and efficiency of old ones. This is as true for the physical therapist teaching amputees and paraplegics to walk again as it is for the physical educator teaching a sport technique. Finally, it must be remembered that the skill itself is of less importance than the one who practices it. Kinesiology serves only half its purpose when it provides information of value for learning or teaching motor skills. It must also serve to lay the foundation for perfecting, repairing, and keeping in good condition that incomparable mechanism—the human body.

COMPONENTS OF A KINESIOLOGICAL ANALYSIS

In any formal field of study, the task of analysis must proceed along a logical and structured plan. This plan must be constructed so that it is both appropriate to the activity and can be readily applied by the practitioner. The teacher, therapist, trainer, athlete, and coach all benefit from knowing how to conduct a kinesiological analysis of a motor skill. The teaching of motor skills, whether it takes place in the clinic, in the fitness club, or on the playing field, consists of presenting a skill and knowing what points to emphasize. It also largely consists of diagnosing difficulties, correcting errors, and eliminating actions that limit performance. The specialist in motor skills must also be aware of the types of injuries that are likely to occur during a particular activity and how to prevent them. To accurately prescribe the movements necessary for rehabilitation, the therapist or trainer must know joint structure and exercise tolerances. An athlete in training must understand the kinesiological factors involved in performance to optimize training effects while guarding against deleterious actions. These tasks that, on the surface, may seem simple can indeed be quite complex, if for no other reason than that motor skills themselves are complex. An effective aid in helping one understand the basic elements and requirements of a motor skill is a systematic kinesiological analysis.

The tools needed for the execution of a detailed kinesiological analysis will be introduced in subsequent chapters. The anatomical components of human movements—the bones, joints, muscles, and related portions of the nervous system—and the mechanical bases for human motion will be presented. The basic movements of the body segments will be described, and it will be shown how the observation of both anatomical and mechanical principles contributes to the efficient use of the body in the performance of motor skills. A kinesiological analysis is the application of this information to assessing the effectiveness of a given motor performance. It consists of

1. *describing* a skill in a logical and systematic fashion by breaking it down into its constituent elements;
2. *evaluating* the performance of the skill by determining whether and how the related anatomical and mechanical principles have been violated; and
3. *prescribing* corrections based on an appropriate identification of the cause or causes.

The basic components for the kinesiological analysis of a motor skill are outlined in table 1.1. In this type of analysis the emphasis is on a qualitative assessment of the performance, which may

TABLE 1.1	Outline for a Kinesiological Analysis

A. Description of the motor skill performance
   1. Primary purpose of the skill
   2. Movement phases
   3. Classification of the skill
   4. Simultaneous-sequential nature of the motion
B. Anatomical analysis
   1. Joint actions and segment motions
   2. Muscle participation and form of contraction
   3. Neuromuscular considerations
   4. Anatomical principles related to effective and safe performance
C. Mechanical analysis
   1. Underlying mechanics objective(s)
   2. Nature of forces causing or impeding motion
   3. Mechanical principles that apply
   4. Violation of principles
      a. Which application(s) of mechanical principles is (are) violated?
      b. What are the errors?
      c. What are the sources of error?
D. Prescriptions for improvement of performance indicate how the performance should be changed so that the principles are no longer violated.

be conducted with the assistance of videotapes, motion pictures, or the naked eye. In any case the analyst must use a systematic approach in the observation of the performance. Have someone demonstrate the movement to be analyzed both before and at frequent intervals throughout the analysis. In lieu of this, motion pictures (preferably slow-motion videos shown on a playback unit that can be stopped at will) are an excellent substitute. If these are not available, a series of still shots or even a single photograph or sketch is helpful. In the initial stages of learning analysis procedures, movement may appear rapid and confusing. With the aid of slow-motion equipment and with much practice, the analyst will gain the skills required for an accurate and systematic approach to observation.

Description of the Motor Skill

The description of the motor skill being analyzed consists of four elements that together help the analyst focus on the essential nature of the skill.

Primary Purpose of a Motor Skill

The first step in the description phase of the analysis is to identify the primary purpose of the movement. Without a clear understanding of why the movement is being performed, it is virtually impossible to evaluate its effectiveness. In this statement of purpose, applicable references to speed, accuracy, form, and distance should be included. For example, the purpose of the 50-meter backstroke is to cover the course in the shortest amount of time. Speed is a major factor. The purpose of swinging an ax is to split a piece of wood. Both speed and accuracy are critical elements if the wood is to be safely split into kindling. The purpose of the springboard dive is to execute the motion according to a prescribed form. Neither speed nor accuracy is stressed; success is measured on appearance alone. The purpose of putting in golf is to sink the ball into the cup from a relatively short distance away. The prime determinant of success in putting is accuracy (figure 1.1).

Movement Phases

It is often beneficial to break down a motion into separate parts, or "phases." Often these phases are fairly obvious, based on the motion. For example, a throw has a windup phase, a throwing phase where the arm comes forward, and a follow-through phase after release (figure 1.2). In some skills, the phases are not as obvious, but to make the analysis manageable, some sort of division should be made.

It is critical that the appropriate starting and ending points for each phase be identified. Two primary factors must be considered in the choice of starting point. The first factor is to consider *when* in the motion the analysis should begin. Many movement skills are discrete, that is, they have a very definite beginning and ending. In such movements the starting point for analysis is fairly obvious—at the beginning of the first phase—as in a throwing skill, which starts with the windup. Other skills are more continuous in nature, either because they are done in a repetitive manner or because one movement flows immediately into the next. Walking is a good example of a cyclical skill, whereas many team sports include movements that change constantly. In a continuous movement situation, the analyst must carefully choose a starting point that will give adequate information about the movement of interest while not ignoring the resultant effects of the previous movement. In walking, many analysts start the first phase of the analysis as the toe leaves the ground and end the last phase when that same toe is about to leave the ground in the next step cycle; others start the phase as the heel strikes the floor and end with the subsequent heel strike.

Classification of the Motor Skills

Motor skills take many forms and are used for many purposes. The therapist is interested in using physical skills and exercise to rehabilitate individuals for independent living or work; the teacher uses motor skills for health, learning, and play; the athlete and coach strive to produce

Figure 1.1   Examples of the primary purpose of a motion: (a) maximum speed; (b) following a prescribed pattern; (c) optimum speed and accuracy; (d) maximum accuracy.

near-perfect performance. Each practitioner requires an understanding of the body and mechanical laws that govern motion. A classification scheme is important because it permits the variety of potential movement skills to be organized into a manageable grouping. This manner of organization facilitates the recognition of commonalities across movements. It also fosters increased understanding by enabling one to focus on either differences or similarities in movement patterns, as the situation demands. Classification of move-

ment patterns and skills provides further clues as to the nature of both the anatomical and mechanical requirements of a particular group of skills.

The following system for classifying motor skills takes into account the objective of the skill, the medium in which the skill occurs, and the nature of the motion.

System for Classification of Motor Skills

I. Maintaining erect posture

II. Movement for exercise and fitness

a.   b.   c.

Figure 1.2   The soccer throw-in can be divided into three phases: (a) windup (preparatory) phase; (b) throwing (propulsion) phase; (c) follow-through phase.

III. Giving motion
   A. To external objects
      1. Pushing and pulling
         a. Lifting and carrying
         b. Punching
      2. Throwing, striking, and kicking
   B. To one's own body
      1. Supported by the ground or other resistant surface
         a. Locomotion on foot
         b. Locomotion on wheels, blades, and runners
         c. Rotary locomotion
      2. Suspended and free of support
         a. Swinging activities on trapeze, flying rings, or similar equipment
         b. Hand traveling on traveling rings or horizontal ladder
         c. Unsupported—i.e., projected into or falling through the air
         d. Weightlessness
      3. Supported by water
         a. Swimming
         b. Aquatic stunts
         c. Boating
IV. Receiving impact
   A. From one's own body in landing from a jump or fall
   B. From external objects in catching, trapping, spotting, or intercepting

The four major headings in this outline are maintaining erect posture, movement for fitness and exercise, giving motion, and receiving impact. Some may question the reason for treating the maintenance of erect posture as a major category instead of including it under giving motion to one's own body. The rationale for this decision is that the emphasis here is on adjusting to the immediate environment rather than on making a movement in the sense that one usually interprets this concept. With one exception, the adjustments are made from a stationary position, the exception being a shift in stance necessitated by standing on a moving base. This action does not involve moving from one place to another but only widening the stance and facing in a different direction to maintain balance. The erect posture then becomes the foundation and starting point for subsequent dynamic postures and motions.

The initial step in the classification of movement is to determine in which major category the skill belongs, and then in which secondary, and possibly tertiary, category. A forehand drive in tennis, for instance, belongs in the primary category of giving motion to an external object and in the secondary one of striking. Turning a cartwheel is a form of giving motion to one's own body while it is supported by the ground and is classified further as rotary locomotion.

In addition to pinpointing the exact categories to which the skill belongs, a number of other factors should be considered. Many skills consist of a series of phases that cut across different categories, and these must be considered separately. The tennis serve, like the forehand drive, is a form of striking, but it also involves tossing the ball, a push pattern skill that should not be overlooked. Vaults over a gymnasium box or horse consist of the approach, the placement of the hands, the momentary support by the hands, and the push-off from the box, followed by the projection of the body together with the necessary adjustments of the bodily segments, and finally the landing, which involves movements of the upper extremities and trunk as well as of the lower extremities. In pole vaulting and rock climbing, there is a smooth transition from pulling to pushing. In hurdling, repeated alternation occurs between the run and the hurdles without any break in rhythm. In many basketball shots for the basket, the shot is accompanied by a jump. All phases of the skill should be included in the analysis.

In many skills, especially those involving either the giving or the receiving of a force of appreciable magnitude, the ability to maintain balance is an all-important feature. Maintaining balance effectively means observing the principles of balance and posture adjustment as well as those relating to the specific form of giving motion or receiving impact. Lifting a heavy weight from the floor or down from a shelf is a good example of a motion-giving activity that depends in large part for its effectiveness on the maintenance of a posture that favors lifting.

The standing long jump shown in figure 1.3 is a skill that belongs in the major category of giving motion to one's own body. The initial phases prior to the takeoff, landing, and recovery phases belong in the secondary category of movement on a solid base, whereas the flight phase is an activity of the unsupported category.

Simultaneous-Sequential Nature of the Motion

Comprised of joints and levers, the body can move in a wonderful variety of ways. To simplify the complexities of such a wide range of possibilities, it is important to understand that when motions are combined, bodily movements may be classified as occurring on a continuum ranging from the *simultaneous* to the *sequential* use of the body segments. The simultaneous use of the body segments, where the various segments move as one, is exemplified by motions such as pushing, pulling, or lifting objects. In a simultaneous movement pattern, all of the movement is directed along a straight line. Simultaneous use of body segments is the only way it is anatomically possible to move the hand or foot in a straight line. This straight-line application of force by the hand or foot is the most advantageous method to use when overcoming heavy or large objects or external forces such as those encountered in pushing file cabinets and lifting weights. In addition, when accuracy is important, such as in putting in golf, lunging in fencing (movement of the arm and weapon), and punching, it is more effective to involve the segments in a simultaneous fashion.

When it is important to have maximum speed at impact or release, a sequential use of

a.

b.

Figure 1.3   Standing long jump: (a) better technique; (b) poorer technique.

| Simultaneous | Combination | Sequential |

Figure 1.4   Examples of skills on the simultaneous to sequential continuum.

the body segments is appropriate. The use of the segments in an orderly sequence so that subsequent segments are accelerated at the appropriate time to create the highest possible speed is critical in activities exemplified by throwing, striking movements such as batting or the golf drive, and kicking. Sequential movements produce forces applied so that the final segment moves along a curved path. The farther this curved path is from the center of the motion, the greater will be the speed of the throwing, striking, or kicking segment.

Motions may occur anywhere along this simultaneous-sequential continuum or may combine the two basic forms (figure 1.4). The skill of putting the shot, for example, involves the sequential use of the lower extremities and trunk followed by the simultaneous use of the upper extremity to safely move the relatively large weight of the shot. For our purposes, simultaneous motions and those combination motions that occur at the simultaneous end of the continuum will be classified as push-pull motions, and those at the other end, the sequential end, will be classified as throwing, striking, and kicking patterns.

To clarify the nature of the motion at any given point in the performance, it is desirable to break the total movement down into phases for analysis. To use the standing long jump (see figure 1.3) as an

example, an analysis of the nature of the motion might be as follows:

1. Preparatory phase—simultaneous motion of the joints of the lower extremity, into a semisquat position.
2. Execution (force) phase—simultaneous extension of the segments in a forward-upward direction.
3. Flight (unsupported) phase—sequential motion of the lower body to "whip" the legs forward.
4. Landing phase—simultaneous flexion of the lower extremity to take up the shock of the landing forces.

Having now described the motor skill by clarifying the primary purpose, classifying the skill and establishing the simultaneous-sequential nature of the skill, *analysis* of the performance is the next, and very critical, step. In evaluating the motion from the starting point, the analyst must then consider to what extent the performer conforms to the anatomical and mechanical requirements necessary to achieve the stated purpose of the motion. Failure to perform in accordance with the principles that govern motion will produce a less than optimal performance. For this reason the analyst should be conversant with the anatomical and mechanical principles that are critical for the movement skill in question.

Anatomical Analysis

The anatomical analysis of a movement should include an examination of the skeletal joint action, a description of segment motion, an account of the muscle participation, and an identification of the neuromuscular mechanisms involved. Anatomical analysis involves analysis of a process rather than a product. That is, it is a review of how the body accomplishes the task rather than an in-depth examination of the results. It should attempt to give specific answers to the following questions:

1. Which joints are involved, and what are their exact movements in the motor skill?

    For each phase of the technique and for each joint participating in the phase, the precise joint action and segment being moved should be identified and recorded as was done for the sample analysis of the force phase of the standing long jump shown in table 1.2.
2. Are any of the joints used to the limit of their range of motion?
3. Which muscles are responsible for the joint actions, and what is the nature of their contraction?

    The muscular action is identified for each joint movement and recorded next to the joint actions on the chart (table 1.2). This implies identifying not only the muscles that are contracting but also their precise function in the movement and the kind of contraction they are undergoing. Identification of the force causing the motion facilitates the subsequent identification of the muscle and type of contraction involved.
4. Which neuromuscular mechanisms are likely to help or hinder the action, and what is the nature of their involvement?

    The muscle-response patterns of well-learned motor skills involve the integrated action of many reflexes and the inhibition of others. After repeated viewing of the performance "live" or on film, the student should name and discuss the reflexes that could be acting at various points in each phase.
5. Which anatomical principles contribute to maximal efficiency and accuracy in the performance of the motor skill?
6. Which principles are directly related to the avoidance of injury?

    In any analysis, a set of anatomical principles governing the safe and effective performance of the movement skill must be considered. These principles take into account the structure and function of the human body, human tolerance of both internal and external stresses, and the efficiency of movement patterns. Hudson (1995) has also suggested that it is critical to examine such core concepts as range of motion, the number of body parts involved, the nature of the body parts involved, and the coordination of the movement. In addition, it is important to look at the alignment of the body, and the reflexes that might be utilized. Anatomical principles of motion then stipulate the way in which each of these core concepts apply to a specific movement. In particular, anatomical principles speak to the qualities associated with each of these concepts.

Mechanical Analysis

In performing a mechanical analysis of a motor skill, the human body is often viewed as a "machine," subject to the same laws and mechanical principles that govern the actions of any other machine. The mechanical analysis of human performance involves the identification of laws and principles that help explain the most appropriate form for the execution of the activity and identify the mechanical reasons for success or failure. To assess the mechanical nature of a technique and use this information in helping performers choose movements that will result in skillful motion, the analyzer should attempt to identify those

TABLE 1.2 Chart for Anatomical Analysis of a Motor Skill

Skill being analyzed: Standing long jump (see figure 1.3).
Phase being analyzed: Force phase

Name of Joint	Starting Position	Observed Joint Action	Segment Being Moved	Force for Movement	Main Muscle Groups Active	Kind of Contraction
Metatarsal-phalangeal	Extended	Hyperextension/flexion	Foot	Muscle	Extensors/flexors	Concentric
Ankle	Dorsiflexed	Plantar flexion	Lower leg	Muscle	Plantar flexors	Concentric
Knee	Flexed	Extension	Thighs	Muscle	Extensors	Concentric
Hip	Flexed	Extension	Pelvis	Muscle	Extensors	Concentric
Pelvis	Decreased tilt	Increased tilt	Trunk	Muscle	Spinal extensors	Concentric
Lumbar spine	Flexion	Extension	Trunk	Muscle	Spinal extensors	Concentric
Thoracic spine	Slight flexion	Extension	Trunk	Muscle	Spinal extensors	Concentric
Cervical spine	Hyperextended	Flexion	Neck	Muscle	Spinal flexors	Concentric
Shoulder girdle	Upward tilt	Upward rotation, abduction	Shoulder girdle	Muscle	Upward rotators / Abductors	Concentric / Concentric
Shoulder joint	Hyperextension, medial rotation	Flexion	Upper extremity	Muscle	Flexors	Concentric
Elbow	Extended	—	—	—	Extensors	Static
Radioulnar	Pronated	—	—	—	—	—
Wrist	Extended	—	—	—	Extensors	Static
Phalanges	Extended	—	—	—	Extensors	Static

Patterned after format presented in P.I. Rasch and R.K. Burke. *Kinesiology and Applied Anatomy.* 6th ed. pp. 339–347. Copyright © 1978 Lea & Febiger, Malvern, PA. Reprinted by permission. This form for recording an anatomical analysis may be reproduced for class use without specific permission.

principles and laws that verify the actions as desirable. Once the movement is classified according to an outline such as that on pages 6–7, the analyst should determine exactly how and when the movements of the performance do or do not satisfy the standards of good performance as explained by the laws and principles of mechanics. Once this process is accomplished, a greater depth of understanding of the skill is achieved, and the basis for making change is founded on sound knowledge and understanding of the reasons "why."

Underlying Mechanics Objective

To explain the mechanical factors that contribute most to performance, it is first necessary to define clearly the purpose or objective of the motion involved. The focus of the statement of mechanical objective will be on the desired outcome of the motion, which is necessary to measure effectiveness. Several systems have been proposed for the classification of mechanical objectives of human movement. A synthesis of many of those systems is presented here as a simplified set of objectives.

The underlying objective of a motion may be

1. Balance
   a. Regain stability
   b. Attain mobility
2. Locomotion
   a. Travel from point to point
   b. Travel a prescribed distance
   c. Travel a prescribed pattern
3. Projection
   a. For maximum height
   b. For maximum range
   c. For maximum accuracy
   d. For optimum speed and accuracy
4. Manipulation
   a. Of objects
   b. To reproduce a pattern
   c. Of a resistance

5. Maximum effort
   a. Maximum speed
   b. Maximum power
   c. Maximum force

Each of these underlying mechanical objectives requires consideration of different but overlapping sets of mechanical factors. The standing long jump, for instance, has the underlying mechanical objective of projection of the body for maximum range (distance). The question now becomes one of determining what must be done in mechanical terms to produce the maximum distance. Because the distance traveled is in the air, the body becomes a projectile, and those factors that cause the projectile to travel the farthest are those that must be considered.

Nature of the Forces Causing or Impeding Motion

To accurately analyze the efficiency with which a motor skill is performed, the analyst must be aware of the kind of motion being performed (classification and simultaneous-sequential nature) and the forces that are acting to cause, modify, or prevent that motion. Pushing and pulling forces, weight and resistance, twisting and turning forces must all be identified, and their effects noted. Muscle force applied through the joints' range of motion to propel the body through the air for maximum distance is a force-causing motion. A force-resisting motion is the resistance force offered by the weight of the jumper. Impact with the ground at the end of the jump will produce a force-stopping motion. Other impeding forces might be produced by lack of strength or limited range of motion.

Mechanical Principles

The identification of the mechanical principles related to the execution of the skill is a first step in establishing the causes of error in the performance of the skill. Focusing on these principles and how they relate to the skill suggests the potential sources of error. Each movement phase must be considered in turn. The core concepts from which these principles are derived include considerations of the speed of the movement, the forces involved in the movement, balance, direction, and timing, and the pressure of air or water. If the motion involves projecting something into the air, the concepts of extension at release (or contact), path of the object, and spin must also be considered. Once again, the primary concern is the quality of each of these factors that is required for an optimum performance. In deriving mechanical principles, one might discuss how much speed or how much force, as well as the direction of the force. It might become important to know how much air pressure is acting or what angle produces the best path of a thrown object.

Violation of Mechanical Principles

Diagnosing the cause of an error is difficult because the cause may be far removed from the observed effect. The purpose in identifying the mechanical principles is to locate potential sources for error. Given the purpose of the skill, which of the principles, if violated, has the greatest potential for limiting performance? How? These are the most troublesome questions to answer. Without quantitative data it is difficult to make any selection with certainty. And even with the support of such data, which indeed can provide us with much useful information, we still cannot be certain. At this time no general method is available to identify and establish the order of importance for those factors that limit performance. One must rely primarily on knowledge of the technique and the principles of mechanics that apply.

Again, using the example of the standing long jump, we know that *speed* and *direction* are the two most important factors in performance. The direction is governed by the direction of the jumper's takeoff. It appears, then,

that direction might be a good place to start to look for errors.

The speed of the jump depends on the speed and force of the push against the ground. The faster the legs can move, the greater will be the push off the ground.

Prescription for Improvement of Performance

After the performance has been described in anatomical and mechanical detail and the causes for error have been identified, the analyst must decide on the appropriate strategy for effecting change in the performance so that it conforms to the anatomical and mechanical ideal. Now the analyst becomes an instructor who must decide not only what must be done but how best to communicate that information to the performer in a manner that will make sense. The task is not unlike that of a physician who uses vast medical knowledge to prescribe bed rest as the best cure for an ailment. The cure may be simple, but the complexities attached to knowing what to do, and why, and then making that information understandable to the patient are far from simple. The instructor of motor skills needs to develop ability as a prescriber as well as an analyst. Both talents will improve with practice. As more systematic analyses are performed, the analyst will become aware of characteristics common to groups of skills. Common errors and their causes will emerge for related skills as well as similar or common prescriptions appropriate for correcting the errors. The important thing to remember is to concentrate on the causes of errors, not on the resultant symptoms. Before the physician can prescribe for a limping gait, the cause must be known and the viable options for treatment identified. Before an instructor of motor skills can prescribe for improvement of a short-standing long jump or any other motor performance, the cause(s) for the error must be known and the valid options for correction determined.

LABORATORY EXPERIENCES

1. Select three motor skills from different sections of appendix H. Identify the underlying mechanics objective for each and classify them according to the outline for classification of motor skills.
2. Using a simple skill of the student's choosing, prepare a qualitative description of a motor skill.

Include a statement of purpose, nature of the motion, and a description of how the motion will be broken into phases.
3. Using the skill from Experience 2, utilize methods of observation and palpation to identify the joints and basic muscle groups involved in the motion.

REFERENCES AND SELECTED READINGS

Adrian, M., and J. M. Cooper. 1994. *Biomechanics of human movement.* 2nd ed. Dubuque, IA: Wm. C. Brown Communications.

Hudson, J. L. 1995. Core concepts of kinesiology. *Journal of Physical Education, Recreation and Dance* 66(5):54–56.

Kirby, R., and J. A. Roberts. 1985. *Introductory biomechanics.* Ithaca, NY: Mouvement Publications.

Kreighbaum, E., and K. M. Barthels. 1994. *Biomechanics.* 4th ed. New York: Allyn & Bacon.

Nordin, M. B., and V. H. Frankel. 1989. *Basic biomechanics of the skeletal system.* Philadelphia: Lea & Febiger.

KEY INTERNET RESOURCES FOR KINESIOLOGY

The two major sites on the World Wide Web which are basic to the study of kinesiology are:

http://www.ncbi.nlm.nih.gov/PubMed/
This is PubMed, the searchable database of the National Library of Medicine. This site is an invaluable tool for locating current research on any topic of interest in medicine, including those topics which are of interest to those studying kinesiology.

http://www.per.ualberta.ca/biomechanics/
Biomechanics World Wide is an excellent starting place for any topic in biomechanics and kinesiology.

Included in this site are links to universities and classes all over the world, instrumentation companies, archives of discussions among biomechanists, and many, many other resources.

In addition to these two most far reaching websites for biomechanics and kinesiology, there are numerous other sites of interest as one studies the anatomical, mechanical, and application aspects of kinesiology. These are listed at the end of the introduction to each part of the text.

Anatomical and Physiological Fundamentals of Human Motion

Introduction to Part I

W here does anatomy end and kinesiology begin? This is a question frequently argued by kinesiologists. Yet, in truth, there is no answer because the question itself is not a valid one. One might as well ask, "Where does the study of words end and the writing of compositions (or articles, or books) begin?" or "Where does the study of building materials end and the designing and erecting of buildings begin?" Just as words are the elements used in all writing, whether creative, factual, or expository, and just as bricks, wood, cement, metal, and glass are some of the elements used in building, so bones, joints, muscles, connective tissue, blood vessels, and nerves are the vital elements of human motion. They are the essential elements used in batting a baseball, passing and carrying a football, shooting a basketball into the basket—in fact, in all running, walking, jumping, throwing, striking, catching, and swimming; likewise, one finds them in keyboarding, manual labor, painting, sewing, knitting, and so forth, almost without end.

One aim of part I is to prepare students of human motion, whether they are in physical education, athletic training, physical therapy, occupational therapy, fitness promotion, or other related professions, to systematically analyze human movements in terms of muscles, joints, and nervous system integration and to apply the knowledge provided to improve performance in motor skills. This section should not be looked upon merely as a review of anatomy but as the very foundation for analysis of human motion. It demonstrates the close relationships between anatomical structure and function, and it provides a body of knowledge that can be utilized in the learning and perfecting of various motor skills. It aims to demonstrate how the bones, joints, and muscles serve as elements in anatomical levers, which act in accord with the laws of mechanics. It also strives to make clear the influences of gravitational and other external forces on muscular actions. For instance, under certain circumstances, these forces may cause an action to be the exact opposite of what one would expect in view of the movement that is being performed. It should be obvious, therefore, that memorizing the actions of muscles will not prepare the student to make accurate analyses. Rather, a true understanding of all the conditions that influence the functions of the muscles is necessary.

A second aim of part I is to equip the future physical education instructor, coach, trainer, therapist, or fitness leader with the anatomical knowledge essential for understanding the nature of common injuries and their prevention or rehabilitation. For this reason, considerable emphasis is placed on the structure of each joint, the factors that contribute to its stability, and the factors that influence the range of motion of each joint. One factor that many seem to be ignorant about is the timetable of ages at which the epiphyseal cartilages become ossified. It should be of interest because it marks the turning point between the period of bone growth and the period of bone maturity. Because of the significance of this information, a schedule of the maturation age of each bone that participates in common activities has been included in the first chapter.

Part I contains eight chapters—two on the musculoskeletal system and its movements, one on the neuromuscular aspects of motion, and five on the anatomy and fundamental movements of specific segments of the body. The order in which these chapters are studied is entirely optional. The authors appreciate the fact that the students who use this text may differ widely in their educational backgrounds. Some may already have completed courses in anatomy, possibly even including the experience of human dissection. Others may have had only brief courses and will feel the need to receive more detailed information. Still others may have had no anatomical instruction whatsoever and may expect none other than what is included in the kinesiology course. In an attempt to meet the needs of all students, whatever their backgrounds, the authors of this text have presented in part I what they consider to be a fairly complete coverage of the aspects of anatomy that relate to movement and, at the same time, have omitted details whose relation to movement seems less significant. Hence, specific muscle attachments and innervation are not included in the main body of the text but may be found in chart form in appendix D at the end of the book for those who want to refer to them. On the other hand, the muscle's line of pull and its relation to the joint at which the motion is occurring are emphasized, because these are considered essential elements of movement.

In the light of the aforementioned aims of part I—to provide the student of human motion with the knowledge necessary for systematically analyzing human motion and applying such an analysis to the improvement of performance in motor skills, and to equip the instructor, therapist, coach, or trainer with the anatomical background for understanding the nature of athletic injuries and their prevention—it might seem that the student should wait until the entire anatomical section has been completed before attempting to analyze movement. On the contrary, the earlier the application of knowledge begins, the better. In fact, attempting to analyze basic movements according to the model presented in chapter 1 as soon as possible serves as a stimulus to the study of anatomy. An example of this situation is given next.

Let us consider starting with the arm in its anatomical position and flexing the forearm at the elbow against the stabilized upper arm. Note that we have already defined the starting position and the movement. We could be even more specific if we wished and state whether the movement was executed quickly or slowly, and whether the movement was performed against resistance as though lifting a weight.

The next step would be to consider the joint itself. The structure of the elbow joint should be reviewed. Because it was stipulated that the movement was made from the anatomical position, it would be advisable to review the radioulnar articulations also, especially the proximal joint because of its close relationship to the elbow joint. It would be helpful to refer to chapter 2 or appendix B to check on the types and characteristics of these joints.

The muscles performing the movement should be considered next with an attempt made to answer such questions as the following: What muscles flex the elbow joint? How are they affected by the starting position and the position of the forearm throughout the movement? Try to discover whether the amount of resistance to this movement affects the participating muscles, but do not overstress this point. Include all the muscles that unquestionably contribute to flexion in this position without being overly concerned at this time as to whether they are "prinicipal" or "assistant" contributors. Review the section on the coordination of the muscular system (see p. 57) and try to identify those muscles serving in the capacity of stabilizers or neutralizers.

Following the procedure described in chapter 1 throughout the study of part 1 will pave the way for the later analysis of more complex movements. Procedural steps for analyzing fitness exercises, sport skills, and other physical activities are presented in chapter 1 (p. 4). For the present, however, it is suggested that the student make simple joint, muscle, and neuromuscular analyses until the process is thoroughly familiar.

Internet Resources

A number of sites on the World Wide Web may be of interest to the student studying the anatomical aspects of kinesiology. Among those that might be most helpful are the following:

http://www.anatomy.gla.ac.uk/fab/index/html
Contains good tutorials on anatomy and gait, primarily lower extremity.

http://www.nlm.nih.gov/research/visible/visible_
      human.html
The Visible Human Project is the most ambitious human anatomy project on the Web, using 3-D imagery of actual slices of a human body. Will require a viewer, several of which are available at this site.

CHAPTER

2

THE MUSCULOSKELETAL SYSTEM

The Skeletal Framework and Its Movements

OUTLINE

■ **The Bones**
Types of Bones
Mechanical Axis of a Bone
Skeletal Changes
■ **Articulations**
Structural Classification
Suggestions for Studying
    Joint Structure
Joint Stability
Factors Affecting the Range
    of Motion
Methods of Assessing a Joint's
    Range of Motion
Average Ranges of Joint Motion
■ *Orientation of the Body*
The Center of Gravity
The Line of Gravity
Orientation Planes of the Body
    and Axes of Motion

Diagonal Planes of Motion
Standard Starting Positions
■ *Fundamental Movements*
of Major Body Segments
Movements in the Sagittal Plane
    about a Bilateral (Frontal-
    Horizontal) Axis
Movements in the Frontal Plane
    about an Anteroposterior
    (Sagittal-Horizontal) Axis
    Movements in the Transverse
    Plane about a Vertical Axis
Movements in a Combination
    of Planes
Naming Joint Actions
    in Complex Movements
Nonaxial Movements
■ *Analyzing Joint Motions*
■ *Laboratory Experiences*

OBJECTIVES

At the conclusion of this chapter, the student should be able to:

1. Classify joints according to structure, and explain the relationship between a joint structure and its capacity for movement.
2. Explain how the schedule of ossification of epiphyseal cartilage is related to the nature of sports suitable for different age groups.
3. Name the factors that contribute to joint range of motion and stability, and explain the relationship that exists between range of motion and stability.
4. Assess a joint's range of motion, evaluate the range, and describe desirable procedures for changing it when indicated.
5. Name and define the orientation positions and planes of the body and the axes of motion.
6. Demonstrate and name fundamental movement patterns using correct movement terminology.
7. Isolate and name single joint actions that are part of complex movements.
8. Perform an anatomical analysis of the joint actions and planes of motion for a selected motor skill.

It is customary—especially for students of human movement and exercise—to begin the study of anatomy with a detailed study of the bones, then to proceed to the joints, and then to the muscles. This path of investigation sometimes dampens the enthusiasm of the students, whose chief focus of interest is movement. Therefore, this chapter and the next emphasize the concept of the total musculoskeletal system as a mechanism for motion. It is hoped that by using this concept the student will find the study of the structural elements of this system more meaningful.

As the phrase implies, the musculoskeletal framework is an arrangement of bones and muscles. Adjacent bones are attached to one another by joints, which provide for the motion of the articulating bones, and the muscles that span the joints provide the force for moving the bones to which they are attached. Mechanically, the total bone–joint–muscle structure is an intricate combination of levers that makes possible a great number of coordinated movements, ranging from the small hand and finger motions used in assembling a television set or playing the piano to the total body movements of a swimmer or a pole vaulter. Any single one of the levers involved in such movements is relatively simple.

In physics we are taught that a lever is defined as a rigid bar that turns about a fulcrum (fixed axis or pivot) when force is applied to it at some specific point. An anatomical lever, therefore, is simply a bone that engages in an angular or turning type of movement when a force is applied to it. This force may be the contracting force of a muscle attached to the bone, or it may be an external force such as gravity or an external weight. If the force is muscle, it is always a pulling force, because muscles, being flexible, are unable to push; they can only pull. If the force is external, such as when a weight is too heavy to be maintained, the muscle force controls the rate at which the lever is allowed to move.

THE BONES

Although anatomy texts give the number of bones in the human skeleton as 206, only 177 of them engage in voluntary movement. The skeleton consists of two major parts, the axial skeleton and the appendicular skeleton (figure 2.1). The axial section comprises the skull, spinal column, sternum, and ribs, and the appendicular section includes the bones of the upper and lower extremities. The bones of the upper extremity include the scapula, clavicle, humerus, ulna, radius, carpal bones, metacarpals, and phalanges, and those of the lower extremity include the three fused bones of the pelvis, the femur, tibia, fibula, tarsal bones, metatarsals, and phalanges. Although the pelvis may be classified with either the axial or the appendicular skeleton, it is actually a link between the axial skeleton and the lower extremity branch of the appendicular skeleton and is functionally as important to one as to the other. The skeleton serves to support weight, as a place for muscles to attach, and to protect critical structures such as the spinal cord, brain, and various organs.

Types of Bones

In spite of the great variety of shapes and sizes of bones, there are only four major bone categories: long, short, flat, and irregular.

Long Bones

Characterized by a cylindrical shaft with relatively broad, knobby ends. The shaft or body has thick walls and contains a central cavity known as a medullary canal. The bones belonging in this category are the clavicle, humerus, ulna, radius, metacarpals, and phalanges of the upper extremity, and the femur, tibia, fibula, metatarsals, and phalanges of the lower extremity.

Short Bones

Relatively small, chunky, solid bones. The carpals and tarsals (wrist and ankle bones) belong to this category.

Flat Bones

Flat, platelike bones. The sternum, scapulae, ribs, pelvic bones, and patellas are examples.

Irregular Bones

The bones of the spinal column. The twenty-four vertebrae, the sacrum, and the coccyx are found in this category.

Mechanical Axis of a Bone

It has already been stated that bones serve as levers. When muscular action is analyzed mechanically, one must know what is meant by the *mechanical axis* of the bone, or the body segment, that is serving as the lever. The student will find it advantageous, therefore, to learn what this term is now while studying the bones. *The mechanical axis of a bone or segment is a straight line that connects the midpoint of the joint at one end with the midpoint of the joint at the other end or, in the case of a terminal segment, with the midpoint of its distal end.* This axis does not necessarily pass lengthwise through the shaft of the bony lever. If the shaft is curved or if the articulating process projects at an angle from the shaft, the greater part of the axis may lie outside the shaft, as in the case of the femur (figure 2.2).

Skeletal Changes

An *epiphysis* is a part of a bone separated from the main bone by a layer of cartilage whose presence in the bone is an indication that the bone has not completed its growth. In the long bones the shaft is separated from the ends and from articulating knobs by epiphyseal cartilages. This is where growth occurs. As growth ceases, the cartilages gradually become ossified (replaced by bone) and, when closure is complete, no more growth can occur. Surprisingly, several epiphyses do not completely ossify until the twentieth, or even the twenty-fifth, year of life. Hence, most high school boys and many college men are engaging in vigorous sports before their bones are fully matured. Physical education instructors,

Figure 2.1   Skeleton. (a) Anterior view. (b) Posterior view.

Mechanical
axis of
femur

Figure 2.2   Mechanical axis of femur.

trainers, and coaches need to be aware of this fact. Although this is not usually harmful in the case of noncontact sports, in violent contact sports like football and boxing the consequences may be extremely serious. Protective devices are helpful, but high standards for these devices must be insisted upon. Even more important, coaches, especially those of young adolescents, must be knowledgeable about anatomy, growth patterns, and safety precautions and conscientious in the application of this knowledge. They must accept their responsibility for the health and safety of each individual player as being of far greater importance than a winning record. The coach who tells a high school boy to aim at the numeral on his opponent's shirt and run full force into him using the top of his helmet (known as "sticking") is either grossly ignorant or callously indifferent.

There is also danger to elementary and junior high school youngsters who are permitted to bear weights that are too heavy for them. "Husky-looking" boys and girls are often mistakenly permitted to form the base of a pyramid, because they give the impression of being strong. If they are on their hands and knees supporting a second and perhaps a third row of youngsters, the weight may be too much for them. This outcome is especially likely if the individuals in the upper rows are careless about where they place their hands and knees. If they are not placed in line with the supporting individuals' arms and thighs, the vertebrae and possibly the arms and thighs will be subjected to rotary stress, which may result in serious injury to the epiphyses of these bones.

The approximate ages at which the ossification of the epiphyseal cartilages is completed are presented in tables 2.1 and 2.2 (Goss 1980). In addition, consideration must be given to the other end of the age spectrum, the elderly, and the concern for osteoporosis. *Osteoporosis* is the loss of calcium, other minerals, and the matrix from the bones, which causes the bones to become porous and brittle. Some of this loss is natural, resulting from the aging process. In serious cases, bones subjected to weight bearing and muscle pull may collapse. In some situations, falling may be the result of bones breaking from their brittleness. At best, osteoporosis negatively affects a person's ability to move. Osteoporosis occurs more often in women than in men. Current research indicates that the negative effects may be reduced through good nutrition and regular exercise throughout life. Moreover, nutrition, hormone regulation, and regular exercise begun late in life also tend to control some of the adverse effects of osteoporosis.

ARTICULATIONS

The structure and function of joints are so interrelated that it is difficult to discuss them separately. Hence, in the discussion of structure, there is much that relates to function and, conversely, much that relates to structure when function is

TABLE 2.1	Approximate Ages of Epiphyseal Closures*	
		Age
Spinal Column		
Vertebrae and sacrum		25
Thorax		
Sternum		25
Ribs		25
Upper Extremity		
Clavicle		25
Scapula		15–17
Humerus		
Head fused with shaft		20
Lateral epicondyle		16–17
Medial epicondyle		18
Ulna		
Olecranon		16
Lower end		20
Radius		
Head and shaft		18–19
Lower end to shaft		20
Lower Extremity		
Pelvic bone		
Inferior rami of pubis and ischium (almost complete)		7–8
Acetabulum		20–25
Femur		
Greater and lesser trochanters		18
Head		18
Lower end		20
Tibia		
Upper end		20
Lower end		18
Fibula		
Upper end		25
Lower end		20

*Listed by body section

Source: Data from Goss, 1980.

TABLE 2.2	Approximate Ages of Epiphyseal Closures*
Approximate Age	
7–8	
Inferior rami of pubis and ischium almost complete	
15–17	
Upper extremity: scapula, lateral epicondyle of humerus, olecranon process of ulna	
18–19	
Upper extremity: medial epicondyle of humerus, head and shaft of radius	
Lower extremity: femoral head and greater and lesser trochanters, lower end of tibia	
About 20	
Upper extremity: humeral head, lower ends of radius and ulna	
Lower extremity: lower ends of femur and fibula, upper end of tibia	
20–25	
Lower extremity: acetabulum in pelvis	
25	
Spine: vertebrae and sacrum	
Upper extremity: clavicle	
Lower extremity: upper end of fibula	
Thorax: sternum and ribs	

*Listed by age

Data from Goss, 1980.

discussed. Careful inspection of the joints depicted in figure 2.3 will give an idea of the relationship between the shape of the joint and the movements it permits. In much the same way that railroad tracks determine the route available to the train, the configuration of the bones that form an articulation, together with the reinforcing ligaments, determine and limit the movements that the involved segment can make.

Structural Classification

There are many different patterns of joint structure, and these form the basis for their classification. The classification found in most anatomy texts, is based on the presence or absence of a joint cavity—that is, a space between the articulating surfaces of the bones. Each type of joint is further classified either according to shape or according to the nature of the tissues that connect the bones. These classifications, with their subdivisions, may be grasped more readily in outline form and in figure 2.3:

	Nonaxial (0 axes)	Uniaxial (1 axis)	Biaxial (2 axes)	Triaxial (3 axes)
	Plane joint	*Hinge joint*	*Condyloid joint*	*Ball and socket joint*
	Carpal joints	Elbow	Metacarpal-phalangeal joints	Hip
		Pivot joint	*Saddle joint*	
		Atlantoaxial joint	Thumb	Shoulder
Planes of motion	None	Sagittal OR Transverse	Sagittal AND Frontal	Sagittal Frontal Transverse
Primary axes	None	Bilateral OR Longitudinal	Bilateral AND Anteroposterior	Bilateral Anteroposterior Longitudinal
Movements	Sliding or gliding	Flexion/Extension OR Rotation Pronation/Supination	Flexion/Extension Abduction/Adduction	Flexion/Extension Abduction/Adduction Rotation

Figure 2.3 Joint Classifications.

Figure 2.4   Frontal section of a diarthrodial joint.

From W. H. Hollinshead and D. B. Jenkins, *Functional Anatomy of the Limbs and Back,* 5th ed. Copyright © 1981 W. B. Saunders, Orlando, FL. Reprinted by permission.

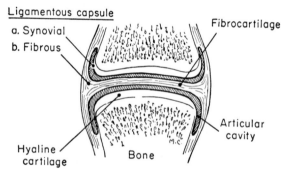

Figure 2.5   Frontal section of a diarthrodial joint having fibrocartilage.

I. Diarthrosis (from the Greek, meaning a joint in which there is a separation or articular cavity) (figures 2.4 and 2.5)

A. Characteristics
   1. An articular cavity is present.
   2. The joint is encased within a sleevelike ligamentous capsule.
   3. The capsule is lined with synovial membrane that secretes synovial fluid for lubricating the joint.
   4. The articular surfaces are smooth.
   5. The articular surfaces are covered with cartilage, usually hyaline, but occasionally fibrocartilage.

B. Classification

   1. Irregular (arthrodial; plane). The joint surfaces are irregularly shaped, usually flat or slightly curved. The only movement permitted is of a gliding nature; hence, it is nonaxial.
   2. Hinge (ginglymus). One surface is spool-like; the other is concave. The concave surface fits over the spool-like process and glides partially around it in a hinge type of movement. This constitutes movement in one plane about a single axis of motion; hence, it is uniaxial. The movements that occur are flexion and extension.

3. Pivot (trochoid; screw). This kind of joint may be characterized by a peglike pivot, as in the joint between atlas and axis, or by two long bones fitting against each other near each end in such a way that one bone can roll around the other one, as do the radius and ulna of the forearm. In the latter type, a small concave notch on one bone fits against the rounded surface of the other. The rounded surface may be either the edge of a disc (like the head of the radius) or a rounded knob (like the head of the ulna). The only movement permitted in either kind of pivot joint is rotation. It is a movement in one plane about a single axis; hence, the joint is uniaxial.

4. Condyloid (ovoid; ellipsoidal). An oval or egg-shaped convex surface fits into a reciprocally shaped concave surface. Movement can occur in two planes, forward and backward, and from side to side. The former movement is flexion and extension, and the latter abduction and adduction or lateral flexion. The joint is biaxial. When these move-ments are performed sequentially, they constitute circumduction.

5. Saddle (sellar; reciprocal reception). This may be thought of as a modification of a condyloid joint. Both ends of the convex surface are tipped up, making the surface concave in the other direction, like a western saddle. Fitting over this is a reciprocally concave-convex surface. This is a biaxial joint, permitting flexion and extension, abduction and adduction, and circumduction. The saddle joint has greater freedom of motion than the condyloid joint.

6. Ball-and-socket (spheroidal; enarthrodial). In this type of joint the spherical head of one bone fits into the cup or saucerlike cavity of the other bone (see figures 5.7, 5.8, 7.8, and 7.9). It is much like the swivel joint on a trailer hitch. It permits flexion and extension, abduction and adduction, circumduction (the sequential combination of the preceding), horizontal adduction and abductions and rotation. It is a triaxial joint, because it permits movements about three axes.

(See appendix C for a more complete chart of diarthrodial joints and their motions.)

II. Synarthrosis (from the Greek, meaning literally "with joint" or, according to our usage, a joint in which there is no separation or articular cavity)
   A. Characteristics
      1. In two of the types (cartilaginous and fibrous), the two bones are united by means of an intervening substance, such as cartilage or fibrous tissue, which is continuous with the joint surfaces.
      2. The third type (ligamentous) is not a true joint but is a ligamentous connection between two bones, which may or may not be contiguous.
      3. There is no articular cavity, hence no capsule, synovial membrane, or synovial fluid.
   B. Classification
      1. Cartilaginous (synchondrosis; from the Greek, meaning "with cartilage"). Only the joints that are united by fibrocartilage permit motion of a bending and twisting nature. Example of fibrocartilaginous type: articulations between the bodies of the vertebrae

(see figure 9.2). Those united by hyaline cartilage permit only a slight compression. Example of hyaline type: epiphyseal unions.

2. Fibrous (suture; from the Latin word meaning "seam"). The edges of bone are united by means of a thin layer of fibrous tissue, which is continuous with the periosteum. No movements are permitted. Only example: the sutures of the skull.

3. Ligamentous (syndesmosis; from the Greek, meaning "with ligament"). Two bodies, which may be adjacent or may be quite widely separated, are tied together by one or more ligaments. These ligaments may be in the form of cords, bands, or flat sheets. The movement that occurs is usually limited and of no specific type. Examples: coracoacromial union (figure 5.9); midunion of radius and ulna (see figures 6.2 and 6.3).

C. Summary

The synarthrodial joints of greatest concern to the kinesiologist are those of the vertebral bodies. The thickness of the intervertebral discs permits a moderate amount of motion simulating that of ball-and-socket joints. The movements are flexion and extension, lateral flexion, circumduction, and rotation.

Suggestions for Studying Joint Structure

To understand thoroughly the structure of a joint and especially the relation of structure to function, the student should supplement book study with firsthand study of a skeleton or of the disarticulated bones that enter into the formation of each major joint. Following this preliminary study, the student may find it helpful to "construct" a joint by taking the two bones (in some cases, three) and fastening them together with pieces of adhesive or masking tape carefully

placed to represent the specific ligaments of the joint. Pieces of thick felt, cut in the proper shape, may be used to represent the fibrocartilage. This technique is particularly helpful in studying the knee, hip, and shoulder joints.

The movements of each joint should be studied both on the skeleton and on the living subject. When using the latter method, it is important to consider all the joints involved in the movement in question. For instance, in studying the movements of the elbow joint, the articulation between the humerus and radius must not be overlooked. The close relationship that exists between certain joints should be noted, for example, the relationship between the elbow joint and proximal radioulnar articulation. The tilting of the pelvis that accompanies many movements of the lower extremity and lumbar spine should be recognized, as should the movements of the shoulder girdle that accompany those of the shoulder joint. A particular pitfall awaits those who study the movements of the shoulder joint only by observing the living subject. If not forewarned, students may overlook the part played by the shoulder girdle. Its movements may be detected by palpating the scapula and clavicle in all movements of the upper arm. To follow the movements of the scapula, the thumb should be placed at the inferior angle, one finger on the root of the scapular spine and another on the acromion process. Firm contact should be maintained as the scapula moves.

A student of movement must always be observant of motion possibilities in all the joints and not limit attention to just one joint. Only through the cooperative involvement of various parts can the total range of movement potential be experienced and understood. Therefore, focusing on one joint would be misleading and would result in misinterpretations of what was being observed.

Joint Stability

The function of the joints is obviously to provide the bones with a means of moving or, rather, of being moved. But because such provisions bring with them a threat of instability, the joints have what might be called a secondary function of providing for stability without interfering with the desired motions.

All the joints of the body do not have the same degree of strength or stability. Some, such as the hip or elbow, are fairly stable. Others, such as the shoulder or knee, are less stable and therefore more easily injured. The strength or degree of freedom of joints follows Emerson's law: "For everything that is given, something is taken." In the shoulder, movement is gained at the expense of stability, whereas in the hip, movement is sacrificed for stability.

By *joint stability* we mean resistance to displacement. Steindler uses the term *cohesion* and suggests four factors that are responsible for this stability: the joint ligaments such as the lateral ligaments of hinge joints, muscle tension (see stabilizing components of muscular force), fascia, and atmospheric pressure (Steindler 1970). The latter is particularly effective at the hip joint. A fifth factor is suggested here—namely, the shape of the bony structure.

Shape of Bony Structure

Shape may refer to the kind of joint, such as hinge, condyloid, or ball-and-socket, but it is even more likely to refer to specific characteristics of the particular joint. Both the shoulder and the hip joints, for instance, are ball-and-socket joints, yet they differ markedly in their stability. The depth of the cuplike acetabulum of the hip joint, in contrast to the small size and shallowness of the glenoid fossa of the shoulder joint, is a case in point. The bony structure of the hip joint obviously gives greater protection against displacement. This difference is reflective of the weight-bearing function of the lower extremity and manipulation function of the upper extremity.

Ligamentous Arrangements

Ligaments are strong, flexible, stress-resistant, somewhat elastic, fibrous tissues that may be in the form of straplike bands or round cords. They attach the ends of the bones that form a movable

joint and help maintain them in the right relationship to each other. They also check the movement when it reaches its normal limits, and they resist movements for which the joint is not constructed. For instance, the collateral ligaments of the knee help prevent any tendency there might be for this joint to abduct or adduct. Likewise, the ulnar and radial collateral ligaments of the elbow prevent abduction and adduction. The ligaments do not always succeed in preventing abnormal or excessive movements because collisions and violent motions may cause them to tear. Also, if they are subject to prolonged periods of stress (a force that deforms), they become abnormally stretched. Because they are not very elastic (i.e., they do not have the capability to return quickly to normal shape) following deformation, ligaments take a long time to recover from a stretch. If overstretched, they may never regain their normal length. Ligaments stretched and damaged in joint injuries should be given plenty of time to heal before being subjected to strenuous activity and strain (deformation). As long as the ligaments remain undamaged, they are an important factor in contributing to joint stability, but once stretched, their usefulness is permanently affected and joint stability is diminished.

Muscular Arrangement

The muscles and muscle tendons that span the joint also play a part in the stability of joints, especially in those joints whose bony structure contributes little to stability. The shoulder joint is a notable example, getting its greatest strength from the shoulder and arm muscles that cross it. (See chapter 5 for an in-depth discussion of the stability of the shoulder joint.)

Of the six muscles that act on the shoulder joint, four of them, known as the rotator cuff (subscapularis, supraspinatus, infraspinatus, and teres minor) are particularly important as stabilizers of this joint. One of their chief functions is protection of the shoulder joint and prevention of displacement of the humeral head. Figure 5.13 shows that all four of these muscles have a strong inward pull on the humeral head toward the glenoid fossa. Likewise, the knee joint depends greatly on the tendons of the quadriceps femoris and hamstring muscles for its strength. A most important defense against joint injury is an increase in the strength of the muscles that support the joint. The role of muscles as stabilizers, as opposed to that of movers or neutralizers, is included in greater detail in chapter 3.

Fascia and Skin

Fasciae consist of fibrous connective tissue that forms sheaths for individual muscles, partitions that lie between muscles, and smaller partitions that separate bundles of muscle fibers within a single muscle. According to their location and function, they may vary in structure from thin membranes to tough, fibrous sheets. In composition they are similar to ligaments in that they are flexible and elastic, within limits, but are susceptible to permanent stretch if subjected to stress that is too intense or too prolonged. The iliotibial tract of the fascia lata and the thick skin covering the knee joint are examples of fascia and skin serving to help stabilize a joint.

Atmospheric Pressure

The importance of atmospheric pressure as a factor in resisting dislocation of a joint was demonstrated many years ago in a unique experiment. First, all of the muscles and then all the ligaments of a hip joint (including the teres femoris ligament) were severed, but surprisingly the head of the femur remained in place because of the atmospheric pressure pushing on the outside of the joint with greater force than the outward pushing force within the joint cavity. Then a hole was drilled through the acetabulum of another hip joint whose ligaments were intact, and immediately thereafter the femoral head separated from the socket as the internal joint suction disappeared with the equalization of internal and external pressure (Steindler 1970).

Factors Affecting the Range of Motion

The simplest way to limit motion is to put an obstacle in the path of the moving object. An obstacle limiting joint motion may be of soft or rigid tissue or both. Consequently, all joints in the same individual do not have the same amount of movement, and the same joints in different individuals do not have the same amount or range of motion (ROM). The ROM depends on several factors. Three factors that affect the stability of a joint are also related to its range of motion. These are the shape of the articular surfaces, the restraining effect of the ligaments, and the controlling action of the muscles.

Muscles and their tendons are undoubtedly the single most important factor in maintaining both the stability and degree of movement in joints. The tightness of the hamstring tendons (behind the knees) is often felt when someone attempts to touch the toes without bending the knees. Many have also discovered that continued practice will stretch these tendons and improve the joint's range of motion appreciably. It is important to remember that flexibility should not exceed the muscles' ability to maintain the integrity of the joints. Exercising the muscles on all sides of a joint can contribute to both flexibility and strength. The apposition of bulky tissue also affects the degree of movement in a joint. Well-developed musculature or excessive fatty tissue will restrict motion. Bulky arm muscles restrict flexion of the forearm at the elbow, and large deposits of abdominal fat limit trunk flexion. Additional factors in the range of motion include gender, body build (both the mesomorph and the ectomorph usually have greater flexibility than the endomorph), heredity (in addition to body build), occupation, personal exercise habits, state of physical fitness, and age.

Any conditions or diseases resulting in a decrease in range of motion may limit one's ability in activities of daily living or participation in physical activity. Reduction in range of motion may result in loss of ability to withstand normal stresses and may result in pain. Therefore, movement opportunities are avoided, resulting in further decreases in joint mobility. This negative cycle often typifies joint disease and injury. One such condition is arthritis, which can affect a person of any age. Regardless of age, maintaining range of movement without pain must be a goal in order to control for other complications. Exercises done in water have been found to be beneficial. The natural resistance of the water combined with its supportive nature provides a fairly comfortable medium for exercising the affected joints.

Methods of Assessing a Joint's Range of Motion

The usual way to assess a joint's range of motion is to measure the number of degrees from the starting position of the segment to its position at the end of its maximal movement. This is the way to measure flexion; extension is usually measured as the return movement from flexion. If the movement continues beyond the starting position, that constitutes hyperextension. Abduction and adduction are either measured separately from the starting position or, if desired, the total range from maximal abduction to maximal adduction is measured.

Measuring ROM can be done in various ways, depending on the joint that is measured. The instrument most commonly used is the double-armed goniometer, with one arm stationary and the other movable (figure 2.6). The pin or axis of the movable arm is placed directly over the center of the joint at which the motion occurs. The stationary arm is held in line with the stationary segment and the movable arm is either held against the segment as it moves or placed in line with the segment after its limit of motion has been reached. At the completion of the movement, the indicator shows the number of degrees through which the segment has moved. When the anatomical landmarks are well defined, and the examiner has identified the joint center properly, the use of the goniometer may be considered accurate, but when the bony landmarks are not well defined because of excess soft tissue coverage or other causes, or the goniometer axis is not properly placed over the joint axis, the goniometer may provide inaccurate information. For enhanced accuracy of the

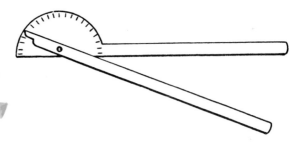

Figure 2.6   Double-armed goniometer.

joint being measured, all other joints and segments should be stabilized. Electronic methods of measuring joint angles are often used in laboratory settings and will be discussed more completely in chapter 23.

A more recent method makes use of film or videotape. Before filming the subject, joint centers are marked so as to be visible in the projected image. Joint angles can then be obtained from the projected images. The range of motion is the difference between the joint angles of two images, one at the start of the movement and the other at its completion (figure 2.7). When this method is used, the segment action must occur in the picture plane (i.e., at a right angle to the camera).

Average Ranges of Joint Motion

Because of the many factors that affect range of motion, including differences in measuring techniques, ranges vary and it is difficult to establish norms. Age, gender, body build, and level of activity may all be factors. Where the extremities are concerned, the individual's opposite is perhaps the best norm. Some averages that may be used as a guide are presented in table 2.3. Illustrations showing joint range of motion for most fundamental movements are found in appendix C.

ORIENTATION OF THE BODY

In preparation for defining the fundamental movements of the major segments of the body and for the analysis of these movements, certain

a.   b.

Figure 2.7   The range of motion at a joint can be determined using film tracings of the joint action. The angles at the knee and ankle joints were measured at the point of the greatest flexion (a) and at the peak of the jump. (b) The difference between the two measures (b minus a) is the range of motion (ROM) for the given joint. The ROM at the knee joint was 177 degrees and at the ankle joint was 78 degrees.

orientation concepts and points of reference need to be established. The essential ones are the center of gravity, the line of gravity, the orientation planes of the body and axes of motion, and the standard starting positions from which the fundamental movements are made.

The Center of Gravity

The *center of gravity* is defined as "an imaginary point representing the weight center of an object"; it is also "that point in a body about which all the parts exactly balance each other" and can be viewed as "the point at which the entire weight

		Sources		
Joint	**1**	**2**	**3**	**4**

TABLE 2.3   Average Ranges of Joint Motion

Joint	1	2	3	4
Elbow				
Flexion	140	145	145	145
Hyperextension	0	0	0	0–10
Forearm				
Pronation	80	90	90	80
Supination	80	85	90	90
Wrist				
Extension	60	70	70	50
Flexion	60	90		60
Radial flexion	20	20	20	20
Ulnar flexion	30	30	35	30
Shoulder				
Flexion	180	170	130	180
Hyperextension	50	30	80	60
Abduction	180	170	180	180
Adduction	50			
Horizontal flexion				135
Horizontal extension				45
Shoulder				
Rotation (arm in abduction)				
Inward	90	90	70	60–90
Outward	90	90	70	90
Hip				
Flexion	100	120	125	120
Hyperextension	30	10	10	30
Abduction	40	45	45	45
Adduction	20		10	0–25
Rotation (in extension)				
Inward	40	35	45	40–45
Outward	50	45	45	45
Knee				
Flexion	150	120	140	130
Ankle				
Plantar flexion	20	45	45	50
Dorsiflexion	30	15	20	20
Spine (cervical)				
Flexion	60			40
Hyperextension	75			40
Lateral flexion	45			45
Rotation	80			50
Spine (thoracic and lumbar)				
Flexion	45–50			45
Hyperextension	25			20–35
Lateral flexion	25			30
Rotation	30			45

Sources: 1. Data from *Guide to the Evaluation of Permanent Impairment.* 1990. 3rd ed. (revised). American Medical Association. Chicago, IL. 2. L. K. Smith and L. D. Lehmkuhl, *Brunnstom's Clinical Kinesiology.* 1983. 4th ed. F. A. Davis, Philadelphia, PA. 3. H. O. Kendall, et al., *Muscles: Testing and Function.* 1971. 2nd ed. Williams & Wilkins, Baltimore. MD. 4. J. J. Gerhardt, and O. A. Russe, *International SFTR Method of Measuring and Recording Joint Motion.* 1975. Hans Huber Publishers, Bern, Switzerland.

of the body may be considered concentrated." In a perfect sphere or cube, the weight center coincides with the geometric center. Its precise location in the human body depends on the individual's anatomical structure, habitual standing posture, current position, and whether external weights are being supported. In a person of average build, standing erect with the arms hanging at the sides, the center of gravity is located in the pelvis in front of the upper part of the sacrum. It is usually lower in women than in men because of women's heavier pelvises and thighs and shorter legs. (See chapter 14 for a more detailed discussion of the center of gravity and related concepts.)

The Line of Gravity

The **line of gravity** is an imaginary vertical line that, by definition, passes through the center of gravity. Hence its location depends on the posi-

tion of the center of gravity, which changes with every shift of the body's position.

Orientation Planes of the Body and Axes of Motion

There are three traditional planes corresponding to the three dimensions of space. Each plane is perpendicular to each of the other two. There are likewise three axes of motion, each perpendicular to the plane in which the motion occurs. The planes and axes of the body are defined as follows.

1. The **sagittal,** or median, **plane** is a vertical plane passing through the body from front to back, dividing it into right and left halves (figure 2.8a)
2. The **frontal,** or coronal, **plane** is a vertical plane passing through the body from side to side, dividing it into anterior and posterior halves (figure 2.8b)

a.   b.   c.

Figure 2.8 The planes of the body: (a) sagittal, or anteroposterior, plane; (b) frontal, or lateral, plane; (c) horizontal, or transverse, plane.

3. The **transverse,** or horizontal, **plane** is a plane that passes horizontally through the body, dividing it into upper and lower halves (figure 2.8c)

Because each plane *bisects* the body, it follows that each plane must pass through the center of gravity. Hence the center of gravity may be defined as the point at which the three planes of the body intersect one another, and the line of gravity as the vertical line at which the two vertical planes intersect each other. When describing a movement in terms of a plane, such as "a movement of the forearm in the sagittal plane," we mean that the movement occurs in a plane parallel to the sagittal plane. It does not necessarily imply that the movement occurs in a plane passing through the center of gravity. If the latter is intended, the term *cardinal plane* is used. Therefore, it may be concluded that there are only three cardinal planes but an infinite number of vertical and horizontal planes parallel to the cardinal planes. Thus, nodding the head is a movement occurring in the cardinal sagittal plane, but movement of either leg or arm forward-upward is movement occurring in the sagittal plane.

Axes

1. The **bilateral** (frontal-horizontal) **axis** passes horizontally from side to side.
2. The **anteroposterior** or **AP** (sagittal-horizontal) **axis** passes horizontally from front to back.
3. The **vertical** (longitudinal) **axis** is perpendicular to the ground.

A rotary movement of a segment of the body occurs *in* a plane and *around* an axis. The axis around which the movement takes place is always at right angles to the plane in which it occurs. One may consider the axis to be an imaginary rod placed in such a position (perpendicular to each plane) so that the segment is permitted to move about this axis. Forward lifting of the leg (flexion) occurs in the sagittal plane about a frontal-horizontal axis, sideward raising of the arm (abduction) occurs in the frontal plane about a

sagittal-horizontal axis, and turning the head to the side (lateral rotation) is movement in the transverse plane about a vertical axis.

An understanding of planes and axes may guide the observer into the best position to observe or record a motion. Movement in a horizontal plane is observed most easily from above or below. Movement within a sagittal plane is best observed from the side. (These positions are parallel to the axis about which the movements are occurring.)

Diagonal Planes of Motion

Noting that many motions used in sports do not follow the traditional planes of motion, Logan and McKinney (1982) codified three **diagonal** (oblique) **planes** of motion to describe these actions. High and low diagonal planes of motion were identified for the shoulder joints, as exemplified by an overarm throw and discus throw, respectively; a low diagonal plane of motion for the hip joint is exemplified by a football punt.

Whatever the degree of obliquity of the plane, the axis for a movement in that plane is always perpendicular to it. Although it is possible to define the obliquity precisely by the number of degrees that it deviates from the cardinal planes, descriptive terms are adequate for general purposes.

Standard Starting Positions
Fundamental Standing Position

In this position the individual stands erect with the feet slightly separated and parallel, the arms hanging easily at the sides with palms facing the body (figure 2.9a). This is the position usually accepted as the point of reference for analyzing all the movements of the body's segments, *except those of the forearm.*

Anatomical Standing Position

This is the position usually depicted in anatomy textbooks. The individual is erect, with the elbows fully extended and the palms facing forward. The

a.   b.

Figure 2.9 Standing positions: (a) fundamental standing position; (b) anatomical standing position.

legs and feet are the same as for the fundamental standing position (figure 2.9b). It is usually accepted as the point of reference for the movements of the forearm, hand, and fingers.

FUNDAMENTAL MOVEMENTS OF THE MAJOR BODY SEGMENTS

Being a multijointed structure, the human body consists of many movable segments. When we watch skillful acrobats, dancers, or basketball players, it might seem like a hopeless task to try to organize their movements into a single, meaningful classification. The task is greatly simplified, however, when we consider one segment at a time and visualize each movement as though it were performed from the *anatomical standing position*. This may take a bit of imagination, but knowing ahead of time the movements of which each joint in the body is capable is nine-tenths of

the battle. These movements are described in chapters 4 through 9 in the systematic discussions of the regions of the body. The following information is basic to an understanding of the movements of specific joints and segments.

Movements in the Sagittal Plane about a Bilateral (Frontal-Horizontal) Axis (Figure 2.10a)
Flexion

The angle at the joint diminishes. Examples include the following:

1. Tipping the head forward.
2. Lifting the foot and leg backward from the knee.
3. Raising the entire lower extremity forward-upward as though kicking.
4. With the upper arm remaining at the side, raising the forearm straight forward (figure 2.10a).
5. With the elbow straight, raising the entire upper extremity forward-upward. The "diminishing angle" is hard to see in this movement until one views the raising of the arm from the shoulder in the same way that the raising of the thigh from the hip joint is viewed. In the latter, one automatically notices the angle that appears between the top of the thigh and the trunk. Similarly, when raising the arm, the angle to look for is the angle between the top of the arm and the neck–head segment, not the angle between the underside of the raised arm and the trunk. One must view the sagittal plane movements of the arm at the shoulder as being similar to those of the thigh at the hip joint.

For general purposes the upper arm may be considered fully flexed when it has reached the overhead vertical position. Later, when the role of the shoulder girdle in arm movements has been studied, it will be seen that the elevation of the

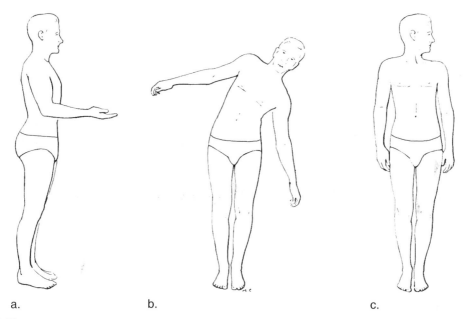

a.   b.   c.

Figure 2.10   Movements of the body in three planes: (a) movement of the forearm in the sagittal plane around a frontal-horizontal axis; (b) movement of the trunk in the frontal plane around a sagittal-horizontal axis; (c) movement of the head in the transverse plane around a vertical axis.

arm does not occur solely at the shoulder joint. The movements of the scapula and clavicle are an important part of the total arm movement. Strictly speaking, the shoulder joint is in a fully flexed position when the humerus is raised until it is parallel with the long axis of the scapula (i.e., when it is in the same plane as the scapula). For the present, however, the upper arm will be considered fully flexed when it has been raised forward-upward until it has reached the vertical position and hyperflexed when it passes beyond this.

Extension

The return movement from flexion.

Hyperflexion

This term refers only to the movement of the upper arm. When the arm is flexed beyond the vertical, it is considered to be hyperflexed. In other joints of the body, flexion is terminated by

contact of the moving segment with another part of the body—for example, the forearm against the upper arm, the lower leg against the thigh, or by structural limitations of the joints themselves (e.g., flexion of the thoracic and lumbar spine).

Hyperextension

The continuation of extension beyond the starting position or beyond the straight line. Examples include the following:

1. Hyperextension of the upper arm is said to occur when the arm is extended backward beyond the body.
2. The forearm is considered to be hyperextended when the angle at the elbow joint has exceeded 180 degrees.

Reduction of Hyperextension

Return movement from hyperextension. This movement could also be called flexion to the starting position—that is, the fundamental or the anatomical starting position, as the case may be.

Movements in the Frontal Plane about an Anteroposterior (Sagittal-Horizontal) Axis (Figure 2.10b)

Viewed from the front or back.

Abduction

Sideward movement away from the midline or sagittal plane or, in the case of the fingers, away from the midline of the hand. This term is used most commonly for sideward movements of the upper arm away from the trunk—in other words, sideward elevation of the arm—and for sideward elevation of the lower extremity. The jumping-jack exercise involves both of these.

Adduction

The return movement from abduction.

Lateral Flexion

This term refers to the lateral bending of the head or trunk. It may also be used for sideward movements of the middle finger, but the more specific terms *radial* or *ulnar flexion* are usually used for these.

Hyperabduction

Like hyperflexion, this term usually refers to the upper arm when the latter is abducted beyond the vertical, as seen from the front or back.

Hyperadduction

The trunk blocks hyperadduction of the upper extremity, and the presence of the supporting lower extremity blocks hyperadduction of the other lower extremity. By combining slight flexion with hyperadduction, the upper extremities can move across the front of the body, and one lower extremity can move across in front of the supporting one.

Reduction of Hyperadduction

The return movement from hyperadduction.

Reduction of Lateral Flexion

The return movement from lateral flexion.

Movements in the Transverse Plane about a Vertical Axis (Figure 2.10c)

Viewed or visualized from overhead or from directly beneath, as through a glass platform. The point of reference for all rotations of the upper extremities is the midposition as in the fundamental (not anatomical) standing position.

Rotation Left and Right

Applies to rotation of the head, neck, or pelvis in such a way that the anterior aspect turns, respectively, to the left or right.

Outward (Lateral) and Inward (Medial) Rotation

Applies to rotation of the thigh, the upper arm, or the upper or lower extremity as a whole in such a way that the anterior aspect of the segment turns laterally or medially.

Supination and Pronation

Apply, respectively, to outward (lateral) and inward (medial) rotation of the forearm.

Reduction of Outward Rotation, Inward Rotation, Supination, or Pronation

Rotation of the segment back to the midposition.

Movements in a Combination of Planes
Circumduction

An orderly sequence of the movements that occur in the sagittal, frontal, and intermediate oblique planes so that the segment as a whole describes a cone is known as *circumduction*. It consists of an axial movement that may occur in any plane. The movement may occur at biaxial or triaxial joints.

Arm circling and trunk circling are examples of circumduction.

Naming Joint Actions in Complex Movements

It is important to note that although all movements do not begin from the anatomical standing position, the joint actions are still named as if they were occurring in the anatomical standing position; however, the plane and axis are identified as those in which the movement actually occurs. An example is flexion and extension of the forearm at the elbow joint. Beginning from the anatomical standing position, this joint action occurs within the sagittal plane about a frontal-horizontal axis. If, however, the elbow movement is preceded by 90 degrees of flexion and inward rotation of the arm at the shoulder joint, elbow flexion and extension are described as occurring within the horizontal plane about a longitudinal axis.

Nonaxial Movements

Movements permitted at any diarthrodial joint except the arthrodial or plane joints are rotary movements and occur in a plane about an axis. Movements in plane joints are nonaxial. An example is the gliding movement that occurs between the articular facets of the spinal column. Nonaxial movements of body segments may occur when they are moved as the result of rotary action of adjacent segments. In a pushing action, the hand moves linearly forward in the sagittal plane because of the axial movements of the arm segments at the shoulder, elbow, and wrist joints. Similarly, in a deep knee bend, the trunk and head move linearly because of the rotary actions of the leg segments.

ANALYZING JOINT MOTIONS

The first four columns of the anatomical analysis model presented in table 1.2 deal primarily with the orientation of the body segments and the patterns of joint motion. For each phase of the tech-

nique and for each joint participating in the phase, the precise joint action and segment being moved should be identified and recorded. The plane of motion for each joint should be stipulated, along with the axis of joint motion. If it seems desirable to measure the range of motion in a given joint, this can be done from sequential motion pictures.

Once the information used in the anatomical model has been collected and examined, the analyst can begin to evaluate the performance in terms of joint motions. This evaluation should take into account some basic anatomical principles. Returning to the long jump example, several joint action principles apply.

Alignment

The proper alignment of segments may differ from movement to movement. The optimum segmental alignment for any skill should be determined based on efficiency, effectiveness, and safety. In the standing long jump example, the joints of the lower extremity need to be fully extended at takeoff to impart maximum jumping force. Because this is a jump for horizontal distance, the joints should be aligned in such a way as to ensure that the center of gravity is in front of the feet at the moment of takeoff.

Range of Motion

Each joint in the body has a limit to its range of motion. The range of motion limitations of the body and the range of motion demands of the activity must be compatible to avoid injury while still producing an effective performance. A limited range of motion in the standing long jump will shorten the amount of extension possible and thereby decrease the length of time over which the push-off force will be applied.

Flexibility

Flexibility reduces the internal resistance to motion. The maintenance of normal flexibility is an important consideration for all. In the jump example, flexibility in the joints of the lower extremity will allow for optimum flexion in the lower extremities while reducing the risk of injury.

LABORATORY EXPERIENCES

1. By studying a skeleton and observing a living subject, classify the following joints without referring to the textbook: hip, elbow, knee, ankle, wrist, radioulnar, metacarpophalangeal joint of finger, shoulder joint. (Do not confuse the motion at the elbow or wrist joints with that of the radioulnar joints.)

2. Take turns with a partner performing simple movements of the head, trunk, upper extremity, and lower extremity, and identify the planes and axes concerned.

3. Construct a simple device to illustrate the planes and axes in relation to the human body.

4. Study the tracing of the soccer throw-in (exercise 5.4 in appendix H). The action between (a) and (b) represents the "force phase," and between (b) and (c) the "follow-through phase." Following the example given for the right metatarso-phalangeal joint, complete the following table for the force phase. Repeat for the follow-through.

5. Measure the joint ranges of motion of 10 to 15 subjects for the movements indicated, using either a goniometer or a flexometer. Compare the results obtained with the averages given in table 2.3. Explain why you think the differences among individuals exist. (The figure numbers refer to appendix C.)

   a. Elbow flexion and hyperextension (figure C.1)
   b. Shoulder flexion and hyperextension (figure C.4b)
   c. Shoulder rotation (figure C.5)
   d. Lateral flexion of trunk (figure C.11b)
   e. Hip flexion (figure C.7)
   f. Medial and lateral hip rotation (figure C.8b)
   g. Plantar flexion and dorsiflexion (figure C.10)

6. Select one or two joint actions (e.g., shoulder flexion and hip flexion). Perform a comparison study of the range of motion for the actions selected using two groups of people, such as the following.

   a. Males versus females
   b. Varsity athletes from different sports (swimming vs. basketball or wrestling vs. gymnastics)
   c. Different age groups (20–30 vs. 50–60)
   d. Joggers versus sedentary people

   Subjects in each group should be matched on the basis of age and gender. Are any "group" differences apparent? Explain your results.

7. Measure the range of motion in one ankle. Tape the ankle and repeat the measurements immediately and then following 10 to 15 minutes of exercise during which the ankle is used (e.g., jogging, basketball, handball). Record your results

Name of Joint	Type of Joint	Starting Position	Observed Joint Action	Plane of Motion	Axis of Motion
R. metatarso-phalangeal	Ellipsoid	Sl. hyper-extension	Hyper-extension	Sagittal	Frontal horizontal
R. ankle					
R. knee					
R. hip					
Lumbar spine					
R. shoulder					
R. elbow					
R. wrist					
R. fingers					

and compare the differences. What effect, if any, did the tape have on range of motion for plantar and dorsiflexion? Inversion and eversion? Using the results of your measurements as the basis, discuss the value of taping as a means of preventing ankle injuries.

8. Measure the ranges of motion at the hip and knee joints during the back somersault depicted in exercise 5.6 in appendix H.

   a. On each tracing, mark the location of the right hip, knee, and ankle joints with a dot. Also place a dot at the midpoint of the waist. Connect the dots with straight lines so as to make a stick figure of the leg.

   b. Using a protractor, measure and record the angles between the trunk and thigh, and the thigh and lower leg, on each tracing.

   c. Determine the range of motion for each joint action from start to end of takeoff [(a) to (c)] and from peak to touchdown [(b) to (e)].

   d. What effect does range of motion in these joints have on skillful performance of this technique? As a coach or teacher, what specific training techniques would you include in the program of the performer to improve the range of motion where needed?

REFERENCES AND SELECTED READINGS

American Medical Association. 1988. *Guide to the evaluation of permanent impairment.* 3rd ed. (revised). Chicago: AMA.

Arnheim, D. D. and W. E. Prentice. 1998. *Essentials of athletic training.* 4th ed. St. Louis: McGraw-Hill.

Enoka, R. M. 1994. *Neuromechanical basis of kinesiology.* 2nd ed. Champaign, IL: Human Kinetics.

Federative Committee on Anatomical Terminology. 1998. *Terminologia Anatomica.* New York: Thieme.

Frankel, V. H., and M. B. Nordin. 1989. *Basic biomechanics of the skeletal system.* 2nd ed. Philadelphia: Lea & Febiger.

Goss, C. M., ed. 1980. *Gray's anatomy of the human body.* 36th ed. Philadelphia: Lea & Febiger.

Logan, G. A., and W. C. McKinney. 1982. *Anatomic kinesiology.* 3rd ed. Dubuque, IA: William C. Brown.

Netter, F. H. 1997. *Atlas of Human Anatomy.* Novartis Medical Education.

Norkin, C., and P. Levangie. 1992. *Joint structure and function: A comprehensive analysis.* 2nd ed. Philadelphia: F. A. Davis.

Roach, K. E., and T. P. Miles. 1991. Normal hip and knee active range of motion: The relationship to age. *Physical Therapy* 71:656–666.

Smith, E. L. W., L. D. Lehmkuhl, and L. K. Smith. 1996. *Brunnstrom's clinical kinesiology.* 5th ed. Philadelphia: F. A. Davis.

Steindler, A. 1970. *Kinesiology of the human body.* Springfield, IL: Charles C Thomas.

3

THE MUSCULOSKELETAL SYSTEM

The Musculature

O U T L I N E

- **Skeletal Muscle Structure**
  Properties of Muscular Tissue
  The Muscle Fiber
  Slow- and Fast-Twitch Fibers
  Muscular Attachments
  Structural Classification
     of Muscles on the Basis
     of Fiber Arrangement
  Effect of Muscle Structure
     on Force and Range of
     Motion
- **Skeletal Muscle Function**
  Line of Pull
  Types of Contraction
  Influence of Gravity
  Length–Tension Relationship
  Force–Velocity Relationship
  Stored Elastic Capabilities

- **Coordination of the Muscular System**
  Roles of Muscles
  Cocontraction
  Action of Biarticular Muscles
  Types of Bodily Movements
- **Methods of Studying the Actions of Muscles**
  Conjecture and Reasoning
  Dissection
  Inspection and Palpation
  Models
  Muscle Stimulation
  Electromyography (EMG)
- **Muscular Analysis**
- **Laboratory Experiences**

OBJECTIVES

At the conclusion of this chapter, the student should be able to:

1. Describe the structure and properties of the whole muscle, fast- and slow-twitch muscle fiber, and the myofibril.
2. Explain how the relationship of the muscle's line of pull to the joint axis affects the movement produced by the muscle.
3. Describe the relationship between the skeletal muscle's fiber arrangement and its function.
4. Define the roles a muscle may play (agonist, antagonist, and synergist), and explain the cooperative action of muscles in controlling joint actions by naming and explaining the muscle roles in a specified movement.
5. Define the types of muscular contraction (concentric, eccentric, and static), and name and demonstrate each type of action.
6. Demonstrate an understanding of the influence of gravity and other external forces on muscular action by correctly analyzing several movement patterns in which these forces influence the muscular action.
7. Describe the various methods of studying muscle action, citing the advantages and disadvantages of each method.
8. State the force–velocity and length–tension relationships of muscular contraction, and explain the significance of these relationships in static and dynamic movements.
9. Identify the muscle groups active in a variety of motor skills.

Body parts are moved by external or internal forces. The internal force responsible for the movement and positioning of the bony segments of the body is the action of skeletal muscles. These muscles are able to serve this function because they can contract, they are attached to the bones, and they cross a joint. In addition, they are constructed of bundles of striated muscle fibers, which differ in both structure and function from the highly specialized cardiac muscle and from the smooth muscle of blood vessels, digestive organs, and urogenital organs.

SKELETAL MUSCLE STRUCTURE

Properties of Muscular Tissue

The properties of striated muscle tissue are extensibility, elasticity, and contractility. The first two enable a muscle to be stretched like an elastic band and, when the stretching force is discontinued, to return again to its normal resting length. Tendons, which are simply continuations of the muscle's connective tissue, also possess these properties. Contractility, the

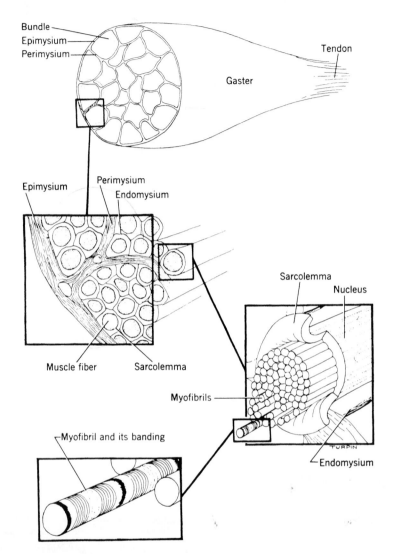

Figure 3.1 Architecture of a skeletal muscle and its fibers.
From T. W. Torrey, *Morphogenesis of the Vertebrates.* Copyright © 1962 John Wiley & Sons, New York.

ability to shorten and produce tension at its ends, is a unique property possessed by muscle tissue only. The average muscle fiber can shorten to approximately one-half its resting length. It can also be stretched until it is approximately one-half again as long as its resting length. The range between the maximal and minimal lengths of a muscle fiber is known as the amplitude of its action. The elongation varies proportionately with the length of the fiber and inversely with its cross section.

The Muscle Fiber

A single muscle cell is a threadlike fiber about 1 to 3 inches in length and containing the cell nucleus, mitochondria (important in cell metabolism), myoglobin (similar to hemoglobin), and

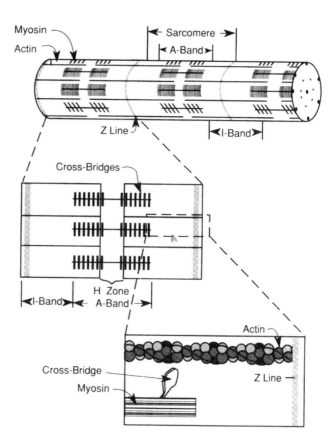

a. Magnification of single muscle fiber showing smaller fibers–myofibrils–in its

b. Myofibril magnified further to show thick and thin filaments composing it and producing its cross-striated appearance; dark A (anisotropic)- bands alternate with light I (isotropic)-bands; H zones, less dense midsections of A-bands; Z lines, more dense

c. Scheme to show how myosin interacts with actin to shorten muscle fibers. The cross-bridges bond to the actin filaments and slide them toward the center of the sarcomere.

Figure 3.2   The single muscle fiber and its myofibrils.

glycogen (form of sugar). In addition, microscopic examination has also revealed that the fiber consists of many hundreds of myofibrils embedded in sarcoplasm, held together by a delicate membrane known as sarcolemma, which has the ability to propagate nerve impulses (figure 3.1). Each fiber is enclosed within a thin connective tissue sheath called endomysium. The microscopic *myofibrils,* which are the contractile elements, are arranged in parallel formation within the fiber and are made of alternating dark and light bands that give the muscle fibers their striated appearance.

The electron microscope has revealed the striations to be a repeating pattern of bands and lines caused by an interdigitating arrangement of two sets of filaments. These myofilaments of contractile proteins, mainly actin (thin ones) and myosin (thick ones), when stimulated, slide past each other. This is due to the coupling and uncoupling of the cross-bridges, which appear as projections (heads) of the myosin filament attaching to the actin filaments. The myofibril is divided into a series of several sarcomeres, with each sarcomere consisting of the portion of the myofibril between two Z lines (figure 3.2). The sarcomere is considered the functional contractile unit of skeletal muscle. A concentric contraction (shortening) occurs when the actin filament slides over the myosin filament, pulling the Z lines toward one another; an eccentric contraction is the reverse, with the actin filament sliding outward, resulting in the return of the sarcomere to its original length or longer. An isometric contraction involving no length change results from the continual breaking and rebuilding of the crossbridges. This is a condensed and highly simplified explanation of contraction, a function that is the unique property of muscle tissue.

The muscle fibers are bound into bundles within bundles (see figure 3.1). Each individual bundle of muscle fibers, called a *fasciculus,* is enclosed in a fibrous tissue sheath called *perimysium;* the group of bundles that constitutes a complete muscle is in turn encased within a tougher connective tissue sheath called *epimysium.* In long muscles whose fibers run parallel to the long axis of the muscle, the bundles form "chains," which function as though the individual fibers ran the entire length of the muscle. Each enclosing sheath (the endomysium, perimysium, and epimysium) is made of connective tissue, which contains elastic fibers arranged both in series (end to end) and parallel (in the same direction) to the contractile elements. The elements that are in series are those which are important in controlling how the tension is applied to the bony levers in moving a load. Those in parallel remain slack in contraction and have a negligible effect during stretching of the muscle fiber.

Slow- and Fast-Twitch Fibers

Although four different fiber types (one slow- and three fast-twitch fibers) have been identified in human skeletal muscle, only the two major categories of slow- and fast-twitch fibers are pertinent for the study of kinesiology. In humans, most limb muscles contain a relatively equal distribution of each muscle fiber type, whereas the muscles of the back (i.e., posture muscles) contain more slow-twitch fibers. Where differences exist, the usual variation may be of the order of 2 percent to 10 per-

cent. However, rare instances of significant variation between fiber types may be found among muscles and individuals, although not between genders.

Fast-twitch muscle fibers are large and pale and have a less elaborate blood supply than slow-twitch muscle fibers. Once stimulated, fast-twitch fibers respond rapidly but fatigue easily. This characteristic makes them suitable for activities requiring intense responses over a short period of time, such as those responses found in sprints or weight-training exercises.

Slow-twitch fibers are small and red and have a rich blood supply. They also contain more myoglobin than fast-twitch fibers. Slow-twitch fibers take relatively longer to reach peak isometric tension (80–100 ms vs. approximately 40–60 ms for fast-twitch fibers), are highly efficient, and do not fatigue easily. Slow-twitch fibers are suitable for activities of long duration, including posture and endurance events.

Research has shown that training does not produce an increase in the number of muscle fibers or major shifts in muscle fiber types. There is evidence that some shift from fast-twitch to slow-twitch fibers can occur with training in animal models, but similar results in humans have not been proven conclusively (McComas 1996). Training does result in muscle fiber hypertrophy and may change some fast-twitch fiber types, but these changes, such as increased endurance and a greater number of capillaries, are reversible when use is discontinued. This is one reason that activity that places demands on the muscle fibers should be done on a lifelong basis.

Muscular Attachments

Muscles are attached to bone by means of their connective tissue, which continues beyond the muscle belly in the form of a tendon (a round cord or a flat band) or an aponeurosis (a fibrous sheet). Historically, anatomy texts designated attachments of the two ends of a muscle as "origin" and "insertion." The origin is usually characterized by stability and closeness of the muscle fibers to the bone. It is usually the more proximal of the two attachments. The insertion, on the other hand, is usually the distal attachment; it frequently involves a relatively long tendon, and the bone into which the muscle's tendon inserts is ordinarily the one that moves. It should be understood, however, that the muscle does not pull in one direction or the other. When it contracts, it exerts equal force on the two attachments and attempts to pull them toward each other. Which bone is to remain stationary and which one is to move depends on the purpose of the movement. A muscle spanning the inside of a hinge joint, for instance, tends to draw the two bones toward one another. However, most precision movements require that the proximal bone be stabilized, whereas the distal bone performs the movement. The stabilization of the proximal bone is achieved by the action of other muscles. Sometimes the greater weight or the more limited mobility of the proximal structure is sufficient to stabilize it against the pull of the contracting muscles.

Reverse Muscle Action

Students often receive the impression that there is some physiological reason for a muscle to pull in a single direction. They fail to grasp the concept of a muscle merely contracting, not realizing that it cannot pull in a predetermined direction. This misconception makes it difficult for students to understand seeming exceptions. Actually, in many movements the insertion or distal attachment of the muscle is stationary and the origin or proximal attachment is the one that moves. Such is the case in the familiar act of performing pull-ups. The movement of the elbow joint is flexion, but it is the upper arm that moves toward the forearm, just the reverse of what happens when one lifts a book from the table. The grasp of the hands on the bar serves to immobilize the forearm, and thus it provides a stable base for the contracting muscles. To avoid the erroneous idea of a muscle always pulling from its insertion toward its origin, the following terminology for muscular attachments is used in this text.

Terminology for Muscular Attachments

Attachments of muscles of the extremities:
    Proximal attachment
    Distal attachment

Attachments of muscles of the head, neck, and trunk:

Upper attachment

> muscles whose line of pull is more or less vertical— that is, parallel with the long axis of the body

Lower attachment

Medial attachment } for muscles whose line of pull is more or less horizontal
Lateral attachment }

Attachments of the diaphragm:
    Peripheral attachment
    Central attachment

Structural Classification of Muscles on the Basis of Fiber Arrangement

The arrangement of the fibers and the method of attachment vary considerably among different muscles. These structural variations form the basis for a classification of the skeletal muscles.

Longitudinal

This is a long, straplike muscle whose fibers lie parallel to its long axis. Two examples are the sartorius, which slants across the front of the thigh, and the rectus abdominis on the front of the abdomen (see figures 7.15 and 9.17).

Quadrate or Quadrilateral
(Figures 3.3e and f)

Muscles of this type are four sided and usually flat. They consist of parallel fibers. Examples include the pronator quadratus on the front of the wrist and the rhomboid muscle between the spine and the scapula.

Triangular or Fan Shaped (*Figure 3.3d*)

This is a relatively flat type of muscle whose fibers radiate from a narrow attachment at one end to a broad attachment at the other. The pectoralis major on the front of the chest is an excellent example.

Fusiform or Spindle Shaped (*Figure 3.3a*)

This is usually a rounded muscle that tapers at either end. It may be long or short, large or small. Good examples are the brachialis and the brachioradialis muscles of the upper extremity.

Unipenniform (*Figure 3.3b*)

In this type of muscle, a series of short, parallel, featherlike fibers extends diagonally from the side of a long tendon, giving the muscle as a whole the appearance of a wing feather. Examples include the extensor digitorum longus and tibialis posterior muscles of the leg.

Bipenniform (*Figure 3.3c*)

This double penniform muscle is characterized by a long central tendon with the fibers extending diagonally in pairs from either side of the tendon. It resembles a symmetrical tail feather. Examples include the flexor hallucis longus and rectus femoris of the leg and thigh, respectively.

Multipenniform

In this type of muscle several tendons are present, with the muscle fibers running diagonally between them. The middle portion of the deltoid muscle of the shoulder and upper arm is a prime example of a multipenniform muscle (see figures 5.11 and 5.14).

Effect of Muscle Structure on Force and Range of Motion

The force a muscle can exert is proportional to its physiological cross section, a measure that accounts for the diameter of every fiber and whose size depends on the number and thickness of the

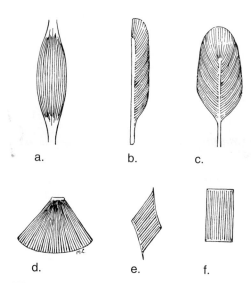

Figure 3.3   Examples of muscles of different shapes and internal structure: (a) fusiform or spindle; (b) penniform; (c) bipenniform; (d) triangular or fan shaped; (e) rhomboidal (quadrate); (f) rectangular (quadrate).

fibers. A broad, thick, longitudinal muscle exerts more force than a thin one, but a penniform muscle of the same thickness as a longitudinal muscle can exert greater force. The oblique arrangement of the fibers in the various classifications of penniform muscle allows for a larger number of fibers than in comparable sizes of the other classifications. Pennate muscles are the most common type of skeletal muscle and predominate when forceful movements are needed.

The range through which a muscle shortens depends on the length of its fibers, with the average muscle fiber capable of shortening to half its resting length. Those long muscles with fibers longitudinally arranged along the long axis of the muscle, such as the sartorius, can exert force over a longer distance than muscles with shorter fibers. Muscles of the pennate type, with their oblique fiber arrangement and short fiber length, can exert their superior force through only a short range.

SKELETAL MUSCLE FUNCTION

The basis for all muscle function is the ability of muscular tissue to contract. This should be kept in mind as various aspects of muscular function are considered.

Line of Pull

The movement that the contracting muscle produces—flexion, extension, abduction, adduction, or rotation—is determined by two factors: the type of joint that it spans and the relation of the muscle's line of pull to the joint. For instance, the contraction of a muscle whose line of pull is directly anterior to the knee joint may cause the joint to extend, whereas a muscle whose line of pull is anterior to the elbow joint may cause this joint to flex. The possible axes of motion are, of course, determined by the structure of the joint itself. It will be recalled that, from the anatomical standing position, hinge joints have only a frontal-horizontal axis, and condyloid (ovoid) joints have both a frontal-horizontal and a sagittal-horizontal axis. Ball-and-socket joints have three axes, frontal and sagittal horizontal and vertical (longitudinal), whereas pivot joints have a vertical axis only.

A muscle whose line of pull is lateral to the hip joint is a potential abductor of the thigh, but muscles whose lines of pull are lateral to the elbow joint cannot cause abduction of the forearm because the construction of the elbow joint is such that no provision is made for abduction or adduction. Because it is a hinge joint, its only axis of motion is a frontal-horizontal one, and the only movements possible are flexion and extension.

The importance of the relation of a muscle's action line to the joint's axis of motion is especially seen in some of the muscles that act on triaxial joints. Occasionally it happens that a muscle's line of pull for one of its secondary movements shifts from one side of the joint's center of motion to the other during the course of the movement. For instance, the clavicular portion of

the pectoralis major is primarily a flexor, but it also adducts the humerus. When the arm is elevated sideward (abducted) to a position slightly above shoulder level, however, the line of pull of some of the fibers of the clavicular portion shifts from below to above the sagittal-horizontal axis of the shoulder joint (figure 3.4). Contraction of these fibers in this position contributes to abduction of the humerus, rather than to adduction. Similarly, several muscles or parts of muscles of the hip joint appear to reverse their customary function. Steindler (1970) pointed out that as the adductor longus adducts the hip joint, it also flexes it until the flexion exceeds 70 degrees. Beyond this point the adductor longus helps extend the hip.

It is not uncommon to classify and name muscles according to the relation of their line of pull to the joint structure. In other words, muscles whose line of pull is such that they produce flexion are called flexors, and those in a position to cause extension are extensors. Similarly there would also be abductors, adductors, and rotators. The difficulty with this type of classification is that it may mislead the student into believing that the muscle is responsible for the related joint action under all circumstances, when in reality this is not the case. The biceps brachii muscle, for instance, is usually listed as a flexor and supinator of the forearm, when in fact the results of electromyographic studies have established that the biceps plays little if any part in flexion of the prone forearm or supination of the extended forearm unless the movements are resisted (Basmajian and DeLuca 1985). This example is not unusual. Many situations occur in which the presence or absence of resistance governs a muscle's participation in a joint action. Other factors, such as the starting position for the joint action, the direction of the movement, and the speed of the movement may also alter a muscle's involvement in the joint action.

Knowing the general location of a muscle with respect to the joint axis—anterior, superior, lateral, or medial—and knowing the line of pull of

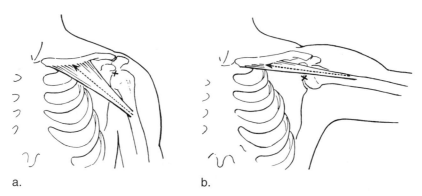

a.   b.

Figure 3.4   The clavicular portion of the pectoralis major muscle reversing its customary function. (a) The line of pull is below the center of the shoulder joint (flexion, adduction). (b) The line of pull is above the center of the shoulder joint (abduction).

the muscle is important information for deducing possible muscle participation during a body movement, but confirmation of those muscle actions must rely on the evidence of electromyography.

Angle of Attachment

The efficiency of a muscle in producing movement at a joint is also affected by the angle of attachment of a muscle to the stationary bone. If the angle of attachment is very shallow (the muscle lies along the line of the bone) most of the tension developed in the muscle will produce a force pulling along the bone. In other words, this muscle will have a very large stabilizing component. Force produced by this muscle will tend to stabilize the joint rather than produce motion. Conversely, a muscle whose angle of attachment is fairly large will have a much larger rotary component of force. The development of tension in this muscle will produce a force which will cause action at the joint. In many muscles the angle between muscle and bone changes as movement occurs. A good example of this is the biceps, whose tendon can be easily palpated where it attaches to the radius. Starting from the neutral position one can feel that the biceps tendon lies almost parallel to the humerus. As the forearm is slowly moved through elbow flexion it is possible to feel the change in the angle between biceps tendon and the radius. When the elbow is

at a 90 degree angle, notice that the biceps tendon forms approximately a 90 degree angle with the radius. In this position, all of the force generated by the biceps can act to produce joint motion. As elbow flexion continues beyond 90 degrees notice that the angle between the biceps tendon and the radius again begins to decrease as the line of pull shifts closer to the bone. As this change occurs the biceps is becoming less efficient at producing joint motion.

Types of Contraction

Because the word *contract* literally means to "draw together" or to shorten, the nature of muscular contraction may cause some initial confusion. A muscle contraction occurs whenever the muscle fibers generate tension in themselves, a situation that may exist when the muscle is actually *shortening, remaining the same length, or lengthening.*

Concentric or Shortening Contraction

Concentric (toward the middle) **contraction** occurs when the tension generated by the muscle is sufficient to overcome a resistance and to move the body segment of one attachment toward the segment of its other attachment. As the arm is raised sideward, the abductor shoulder muscles shorten to overcome the resistance of the arm. The muscle ac-

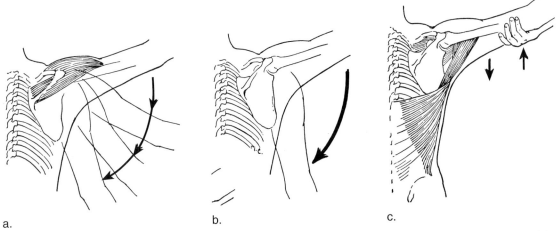

a.   b.   c.

Figure 3.5   Influence of gravitational force on muscular action in sideward depression of the arm (adduction of the humerus): (a) eccentric contraction of the abductors in slow lowering of the arm; (b) absence of muscular action when the arm dropped to the side; (c) concentric contraction of the adductors when the movement is performed against resistance.

tually shortens and, when one end is stabilized, the other pulls the bone to which it is attached and turns it about the joint axis (figure 3.5c).

Eccentric or Lengthening Contraction

When a muscle slowly lengthens as it gives in to an external force (such as gravity) that is greater than the contractile force it is exerting, it is in *eccentric* (away from the middle) *contraction.* The term *lengthening* is misleading, because in most instances the muscle does not actually lengthen. It merely returns from its shortened condition to its normal resting length (figure 3.5a). The abductor shoulder muscles are in eccentric contraction when the arm is slowly lowered from an abducted position. In most instances in which muscles contract eccentrically, the muscles are acting as a "brake," or resistive force, against the moving force of gravity or other external forces. When the muscles contract in this manner, they are said to perform negative work.

Isometric or Static Contraction

Isometric means "equal length." Tension of the muscle in partial or complete contraction without

any appreciable change in length is *isometric* contraction. Isometric contraction is likely to occur under two different conditions.

1. Muscles that are antagonistic to each other contract with equal strength, thus balancing or counteracting each other. The part affected is held tensely in place without moving. Tensing the biceps to show off its bulge is an example of this. The contraction of the triceps prevents the elbow from further flexing.
2. A muscle is held in either partial or maximal contraction against another force, such as the pull of gravity or an external mechanical or muscular force. Examples of this are holding a book with outstretched arm, a tug of war between two equally matched opponents, and attempting to move an object that is too heavy to move.

Isotonic Contraction

Isotonic means "equal tension." *Isotonic* contraction is a contraction in which the tension remains constant as the muscle shortens or lengthens. It is commonly, although erroneously, used as a

synonym for either eccentric or concentric contraction. The latter terms, however, do not indicate the degree of tension; they merely indicate
an increase or decrease in length.

Isokinetic Contraction

Literally, isokinetic means "equal or same motion" (*iso + kinetic*). Through the use of special
equipment, it is possible to have maximum muscle effort at the same speed throughout the entire
range of motion of the related lever. The response
of the muscles in maximum contraction to the
"accommodating resistance" of the machinery is
called *isokinetic* contraction.

Influence of Gravity

Movements of the body or its segments may be
in the direction of gravitational forces (downward), opposing gravity (upward), or perpendicular to gravity (horizontal). It is essential to consider the direction and speed of the movement
when identifying the nature of the muscular involvement of any movement. The muscles may
be contracting, either to provide the force for a
movement or the force to resist and control the
movement, or they may be completely relaxed
(figure 3.5). It may surprise the student to learn
that the muscles used when placing a book on a
low table or a suitcase on the floor are the same
as those used for lifting it. They are used in a different way, however. When the book or suitcase
is lifted, the muscles provide the force, and the
weight of the object (gravity) is the resistance. In
this case the muscles shorten in concentric contraction. When the object is slowly lowered, however, the muscles lengthen in eccentric contraction as they resist, but gradually give in to, the
force of gravity. Without the muscular resistance,
the force of gravity would lower the object at a
far more rapid rate! Another example of the influence of gravity on muscular action is the action of
the lower extremity muscles when one lowers the
body weight by bending the knees to assume a
squat or semisquat position and then returns to the
erect position. As the body is lowered the extensor

muscles of the hips and knees are undergoing eccentric contraction. They are indeed lengthening
in this instance, yet their tension is increasing as
they assume the burden of the body weight and
gradually allow it to lower in a controlled manner.
When the joint action is reversed and the body
weight is lifted, the extensor muscles are contracting concentrically until the hips and knees are
straight and the body is erect.

As has been demonstrated, any slow, controlled movement in the downward direction of
gravity's force uses the same muscles in eccentric
contraction that would be used in concentric contraction to perform the opposite upward movement (against gravity). Slow lowering of the forearm from a flexed position to one of extension is
controlled by eccentric contraction of the elbow
flexors, the same muscles that, by contracting
concentrically, cause flexion. A forceful movement downward does not follow this pattern,
however. When done forcefully, as in the downswing of a golf swing, the same movement of
elbow extension uses the elbow extensors in concentric contraction, because gravitational pull is
now being exceeded (figure 3.6).

Muscular involvement in movements performed horizontally is not affected by gravity in
the manner just described. Regardless of the force
or speed of the movement, the muscle force for
extension of the forearm at the elbow in the transverse plane is provided by the elbow extensors.
The only exception to this is seen when one is opposing an external force other than gravity, and it
proves to be too strong. In a tug of war, for instance, the weaker opponents will find their elbows being pulled out straight in spite of themselves. The elbow flexor muscles are in eccentric
contraction as they attempt to resist the force
causing the extension at the elbow.

The elbow flexor muscles are in eccentric
contraction as they attempt to resist the force
causing the extension at the elbow. Finally, at
times the movement of the body or its segments
occurs without muscular action. In these instances
the external force causing the movement is not resisted by eccentric muscle action. Examples are

Figure 3.6   Example of a rapid downward action utilizing a concentric muscle contraction.

allowing the force of gravity to cause the arm to drop to the side from a flexed or abducted position (figure 3.5b) and the passive moving of a body segment by another person.

Length–Tension Relationship

There is an optimum length at which a muscle, when stimulated, can exert maximum tension. This length varies somewhat according to both the muscle's structure and its function but, as a general rule, it is slightly greater than the resting length of the muscle. Lengths that are either greater or less produce less tension. This relationship applies for all three types of contraction: isometric, concentric, or eccentric. A typical length–tension curve is depicted in figure 3.7. The maximum resting length occurs at 100 percent. Curve 1 represents the tension generated when the muscle is passively stretched, and curve 2 represents the total tension

generated in the muscle. The active tension of the muscle would thus be the difference between the passive and the total tension, curve 2 minus curve 1. This relationship suggests that when maximum force is desired, the muscle should be longer than the resting length. However, other factors such as the muscle's angle of pull must be considered. It is rare for the angle of pull for optimum force application to occur when the muscle is in the resting position.

Force–Velocity Relationship

As the speed of a muscular contraction increases, the force it is able to exert decreases. The velocity of contraction is maximal when the load is zero, and the load is maximal when the velocity is zero (figure 3.8). For any given load there is an optimum velocity that is somewhere between the slowest and fastest rates. As the load increases, the optimum rate decreases. So does the need for more cross-bridges. Because it takes time for the cross-bridge sites to establish or break down, the inverse relationship between load and rate is readily understood. Thus, if an activity requires the development of large forces, only a small amount of muscle shortening should be expected. If, on the other hand, high limb or implement velocities are needed, then little force should be expected from the contracting muscles.

Stored Elastic Capabilities

It has been established under controlled experimental conditions that when concentric contraction is preceded by a phase of active stretching, elastic energy, stored in the stretch phase, is available for use in the contractile phase. The work done by muscles shortening immediately after stretching was found to be greater than that done by those shortening from a resting state or from an isometric contraction. In addition, this work increased with the speed of stretching and shortening. This enhanced potential for work is attributed to a combination of the series elastic components and the stretch reflex. Common

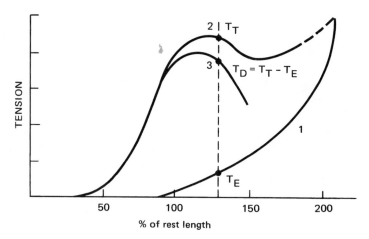

Figure 3.7   Length–tension curves for isolated muscle. Curve 1, passive elastic tension (T_E) in a muscle passively stretched to increasing lengths. Curve 2, total tension (T_T) exerted by muscle contracting actively from increasingly greater initial lengths. Curve 3, developed tension calculated by subtracting elastic tension values on Curve 1 from total tension values at equivalent lengths on Curve 2; i.e., $T_D = T_T - T_E$.

From B. Gowitzke and M. Milner. *Scientific Bases of Human Movement.* 3rd ed. Copyright © Williams & Wilkins, Baltimore, MD. Reprinted by permission.

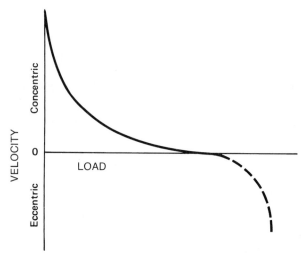

Figure 3.8   Force–velocity relationship. As the velocity of concentric contraction increases, the force that can be exerted decreases. When the velocity drops to zero, the contraction is isometric. In eccentric contraction, tension increases with the increased speed of lengthening.

movement patterns in sports often consist of a stretch before a counterconcentric contraction. The back swings for a kick, tennis drive, or pitch not only provide more distance through which the foot, racket, or hand can develop speed but also put the anterior hip and shoulder muscles on a stretch just prior to their contraction in the forward force phase (Plummer 1986). This pre-stretch makes use of the stretch-shortening cycle to produce a more efficient movement.

COORDINATION OF THE MUSCULAR SYSTEM

An effective, purposeful movement of the body or any of its parts involves considerable muscular activity in addition to that of the muscles that are directly responsible for the movement itself. To begin with, the muscles causing the movement must have a stable base. This means that the bone (or bones) not engaged in the movement but providing attachment for one end of such muscles must be stabilized by other muscles. In some movements, such as those in which the hands are used at a high level, the upper arms may need to be maintained in an elevated position. This necessitates contraction of the shoulder muscles to support the weight of the arms. Many muscles, especially those of biaxial and triaxial joints, can cause movements involving more than one axis, yet it may be that only one of their actions is needed for the movement in question. A similar situation exists in regard to the muscles of the scapula. A muscle cannot voluntarily choose to effect one of its movements and not another; it must depend on other muscles to contract and prevent the unwanted movement. Even a simple movement such as threading a needle or hammering a nail may require the cooperative action of a relatively large number of muscles, each performing its own particular task in producing a single, well-coordinated movement.

Roles of Muscles

Muscles have various roles. What their particular roles are in a given movement depends on the requirements of that movement. These roles are designated prime movers, antagonists, and synergists. Furthermore, if one concedes that the negative function of remaining relaxed can be viewed as a role, then the muscles that are antagonistic to the movers may also be included as participants in the total cooperative effort. The definitions of these roles are as follows.

Movers, or Agonists

A mover is a muscle that is directly responsible for producing a movement. In the majority of movements there are several movers, some of them of greater importance than others. These are the principal, or prime, movers. The muscles that help perform the movement but seem to be of less importance, or contract only under certain circumstances, are the assistant movers. Muscles that help only when an extra amount of force is needed, as when a movement is performed against resistance, are sometimes called emergency muscles. This distinction between the various muscles that contribute to a movement is an arbitrary one. There may well be some difference of opinion as to whether a muscle is a prime or an assistant mover in a given movement.

Synergists

The term synergy is often used to describe muscles in various ways, from mutual neutralizer to stabilizer. In this text, synergistic muscle action will be used to indicate cooperative muscle functioning in various roles. Muscles acting as synergists may fill one of several roles. The way in which a muscle aids in the production of the desired motion determines its synergistic role. Muscles may act as stabilizers or neutralizers.

Stabilizing, fixator, and supporting muscles

This group includes the muscles that contract statically to steady or support some part of the body against the pull of the contracting muscles, against the pull of gravity, or against the effect of momentum and recoil in certain vigorous movements. One of the most common functions of stabilizers is steadying or fixating the bone to which a contracting muscle is attached. It is only by the stabilizing of one of its attachments that the muscle is able to cause an effective movement of the bone at which it has its other attachment (figure 3.9). The term supporting may be used when a limb or the trunk must be supported against the pull of gravity while a distal segment such as the

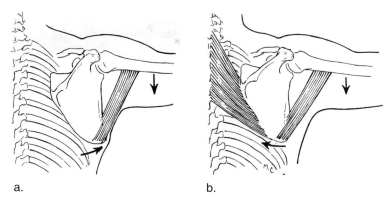

a.   b.

Figure 3.9   If the scapula were not stabilized, the teres major would increase the upward rotation of the scapula as it adducted the humerus. This dual action on the humerus and scapula is shown in (a). In (b) the scapula is stabilized by the scapular adductors and downward rotators. This permits the teres major to concentrate its force on the adduction of the humerus.

hand, foot, or head is engaging in the essential movement.

Neutralizers   A neutralizer is a muscle that acts to prevent an undesired action of one of the movers. Thus, if a muscle both flexes and abducts, but only flexion is desired in the movement, an adductor contracts to prevent the abduction action of the mover.

Occasionally two of the movers have one action in common but can also perform second actions that are antagonistic to each other. For instance, one muscle may upward rotate and adduct while the other may downward rotate and adduct. When they contract together to cause adduction, their rotary functions counteract each other (figure 3.10). Muscles that behave this way in a movement are mutual synergists as well as movers.

Antagonists

Muscles that have an effect opposite to that of movers, or agonists, are labeled antagonists. Because they are located on the opposite side of the joint from the movers they are also called contralateral muscles. The elbow flexors, located on the anterior arm, are antagonistic to the elbow ex-

tensors located on the posterior arm. When the forearm is extended at the elbow, as in doing a push-up, the extensors are the movers and contract concentrically to provide the force for the movement. The flexors are the antagonists and are relaxed. In the return movement, the letdown, the joint action at the elbow is flexion but the flexors do not contract—they remain relaxed. The contracting muscles, once again, are the extensors, but now they are contracting eccentrically to resist gravity and control the speed of the elbow flexion. When a body segment is moved by muscular effort, the contracting muscles are the movers in concentric contraction. When movement of a segment is effected by the force of gravity and resisted by muscle force, the contracting muscles are the antagonists in eccentric contraction.

Now that the general rule has been stated, it is necessary to describe what may at first appear to be a contradiction. If a movement performed with great force and rapidity is not checked, it will subject the ligamentous reinforcements of the joint to sudden strain. The tissues would probably be severely damaged. This is particularly true of quick movements of the arm or leg because of the tremendous momentum that can be developed in a long lever. This is often referred to as a ballistic

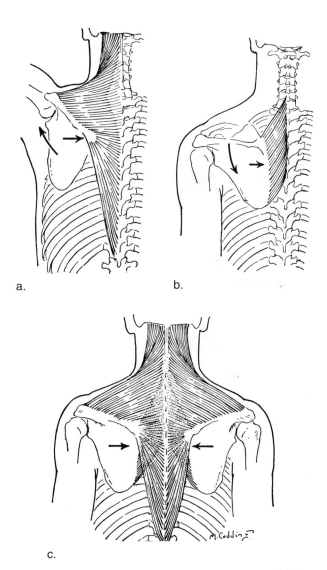

Figure 3.10   The trapezius and rhomboids as mutual movers and neutralizers. (a) The trapezius alone adducts the scapula and rotates it upward. (b) The rhomboids alone adduct the scapula and rotate it downward. (c) Together the trapezius and rhomboids adduct the scapula without rotating it either upward or downward.

movement, which by definition is a movement carried on by its own momentum. To prevent injury from the momentum of the limbs, the muscles that are antagonistic to the movers contract momentarily to check the movement. As they contract, the movers relax, if indeed they have not already relaxed, allowing momentum to complete the movement. The situation is a little like taking the foot off the accelerator to put it on the brake. At the moment when the movement is being checked, the so-called antagonistic muscles are not truly antagonistic. In a vigorous movement, the antagonistic muscles may be said to perform two functions. Their first function is to relax in order to permit the movement to be made without hindrance; their second function is to act as a brake at the completion of the movement and, by doing so, to protect the joint.

Summary of Muscle Classification Based on Role in Total Movement

Mover or agonist: A muscle that is directly responsible for effecting a movement.

Synergist:

Fixator, stabilizer, supporting muscle: Muscles that contract statically to steady or to support some part of the body against the pull of contracting muscles, the pull of gravity, or any other force that interferes with the desired movement.

Neutralizer: A muscle that acts to prevent an undesired action of one of the movers.

Antagonist: A muscle that causes the opposite movement from that of the movers.

Example of the Different Roles of Muscles in a Total Movement

Let us consider the movement of the right upper arm when playing shuffleboard (pushing a disk with a cue). The movement of the humerus at the shoulder joint is flexion, and this is accompanied by slight upward rotation and abduction of the scapula. The *movers of the humerus* are the anterior deltoid, the clavicular portion of the pectoralis major, and the coracobrachialis. (Look these terms up if you are not yet familiar with them.) The two former muscles are also inward rotators of the humerus, but because this movement is not desired, it must be prevented. The infraspinatus and the teres minor take care of this. Therefore, they are serving as *neutralizers* in this pushing action. Meanwhile, the scapula is rotating upward through the action of the serratus anterior and trapezium II and IV, which are serving as *shoulder girdle movers.* Trapezius II, which is an elevator as well as an upward rotator of the scapula, and trapezium IV, which is a depressor

as well as an upward rotator, mutually neutralize each other with respect to elevation and depression while they are cooperating in rotating the scapula upward. Hence they are both *movers* and *mutual neutralizers.*

Consider the movers of the humerus once again, keeping in mind that muscles tend to pull both their distal and proximal ends toward each other. Note that the proximal attachments of both the anterior deltoid and the pectoralis major are side by side on the anterior border of the clavicle. As they contract, they not only raise the humerus forward but also tend to pull the clavicle laterally, a movement that would put a strain on the sternoclavicular joint. They are prevented from doing this by the action of the subclavius muscle, which pulls the clavicle medially and thus serves as a stabilizer. So in this simple pushing movement we see that we have muscles acting as movers, neutralizers, and stabilizers, which, by their cooperative action, ensure an efficient movement.

Cocontraction

This action of muscles is usually defined as the simultaneous contraction of movers and antagonists. This sounds simple and straightforward, but nevertheless it requires interpretation. In any given movement, even the simplest, several muscles other than the movers are likely to be involved. There are neutralizers and mutual neutralizers whose function it is to counteract an additional function of a mover that is not desired in the present movement (see figure 3.10). There are also many movements that require the action of stabilizers. These may be for stabilizing a weight-bearing segment against gravity, or for the stabilization of a freely movable bone that provides for the proximal attachment of one of the movers (see figure 3.9).

The patterns of muscle activation that can occur in the production of human movement are vast in number. Recent research in muscle activation has shown that the relationships between muscle actions is, by nature, task dependent. That is, the relationships will depend on the nature of the motion to be produced. With this in mind, it is perhaps best to examine muscle activation patterns in terms of synergy rather than coactivation or cocontraction (Zajac and Gordon 1989).

Action of Biarticular Muscles

Another type of coordination of the muscular system may be seen in the so-called tendon action of the biarticular muscles—that is, the muscles that pass over and act on two joints. Examples of these are the hamstrings (the semitendinosus, the semimembranosus, and the biceps femoris), which flex the leg at the knee and extend the thigh at the hip; the rectus femoris, which flexes the thigh and extends the leg; the sartorius, which flexes both the thigh and the leg; the gastrocnemius, which helps flex the leg in addition to its primary function of extending the foot; and the long flexors and extensors of the fingers. The latter are actually multijoint muscles, because they cross the wrist and at least two of the joints of the fingers. A characteristic of all these muscles, whether they act on joints that flex in the same direction, as in the case of the wrist and fingers, or in the opposite direction, as in the case of the knee and hip, is that they are not long enough to permit complete movement in both joints at the same time. This results in the tension of one muscle being transmitted to the other, in much the same manner that a downward pull on a rope that passes through an overhead pulley is transmitted in the form of a pull in the reverse direction to the rope on the other side of the pulley. Thus, if the hamstrings contract to help extend the hip, tension in the form of a stretch is placed on the rectus femoris, causing it to extend the knee. Or if the rectus femoris contracts to help flex the hip, tension in the form of a stretch is placed on the hamstrings, causing them to flex the knee. This is a simplified version of what in actuality is a rather complex coordination.

When monoarticular (one-joint) muscles contract, their shortening is accompanied by a corresponding loss of tension. In quick movements of the limbs, monoarticular muscles rapidly lose their tension. The advantage of biarticular muscles is that they can continue to exert tension without shortening. The biarticular muscles have two different patterns of action, described as *concurrent* and *countercurrent* movements.

An example of concurrent movement is seen in the simultaneous extension of the hip and knee and also in the simultaneous flexion of these joints. As the muscles contract, they act on each other in such a way that they do not lose length; thus their tension is retained. It is as though the pull traveled up one muscle and down the other in a continuous circuit. In simultaneous extension of the hip and knee, for instance, the rectus femoris's loss of tension at the distal or knee end is balanced by a gain in tension at the proximal or hip end. Similarly, the hamstrings, which are losing tension at their proximal end, are gaining it at their distal end.

The countercurrent pattern presents a different picture. In this type of movement, while one of the biarticular muscles shortens rapidly at both joints its antagonist lengthens correspondingly and thereby gains tension at both ends. An example of this action is seen in the rapid loss of tension in the rectus femoris and corresponding gain of tension in the hamstrings when the hip is flexed and the knee is extended simultaneously. A vigorous kick is a dramatic illustration of this kind of muscle action. The backward swing of the lower extremity preparatory to kicking is a less spectacular but equally valid example. The forward swing in walking is another. In both patterns of movement the monoarticular and biarticular muscles appear to supplement each other and thus, by their cooperative action, produce smooth, coordinated, efficient movements (figure 3.11).

When a biarticular muscle contracts it acts on both joints it crosses. If action is desired in only one joint, the other joint must be stabilized by another muscle or by some external force. In such circumstances, Fujiwara and Basmaiian (Basmajian and DeLuca 1985) found that the rectus femoris shows maximum activity in either pure hip flexion or pure knee extension, and the medial

a.   b.

Figure 3.11   (a) A concurrent muscle action of the rectus femoris on top of the thigh and the hamstrings on the underside of the thigh occurs when each of the antagonist muscles lengthens at one joint and shortens at the other. (b) A counter-current muscle action occurs as the rectus femoris shortens concentrically at both joints while the hamstrings are stretched at both joints.

hamstrings, similarly, are most active in either hip extension or knee flexion. In the biarticular countercurrent movements of hip flexion and knee extension, the rectus femoris exhibited strong activity. The medial hamstrings exhibited similar strong activity during hip extension and knee flexion. When the movement was concurrent hip flexion and knee flexion, however, the rectus femoris showed no activity, but the hamstring did. Similarly, during knee extension and hip extension, the hamstrings were inhibited and the rectus femoris was active. The activity of the rectus femoris and hamstrings was thus inhibited when they were antagonists.

Types of Bodily Movements

Movements may be passive or active, and if active, they may be slow or rapid. They may in-

volve the constant application of force, or after the initial impetus has been given, they may continue without further muscular effort.

A *passive* movement requires no effort on the part of the person involved. It is performed by another person such as a therapist giving a treatment or an instructor or partner stretching tight ligaments, fascia, and muscles in an attempt to increase the range of motion of a particular joint. In some cases, it is a movement that has been started by the subject's own effort but is continued by momentum. It might also be caused by the force of gravity if the subject remained relaxed and used no muscular effort to aid, restrain, or guide the moving part. To avoid injury, care must be taken that the subject does not resist the movement and that the person applying the force to cause the movement is not too aggressive.

An *active* movement is produced by the subject's own muscular activity. It is usually performed volitionally, but it may be a reflex reaction to an external or internal stimulus. It may be rapid or slow. In slow movements muscular tension is maintained throughout the range of motion. Pushing a heavy piece of furniture across the room is an example of this type of movement. In *rapid* movements, tension could also be maintained throughout the range of motion, but this would be an inefficient way of performing. For efficiency, rapid movements should be performed ballistically. The concept of *ballistic* movement was introduced a number of years ago by experimental psychologists. They used the term for movements that were initiated by vigorous muscular contraction and completed by momentum. This type of movement is characteristic of throwing, striking, and kicking. It is also seen in the finger movements used for typing and piano playing. When such movements are performed nonballistically—that is, with constant muscular contraction—they are uneconomical and hence not skillful. In fact, they are characteristic of the way in which beginners tend to attempt new coordinations, especially if they are concentrating on accuracy of aim rather than on a ballistic type of motion. They need to be encouraged in the early stages of learning a skill to concentrate on form rather than accuracy if they are to master the skill of moving ballistically.

Ballistic movements may be terminated by one of three methods: (1) by contracting antagonistic muscles, as in the forehand drive in tennis; (2) by allowing the moving part to reach the limit of motion, in which case it will be stopped by the passive resistance of ligaments, other tissues, or the braking action of antagonistic muscles, as in the case of the forceful overarm throw; or (3) by the interference of an obstacle, as when chopping wood.

In many movements found in both sports and activities of living, three types of muscular action cooperate to produce a single act. This kind of cooperation is seen especially in striking activities that require the use of an implement, such as a tennis racket, golf club, or ax. Movements such as these involve (1) fixation to support the moving part and to maintain the necessary position, (2) ballistic movement of the active limb, and (3) fixation in the fingers as they grasp the implement.

METHODS OF STUDYING THE ACTIONS OF MUSCLES

In addition to the obvious method of studying the actions of muscles in a textbook, there are a number of procedures that may be more meaningful to the student.

Conjecture and Reasoning

Using knowledge of the location and attachments of a muscle and the nature of the joint or joints it spans, one can deduce a great deal about a muscle's actions. Conjecture and reasoning is a method that is valuable to use in conjunction with other methods. Although the use of this method does not identify which muscles are actually contracting in a given action, a careful study of the muscles' attachments and line of pull (figure 3.12) will enable one to see what movements a muscle is *capable* of causing.

Dissection

An excellent way of studying the location and attachments of a muscle and its relation to the joint it spans is dissection. This method provides a more meaningful basis for visualizing the muscle's potential movements, but it sometimes leads to misinterpretations and erroneous conclusions.

Inspection and Palpation

Even though its use is limited to superficial muscles, inspection and palpation of normal living subjects is a valuable method, as far as it goes. Much of the information in early anatomy

Figure 3.12   Locating a muscle's line of pull by placing ends of a string or elastic at the location of the muscle's attachment. The line of pull of the sternocleidomastoid is located using this procedure.

textbooks was based on the combination of dissection of the cadaver and inspection and palpation of living subjects. Before the days of electromyography these were the chief methods of determining the actions of the muscles. There is a possibility of misinterpretation, however, against which students should be warned. When the force of a muscle contraction is weak, it is sometimes difficult to feel its contraction. If the subject repeats the action against greater resistance, the contraction may be stronger and more easily felt. The conclusion may be drawn erroneously that the muscle is a major mover for the action involved, when in fact it comes into action only as an assistant under conditions of heavy resistance.

Models

Numerous devices, both commercial and homemade, can be used for demonstrating and studying the actions of muscles. Probably the most commonly used device is the simplest of all— a long rubber band (or chain of short ones) held against the bones of a skeleton in such a way as to represent a single muscle. The movement is

demonstrated by holding the elastic on a stretch with one end representing the proximal attachment and the other the distal attachment. The tendency of both bones to move toward each other can easily be demonstrated, as well as the necessity for stabilizing one bone so that the muscle can be effective in moving the other bone.

Muscle Stimulation

To most kinesiologists the term "muscle stimulation" means G. B. Duchenne, the pioneer in the use of electrical stimulation as a means of studying the actions of the muscles and the author of *Physiologie des Mouvements*. This classic work was translated into English and published in 1949. It made a tremendous contribution to the science of kinesiology, yet its limitations must be recognized. It demonstrates the contraction of individual muscles when they are stimulated electrically. Unfortunately, it cannot analyze the sequence of muscular actions that occur in an everyday act such as walking, lifting a package, or working with a common tool. Neither can it reveal the complex combinations of muscular actions in ordinary sport techniques.

   In spite of its limitations, muscle stimulation is being used in many modem kinesiology laboratories as a device for studying the responses of individual muscles to electrical stimulation and to rehabilitate muscles. One of the more promising areas of research in the rehabilitation field has been that of functional electrical stimulation (FES). FES combines electrical stimulation with computer control systems to offer some movement in muscles that have no functional nerves. The development of FES technology is aimed at providing mobility to disabled individuals. At this writing, much work remains to be done. FES systems have been used with some success in a number of settings, but the complexity of human movement, even the simple act of walking, has made the task of programming computers to stimulate the appropriate muscles in the appropriate sequence a daunting one. It is possible, however, that in this century, disabled individuals may be

Figure 3.13   Electromyography is a valuable tool for studying muscle activity.

able to walk with the aid of electrical stimulation and computer control.

Electromyography (EMG)

Although few undergraduate students may have the opportunity of personal experience with electromyography, all may benefit by reading the reports of EMG investigations. A wealth of information concerning muscular action is available in such reports. Electromyography is based on the fact that contracting muscles generate electrical impulses. It is a technique of recording such impulses or action potentials, as they are also called (figure 3.13). It provides specific information about muscular actions that we have only been able to guess at in the past, information that has proved much of our guessing to be inaccurate. The unique advantages of EMG are that it reveals both the intensity and duration of a muscle's action and, in fact, discloses the precise time sequences of muscular activity in a movement.

Furthermore, it reveals the actions not only of the agonists and antagonists but also of the muscles serving as stabilizers and neutralizers. Perhaps its greatest contribution to our knowledge of muscular action is its ability to record the impulses of deep as well as superficial muscles. Basmajian, the apostle of electromyography, says that it surpasses all the older methods of studying muscular action in that it reveals what the individual muscles are actually doing, not just what they *can do* or *probably do* (Basmajian and DeLuca 1985).

Muscular Analysis

The approach to the analysis of the muscle participation in a given motion is exactly the same as that used for joint action. Using the same anatomical analysis model (table 1.1), the analyst adds a description of muscular involvement to the previously completed analysis of joint and segment involvement. The muscular action is identified for each joint movement and recorded next to the joint actions on the chart (see table 1.2). This implies identifying not only the muscle groups (flexors, extensors, abductors, adductors, etc.) that are contracting but also their function in the movement and the kind of contraction they are undergoing (concentric, eccentric, or static). Identification of the force causing the motion facilitates the subsequent identification of the muscle and type of contraction involved. In those instances where

the force causing the motion is gravity, the muscle contraction type is most likely to be eccentric. If muscle is the force causing the motion, the contraction is concentric. It is critical to remember the influence of gravity during this portion of the analysis. When gravity is the force producing motion, the muscle group that is active will be that which is antagonistic to the *observed* motion. In other words, extension produced by the pull of gravity is controlled by eccentric contraction of the *flexor* muscles.

Any of the methods described for studying muscle actions may be used to determine which muscle groups are active during a performance. Once the general muscle groups have been identified, the analyst may wish to identify specific prime movers (agonists) and synergists. Chapters 5 through 9 will provide knowledge required concerning individual muscles and their actions.

A condition of efficient movement is to use only those muscles that are appropriate to the motion. Tension in muscles that are not active in the skill produces fatigue and often a performance that is both inefficient and ineffective. Failure to use all requisite muscle groups can also seriously impair movement. A common fault in unskilled jumpers, for example, is tension in the anterior muscles of the lower leg (the ankle dorsiflexors). This tension can restrict the forceful plantar–flexion muscle action and related ankle motion necessary for an efficient and effective jump.

LABORATORY EXPERIENCES

1. Take two sticks that are joined at one end by a hinge. Attach a single piece of elastic or a long rubber band to the opposite ends of the two sticks.
   a. Separate the ends of the sticks as far as the elastic will permit and then demonstrate the way the elastic will pull both sticks together.
   b. Demonstrate the way in which the elastic will move only one of the sticks if the other one is stabilized.
   c. Repeat both a and b, using the arm of the skeleton instead of the sticks.
2. Get a subject to hold a heavy dumbbell in the right hand and slowly raise the arm sideward/upward without bending the elbow. Keep your fingers on

the clavicular portion of the pectoralis major. Does it contract? If so, at what position of the arm does it begin?

3. Flex the fingers hard. Keep them flexed and flex the hand at the wrist as far as possible. What happens to the fingers? Explain.

4. Extend the fingers, and then hyperextend the hand at the wrist as far as possible. What happens to the fingers? Explain.

5. Get a subject to lie on the left side with the hip and knee in a partly flexed position and the right leg fully extended. The right thigh should now be flexed passively by an operator. The subject should attempt to keep the knee straight but not to the point of interfering with the hip flexion. What happens? Where does the subject feel discomfort? Explain.

6. Have the subject, in the same starting position as in Lab Experience 5, flex both the right thigh and right leg completely. The right thigh should now be passively extended by an operator, with the subject attempting to keep the leg flexed at the knee. As the thigh becomes fully extended, what happens to the knee? Where does the subject feel discomfort? Explain.

(Caution: Do not use an acrobat or acrobatic dancer as a subject for Lab Experience 5 or 6, or the experiments may not work. Why?)

7. Have a subject lie supine on a table with the knees at the edge and the lower legs hanging down. Ask the subject to extend one leg at the knee while you attempt to stop the motion by applying strong resistance at the front of the ankle. Note the amount of resistance you have to apply. Now ask the subject to flex the leg at the knee while you attempt to stop the movement by resisting at the rear of the ankle. Which action requires more resistance on your part?

Now ask the subject to sit up and flex the trunk well forward from the hips. Repeat the same two actions of knee flexion and extension against resistance. Which action requires more effort on your part this time? How does this compare with the first result? Explain.

It may help you to know that the rectus femoris crosses the front of the hip joint and the front of the knee joint. Hence, it is a flexor of the hip and an extensor of the knee. The biceps femoris is located on the back of the thigh and therefore is an extensor of the hip and flexor of the knee. Note: Laboratory exercises on the action of muscles as movers, stabilizers, and neutralizers are not included here because, in order to do them, it is necessary to know the individual muscles. They will be found in the laboratory sections of chapters 5 through 9.

8. Following the analysis model presented in table 1.2, do an analysis of the muscle groups (i.e., flexors, extensors, etc.) active in the performance of a motor skill that involves a number of joints.

REFERENCES AND SELECTED READINGS

Basmajian, J. V., and C. J. DeLuca. 1985. *Muscles alive.* 5th ed. Baltimore: Williams & Wilkins.

Enoka, R. M. 1988. Muscle strength and its development: New perspectives. *Sports Medicine* 6:146–68.

Foss, M. L., S. J. Keteyian, and E. L. Fox. 1998. *Fox's physiological bases of physical education and athletics.* 6th ed. St. Louis: McGraw-Hill.

Gowitzke, B., and M. Milner. 1988. *Understanding of scientific bases of human movement.* 3rd ed. Baltimore: Williams & Wilkins.

McComas, A. J. 1996. *Skeletal muscle.* Champaign, IL: Human Kinetics.

Morrissey, M. C. 1988. Electromyostimulation from a clinical perspective: A review. *Sports Medicine* 6:29–41.

Plummer, L. A. 1986. The influence of muscle elasticity and reflex response on force production characteristics during a stretch-shortening cycle. Master's thesis. University of Illinois, Urbana champaign.

Rasch, P. J. 1989. *Kinesiology and applied anatomy.* 7th ed. Philadelphia: Lea & Febiger.

Rogers, M. M., and P. Cavanagh. 1984. Glossary of biomechanical terms, concepts, and units. *Physical Therapy* 64:1886–902.

Saltin, B., and P. D. Gollnick. 1983. Skeletal muscle adaptability: Significance for metabolism and performance. *Handbook of physiology,* Sec. 10, pp. 555–631. Bethesda, MD: American Physiology Society.

Steindler, A. 1970. *Kinesiology of the human body.* Springfield, IL: Charles C Thomas.

Zajac, F. E., and M. E. Gordon. 1989. Determining muscle's force and action in multiarticular movement. *Exercise and Sport Sciences Review* 17:187–230.

THE NEUROMUSCULAR BASIS OF HUMAN MOTION

OUTLINE

- **The Nervous System and Basic Nerve Structures**
  Neurons
  Nerves
  The Synapse
- **The Motor Unit**
  Gradations in the Strength
    of Muscular Contractions
- **Sensory Receptors**
  Proprioceptors
- **Reflex Movement**
  Exteroceptive Reflexes
  Proprioceptive Reflexes
  Posture and Locomotor
    Mechanisms
- **Volitional Movement**
  Central Nervous System:
    Levels of Control
  Kinesthesis
  Reciprocal Inhibition
    and Coactivation
- **Neuromuscular Analysis**
- **Laboratory Experiences**

OBJECTIVES

At the conclusion of this chapter, the student should be able to:

1. Name and describe the functions of the basic structures of the nervous system.
2. Explain how gradations in strength of muscle contraction and precision of movements occur.
3. Name and define the receptors important in musculoskeletal movement.
4. Explain how the various receptors function, and describe the effect each has on musculoskeletal movement.
5. Describe reflex action, and enumerate and differentiate among the reflexes that affect musculoskeletal action.
6. Demonstrate a basic understanding of volitional movement by describing the nature of the participation of the anatomical structures and mechanisms involved.
7. Perform an analysis of the neuromuscular factors influencing the performance of a variety of motor skills.

The role of the bones, joints, and muscles in human movement were presented in the previous two chapters. The appropriate function of these systems requires an intact nervous system. Therefore, this chapter takes up the role of the nervous system in initiating, modifying, and coordinating muscular action.

Loofbourrow (1973) presented this topic so succinctly and vividly that his classic and still applicable introductory paragraph is quoted here in full as an introduction to this chapter:

> The forces which move the supporting framework of the body are unleashed within skeletal muscles on receipt of signals by way of their motor nerves. In the absence of such signals, the muscles normally are relaxed. Movement is almost always the result of the combined action of a group of muscles which pull in somewhat different directions, so the control of movement involves a distribution of signals within the central nervous system (CNS) to appropriate motor nerves with precise timing and in appropriate number. In order for movements to be useful in making adjustments to external situations, it is necessary for the central nervous system to be appraised of these situations, which are continually changing. A means of providing this information promptly exists in a variety of receptors sensitive to changes in temperature, light, pressure, etc. These receptors are signal generators which dispatch signals (nerve impulses) to the CNS over afferent nerve fibers. The CNS receives these signals together with identical ones from within the muscles, joints, tendons, and other body structures and is led thereby to generate and distribute in fantastically orderly array myriads of signals to various muscles. This, despite the enormous complexity of the machinery involved, enables the individual to do one main thing at a time. This is integration. It is what Sir Charles Sherrington meant by "the integrative action of the nervous system."

The following discussion does not presume to be an exhaustive treatise on neuromuscular mechanisms. It attempts rather to present as simply as possible those mechanisms that are pertinent to the study of kinesiology. Because of techniques made possible by electronic sensing devices, great strides have been made in acquiring more accurate information concerning the intricacies of muscular function.

THE NERVOUS SYSTEM AND BASIC NERVE STRUCTURES

It is assumed that the kinesiology student is already familiar with the general plan of the nervous system; hence, it will not be described in full here. Only a brief outline of the major divisions will be presented to give the reader a framework for the topics selected for discussion:

I. Central nervous system
  A. Brain
  B. Spinal cord

II. Peripheral nervous system
  A. Cranial nerves (12 pairs)
  B. Spinal nerves (31 pairs)

III. Autonomic nervous system (sympathetic and parasympathetic)

The autonomic nervous system is not a distinct system based on structure and geographic location, as are the central and peripheral systems, but is rather a functional division that overlaps with those in specific areas. It includes those portions of the brain, spinal cord, and peripheral nervous system that supply cardiac muscle, smooth muscle, and gland cells.

Neurons

A neuron, the structural unit of the nervous system, is a single nerve cell consisting of a cell body and one or more projections. Three kinds of neurons propagate impulses. Two kinds of neurons whose long fibers constitute the peripheral nervous system are the sensory (or afferent) and motor (or efferent) neurons (figure 4.1). There are also numerous connector neurons located only within the central nervous system.

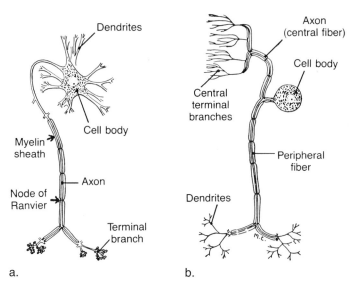

Figure 4.1   Neurons: (a) motor neuron; (b) sensory neuron.

The cell bodies of the majority of efferent, or motor, neurons are situated within the anterior horns of the spinal cord. (Some also exist in the brainstem and sympathetic ganglia.) Many short, threadlike extensions of the cell body, known as dendrites, synapse with the axons of other cells, the latter being either sensory or connector neurons.

Each motor and connector neuron has a specialized process termed an axon. The axon of the motor neuron emerges from the spinal cord in a ventral root. It then travels by way of a peripheral nerve to the muscle that it helps activate. There it divides and subdivides into smaller and smaller branches, the most distal being known as the terminal branches. Each terminal branch ends within a single muscle fiber in the structure called the motor endplate or neuromuscular junction.

The cell body of a spinal afferent, or sensory, neuron, unlike that of a motor neuron, is situated in a dorsal root ganglion just outside the spinal cord. (The cell bodies of cranial sensory neurons are in cranial nerve ganglia.) The neuron has a single short process that projects from the cell body and then bifurcates into two branches that go in opposite directions. One, the so-called central fiber, travels in the dorsal root of the nerve to

the posterior horn of the spinal cord, where it divides into numerous branches. It may terminate in the cord, or it may ascend in the cord to the brain and terminate there. The other branch of the afferent neuron is the long peripheral fiber, which comes from a receptor. It travels in a nerve trunk (peripheral nerve) to the vicinity of the appropriate dorsal root ganglion, where it unites with the cell body via the short stemlike process mentioned earlier (figure 4.1b).

Authorities differ in their choice of nomenclature for the parts of a sensory neuron. Some apply the term *axon* to the short stemlike process; others apply this term to the central fiber—the branch that enters the spinal cord. This text adopts the latter use of the term, because it is in keeping with a commonly accepted definition—namely, that an axon is the fiber over which impulses are conducted *away from* the cell body, as opposed to dendrites, which convey impulses toward the cell body. When referring to a sensory neuron, the term *dendrite* is applied not to the long fiber that conveys impulses from peripheral regions to the cell body, but rather to its branches. The long sensory fiber itself is known simply as the peripheral fiber.

It was noted earlier that the dendrites of efferent (motor) neurons make contact within the spinal cord, either with the terminal branches of afferent (sensory) neurons or with connector neurons. Connector neurons, also known as internuncial neurons, are a third type of nerve cell. They exist completely within the central nervous system and serve as connecting links. They may vary from a single small neuron, connecting a sensory neuron with a motor neuron, to an intricate system of neurons whereby a sensory impulse may be relayed to many motor cell bodies. We know from common experience that a complex motor act may result from a single sensory impulse. For instance, a sudden loud noise may cause us to jump, turn around, and tense nearly every muscle in our body. The connector neurons are responsible for this widespread response to the single sensory impulse. Thus only one connector neuron may be participating in a movement, or there may be an intricate network making possible an almost limitless number of connections with other neurons.

Nerves

Just as an electric cable is an insulated bundle of wires for the transmission of electric currents, so a nerve is a bundle of fibers, enclosed within a connective tissue sheath, for the transmission of impulses from one part of the body to another. A nerve, or nerve trunk as it is frequently called, may consist entirely of outgoing fibers from the central nervous system to the muscles and other tissues, or it may consist only of incoming fibers from the sensory organs to the central nervous system. The typical spinal (peripheral) nerve, however, is mixed; that is, it contains both outgoing and incoming fibers. Each spinal nerve is attached to the spinal cord by an anterior (motor) root and a posterior (sensory) root (figure 4.2). The posterior root bears a ganglion (a collection of cell bodies), and it is just beyond the ganglion that the two roots unite to form the spinal nerve. Once outside the vertebral canal, each spinal nerve divides into an anterior and a posterior branch, each of which contains both motor and

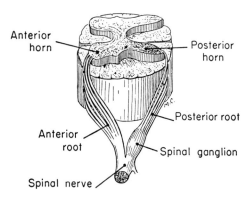

Figure 4.2   Section of the spinal cord showing the anterior and posterior roots of a spinal nerve.

sensory fibers. The anterior branches supply the trunk and limbs, the posterior branches the back. Motor nerves that activate skeletal muscle fibers are referred to as the alpha motor system.

The 31 pairs of mixed peripheral nerves exit from both sides of the vertebral column between every two vertebrae, with the first spinal nerve exiting from between the skull and the first cervical vertebra. Therefore, there are 8 cervical, 12 thoracic, 5 lumbar, 5 sacral, and 1 coccyx spinal nerves. Specific areas of the body are activated by fibers from specific peripheral nerves. Table 4.1 outlines the spinal nerve innervation patterns.

The Synapse

Synapses are connections between and among neurons and occur only within the central nervous system (figure 4.3). A synapse, and there may be thousands between any two neurons, is a proximity of the membrane of an axon and the membrane of a dendrite or a cell body. No physical union occurs between or among neurons. Conduction of impulses takes place in one direction only, from the axon of one neuron to the dendrites, cell body, or, rarely, to the axon of another. Synapses are influenced by use and disuse. The more often one is crossed, the easier it becomes for signals to pass through it. Conduction velocity is very rapid along the nerve fiber. Whenever there is a delay, it occurs at the

TABLE 4.1	Peripheral Nerve Innervation Pattern		
Vertebrae	**Peripheral Nerves**	**Plexus**	**General Innervation**
Cervical (7)	8 pairs (between skull and C1)	Cervical (C1–C4)	Head and neck
		Brachial (C5–T1)	Upper extremities
Thoracic (12)	12 pairs		Trunk, including abdomen
Lumbar	5 pairs	Lumbar (L1–4)	Lower extremities Pelvis
		Lumbosacral (L4–S3)	Lower extremities
Sacral (5 fused)	5 pairs	Sacral (S1–5)	Pelvis and lower extremities
Coccyx	1 pair	Coccygeal (S4–C)	Coccyx

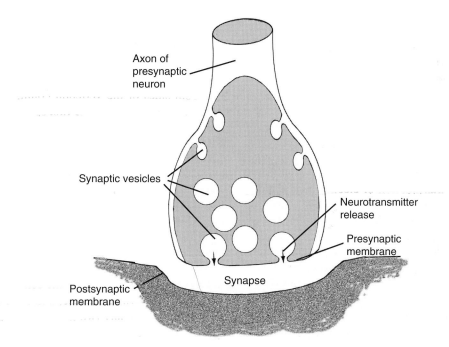

Figure 4.3   Nerve ending and synapse.

synapses. The greater the number of synapses from receptor to effector, the longer the time from stimulus to response.

The transmission of an impulse across a synapse depends on the release of a chemical transmitter substance by the axon. This substance diffuses throughout the membranes, and an action potential is created in the postsynaptic neuron. The action potential may be excitatory or inhibitory. Threshold level is the minimum level of stimulus (chemical transmitter) necessary to result in the initiation or propagation of a signal. Too little transmitter results in no impulse being carried to the next neuron, but an increase in this transmitter beyond the threshold level produces a response equal to but not greater than that needed for the threshold level. It must be remembered that it is at the synapse where facilitation (making it easier) or inhibition (making it more difficult) occurs. If the threshold level is altered so that only a small amount of additional neurotransmitter needs to be released for the threshold level to be achieved, facilitation will occur. Conversely, if a larger quantity of the chemical is needed before threshold level is reached, inhibition will occur. The student is reminded that more than one motor neuron may attach to a single muscle fiber, and therefore neurotransmitters released from several neurons simultaneously may have an additive or inhibitory effect.

THE MOTOR UNIT

The structural units of the nervous and motor systems are, respectively, the neuron and the muscle fiber. Functionally, the two systems combine to form the neuromuscular system. The functional unit of the neuromuscular system is the *motor unit,* and it consists of a single motor neuron (see figure 4.1a), together with all of the muscle fibers that its axon supplies (figure 4.4). All muscle fibers activated by the same motor neuron are of the same muscle fiber type.

Motor units vary widely in the number of muscle fibers supplied by one motor neuron. Some motor units may have as many as 2000 or more muscle fibers (gastrocnemius); others may have fewer than 10 (eye muscles). A muscle that has a small ratio of muscle fibers to alpha motor neurons is capable of more precise movements than is the muscle with a small number of motor neurons for the same number of muscle fibers. Hence the ratio of muscle fibers to motor neurons has a direct bearing on the precision of the movements executed by the muscle. For example, the small muscles of the thumb and index finger are capable of movements of great precision because their motor units have such a low ratio of muscle fibers to motor neurons or, to state it differently,

such a large number of motor neurons per muscle. By way of contrast, the gluteus maximus has a relatively small number of motor neurons for its size, hence a large number of muscle fibers per neuron. It does not need to be pointed out that the movements for which the gluteus maximus is responsible can scarcely be described as precise.

Gradations in the Strength of Muscular Contractions

Common experience indicates that the same muscles contract with various gradations of strength according to the requirements of the task. The elbow flexors, for example, are able to contract just enough to enable the hand to lift a piece of paper from the desk; they can also contract forcefully enough to lift a 15-pound briefcase. How do they adjust to such extremes? Two major factors influence the gradation of contraction. These are (1) the number of motor units that participate in the act and (2) the frequency of stimulation. If the stimulus is of threshold value, all the muscle fibers in the motor unit will contract maximally. If the stimulus is subliminal, in other words, below threshold value, none of the muscle fibers in the unit will contract at all. This characteristic is known as the *all-or-none principle of muscular contraction.* It must be emphasized that the principle applies only to individual motor units, not to entire muscles. To reiterate, if the stimulus is of threshold value, each muscle fiber in the participating unit whose threshold level has been reached will contract. Hence, it follows that, other things being equal, the more motor units that contract, the greater will be the total strength developed.

There is an orderly sequence to the recruitment of motor units. Innervation begins with the recruitment of the smaller slow-twitch fiber motor units, which have lower thresholds. They are followed by the larger fast-twitch motor units, which have high threshold levels. The sequence of recruitment is reversed with the release of tension—that is, "last on" is "first off."

If stimuli are discharged at low frequency, the muscle fibers will partially relax between im-

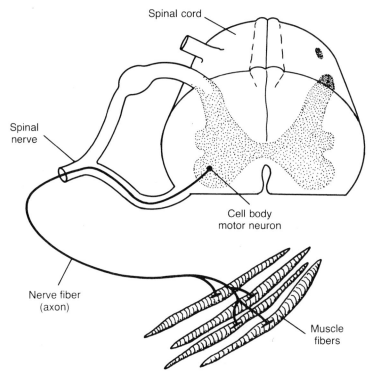

Figure 4.4   The organization of a motor unit.

Adapted from J. V. Basmajian and C. DeLuca, *Muscles Alive,* 5th ed. Copyright © 1985 Williams & Wilkins, Baltimore, MD. Reprinted with permission.

pulses, but if the stimuli are discharged at high frequency, the fibers will have insufficient time to relax and the result is summation or maximal contraction. If these two factors are combined—that is, if the maximum number of fibers are stimulated with the impulses being discharged at high frequency—the resulting contraction is of maximal strength.

It should be noted that motor unit areas overlap, with a single muscle fiber often belonging to more than one motor unit. It takes a number of motor units firing to result in joint angle changes. The ability of a single muscle fiber to respond to more than one motor unit also becomes important with aging; there is evidence to suggest that with age, the number of active motor units decreases (Doherty, Vandervoort, and Brown 1993). With appropriate equipment (electromyography and

audio feedback), it is also possible to learn how to control single motor unit firing. This phenomenon has played an important role in research, biofeedback, and control of some prosthetic devices.

SENSORY RECEPTORS

Most activities of the nervous system begin with stimuli that activate sensory nerve terminals. Whereas motor nerves end on muscle fibers, forming motor units, sensory nerves are attached to specialized endings referred to as receptors. These receptors are specialized cells or organs that are selective in their response to different types of stimuli, although they often respond to more than one type of stimulus. There are two major classfications, exteroceptors and interoceptors.

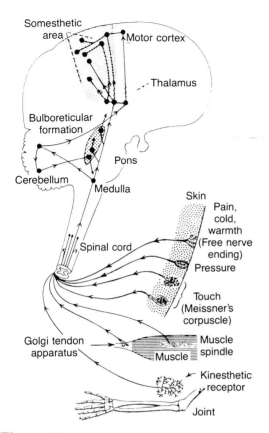

Figure 4.5   Transmission of proprioceptive sensations to the brain, showing the sensory receptors and the nerve pathways for transmitting these sensations into the brain.

From A. C. Guyton, *Textbook of Medical Physiology,* 5th ed. Copyright © 1976 W. B. Saunders, Orlando, FL. Reprinted by permission.

Exteroceptors are located at or near a body surface and receive and transmit stimuli that come from outside the body, including the receptors of the familiar five senses: sight, hearing, smell, taste, and touch. Interoceptors include the receptors for other cutaneous sensations, such as heat, cold, pain, and pressure (figure 4.5).

The interoceptors may be subdivided into receptors that receive impulses from the viscera and those that receive impulses from the tissues directly concerned with musculoskeletal movements and positions. The former are known as visceroceptors, and the latter are called proprioceptors.

Proprioceptors

Students of motor activity and posture find the proprioceptors of special interest, for these are the receptors that receive impulses that occur because of body movements or positions. They are located in the muscles, tendons, and joints, including the surrounding and protective tissues such as capsules, ligaments, and other fibrous membranes, and in the labyrinth of the inner ear. The proprioceptors are stimulated by motions of the body and in turn are responsible for transmitting a constant flow of information from these structures to the central nervous system. This information involves the appropriateness of the response in regard to the degree, direction, and rate of change of body movements. Without these sensory reports, effective coordination in motor patterns would not occur. Information from the receptors is directed both to the conscious and unconscious levels and, in addition to giving us a sense of awareness of body and limb positions, provides us with automatic reflexes. Proprioceptors are classified as muscle proprioceptors (muscle spindles and Golgi tendon organs), joint and skin proprioceptors (Ruffini endings and pacinian corpuscles), and labyrinthine and neck proprioceptors (figures 4.5 and 4.6).

Muscle Proprioceptors

An abundance of two types of receptors are located within muscles and tendons. Both are responsive to stretch tension. The *muscle spindle* detects relative muscle length and the *Golgi tendon organ* (GTO) detects muscle tension and active contraction.

Muscle spindles   The muscle spindles are scattered throughout the muscle but predominate in the belly of the muscle, lying between the muscle fibers and parallel with them. More spindles are located in muscles controlling precise movements than are located in postural muscles. When the spindle is stretched, a sensory nerve located in its center sends impulses to the CNS, which in turn activates the motor neurons innervating the mus-

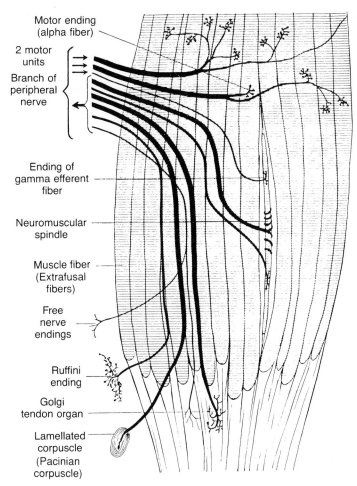

Motor ending
(alpha fiber)

2 motor
units

Branch of
peripheral
nerve

Ending of
gamma efferent
fiber

Neuromuscular
spindle

Muscle fiber
(Extrafusal
fibers)

Free
nerve
endings

Ruffini
ending

Golgi
tendon organ

Lamellated
corpuscle
(Pacinian
corpuscle)

Figure 4.6   Schematic representation of a muscle and its nerve supply.
From E. Gardner, *Fundamentals of Neurology,* 6th ed. Copyright © 1975 W. B. Saunders, Orlando, FL. Reprinted by permission.

cle, thus causing it to contract. The muscle spindle is responsive to both length (tonic response)
and rate of change in length (phasic response). A
single spindle is a tiny capsule (about 1 mm
long), filled with fluid and containing some specialized muscle fibers known as intrafusal
(fusimotor) fibers, to distinguish them from the
extrafusal (skeletomotor) or "regular" muscle
fibers (figure 4.7). There are two kinds of intrafusal fibers, nuclear bag fibers and nuclear chain
fibers. They are similar in that they both have
central noncontractile areas in which the nuclei

are situated, and both have polar ends that are
contractile. They differ in size and in the arrangement of the nuclei. The nuclear bag fiber is the
larger of the two, and the nuclei appear crowded
into the baglike central area, which gives the fiber
its name. The small nuclear chain fiber is named
for the single line, chainlike arrangement of the
nuclei in its slim, noncontractile central portion.
There are differences also in the intricate system
of innervation.

Each spindle is supplied with a type Ia afferent neuron that has a characteristic ending known

Figure 4.7   A muscle spindle containing two nuclear bag intrafusal fibers and three nuclear chain fibers, shown as it lies in parallel with the contractile (extrafusal) fibers of the muscle. Innervation is omitted.

From E. B. Gardner, "Proprioceptive reflexes and their participation in motor skills" in *Quest* XII:4. Copyright © 1969 Human Kinetics Publishers, Champaign, IL. Reprinted by permission.

as the *primary,* or *annulospiral,* ending. This ending is divided into as many branches as there are intrafusal fibers, and each branch is coiled around the noncontractile midsection of the intrafusal fiber. The annulospiral (AS) ending is highly sensitive to the velocity of changes in fiber length (phasic response), but only while the change is occurring. It also reacts to static (tonic) or length responses but with a sharp decline in frequency of impulse.

Most muscle spindles also have from one to five sensory endings that, because of their appearance, are given the picturesque name of *flower-spray* (FS) endings. Each FS ending has its own sensory (type II) fiber. The FS endings (also called secondary endings) are found at either end of the noncontractile midsection of the intrafusal fibers. They are believed to register static muscular length only (tonic response). The impulses transmitted by the FS endings increase almost directly in proportion to the amount of stretch and continue for a prolonged period of time. The FS endings are less sensitive to muscle stretch than the AS endings and therefore require a greater stimulus before responding. Because both the AS and FS endings activate the nuclear chain fibers, it is assumed that these fibers are responsible for the static response of both AS and FS endings. In contrast, only the AS endings activate the nuclear

bag fibers. These fibers, then, must be responsible for the strong phasic response of the AS endings (Gowitzke and Milner 1988; Park, Toole, and Lee 1999).

Muscle spindles are also supplied with their own small efferent fibers. To differentiate these fibers from the motor neurons of the "regular" muscle fibers, they are termed *gamma fibers,* in contrast to the "regular" motor neurons whose axons are termed *alpha fibers* (see figure 4.6). As a group, the gamma fibers form a *gamma fiber system.* Approximately one-third of the fibers in the peripheral nerve are gamma fibers. Impulses conveyed by gamma fibers (also called gamma efferents) cause the intrafusal muscle fibers to contract. This shortening of the spindle muscle fibers stretches their central noncontractile region where the AS endings are situated, and this stimulates them, causing their rate of firing to increase. Hence the effect of the gamma system is to control the sensitivity of the spindle afferents (gamma bias). The AS endings can be caused to fire, not only by passive stretch of the muscle as a whole, but also in the absence of such stretch by the function of the gamma system.

An exaggerated but familiar example of a simple adjustment of this nature is seen when picking up an object that is thought to be heavy. When the opposite proves to be the case, the cor-

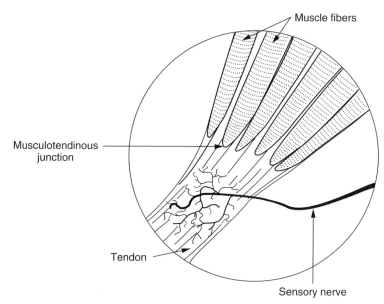

Muscle fibers

Musculotendinous
junction

Tendon

Sensory nerve

Figure 4.8   Golgi tendon organ located in series at the musculotendinous junction.
From E. L. Fox, R. W. Bowers, and M. L. Foss, *The Physiological Basis of Physical Education and Athletics,* 4th ed. Copyright © 1988
W. B. Saunders Company. Reprinted by permission of Times Mirror Higher Education Group, Inc., Dubuque, IA. All rights reserved.

rection in muscular effort is almost instantaneous. Less spectacular examples of this kind of coordination occur in all movements all the time. The gamma system provides a means of maintaining a position regardless of the tension put on it and enables smooth rather than jerky muscle response.

In summary, a muscle spindle can be stimulated in two different ways: (1) by stretching the whole muscle, causing the spindle to stretch; and (2) by contracting the ends of the intrafusal fibers via the gamma efferent system, thus stretching the center receptor portion of the spindle. The muscle spindle response is *tonic* in reacting to a static length and *phasic* in reacting to the rate at which length changes. Primary (AS) endings are sensitive to both tonic and phasic stretches, but secondary (FS) endings respond only to tonic stretch. Muscle spindles are very complex organs that are responsible for controlling the coordination of our muscular behavior. The feedback, which they supply continually, ensures a constant adjustment of muscular contraction.

Golgi tendon organ   In contrast to the muscle spindle, the *Golgi tendon organ,* when stretched, sends signals to the central nervous system and causes the muscle to relax rather than contract. It consists of a mass of nerve endings, which are enclosed within a connective tissue capsule and embedded in a muscle tendon (figure 4.8). It is situated close to the junction of the tendon with the fleshy part of the muscle in such a way that it has an end-to-end relationship with the muscle fibers. It is said to be "in series" with the muscle fibers. As the muscle shortens in contraction, the tension in the tendon increases and the Golgi tendon organs are stretched and activated. They are much less sensitive to stretch than spindles and require a stronger stretch to be activated. When the stress is greater than the Golgi tendon organ stretch threshold, the reflex contraction that is due to spindle stimulation is overridden and the muscle relaxes. The Golgi tendon organ provides instantaneous information about the degree of tension on each small segment of muscle. It is therefore a protective mechanism, and when the tension is extreme, its inhibitory effect can be great enough to effect a whole muscle relaxation.

Joint and Skin Proprioceptors

Two important receptors located in the joints or skin are the pacinian corpuscles and the *Ruffini endings*. Pacinian corpuscles are found beneath the skin, concentrated in regions around the joint capsules, ligaments, and tendon sheaths. They are large end organs consisting of a tip of nerve fiber surrounded by many concentric layers of capsule. They are activated by rapid joint angle changes and by pressure that compresses and distorts the capsule, but only for a very brief period of time. Consequently, they are important for detecting rapid changes in pressure but useless for constant pressure awareness. In running, the information provided by the pacinian corpuscles allows the nervous system to predict where the feet will be at any time so that appropriate adjustments in limb position can be anticipated and effected as needed. Ruffini endings are also activated by mechanical deformation but, in contrast to the pacinian corpuscles, are important for signaling continuous states of pressure. They adapt slowly at first but then transmit a steady signal thereafter. Ruffini endings are located in the deep layers of the skin and are scattered throughout the collagenous fibers of the joint capsules. They are stimulated strongly by sudden joint movements and are thus important in sensing joint position and changes in joint angle of as little as 2 degrees. Each joint receptor monitors a specific section of the total range of motion of the joint. By knowing which receptor is stimulated, the brain can tell how far the joint is bent. The sensing of the complete movement by the central nervous system is the result of the integration of the stimuli received from the individual receptors.

Although *cutaneous* receptors are fundamentally exteroceptors, the ones that receive stimuli from touch (Meissner corpuscles), pressure (pacinian corpuscles), and pain (free nerve endings) serve as proprioceptors when they show sensitivity to texture, hardness, softness, and shape and when they participate in the extensor thrust reflex, pain, or flexion withdrawal reflex.

Labyrinthine and Neck Proprioceptors

These proprioceptors detect sensations concerned with determination of body position and changes in position as they relate to equilibrium. The labyrinths detect orientation and movements only in the head, whereas the neck proprioceptors inform the nervous system of the orientation of the head in relation to the body.

The labyrinths of the inner ear consist of the cochlea, the three semicircular canals, and the utricle and saccule (figure 4.9). The cochlea is concerned with hearing, but the rest of the labyrinth is concerned with the sense of balance, or equilibrium. Each of the canals contains a membranous tube, and the bony spaces for the macule of the utricle and the saccule contain membranous sacs correspondingly named. The entire membranous labyrinth is filled with fluid called endolymph and is lined with hair cells that are sensitive to the movement of the fluid as the head moves. These hair cells are intimately related to branches of the eighth cranial nerve. Thus, movement of the head is translated into nerve impulses that reach the brain.

In addition to hair cells located throughout the labyrinth, there is a gelatinous substance in which otoliths (small carbonate of lime crystals) are embedded. The otoliths accentuate the effects of gravity on the hair cells and thus are able to detect changes in position that upset static equilibrium. They are also sensitive to linear acceleration by the head.

The semicircular canals are each in a different plane at right angles to each other. When the head turns, the canals move with it, but at first the fluid in them tends to remain stationary owing to inertia. When the head stops, the canals do also, but again, because of inertia, the fluid does not stop moving immediately. Relative motion in the endolymph produces motion in the hair cells, triggering impulses to the cranial nerve. This process

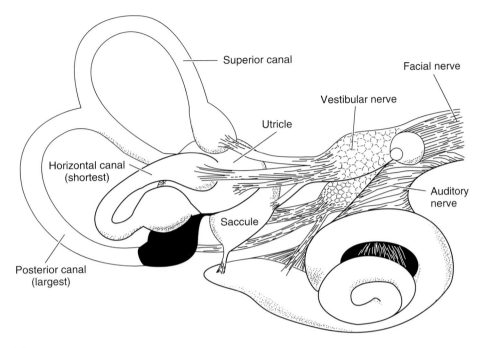

Figure 4.9   The labyrinthine system of the inner ear.

From B. A. Gowitzke and M. Milner, *Scientific Bases of Human Movement.*, 3rd ed., p. 290. Copyright © 1988 Williams & Wilkins, Baltimore, MD. Reprinted by permission.

enables the canals to detect any changes in angular velocity of the head. The anatomical arrangement of the entire labyrinth is such that some part of it is especially sensitive to any position or direction of movement of the head with respect to gravity.

The most important proprioceptive information needed for the maintenance of equilibrium is that provided by the joint (ligament) receptors of the neck (C1–C3), because they are sensitive to the angle between the body and the head. When the head is bent in one direction, the impulses from the neck prevent the labyrinthine proprioceptors from producing a feeling of imbalance. They do this by sending signals exactly opposite to those transmitted by the labyrinth. If the entire body's orientation with respect to gravity is altered, however, the neck receptors do not counteract the labyrinthine receptors, and change in equilibrium is sensed.

REFLEX MOVEMENT

Reflexes are integrated at various levels of the nervous system. A reflex movement is a specific pattern of response that occurs without volition and without the need of direction from the cerebrum. The anatomical basis for a reflex act is the reflex arc (figure 4.10). This consists of an afferent neuron that comes from a receptor organ, enters the spinal cord, and there makes a synaptic connection either directly with the dendrites and the cell body of an efferent neuron or indirectly through one or more connector neurons. The axon of the efferent neuron extends from the cord to the muscle, where its distal branches terminate in muscle fibers. The point of contact between an axon and a muscle fiber is known as a myoneural junction, or motor endplate. The number of reflex arcs and the number of motor units involved depend both on the nature of the reflex and on the

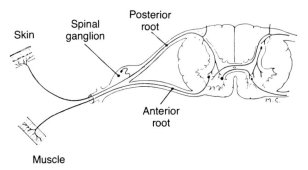

Figure 4.10   Reflex arc mechanism.

extent of muscular activity needed. Automatic reflex motions accompany all normal voluntary motion. Indeed, very few muscles in most movement patterns are under conscious control.

Exteroceptive Reflexes

Although some overlap occurs, as could be inferred from the discussion of receptors, two main classes of reflexes are related to skeletal movements—namely, exteroceptive and proprioceptive. Many of the exteroceptor reflexes exhibited by animals and human beings are familiar to us. A horse will twitch its skin when flies alight on it; a dog will scratch when its skin is irritated by a flea, or perhaps tickled by a person. A human jumps upon hearing a sudden loud noise. A person also blinks when a foreign body strikes the eyeball, or even threatens to strike it. Three exteroceptive reflexes that may be of special interest are the extensor thrust, flexor, and crossed extensor reflexes.

Extensor Thrust Reflex

Pressure against the sole of the foot stimulates the pacinian corpuscles in the subcutaneous tissue and elicits the reflex contraction of the extensor muscles of the lower extremity. When the weight is supported by the feet, the pressure of the floor is sufficient to bring about this reaction. As the weight is shifted to the balls of the foot in preparation for a jump, or to the palms of the hand in preparation for a handspring the pressure

results in the extensor thrust reflex facilitating the contractions of the extensor muscles of the legs or arms, respectively, thus assisting the push-off from the floor (Deutsch et. al. 1987; Gowitzke and Milner 1988) (figure 4.11). Similarly in archery, the pacinian corpuscles in the bow hand are stimulated, and facilitation of the extensor muscles of the bow arm occurs. However, in this instance, the archer must counteract this reflex action and prevent full extension at the elbow or suffer a painful lesson of being whipped by the released strings. The extensor thrust reflex is often included as a proprioceptive reflex in some classifications.

Flexor Reflex

The flexor reflex most frequently operates in response to pain and is a device for self-protection. Because of the flexor reflex, we quickly withdraw a part of the body the instant it is hurt. If a finger is pricked by a pin or if it inadvertently touches a hot pan, we do not have to decide to remove our hand from the source of pain; we jerk it back even before we realize what happened to it. Furthermore, all the necessary muscles for withdrawing it are activated promptly, not just those in the immediate vicinity of the injury. Although we are all too aware of the pain, this awareness occurs after the withdrawal and plays no part in the reflex action. The value of the awareness is rather in teaching us to avoid repeating the act that caused the pain. This reflex is also called the withdrawal reflex.

Figure 4.11   Extensor thrust reflex. As the weight is transferred to the ball of the foot in preparation for the hurdle, the concentrated pressure on the ball of the foot may enable the extensor thrust reflex to facilitate the push-off from the ground.

Crossed Extensor Reflex

This reflex functions cooperatively with the flexor reflex in response to pain in a weight-bearing limb. For instance, when an animal injures its paw, the flexor reflex causes it to withdraw the paw. Simultaneously, owing to the crossed extensor reflex, the extensor muscles of the opposite limb contract to support the additional weight thrust upon it. Similarly, if a person who is barefoot happens to step on a tack with the right foot, the body weight quickly shifts to the left foot and the right foot is withdrawn from the floor. As the flexors of the right limb contract to enable the lifting of the right foot, the extensors of the left limb contract more strongly to support the weight of the entire body.

Applications of the crossed extensor reflex have also been made to a non-weight-bearing limb. When a pain stimulus is applied to one hand, at the same moment that the hand is withdrawn the opposite arm will extend as though to push the body away. Some individuals have also suggested that walking may reflect an application of the crossed extensor reflex. Release of pressure from the sole of the back foot results in facilitation of the extensor muscles of the front leg to accommodate the shift in weight over that foot.

Proprioceptive Reflexes

Earlier in this chapter receptors were classified as exteroceptors and interoceptors, the latter being subdivided into visceral receptors and proprioceptors. Proprioceptive reflexes are generally described as those reflexes that occur in response to stimulation of receptors located in the skeletal muscles, tendons, joints, and labyrinths of the inner ear. According to this interpretation, the proprioceptive reflexes are those interoceptors related to motions and positions of the body. The stretch, or myotatic, reflex is always included among these. Some classifications also include the extensor thrust, the labyrinth and neck, and the tendon organ reflex.

Stretch Reflex

The stretch reflex is so named because stretch on the muscle stimulates the muscle spindle, resulting in the reflex contraction of the stretched muscle and its synergists and relaxation of its antagonists. The muscle spindle picks up the stretch stimulus and transmits it by way of the afferent neuron to the spinal cord. There the central terminal branches of the sensory neuron synapse directly with the dendrites of the motor neuron, which activates the same muscle fibers that were stretched. These fibers then contract. This two-neuron reflex arc is the simplest type of reflex arc, consisting of a single sensory neuron and single motor neuron, which may involve one or more synapses. The important characteristic of this type of reflex arc is that it does not make use of connector neurons in the spinal cord.

There are two responses to the stretch reflex—phasic or tonic—depending on the velocity at which the stretch occurs. The frequency of discharge from the primary endings of the muscle spindle is directly related to the velocity at which the muscle fibers are being stretched. The greater the frequency of these impulses, the greater will be the resulting muscle fiber contraction.

The phasic type includes familiar clinical tests, such as the knee jerk. Reflexes of this type are extremely rapid and the contraction is of brief duration. The word "jerk" gives an accurate picture. Although it is true that the cause of the stimulus in this instance is exteroceptive in nature (a rubber-headed hammer or the edge of the hand), it is nevertheless classed as a proprioceptive reflex. If the stretch is sudden and sufficiently strong, the stretched muscle contracts quickly and forcefully because of the response of the primary endings of the muscle spindles.

A slow stretch, such as is elicited in postural sway, will result in a tonic response (figure 4.12). Another demonstration of this reflex may be observed when a weight is placed in the hand, with the forearm in 90 degrees of flexion at the elbow

joint. The result is likely to be a subtle depression of the hand and forearm (slight extension at the elbow) immediately followed by a return movement to compensate.

Movements that put muscles on a stretch in the backswing or preparatory phase can take advantage of the stretch reflex. If the desired outcome is a strong application of force, the preparatory movement should be rapid, to benefit from the phasic increase in spindle discharge, and long, to increase the tonic response. The backswing in forceful striking and throwing patterns, the crouch before a vertical jump, and the stretch before a tuck dive are all examples (figure 4.13a). If, however, the desired outcome is accuracy, as in a badminton low serve or a golf putt, the backswing should be short and slow, with a pause before the force application (figure 4.13b). This approach allows the phasic frequencies of the primary endings to slow down to tonic level (Gowitzke and Milner 1988).

In the static type of stretch reflex, the muscle is stretched slowly. This causes primary and secondary endings of several spindles to be stimulated and results in a more sustained muscular contraction. The importance of the static stretch is that it causes muscle contraction as long as a muscle is put on excessive stretch. When such a reflex is elicited by the stretch caused by the tendency of weight-bearing joints to flex, the response of the extensor muscles is commonly referred to as the *antigravity reflex.* Some also use this term to include the response of lower extremity and trunk muscles to the involuntary forward-backward swaying that usually occurs when a person stands in one position for a long time.

The gamma efferent system functions to adjust the muscle spindle length by causing the intrafusal fibers to contract (see p. 78). This mechanism receives signals whenever the alpha motor system stimulates the extrafusal (skeletal muscle) fibers. Thus a balance between the length of the skeletal and spindle fibers is maintained. In addition, the gamma efferent system is under voluntary control (gamma bias). For example, this mechanism is at work when a subject anticipates

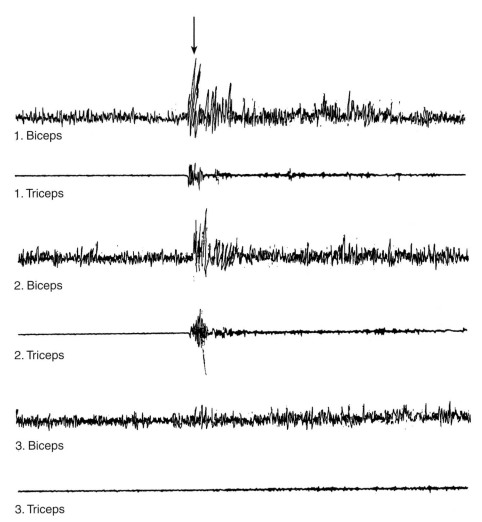

1. Biceps

1. Triceps

2. Biceps

2. Triceps

3. Biceps

3. Triceps

Figure 4.12   Electromyograms: Stretch reflex. Subject is maintaining the elbow joint at 90 degrees of flexion while holding a bucket. Arrow (↓) indicates loading the bucket. Tracings 1 and 2 show the biceps and triceps muscle activity when the load is dropped from decreasing heights (phasic response). Tracing 3 shows muscle activity when the load is placed into the bucket (tonic response).

receiving a weight. Impulses are sent along the gamma system, adjusting the threshold level of the muscle spindle so that as soon as any change occurs, a reflex contraction results. Remember what happens when lifting an empty box after thinking it would be weighted.

The flower-spray endings, or secondary afferents, are less sensitive to stretch and only result in the tonic response. Therefore, a greater or prolonged stretch is necessary to stimulate the secondary endings. Whereas the primary endings always facilitate the contraction of the muscle in which they are located, the influence of the secondary afferents depends on the type of muscle in which it is located. Secondary afferents facilitate flexor muscles and inhibit extensor muscle

a.   b.

Figure 4.13   (a) The phasic type of stretch reflex will facilitate force development if the backswing is long and rapid with little pause between the backswing and force phase as demonstrated in a forceful overarm throw. (b) To take advantage of the tonic type of stretch reflex when accuracy is desired, the backswing should be short and slow, with a pause before the force phase. An example is the golf putt.

contraction. Therefore, the secondary afferent response would reinforce the primary afferent response if the stimulated spindle was located in a flexor muscle but would result in a cocontraction if the stimulated spindle were in an extensor muscle. This would be due to the reflex contraction facilitated by the primary endings in the extensor muscle and the facilitation of the flexor muscle by the secondary ending. Two joint muscles respond to secondary afferent stimulation as though they are flexor muscles.

Spindles may also be stimulated by pressure and vibration. This fact is important whenever pressure must be placed on another individual. In gymnastics, if pressure is placed on flexor muscles, the gymnast may fall rather than be helped to hold a position. Similarly, pressure on the extensor muscles when working in rehabilitation may inhibit elbow flexion. Use of this technique

may provide additional variations to the rehabilitation setting.

In some instances it would be desirable to minimize the effect of the stretch reflex, as in flexibility exercises. This can be done if the stretch is done slowly and is held, as in static stretching. A quick stretch or bounce will evoke a stronger, phasic, reflex contraction.

Tendon Reflex

The second muscle proprioceptor, the *Golgi tendon organ* (GTO), is located in series at the musculotendinous junction. It too is stimulated by tension, but because of its location, the stretch may be induced on the tendon when the muscle contracts as well as when the muscle is stretched. The threshold of the GTO to muscle stretch is higher than that of the muscle spindle. That is, if the stimulus is strong enough to stimulate the

GTO, the muscle spindle response is overridden. On the other hand, the GTO is very sensitive to tension when it is produced by tendon stretch resulting from muscle contraction. In either case, the reflex effect is to inhibit impulses from the motor nerve to the muscle and its synergists, thus causing the muscle to relax. Simultaneously, the antagonist contracts from being facilitated.

When tension on the muscle is extreme, the Golgi tendon organs' inhibiting action results in sudden relaxation of the muscle. This effect is called the *lengthening reaction* and undoubtedly serves as protection for muscles or tendons that could be torn or ruptured by the strong contractile force. Guyton (2000) has suggested that the tendon reflex serves as a feedback mechanism to control the tension in the muscle. If the tension in the muscle became too great, the inhibiting action of the receptors would cause relaxation. If the muscle tension became too little, the receptors would stop firing, and the muscle tension would be able to increase.

The behavior of the tendon reflex in the performance of some skills by beginners is also a matter of interest. It may be that the reason beginners do not follow through has to do with the fact that the tendon reflex causes relaxation of vigorously contracting muscle. It is suggested that until an increase in the Golgi tendon organ threshold develops with learning, beginners may need voluntary effort to counteract the inhibitory effect of the tendon reflex.

Labyrinth and Neck Reflexes

Newborn infants start out with very simple reflexes, which in the process of normal motor development are suppressed or modified. This phenomenon is especially evident in the labyrinth and neck reflexes. The tonic labyrinth reflexes emanate from utricle and semicircular canal receptors, which are sensitive to changes in position of the head with respect to gravity. Because of the primitive tonic labyrinth reflex present in the newborn child, a supine position of the head facilitates extension of the extremities, whereas a prone position inhibits extension and facilitates flexion. At a few months of age or more, this primitive reflex is suppressed, and the labyrinth righting reflex is evident. In cooperation with other righting reflexes of the neck and eyes, it evokes muscular responses to restore the body to a normal upright position.

Righting reflexes can be demonstrated in adults. They respond to any body-tilting action by attempting to restore balance through facilitating limb actions, such as an arm or leg being thrust out. In spinning, the limbs facilitate restoration of the normal head position by actions that inhibit the rotation. The arm on the same side as the direction of the spin is thrust out during the spin, and the opposite arm is thrust out at the termination of the spin. This latter action is probably a response to the imbalance caused by the dizziness experienced at the conclusion of the spin because of the continuation of movement (inertia) of the fluid and resulting stimulation of the hair cells.

Tonic neck reflexes are evident when the joint receptors in the neck are stimulated by any movement in the neck. They are also present at birth, and even though they are masked by further development, they remain in adults. Like the tonic labyrinth reflex, they can also be demonstrated in adults. Actions due to tonic neck reflexes in the primitive infant form are predictable. If the head is flexed, flexion will occur in the upper extremities and extension in the lower ones. With head extension, the opposite occurs— extension in the upper extremities and flexion in the lower ones. Rotation of the head to the right is accompanied by extension and abduction of the limbs on the chin side, and flexion and adduction on the opposite side.

Tonic neck and tonic labyrinth reflexes become most apparent in adults in stressful situations. They are hard to distinguish from each other because movements of the head and neck occur together and labyrinth and neck receptors are stimulated simultaneously. In some instances they reinforce each other in their effect on joint actions of the extremities, and in some instances they oppose each other. There are times when we should take advantage of them to facilitate actions and other times when it would be beneficial to suppress them.

Fukuda (1960) and Gardner (1969) have stated that the neck reflexes are more effective in modifying upper extremity actions and the labyrinthine in modifying those of the lower extremities, and these results are still accepted. There is no question that head position influences the actions of the arms. When a strong pulling action is required, flexion of the head will facilitate it to some extent. On the other hand, the neck reflex facilitation suggests that the head should be extended for strong pushing actions. For facilitating a one-armed pull, the head should be turned away in addition to being flexed and, in a one-armed push, the head should be turned toward the pushing arm. Other examples of reflex facilitation include extension of the head in a handstand to reinforce extension in the arms, flexion of the head to reinforce trunk, arms, and leg flexion in forward or backward rolls, and head rotation in archery to facilitate bow arm pushing on the chin side and bowstring arm pulling by the opposite side (Deutsch et al. 1987; Gowitzke and Milner 1988; Le Pellec and Maton 1993).

Undoubtedly one of the difficulties in learning new motor skills is the failure to suppress reflex responses. In falling backward, our natural reaction is to extend the arms and throw the head forward. If a beginner did this in attempting a back dive, the entry into the water would be uncomfortable, to say the least. The labyrinth righting reflex must be suppressed consciously so that the head may be extended back and the body follow. Belly flops in front dives can also be attributed to the labyrinth righting reflex.

Posture and Locomotor Mechanisms

Whether because of reflex action or to some other mechanism, it seems apparent that the human body has certain provisions for remaining more or less erect and for engaging in locomotion and that these follow the general pattern of reflex behavior. The coordinated efforts of the body to resist the downward pull of gravity include the extensor thrust reflex, the static type of stretch reflex in response to gravitational pull, the muscular action evoked by forward-backward swaying, and the various mechanisms for preserving equilibrium, including visual orientation and labyrinthine reflexes.

In regard to locomotion, the action of the legs of a four-footed animal has been attributed to reflex action. Some classify this reflex as a division of the crossed extensor reflex (Ruch and Patton 1979). Because research in this area has been done primarily on dogs and cats it has been suggested that this reflex exists only in quadrupeds. Nevertheless, it is logical to assume that it exists also in humans inasmuch as the early forms of locomotion—creeping and crawling—resemble the locomotion of quadrupeds. Even after the erect position is assumed, the swing of the arms in opposition to the lower extremities reflects the earlier four-footed gait.

VOLITIONAL MOVEMENT

This topic involves such an extensive and complex body of knowledge that only the bare essentials and a few concepts can be touched on here. The chief anatomical structures concerned with volitional movement, in addition to those mentioned earlier (skeletal muscle, basic nerve structures, motor units, and sensory receptors), are the cerebral cortex, the cerebellum, the brainstem, spinal cord, and the numerous motor pathways, both pyramidal (corticospinal tracts) and extrapyramidal tracts.

Volitional movement is goal directed where the higher centers of the brain have the most general control, with each succeeding level having more specific control. The central nervous system is often divided into five levels in hierarchical order.

Central Nervous System: Levels of Control

The *cerebral cortex* (figure 4.14) is the first and highest level of control. It is the level at which consciousness occurs and the level responsible

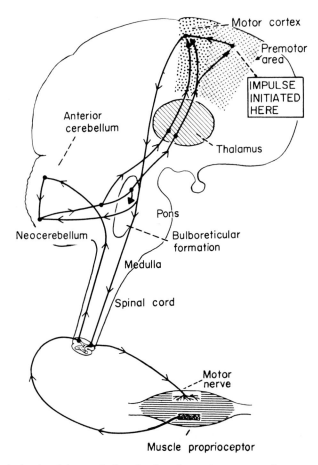

Figure 4.14   Feedback circuits of the cerebellum for damping motor movements.
From A. C. Guyton, *Function of the Human Body,* 4th ed. Copyright © 1974 W. B. Saunders, Orlando, FL. Reprinted by permission.

for the initiation of voluntary movement. The cerebral cortex contains a motor area situated in front of the transverse central fissure known as the precentral gyrus. Within this area, all body parts are represented by an area whose size correlates with the complexity or precision of the body part. Therefore, the area representing the thumb and fingers requires a larger area than that representing the foot. Movements, not muscles, are represented here. The premotor area located in front of the motor cortex is responsible for learning complex acts.

The basal ganglia area is the second level of control. This area is located at the thalamus level and is often identified as containing the subcortical nuclei. The basal ganglia area is responsible for homeostasis, that is, for maintaining a level of constancy within prescribed ranges before adjustments are made. It is responsible for the coordination and control of some learned acts involving posture and equilibrium, including the sensory integration for the righting reflexes.

Level three is in the cerebellum (figure 4.14). The cerebellum is often referred to as the "little brain." It plays a key role in sensory integration, receiving diverse inputs and acting as a feedback center comparing what should have been with the motion that occurred. The cerebellum is a vital center for regulating the timing and intensity of muscle activity to produce smooth, precise movement.

The pons–medulla area, known as the *brainstem* (figure 4.14), is level four of the central nervous system. This area contains the reticular formation, which encompasses numerous neurons and nuclei and houses important centers for arousal and monitoring of physiological parameters from the cardiorespiratory mechanisms. The brainstem also contains key facilitory and inhibitory centers, thereby having a direct effect on muscle sensitivity.

The lowest level of control of the central nervous system, level five, is the *spinal cord* (figure 4.14), containing cell bodies of the lower motor neurons that control the skeletal muscles. It has the most specific control and is the common pathway between the central and peripheral nervous systems. Because signal integration occurs at synapses, and all synaptic connections between and among neurons occur within the central nervous system, the spinal cord is the final point for nerve impulse integration and control.

Although reported as discrete levels and areas with specific functions, functions of the five levels and areas of the central nervous system overlap depending on the classification scheme used. It is true, however, that higher centers may override lower centers, but the reverse is not true. For accurate volitional movement to occur, sensory information is imperative, and continuous sensory stimulation is necessary for accurate volitional action. Moreover, the response of the central nervous system depends on the initial position of the segment or limb (joint angle) for the intensity of muscle contraction.

Pyramidal and Extrapyramidal Tracts

Tracts are bundles of fibers. The pyramidal and extrapyramidal tracts are two tracts originating from the cerebral cortex and ending at the spinal cord. Together, these two tracts play a vital role in a person's ability to initiate fine coordinations representative of skilled movement. The corticospinal, or pyramidal, tract is predominantly comprised of axons from motor neurons, which originate in the cerebral cortex and end in the spinal cord on other motor neurons. Because there is only one synapse, this is a very fast system. During the descent, the majority of the fibers cross on a level with the medulla. The fibers pass in the anterior portion of the medulla, forming the pyramids, and thus this tract is referred to as the pyramidal tract. Because the majority of its fibers cross, fibers originating on the right side control the limb muscles on the left side. Specifically, this tract controls muscles for precision. Because myelination of the axons occurs with maturity, it is reasonable that young children would have difficulty with skills requiring fine coordination. Disruption of this system results in weakness and difficulty in initiating voluntary movements.

Structurally, the extrapyramidal system also originates at the cerebral cortex and ends at the spinal cord, but during its descent the axons have many important synaptic connections with all levels of the central nervous system. These communication links are named for their connections. There are, for instance, the vestibulospinal, reticulospinal, and rubrospinal pathways. There are also many significant connections with the cerebellum. Fibers from the extrapyramidal tract cross just above the medulla and travel outside the pyramids. This system predominates in young children. Its function is one of stabilization and control of posture as well as general movement patterning.

Kinesthesis

The conscious awareness of position of body parts and the amount and rate of joint movement is known as kinesthesis. Kinesthetic sensations originate primarily in the sensory receptors of the joint capsules and ligaments and include the Ruffini endings, pacinian corpuscles, and Golgi tendon organs. Signals from these receptors are transmitted rapidly to the cord and brain in beta type A nerve fibers so that the central nervous system is instantaneously aware (at the cerebral cortex level of conscious awareness) of the exact position of the body parts. Without this rapid transmission and processing of information, accurately controlled movements could not proceed. Kinesthetic perception and memory are the basis of voluntary movement and motor learning. This perception and memory enable the performer to initiate a whole movement pattern or modify a part of it, such as the elimination or addition of a joint action, or a change in timing or speed of an action.

Reciprocal Inhibition and Coactivation

One of the mechanisms that provides for economical and coordinated movement is the one known as reciprocal inhibition. According to this concept, when motor neurons are transmitting impulses to muscles, causing them to contract, the motor neurons that supply their antagonists are simultaneously and reciprocally inhibited. The antagonistic muscles, therefore, remain relaxed and the movers, or agonists, contract without opposition. The relaxation occurs to the degree to which the agonists are activated. Reciprocal inhibition operates automatically in movements elicited by the stretch reflex and also in familiar volitional movements. In more complicated and in less familiar coordinations its operation depends on the degree of skill developed by the performer.

Coactivation, or reciprocal activation, most frequently appears in movement when there is uncertainty about the movement task. As practice or training increases familiarity with the movement, coactivation decreases in favor of reciprocal inhibition. In this way efficiency of movement also increases. There is further evidence which suggests that coactivation also occurs in order to maintain joint stiffness, especially when faced with an unstable or perturbed posture (Enoka 1997; Park, Toole, and Lee 1999).

NEUROMUSCULAR ANALYSIS

The muscle-response patterns of well-learned motor skills involve the integrated action of many reflexes and the inhibition of others. After repeated viewing of the performance "live" or on film, the student should name and discuss the reflexes that could be acting at various points in each phase. The reflexes that should be considered are spindle reflexes (stretch reflex), the Golgi tendon organ reflex, joint reflexes, cutaneous responses, labyrinthine reflexes, neck reflexes, and visual righting reflexes. For each reflex, the receptors involved should be identified, the expected action facilitated by the reflex described, and the actual results explained. To return to the standing long jump in figure 1.3, the following reflex actions are plausible examples of reflex action:

1. Reflex: Labyrinthine head righting reflex is present.
   Receptor: Labyrinthine system—inner ear.
   Time: Preparation for takeoff.
   Evidence: As the trunk leans farther forward, the head and neck become more hyperextended.
2. Reflex: Stretch reflexes in extensors of hip, knee, and ankle are present.
   Receptor: Muscle spindle.
   Time: Early preparation for takeoff (crouch).
   Evidence: The stretch reflexes are activated in the extensors as flexion occurs in the hips, knees, and ankles. The result is facilitation of contraction of the extensor muscles.
3. Reflex: Extensor thrust reflexes.
   Receptor: Pacinian corpuscles (soles of the feet).
   Time: As force is applied to the floor for takeoff.
   Evidence: Pressure facilitates extensor muscle contraction of the lower extremities.

LABORATORY EXPERIENCES

1. Engage a partner in arm wrestling until one of you loses. Explain the sudden cessation of muscle tension in the loser that resulted in the end of the contest.

2. Record and explain what happens neurologically when an individual is upset from a blow in front of the knees as opposed to behind them.

3. Explain what happens neurologically when an individual pushes a door at the same time a person on the other side pulls it open.

4. Ask your partner to stand facing you with eyes closed. By moving body segments, place your partner in some novel pose. Ask your partner, with eyes still closed, to describe the position exactly. After once again assuming the original standing position, ask your partner to reproduce the novel position. Explain the neuromuscular mechanisms that enable your partner to sense and reproduce the movement.

5. Record the distance of your best of three standing broad jumps. Repeat the jumps, but this time flex the head and neck vigorously as the legs are extended. After a few practice trials record the distance of the three jumps, which incorporate the reflex pattern. Compare your results with those of others in the class. What effect did the reflex pattern have? Explain.

6. Stand in a doorway with your arms at your side. Now press the backs of your hands strongly against the door jambs. Hold this position for at least 30 seconds. Step clear of the doorway and turn your head to the right. What happens to your arms? Explain.

7. Look at the sequence of film tracings for the backward somersault depicted in exercise 5.6 in appendix H. Which proprioceptive reflexes could be present in the position represented in frame (a)? For each reflex named, state the evidence that would suggest the presence of the reflex, the expected effect the reflex could have on the movement, and the verification of the effect as shown by the action in the next frames. Were there any expected reflex actions that apparently did not occur? Explain.

REFERENCES AND SELECTED READINGS

Basmajian, J. V., and C. J. DeLuca. 1985. *Muscles alive.* 5th ed. Baltimore: Williams & Wilkins.

Burne, J. A., and O. C. J. Lippold. 1996. Reflex inhibition following electrical stimulation over muscle tendon in man. *Brain* 119:1107–14.

Deutsch, H., H. Kilani, E. Moustafa, N. Hamilton, and J. Herbert. 1987. Effect of head–neck position on elbow flexor muscle torque production. *Physical Therapy* 67:517–21.

Doherty, T. J., A. A. Vandervoort, and W. F. Brown. 1993. Effects of aging on the motor unit: A brief review. *Canadian Journal of Applied Physiology* 18:331–58.

Enoka, R. M. 1994. *Neuromechanical basis of kinesiology.* 2nd ed. Champaign, IL: Human Kinetics.

Enoka, R. M. 1997. Neural adaptations with chronic physical activity. *Journal of Biomechanics* 30(5):447–55.

Fukuda, T. 1960. Studies on human dynamic postures from the viewpoint of postural reflexes. *Acta Oto Laryngologica* Supplementum 161:5–52.

Gardner, E. B. 1969. Proprioceptive reflexes and their participation in motor skills. *Quest,* Monograph XII, 1:25.

Gowitzke, B. A., and M. Milner. 1988. *Understanding the scientific bases of human movement.* 3rd ed. Baltimore: Williams & Wilkins.

Guyton, A. C. 2000. *Textbook of medical physiology.* 10th ed. Philadelphia: Saunders.

Hamill, J., and K. M. Knutzen. 1995. *Biomechanical basis of human movement.* Philadelphia: Williams & Wilkins.

Kandel, E. R., and J. H. Schwartz, eds. 1985. *Principles of neural science.* 2nd ed. New York: Elsevier.

Le Pellec, A., and B. Maton. 1993. The influence of tonic neck reflexes on voluntary fatiguing elbow movements in humans. *European Journal of Applied Physiology* 67:237–38.

Loofbourrow, G. N. 1973. Neuromuscular integration. In *Science and medicine of exercise and sports.* 2nd ed., edited by W. R. Johnson and E. Buskirk. New York: Harper & Row.

Myklebust, B. M. 1990. A review of myotatic reflexes and the development of motor control and gait in infants and children: A special communication. *Physical Therapy* 70:188–203.

Nichols, T. R., T. C. Cope, and T. A. Ablew. 1999. Rapid spinal mechanisms of motor coordination. *Exercise and Sport Sciences Reviews* 27:255–84.

Park, S., T. Toole, and S. Lee. 1999. Functional roles of the proprioceptive system in the control of goal-directed movement. *Perceptual and Motor Skills* 88:631–47.

Winter, J. M. and P. E. Crago, eds. 2000. *Biomechanics and neural control of posture and movement.* New York: Springer.

5

THE UPPER EXTREMITY:

The Shoulder Region

OUTLINE

■ *The Shoulder Girdle*
  (Acromioclavicular and
  Sternoclavicular Articulations)
  Structure of Acromioclavicular
    Articulation
  Structure of Sternoclavicular
    Articulation
  Movements
■ *Muscles of the Shoulder Girdle*
  Location
  Characteristics and Functions
    of Shoulder Girdle Muscles
■ *The Shoulder Joint*
  (Glenohumeral Articulation)
  Structure
  Ligamentous and Muscular
    Reinforcements
   Movements
■ *Muscles of the Shoulder Joint*
  Location
  Characteristics and Functions

■ *Joint and Muscular Analysis*
  of the Fundamental Movements
  of the Arm on the Trunk
  Movements in the Frontal Plane
  Movements in the Sagittal Plane
  Movements in the Horizontal
    Plane
  Diagonal Movements
  Shoulder Girdle Movements Not
    Involving the Arm
■ *Common Injuries*
  of the Shoulder Region
  Acromioclavicular Sprain
  Fracture of the Clavicle
  Dislocation of the Shoulder
  Chronic Dislocation
    of the Shoulder
  Rotator Cuff Strains
■ *Laboratory Experiences*

OBJECTIVES

At the conclusion of this chapter, the student should be able to:

1. Name, locate, and describe the structure and ligamentous reinforcements of the articulations of the shoulder region.
2. Name and demonstrate the movements possible in the joints of the shoulder region regardless of starting position.
3. Name and locate the muscles and muscle groups of the shoulder region, and name their primary actions as agonists, stabilizers, neutralizers, or antagonists.
4. Analyze the fundamental movements of the arm and trunk with respect to joint and muscle actions.
5. Describe the common injuries of the shoulder region.
6. Perform an anatomical analysis of the shoulder region in a motor skill.

Anatomical cooperation is beautifully illustrated in the movements of the arms on the trunk. The arm travels through a wide range of movements, and in each of these the scapula cooperates by placing the glenoid fossa in the most favorable position for the head of the humerus. This is known as *scapulohumeral rhythm.* When the arm is elevated sideward (abducted), for instance, the scapula rotates upward; when it is elevated forward (flexed), the scapula not only rotates upward but it tends to slide partially around the rib cage (abducted). Although occasionally movement of the scapula is deliberately repressed (as in some stylized dance movements, and in some posture exercises), in all natural movements, the scapula shares with the humerus in the movements of the arm on the trunk. In abduction of the arm, for instance, the movements of the scapula and humerus are continuous throughout the movement, with the humeral movement accounting for approximately two-thirds of the total movement and the scapular movement for one-third. It is important to remember, however, that this cooperative scapulohumeral rhythm is not a linear relationship. It varies with individuals and with the phase of the movement.

The upper extremity is suspended from the axial skeleton (head and trunk) by means of the shoulder girdle. The latter consists of the sternum and two clavicles in front, and two scapulae in back. The sternoclavicular joints connect the sternum and each clavicle, and the acromioclavicular joints connect the acromion process of each scapula with the corresponding clavicle. Because there is no union between the two scapulae in back, this is an incomplete girdle. The upper extremity's connection with the shoulder girdle is made through the glenohumeral joint, the joint between the head of the humerus and the glenoid fossa of the scapula, better known as the shoulder joint.

The sternoclavicular joint is an exceedingly small one, about the size of the joint between the great toe and the first metatarsal bone, yet it is the sole skeletal connection between the upper extremity and the trunk. This anatomical arrangement accounts for the extensive freedom of motion enjoyed by the upper extremity and is a vital factor in the superb cooperation that exists between the shoulder joint and the shoulder girdle. The upper arm has a remarkably wide range of motion owing largely to its ball and shallow socket construction. Its movements are further amplified by the cooperative actions of the shoulder girdle, as just described.

To understand and appreciate the great variety of movements of the arm on the trunk, it is essential that one be thoroughly familiar with the structure and function of each joint involved and be able to distinguish between the contributions of each in any given movement.

THE SHOULDER GIRDLE (ACROMIOCLAVICULAR AND STERNOCLAVICULAR ARTICULATIONS)

Structure of Acromioclavicular Articulation

The articulation between the acromion process of the scapula and the outer end of the clavicle (figure 5.1) belongs to the diarthrodial classification. Within this group it is further classified as an irregular (arthrodial) joint. A small wedge-shaped disc may be found between the upper part of the joint surfaces, but this is frequently absent. The articular capsule is strengthened above by the acromioclavicular ligament, which passes from the upper part of the outer end of the clavicle to the upper surface of the acromion process. The joint is strengthened behind by the aponeurosis of the trapezius and deltoid muscles. The clavicle is further stabilized by means of the coracoclavicular ligament (actually two ligaments, the conoid and the trapezoid), which, as the name suggests, binds the clavicle to the coracoid process.

The conoid ligament passes from the base of the coracoid process to the conoid tubercle on the underside of the clavicle. The trapezoid ligament extends from the top of the coracoid process to the trapezoid ridge on the underside of the clavicle.

Structure of Sternoclavicular Articulation

The sternal end of the clavicle articulates with both the sternum and the cartilage of the first rib (figure 5.2). It is classified as a double arthrodial joint because there are two joint cavities, one on either side of the articular disc. This round flat disc of white fibrocartilage is attached above to the upper, posterior border of the articular surface of the clavicle and below to the cartilage of the

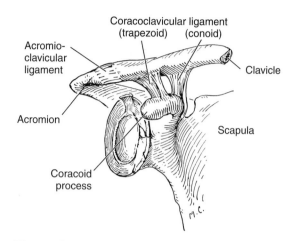

Figure 5.1   Anterior view of acromioclavicular articulation.

first rib near its junction with the sternum. The articular capsule is thin above and below but is thickened in front and behind by bands of fibers called the anterior and posterior sternoclavicular ligaments.

The sternoclavicular articulation is of great importance in the movements of the shoulder girdle and of the arm as a whole, because it is the only bony connection between the humerus and axial skeleton. It permits limited motion of the clavicle in all three planes and, because of the bone's attachment to the scapula at its distal end, is partially responsible for the latter's movements. It is reinforced by four ligaments: the anterior sternoclavicular, a band of fibers blending with the anterior fibers of the articular capsule limiting anterior clavicular motion; the posterior sternoclavicular, which blends with the posterior fibers of the articular capsule limiting posterior clavicular motion; the interclavicular, consisting of a flat band that passes across the upper margin of the sternum and attaches to the sternal end of each clavicle and limits downward clavicular motion; and the costoclavicular, a short strong band of fibers that connects the upper border of the first costal cartilage with the costal tuberosity on the underside of the clavicle and restricts clavicular elevation, protraction, and retraction.

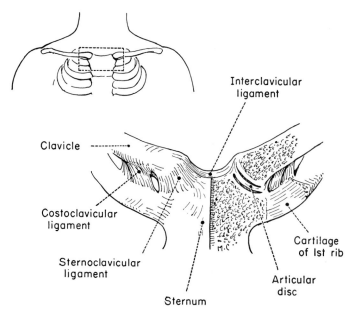

Figure 5.2   Anterior view of sternoclavicular articulation.

The movements of the clavicle at the sternoclavicular joint are as follows: elevation and depression, which occur approximately in the frontal plane about a sagittal-horizontal axis; horizontal forward-backward (protraction and retraction) movements, which occur in the horizontal plane about a vertical axis; and a limited degree of forward and backward rotation, which occurs approximately in the sagittal plane about the bone's own longitudinal axis. (In forward rotation the top of the clavicle revolves forward-downward.)

Movements

It is customary to define the movements of the shoulder girdle (figure 5.3) in terms of the movements of the scapulae. In doing this, there is some danger that the reader will visualize the movement as taking place solely in the joint between the scapula and the clavicle. It is well to emphasize the fact that every movement of

the scapula involves motion in both joints, the acromioclavicular and the sternoclavicular. The movements of the shoulder girdle expressed in terms of the composite movements of the scapula are as follows.

Elevation

An upward movement of the scapula (figure 5.3a), with the vertebral border remaining approximately parallel to the spinal column. The elevation of the scapula is the direct result of elevation of the outer end of the clavicle, a movement that takes place at the sternoclavicular joint. This movement occurs to a slight extent during elevation of the humerus and to a greater extent in lifting the shoulders in a hunching gesture. The farther the clavicles depart from the horizontal position, the closer the scapulae move toward each other. The latter movement might well be called passive adduction, because it is caused by the movement of the clavicles rather than by the adductor muscles of the scapulae.

a.

b.

c.

d.

Figure 5.3   Movements of the shoulder girdle: (a) elevation; (b) abduction (combined with lateral tilt and upward rotation); (c) upward rotation; (d) upward tilt.

Depression

The return from the position of elevation. There is no depression below the normal resting position.

Abduction, or Protraction

A lateral movement of the scapula away from the spinal column with the vertebral border remaining approximately parallel to it (figure 5.3b). Pure abduction of the scapula is a hypothetical movement. Actually, because of two factors, the rounded contour of the thorax and the forward movement of the clavicle about a vertical axis at the sternoclavicular joint, a pure lateral movement of the scapula in the frontal plane is im-possible. As the scapula abducts, it turns slightly about its vertical axis in a movement known as a lateral tilt. This turning is characterized by a slight backward movement of the vertebral border and a corresponding forward movement of the axillary border. This movement causes the glenoid fossa to face slightly forward and the arms, if relaxed, to hang in a more forward position and in slight inward (medial) rotation.

Adduction, or Retraction

A medial movement of the scapula toward the spinal column combined with a reduction of lateral tilt.

Upward Rotation

A rotation of the scapula in the frontal plane so that the glenoid fossa faces somewhat upward (figure 5.3c). The movement occurs largely at the acromioclavicular joint but is accompanied by elevation of the outer end of the clavicle. Upward rotation is always associated with elevation of the humerus, either sideward or forward. This scapular motion puts the glenoid fossa in a favorable position for upper extremity movement, positioning the small glenoid fossa beneath the larger head of the humerus and contributing significantly to the stability of the shoulder joint as well

as maintaining the position of the deltoid muscle for effective action.

Downward Rotation

The return from the position of upward rotation. There may be slight downward rotation beyond the normal resting position so that the glenoid fossa faces slightly downward.

Upward Tilt

A turning of the scapula on its frontal-horizontal axis so that the posterior surface faces slightly upward and the inferior angle protrudes from the back (figure 5.3d). This action is accompanied by a rotation of the clavicle about its mechanical axis so that the superior border turns slightly forward-downward, and the inferior border turns backward-upward. It occurs only in conjunction with hyper-extension of the humerus.

Reduction of Upward Tilt

The return movement from upward tilt.

MUSCLES OF THE SHOULDER GIRDLE

Location

The muscles of the shoulder girdle are classified as anterior or posterior muscles according to their location on the trunk.

Anterior	Posterior
Pectoralis minor	Levator scapulae
Serratus anterior	Rhomboids
Subclavius	Trapezius (4 parts)

Characteristics and Functions of Shoulder Girdle Muscles

Pectoralis Minor

This muscle (figure 5.4) participates in several movements of the *scapula—downward rotation, upward tilt, depression,* and the combined movements of *abduction* and *lateral tilt.* In addition to

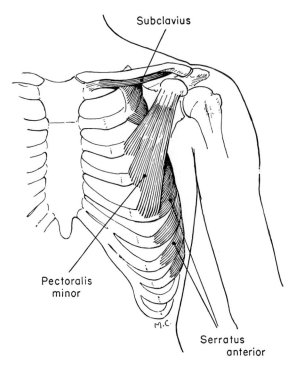

Figure 5.4 Anterior muscles of shoulder girdle.

its action on the scapula, an important function of the pectoralis minor is its lifting effect on the ribs, both in forced inspiration and in maintaining good chest posture. When the scapulae are stabilized by the adductors, contraction of the pectoralis minor *elevates* the third, fourth, and fifth ribs. Even without contracting, it exerts a slight upward and outward pull on these ribs if the muscle is well developed. The pectoralis minor can therefore contribute either to good or to poor posture, depending on whether its more effective pull is on the ribs or on the scapula. The key to its function as a muscle influencing good posture is stabilization of the scapulae by the adductors—that is, the rhomboids and the middle trapezius. The pectoralis minor may be palpated midway between the clavicle and the nipple when the arm is elevated backward against resistance, provided the pectoralis major is relaxed, and also when the subject sits with the forearm resting on a table and pushes both downward and laterally simultaneously.

Serratus Anterior

The upper portion causes *abduction* and *lateral tilt* of the scapula close to the ribs (see figures 5.4 and 5.16). The upper and lower portions of the serratus anterior and trapezius combine to form a force couple for upward rotation of the scapula. Activity of these muscles is especially evident during elevation of the arm, with the lower trapezius the more active of the two during abduction and the serratus anterior the more active during flexion. This muscle is important in reaching and pushing. A paralyzed serratus anterior prevents elevation of the arm above 100 degrees.

The muscle may be palpated on the anterior-lateral surface of the upper thorax, especially on a thin, muscular subject.

Subclavius

The pull of this muscle (see figure 5.4), which is slightly downward and strongly toward the sternum, suggests that its chief function is to protect

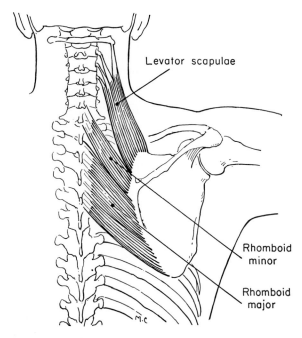

Figure 5.5   Posterior muscles of shoulder girdle, deep layer.

and stabilize the sternoclavicular articulation. It is also in a position to depress the scapula. It is not possible to palpate this muscle.

Levator Scapulae

This muscle is also listed with the muscles of the neck. As a muscle of the shoulder girdle, the levator scapula (figure 5.5) causes elevation and downward rotation of the scapula when the trunk is in the erect position. The weight of the arm at the acromial end of the scapula pulls that end down at the same time that the levator is lifting the medial angle. These two forces act as a force couple to rotate the scapula.

Basmajian and DeLuca (1985) and Rasch (1989) agree in attributing the levator scapula's movement of downward rotation to the weight of the arm and to the scapula's consequent need of postural support. Brunnstrom (Smith et al. 1996) claims that the levator, together with the rhomboid minor, tends to rotate the scapula downward in the early phase of contraction, preliminary to elevating it.

If the levator scapula rotates the scapula downward only when the weight of the arm prevents it from adducting the scapula, it would be assumed that the trunk must be in the erect position for gravity to have this effect. In other positions, as in swimming, one would expect the levator to adduct as well as to elevate the scapula. This muscle is a difficult one to palpate successfully.

Rhomboids, Major and Minor

Functionally, the rhomboids may be regarded as one muscle (figure 5.5). They cause downward rotation, adduction, and elevation of the scapula. Their cooperative action with trapezius III (see next section) is an important factor in the maintenance of good shoulder posture. When the tonus of these two muscles is deficient, the unbalanced pull of the pectoralis minor and the serratus anterior results in habitually abducted and tilted scapulae (round shoulders). This in turn results in the failure of the pectoralis minor and serratus anterior to hold the chest in good posture. Thus, one

Figure 5.6   Trapezius.

weak link in the chain of postural relationships leads to another. The rhomboids are also most active with the middle trapezius in stabilizing the scapula during abduction of the arm. Little activity occurs in these muscles during arm flexion until 150 degrees of flexion is reached, when activity increases markedly (Basmajian and DeLuca 1985).

These muscles are difficult to palpate, because they are completely covered by the trapezius. The technique suggested by Smith et al. (1996) is recommended.

Trapezius

The trapezius (figure 5.6) is a fascinating muscle to study. Because it is located directly under the skin, it is easy to palpate. Although some anatomists treat the muscle in three parts, it is more accurate to consider the four parts shown in figure 5.6 separately. Parts I and II compose the upper trapezius, part III the middle, and part IV the lower. Its actions include the following:

Part I.   Elevation.

Part II.   Elevation; upward rotation; adduction.

Part III.   Adduction.

Part IV.   Upward rotation; depression; adduction.

The trapezius shows definite activity during both elevation and adduction (retraction) of the scapula. In elevation the upper portion shows the greatest activity, and in retraction the middle and lower portions are most active. During abduction of the humerus and the accompanying upward rotation of the scapula, the lower two-thirds of the trapezius is most active, and during flexion of the humerus the lower third is most active. The greatest activity of the muscle as a whole is seen in the upward rotation of the scapula accompanying abduction of the humerus (Basmajian and DeLuca 1985).

The relation of the trapezius to the rhomboids and serratus anterior is interesting. The rhomboids and part III of the trapezius both adduct the scapulae and have similar activity patterns during elevation of the arm. In these actions they are partners. Parts II and IV, however, rotate the scapulae upward; the rhomboids rotate them downward. In this respect, then, they are antagonists.

Trapezius III and the upper serratus anterior are antagonistic, the former adducting and the latter abducting the scapulae. But trapezius II and IV are partners with the lower serratus because they act on the scapula as a force couple to rotate the scapula upward, with part II pulling up on the acromial end of the scapular spine and part IV and the serratus anterior pulling down on the medial end or root. (See the discussion of a force couple on pp. 344–345 and figure 13.7.) This action facilitates elevation of the arm. The lower and middle parts of the trapezius are quite active during the entire range of abduction. They are less active during the early stages of flexion when the scapula is being abducted. It is here that the serratus anterior, a scapular abductor as well as rotator, dominates.

Trapezius I and II have one important function that may be overlooked because little, if any, actual movement is involved. This is support for the distal end of the clavicle and the acromion process of the scapula when a heavy weight is held by the hand with the arm down at the side. Anyone who has carried a heavy suitcase for a long distance has doubtless experienced tension and subsequent soreness in these parts of the muscle. When no weight is carried, however, the capsule of the sternoclavicular articulation provides all the support necessary

for the fully depressed clavicle (Norkin and Levangie 1992).

These various combinations of function are an excellent illustration of the cooperative action of the muscles and of the astonishing versatility of the musculoskeletal mechanism.

THE SHOULDER JOINT (GLENOHUMERAL ARTICULATION)

Structure

The shoulder joint is formed by the articulation of the spherical head of the humerus with the small, shallow, somewhat pear-shaped glenoid fossa of the scapula (figure 5.7). It is a ball-and-socket joint. The structure of the joint and the looseness of the capsule (permitting between 1 and 2 inches of separation between the two bones) account for the remarkable mobility of the shoulder joint. Both the humeral head and the glenoid fossa are covered with hyaline cartilage. The cartilage on the head of the humerus is thicker at the center, whereas that which lines the cavity is thicker around the circumference. The glenoid fossa is further protected by a flat rim of white fibrocartilage, also thicker around the circumference. Called the glenoid labrum, this cartilage serves both to deepen the fossa and to cushion it against the impact of the humeral head in forceful movements (figure 5.8).

The joint is completely enveloped in a loose sleevelike articular capsule that is attached proximally to the circumference of the glenoid cavity and distally to the anatomical neck of the humerus. The capsule is lined with synovial membrane that folds back over the glenoid labrum, covers all but the upper portion of the anatomical neck of the humerus, and extends through the intertubular or bicipital groove in the form of a sheath for the tendon of the long head of the biceps. There are several bursae in the region of the shoulder joint. Among the larger are

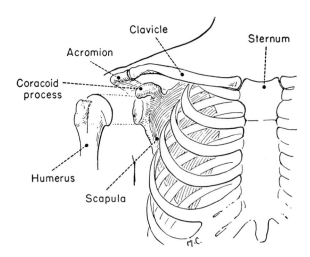

Figure 5.7   Anterior view of shoulder joint and shoulder girdle.

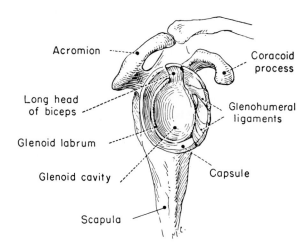

Figure 5.8   Lateral view of right scapula showing glenoid cavity.

the one between the deltoid muscle and the capsule and the one on top of the acromion process.

Ligamentous and Muscular Reinforcements

The shoulder joint is protected and stabilized by both ligaments and muscles. Inspection of the illustrations on these pages (supplemented by study of the table of muscular attachments in ap-

pendix D) will help the reader understand the relationships of the ligaments and muscles to the joints they reinforce.

The coracohumeral ligament, the three bands of the glenohumeral ligament, and the bridgelike coracoacromial ligament constitute the *ligamentous reinforcements* of the shoulder joint (figure 5.9). Muscular reinforcement is provided above by the supraspinatus muscle and the long head of the biceps brachii, below by the long

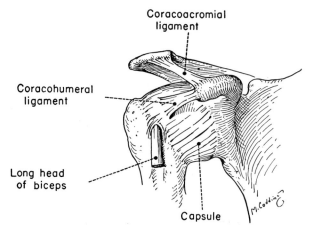

Figure 5.9   Anterior view of shoulder joint showing ligaments.

head of the triceps brachii, in front by the subscapularis muscle and the fibrous prolongations of both the pectoralis major and teres major muscles, and behind by the infraspinatus and teres minor muscles (see figures 5.11 through 5.15).

Apparently these reinforcements alone do not prevent downward dislocation, however. In 1959 Basmajian and Bazant investigated the muscles whose fibers cross the shoulder joint vertically, as compared with those whose fibers cross it horizontally. To their surprise, they discovered that it was the horizontal fibers and not the vertical that were active in preventing downward dislocation of the humerus. After doing a dissection of the shoulder joint, they agreed that the slope of the glenoid fossa was an important factor. Because of this slope, the head of the humerus was forced laterally as it was pulled downward, and it took the horizontally directed muscle fibers to check this lateral movement which, in turn, stopped the downward movement. A number of investigators have studied the mechanisms of stability in downward motion. They concluded that downward dislocation of the humerus is prevented primarily by four factors: (1) the slope of the glenoid fossa; (2) the tightening of the upper part of the capsule and of the coracohumeral ligament; (3) the activity of the supraspinatus muscle and, to a lesser

extent, of the posterior fibers of the deltoid; and (4) the combined actions of the infraspinatus, teres minor, and subscapularis, which compress the head of the humerus into the glenoid fossa, adding to vertical stability (Basmajian and DeLuca 1985; Norkin and Levangie 1992; Bigliani et al. 1996).

The shoulder joint therefore is stable when in extension but very vulnerable when flexed. That is why it is dangerous in sports to have force applied when the arm is raised overhead, such as when the quarterback is throwing a pass.

Movements

The movements of the humerus, all of which take place at the glenohumeral articulation, are illustrated in figure 5.10. The expected average ranges of these movements are summarized in table 2.3. They are defined as follows.

Flexion and Hyperflexion

A forward-upward movement in a plane at right angles to the plane of the scapula (sagittal plane). If the movement exceeds 180 degrees, it is hyperflexion.

Extension

Return movement from flexion (sagittal plane).

Figure 5.10 Movements of the humerus: (a) flexion, extension, hyperextension, circumduction; (b) abduction and adduction; (c) horizontal adduction and abduction; (d) diagonal adduction and abduction; (e) inward and outward rotation.

Hyperextension

A backward movement in a plane at right angles to the plane of the scapula (sagittal plane).

Abduction

A sideward-upward movement in a plane parallel with the plane of the scapula (frontal plane).

Adduction

Return movement from abduction (frontal plane).

Outward (Lateral) Rotation

A rotation of the humerus around its mechanical axis so that when the arm is in its normal resting position, the anterior aspect turns laterally (horizontal plane).

Inward (Medial) Rotation

A rotation of the humerus around its mechanical axis so that when the arm is in its normal resting position, the anterior aspect turns medially (horizontal plane). The full range of inward and outward rotation is best observed when the forearm is held in 90 degrees of flexion and the humerus is held in 90 degrees of abduction.

Horizontal Adduction

A forward movement of the abducted humerus in a horizontal plane (i.e., from a plane parallel to the plane of the scapula to a plane at right angles to it). Sometimes identified as *horizontal flexion* in other textbooks.

Horizontal Abduction

A backward movement of the flexed humerus in a horizontal plane (i.e., from a plane at right angles to the plane of the scapula to a plane parallel to it). Sometimes called *horizontal extension* in other texts.

Circumduction

A combination of flexion, abduction, extension, hyperextension, and adduction performed sequentially in either direction so that the extended arm describes a cone and the fingertips a circle.

MUSCLES OF THE SHOULDER JOINT

Location

The muscles of the shoulder joint are listed according to their position in relation to the joint. This position is not always apparent, as a look at the illustrations will show. All muscles in this classification pass either from the trunk or the scapula to the arm.

Anterior	**Posterior**
Pectoralis major	Infraspinatus
Coracobrachialis	Teres minor
Subscapularis	
Biceps brachii	

Superior	**Inferior**
Deltoid	Latissimus dorsi
Supraspinatus	Teres major
	Triceps brachii, long head

Charateristics and Functions
Pectoralis Major

This large fan-shaped muscle of the chest (figure 5.11) converges to a flat tendon, which, like that of the latissimus dorsi, twists on itself so that the lowest fibers become the uppermost at its point of attachment. The muscle is divided functionally into two parts, clavicular and sternal (or sternocostal). The clavicular portion lies close to the anterior deltoid muscle and acts with it in flexion, horizontal adduction, and inward rotation of the humerus.

Ordinarily the line of pull of the clavicular portion of the pectoralis major lies below the axis of the shoulder joint. However, when the arm is raised sideward well above the horizontal, the line of pull of the upper clavicular fibers shifts above the center of the shoulder joint, and these fibers then cease to adduct and become abductors of the humerus (see figure 3.4). The clavicular fibers of the pectoralis major are significantly active in abduction at the level of 110 degrees. The sternocostal portion is generally antagonistic

Figure 5.11   Anterior view of muscles of shoulder joint, superficial layer.

to the clavicular portion in its actions in the sagittal plane. It acts in downward and forward movements of the arm and in medial rotation when accompanied by adduction. The pectoralis major as a whole is most powerful for actions in the sagittal plane and is particularly important in all pushing, throwing, and punching activities. The clavicular portion may be palpated just below the medial two-thirds of the clavicle, the sternal portion just lateral to the sternum and below the clavicular part, and the muscle as a whole at the anterior border of the axilla.

Coracobrachialis

The muscle's line of pull passes in front of the shoulder joint (figure 5.12), which suggests that it participates in *forward movements of the humerus.* Because the proximal attachment and line of pull of the coracobrachialis and the long head of the biceps are so similar, it has been difficult to determine the specific actions of the cora-

cobrachialis. However, Stevens, Rosselle, and Michels (1976) were successful in isolating and recording activity in the coracobrachialis, confirming that it serves as a main force in horizontal adduction movements. Their research also verified the belief that this muscle, the middle deltoid, and the long head of the triceps, acting like guy wires on a mast, serve to stabilize the shoulder joint. It may be palpated on the front of the upper arm between the anterior deltoid and the pectoralis major, but it is a difficult muscle to identify.

Subscapularis

As one of the *rotator cuff* muscles, the subscapularis (figures 5.12 and 5.13a) contributes significantly to stabilization of the glenohumeral joint, especially in the prevention of dislocation during forced lateral rotation of the abducted arm. It is also one of the depressors of the humeral head during abduction and flexion of the arm. Its chief

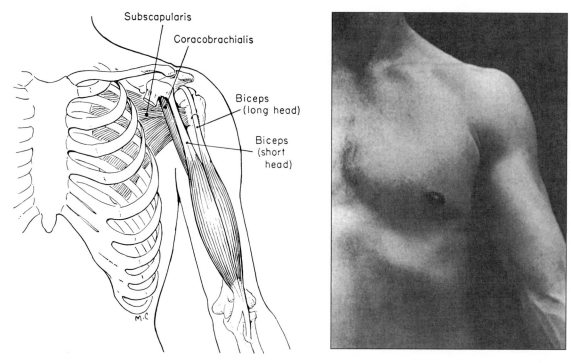

Figure 5.12   Anterior view of muscles of shoulder joint, deep layer.

action as a mover is inward rotation, which it performs most effectively when the arm is at the side or is elevated posteriorly. It has also shown significantly more electrical activity in horizontal abduction than in horizontal adduction.

Biceps Brachii

Although essentially a muscle of the elbow joint, the biceps (see figure 5.12) crosses the shoulder joint and is active in some of the movements of the humerus. Both heads are always active in flexion and in abduction with resistance when the elbow is straight. The muscle is also active in horizontal adduction and the short head sometimes participates in adduction against resistance and in medial rotation.

Deltoid

The complex structure of the deltoid (figures 5.11 and 5.14), with the multipenniform arrangement of the bundles making up the middle portion,

gives it a potential for great strength without undue bulk. The middle portion of the muscle is a *powerful abductor of the humerus,* its greatest activity occurring when the humerus is raised between 90 and 120 degrees. It is capable of supporting the weight of the upper extremity for long periods while the hand is working at a height. The multipenniform arrangement of fibers compensates for the middle deltoid's rather poor angle of pull. The angle of pull, however, serves the useful purpose of providing the muscle with a strong stabilizing component force. This is fortunate because, in the raised position, the shoulder joint depends more on its muscles than on its ligaments for holding the head of the humerus on the glenoid fossa. The middle portion has also been found to be active in horizontal abduction.

The anterior portion of the deltoid aids in all *forward movements* of the arm and in *inward rotation* of the humerus. It is also active in abduction.

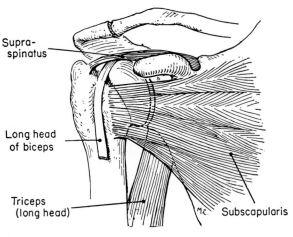

Supra-spinatus

Long head of biceps

Triceps (long head)

Subscapularis

a.

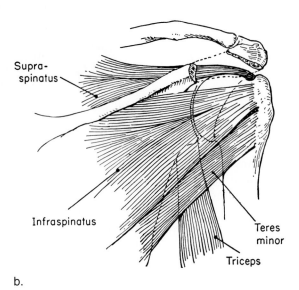

Supra-spinatus

Infraspinatus

Teres minor

Triceps

b.

Figure 5.13   Muscular reinforcement of shoulder joint: (a) anterior view; (b) posterior view.

There is disagreement in the literature concerning the movements effected by the posterior deltoid, but there seems to be sufficient evidence to conclude that, in addition to extension and lateral rotation, the lowest fibers, being situated below the axis of motion, assist in forceful adduction of the humerus from an overhead position. On the other hand, some of the upper fibers (those closest to

the middle deltoid) probably act with the latter in contributing to abduction.

Supraspinatus

This muscle (figures 5.13 and 5.15) acts together with the deltoid in abduction of the arm throughout the entire range. It also acts in flexion and horizontal extension. Action potentials reach their

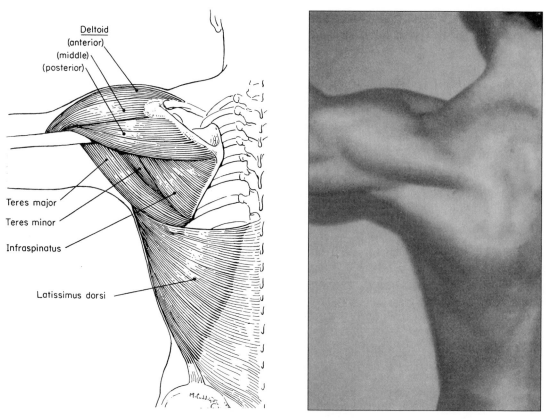

Figure 5.14   Posterior view of muscles of shoulder joint, superficial layer.

maximum when the arm is at 100 degrees of flexion. As part of the rotator cuff it plays a significant part in the stability of the shoulder joint and is important in preventing downward dislocation (Basmajian and DeLuca 1985). It may be palpated above the spine of the scapula, provided that the scapula is supported, as when the armpit rests over the back of a chair.

Infraspinatus and Teres Minor

In addition to their outward rotary action, these two muscles (see figures 5.13b, 5.14, and 5.15), which seem to act as one, have two additional noteworthy functions. Together with the subscapularis they depress the head of the humerus and thus prevent it from jamming against the

acromion process during flexion and abduction of the arm. They are also part of the rotator cuff muscles (infraspinatus, teres minor, subscapularis, and supraspinatus), whose important function it is to aid materially in holding the head of the humerus in the glenoid fossa. Their important function in this capacity is to prevent dislocation of the shoulder joint, especially when the humerus is in the abducted position. They may be palpated on the posterior surface of the scapula, medial to and below the posterior deltoid muscle.

Latissimus Dorsi

This is a broad sheet of muscle (see figure 5.14) that covers the lower and middle portions of the back. Coming mainly from the lower half of the thoracic spine and the entire lumbar spine, the fibers gradually converge as they pass upward and laterally toward the axilla. Here the fibers twist on themselves in such a way that the lowest fibers become the uppermost. They end in the narrow flat tendon of the distal attachment. The muscle has a favorable angle of pull for extension and adduction of the arm, particularly when the latter is raised between 30 and 90 degrees. EMG has confirmed the action of the latissimus dorsi in extension and adduction during static and dynamic, resisted and unresisted movements. Although controversy exists, recent electromyographic evidence confirms that the latissimus dorsi muscle is active during inward rotation of the humerus (Basmajian and DeLuca 1985). The muscle may be palpated on the posterior border of the axilla just below the teres major.

Teres Major

Structurally this muscle (see figures 5.14 and 5.15) appears to be in a favorable position to work with the latissimus dorsi in *downward and backward movements* of the humerus and also in *inward rotation,* but Basmajian and DeLuca (1985) detected no sign of activity in this muscle during these movements unless external resistance was applied. Against active resistance, activity was evident during inward rotation, adduction, and extension. No added resistance is needed, however, for the teres major to be active during hyperextension and adduction when the arm is behind the back.

Triceps Brachii

Although primarily a muscle of the elbow joint, the triceps (see figures 5.13 and 5.15) is active

Figure 5.15   Posterior view of muscles of shoulder joint, deep layer.

in movements of the humerus because its long head crosses the shoulder joint. It assists in adduction, extension, and hyperextension of the humerus.

JOINT AND MUSCULAR ANALYSIS OF THE FUNDAMENTAL MOVEMENTS OF THE ARM ON THE TRUNK

As stated earlier, the movements of the arm on the trunk involve the cooperative action of the shoulder girdle and the shoulder joint, the former including both the acromioclavicular and the sternoclavicular joints. To correctly analyze the great variety of movements of the upper extremity, it is essential to understand this cooperative action of the three joints and their muscles. The fundamental movements of the arm on the trunk, together with the anatomical analysis of each, are presented next.

Movements in the Frontal Plane
Abduction

This movement may occur from any distance up to the vertical (figure 5.16).

Shoulder joint *Abduction* of the humerus by the deltoid and supraspinatus accompanied by slight depression of the humeral head because of the action of the subscapularis, infraspinatus, and teres minor. This is the least forceful of shoulder joint actions. True humeral abduction is the sideward elevation of the humerus in a plane parallel with the scapula. Hence, if the scapulae were slightly abducted and laterally tilted from poor posture, for instance, the abducted humeri would not be strictly in the frontal plane of the body but would be moving in an oblique plane, slightly anterior to the frontal plane.

Outward or *lateral rotation* by the infraspinatus and teres minor when palms are turned

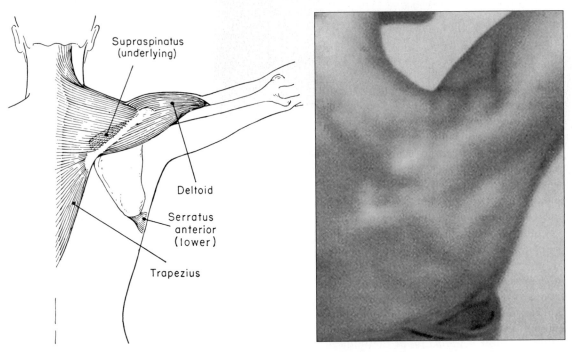

Figure 5.16   Muscles that contract to produce abduction of the upper extremities.

Figure 5.17 Adduction of the upper extremity against resistance. The latissimus dorsi, teres major, and rhomboids are in strong contraction.

either out or up. Possible abduction by the biceps when the arm is in complete outward rotation.

Shoulder girdle *Upward rotation* of the scapula by the serratus anterior and trapezius II and IV.

Adduction

This movement may occur from any degree of sideward elevation, either against resistance or in any position that rules out the help of gravitational force (figure 5.17).

Shoulder joint *Adduction* of the humerus by the latissimus dorsi, the teres major (against resistance), sternal portion of the pectoralis major, and

probably the lowest fibers of the posterior deltoid. Reduction of outward rotation mainly by the subscapularis and the teres major. The teres major is also active in adduction when the arm moves behind the back.

Shoulder girdle *Reduction of upward rotation* by the rhomboids and pectoralis minor, with help from the levator scapulae.

Movements in the Sagittal Plane
Flexion

This movement may occur up to the horizontal (figure 5.18).

Figure 5.18   Flexion of the upper extremity against resistance. The anterior and middle deltoid, upper trapezius, and serratus anterior are in strong contraction.

Shoulder joint   *Flexion* of the humerus by the anterior deltoid and clavicular portion of the pectoralis major, probably with some participation of the coracobrachialis (against resistance) and biceps brachii.

Slight outward rotation by the infraspinatus and teres minor.

Shoulder girdle   *Upward rotation* of the scapula by the serratus anterior and trapezius II and IV (slight).

Abduction and lateral tilt of the scapula by the serratus anterior and pectoralis minor, unless intentionally inhibited.

Continued Flexion

This movement may occur from the horizontal to the vertical and beyond.

Shoulder joint   *Flexion* of the humerus by the same muscles as above; hyperflexion if the humerus moves beyond the vertical.

Continued *outward rotation* by the infraspinatus and teres minor if the palms turn to face each other when the arms reach the vertical.

Shoulder girdle   *Upward rotation* of the scapula by the serratus anterior and trapezius II and IV (increased).

Slight to moderate *elevation* of the scapula by the levator scapulae, trapezius I and II, and rhomboids, unless effort is made to inhibit elevation. This action would be evident in reaching activities such as the high jump, long jump, or the pushing phase of the pole vault.

Reduction of abduction and lateral tilt mainly by virtue of the overhead position.

Figure 5.19 Extension of the upper extremity against resistance. The latissimus dorsi and teres major are in strong contraction.

Extension

This movement may occur from the overhead vertical to the starting position, either against resistance or in a position that rules out the help of gravitational force (figure 5.19).

Shoulder joint *Extension* of the humerus by the sternal portion of the pectoralis major (diminishing as the movement progresses), teres major (against resistance), latissimus dorsi (especially during the lower 60 degrees of motion), and possibly the posterior deltoid and the long head of the triceps brachii. Extension is the most powerful of shoulder movements.

Reduction of outward rotation, probably by relaxation of outward rotator muscles but possibly aided by the subscapularis, teres major, latissimus dorsi, and pectoralis major.

Shoulder girdle *Reduction of elevation and upward rotation* by relaxation of muscles. If the movement is performed against resistance, the pectoralis minor, trapezius IV, subclavius, and rhomboids would doubtless be active. In pulling movements like a chin-up, strong adduction of the middle trapezius and rhomboids and strong depression by the pectoralis minor and lower trapezius would also be evident.

Hyperextension *(Figure 5.20)*

Shoulder joint *Hyperextension* of the humerus by the posterior deltoid, latissimus dorsi, and teres major.

Shoulder girdle *Upward tilt* of the scapula by the pectoralis minor.

Elevation if movement is carried to the extreme. Possibly the hyperextension of the humerus pushes the scapula into a position of slight elevation. If any scapular muscles are acting, they would probably be the levator scapulae, trapezius I and II, and rhomboids, with possibly the clavicular portion of the sternocleidomastoid (a neck muscle) helping.

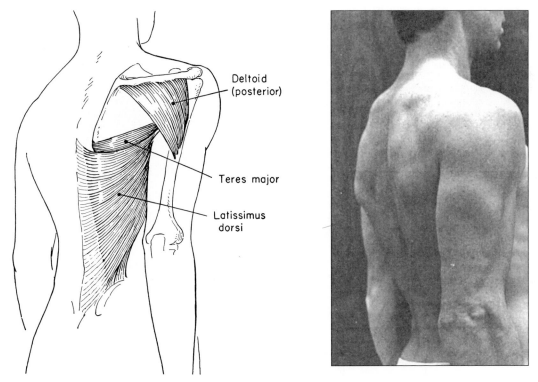

Figure 5.20 Muscles that contract to produce hyperextension of the upper extremity.

Movements in the Horizontal Plane

Outward Rotation *(Figures 5.21 and 5.22)*

Shoulder joint *Outward rotation* of the humerus by the infraspinatus and teres minor with the posterior deltoid acting only if the humerus is also being adducted and extended, as in a calisthenic or postural exercise.

Shoulder girdle *Adduction* of the scapulae and *reduction of any lateral tilt,* which may have been present by the rhomboids and trapezius III, with some involvement of trapezius II and IV.

Inward Rotation

Shoulder joint *Inward rotation* of the humerus by the subscapularis, teres major (against resistance), latissimus dorsi, anterior deltoid, and pectoralis major. If the upper extremity is in a position of outward rotation to start with,

the coracobrachialis and short head of the biceps would be active in the first part of the movement.

Shoulder girdle *Abduction and lateral tilt* by the serratus anterior and pectoralis minor, with a tendency toward elevation by the levator scapulae, trapezius I and II, and rhomboids.

Horizontal Adduction

Shoulder joint *Horizontal adduction* of humerus by the pectoralis major, anterior deltoid, and coracobrachialis, with the short head of the biceps helping if the forearm is extended.

Shoulder girdle *Abduction and lateral tilt* of scapula, unless deliberately inhibited. The movement is produced by the serratus anterior and pectoralis minor.

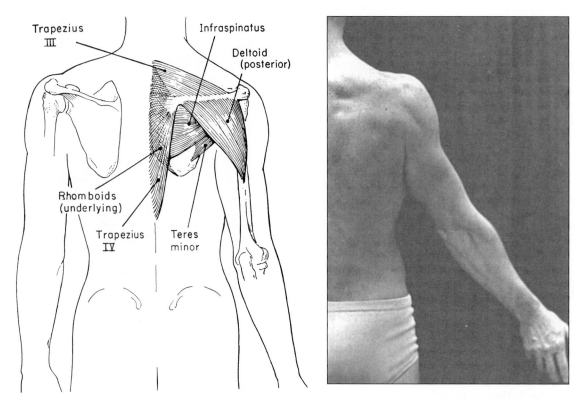

Figure 5.21 Muscles that contract to produce outward rotation of the arm and accompanying adduction of the scapula.

Horizontal Abduction

Shoulder joint *Horizontal abduction* of the humerus by the posterior deltoid, posterior portion of middle deltoid, infraspinatus, teres minor, and long head of the triceps.

Shoulder girdle *Adduction and reduction of lateral tilt* of scapula by the rhomboids and trapezius III in particular, with II and IV also participating.

Diagonal Movements

Unless performing calisthenic or gymnastic exercises, one rarely performs pure fundamental movements of the arm on the trunk. Most athletic and everyday movements are "in-between" or combination movements. To analyze these in

terms of their muscular action, it is necessary to estimate the approximate proportions of the fundamental joint motions. For instance, the follow-through on a tennis serve might involve extension (forward-downward depression) of the arm (see shoulder joint and shoulder girdle analysis), or it might consist of extension combined with a slight amount of "horizontal" adduction swing. In other words, this could be described as a diagonal forward-downward and slightly inward movement of the arm, consisting mainly of extension of the humerus combined with a slight degree of adduction. An appropriate term proposed by is *diagonal adduction* (figures 5.10 and 5.23). After the server's racket is moved forward-upward to ball contact by inward rotation of the humerus at the shoulder and extension at the elbow, the arm movement is diagonally down and

a.   b.

Figure 5.22   (a) Outward rotation of the arm against resistance. The posterior deltoid, infraspinatus, and teres minor are in strong contraction. (The hyperextension and lateral flexion of the trunk are caused by the extreme effort. The latissimus is contracting because he is pushing his elbow down.) (b) Inward rotation. The pectoralis major, anterior deltoid, teres major, and latissimus dorsi are in strong contraction.

across the body in a combination of extension and adduction—that is, diagonal adduction.

A true forehand drive might well consist of a pure horizontal forward swing from a side horizontal position (horizontal adduction of the humerus and abduction of the scapula), but the arm is more likely to start slightly above or below the horizontal and to move in a diagonal path.

An underhand volleyball serve or the motion of a snow shovel, which are likely to have an upward as well as a forward component, would consist of a horizontal forward swing from the side horizontal position of the arm combined with a slight amount of forward-upward elevation. This would involve slight shoulder joint flexion accompanied by a combination of abduction, lateral tilt, and upward rotation of the shoulder girdle.

Shoulder Girdle Movements Not Involving the Arm

In addition to these coordinated movements of the arm on the trunk, there are three movements of the shoulder girdle in which movements of the arm are passive because they are produced by the changes in position of the shoulder girdle from which they are suspended. These are (1) a lifting or hunching of the shoulders, (2) protraction of the shoulders, and (3) retraction of the shoulders.

Shoulder Lifting or Hunching
Shoulder girdle   *Elevation* by the levator scapulae, trapezius I and II, and rhomboids, with assistance by the sternocleidomastoid if the movement is performed against resistance. Reduction of the

Figure 5.23 A tennis serve showing diagonal adduction of arm at shoulder joint during follow-through. Courtesy of H. E. Edgerton.

elevation is achieved by relaxing the muscles and letting the force of gravity have its way.

Shoulder Protraction
Shoulder girdle *Forceful abduction and lateral tilt* of scapula by the serratus anterior and pectoralis minor.

Shoulder joint Slight *passive inward rotation*. Reduction of the movement is achieved by relaxation of the muscles but may be followed by slight retraction.

Shoulder Retraction
Shoulder girdle *Adduction and reduction of lateral tilt* by the rhomboids, trapezius III, and possibly II and IV.

COMMON INJURIES OF THE SHOULDER REGION

Acromioclavicular Sprain

This injury occurs if the acromioclavicular joint is forced beyond its normal range of motion, such as from a downward blow against the outer

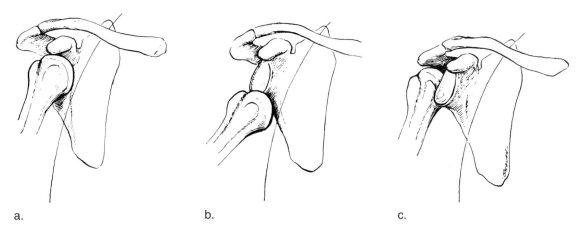

a.   b.   c.

Figure 5.24   Dislocations of the shoulder: (a) typical subcoracoid dislocation; (b) subglenoid dislocation; (c) posterior dislocation.
From D. H. O'Donoghue, *Treatment of Injuries to Athletes,* 3rd ed. Copyright © 1976 W. B. Saunders, Orlando, FL. Reprinted by permission.

end of the shoulder, causing the acromion to be driven downward away from the clavicle. It is also caused by a fall in which the person lands on an outstretched hand or flexed elbow when the arm is in a vertical position and at an angle of 45 to 90 degrees of flexion or abduction from the trunk. The damage consists of the tearing or severe stretching of the acromioclavicular ligaments.

Fracture of the Clavicle

A fracture of the clavicle in its middle third may result from the same type of injury that causes acromioclavicular sprains—namely, either a direct downward blow to the acromion process, or, more commonly, landing on the hand from a fall with the arm rigidly outstretched. Such a fracture may be recognized or at least suspected if the injured person tends to support the injured arm with the good arm and carries the head tilted toward the injured side with the face turned to the opposite side. Teenagers and preteenagers are more likely to have a greenstick fracture from such injuries (Arnheim and Prentice 1998).

Dislocation of the Shoulder

There are three types of these dislocations: forward or subcoracoid (figure 5.24a); downward or subglenoid (figure 5.24b); and posterior (figure 5.24c). The most common type among young athletes is the forward (subcoracoid) type, which is most likely to occur when the humerus is abducted and laterally rotated or when the pectoralis major is forcefully contracting. In this circumstance, the head of the humerus, having slipped forward out of the glenoid fossa, comes to rest beneath the coracoid process (figure 5.24a). The injured arm is usually held out from the side in a position of slight abduction and lateral rotation. The shoulder is well protected from downward dislocations because of the upward tilt of the glenoid fossa and the effectiveness of the supraspinatus, posterior deltoid, and the superior part of the capsule in tightening to hold the humeral head in the socket. When these dislocations do occur, they are caused by a blow from the top of the shoulder and happen more easily when the arm is slightly abducted.

Chronic Dislocation of the Shoulder

This dislocation is usually forward and results either from a congenital abnormality or from repeated acute dislocations in an otherwise normal joint. With proper care following an acute dislocation there should be no recurrences. Congenital abnormalities resulting in dislocations are likely to require surgery.

Rotator Cuff Strains

The supraspinatus muscle is the rotator cuff muscle most often injured. Strains or tearing of the rotator cuff may be caused by overuse, falling on an outstretched arm, and violent, fast arm motions.

LABORATORY EXPERIENCES

Joint Structure and Function

1. Facing your partner's back, hold your thumb against the inferior angle of one scapula and your index or middle finger against the root of the spine at the scapula. Try to follow the movements of the scapula as your partner performs all the fundamental movements of the arm on the body.

2. Study the movements of the glenohumeral, acromioclavicular, and sternoclavicular articulations. Classify each joint according to structure (see pp. 26–30). For each joint, name and describe briefly the articulating processes and surfaces, ligaments and cartilages. Explain how the joint structure influences the ranges of identified motions and prevents motions not observed.

3. In five different subjects measure the amount of abduction that occurs in the shoulder girdle (i.e., the separation of the scapulae) when the arms are flexed 90 degrees at the shoulder joint. How much can this vary in one individual? In measuring the distance between the scapulae, measure the horizontal distance between the midpoints of the vertebral borders.

4. Using a protractor or goniometer, measure the amount of upward rotation of the scapula that occurs when the arm is abducted to the overhead position. To make this measurement, center the instrument over the medial angle of the scapula and adjust one of its arms in line with the normal resting position of the inferior angle and the other in line with the inferior angle after maximum upward rotation of the scapula has taken place.

Muscular Action

Directions: Work in groups of three, with one person serving as the subject, the second as an assistant helping to support or steady the stationary part of the body and giving resistance to the moving part, and the third palpating the muscles and recording the results according to the format used in table 1.2.

5. **Abduction of the Arm.** Shoulder joint: abduction and possibly outward rotation; shoulder girdle: upward rotation.
   Subject: In erect position, abduct the arm to shoulder level, keeping the forearm extended.
   Assistant: Resist movement by exerting pressure downward on subject's elbow. See to it that subject does not elevate shoulder.
   Observer: Palpate the three portions of the deltoid and tell which portions contract. Palpate the four parts of the trapezius. Which parts contract? Does the pectoralis major contract during any part of the movement?

6. **Adduction of the Arm** (see figure 5.17). Shoulder joint: adduction and possibly reduction of outward rotation; shoulder girdle: downward rotation.
   Subject: In erect position with arm abducted to shoulder level, lower arm until 45 degrees from side.
   Assistant: Place hand under subject's elbow and resist movement. (If no resistance is given, the muscle action will be the same as in abduction, except that the contraction will be eccentric instead of concentric.)
   Observer: Palpate the latissimus dorsi, teres major, pectoralis major, and posterior deltoid. Do they each contract and, if so, during which part of the movement?

7. **Flexion of the Arm** (see figure 5.18). Shoulder joint: flexion; shoulder girdle: upward rotation and probably abduction.

   Subject: In erect position, flex arm to shoulder level, keeping elbow extended.

   Assistant: Resist movement by exerting pressure downward on the subject's elbow. See that subject does not elevate shoulder.

   Observer: Palpate the anterior deltoid and the pectoralis major. Do both the sternal and clavicular portions of the latter muscle contract?

8. **Extension of the Arm** (see figure 5.19). Shoulder joint: extension; shoulder girdle: downward rotation and probably adduction.

   Subject: In erect position with arm flexed to shoulder level, lower it until 45 degrees from side.

   Assistant: Resist movement at underside of elbow.

   Observer: Palpate the latissimus dorsi and the pectoralis major. Do they contract with equal force throughout the movement?

9. **Hyperextension of the Arm** (see figure 5.20). Shoulder joint: hyperextension; shoulder girdle: upward tilt.

   Subject: Either in erect position or lying face down: hyperextend upper extremity, keeping elbow extended.

   Assistant: Place hand over subject's elbow and resist movement.

   Observer: Palpate the posterior deltoid, latissimus dorsi, and teres major.

10. **Horizontal Abduction of the Arm** (from horizontal adduction). Shoulder joint: horizontal abduction and slight outward rotation; shoulder girdle: adduction and reduction of lateral tilt.

    a. *Subject:* In erect position with arms flexed to shoulder level, palm down, horizontally abduct the arms as far as possible.

    Assistant: Stand facing subject between the arms and resist movement by grasping the outstretched elbows.

    Observer: Palpate the posterior deltoid and latissimus dorsi. What other muscles can be palpated?

    b. *Subject:* Lying face down on narrow plinth or on table close to edge with arm hanging straight down (flexed), horizontally extend the arms as far above the horizontal as possible.

    Assistant: Resistance may be given at elbow but is not necessary, because gravity furnishes sufficient resistance.

    Observer: Same as in a.

11. **Horizontal Adduction of the Arm** (from abducted position). Shoulder joint: horizontal adduction and slight inward rotation; shoulder girdle: abduction and lateral tilt.

    a. *Subject:* In erect position with arm abducted to shoulder level, palm down, horizontally adduct the arms.

    Assistant: Stand behind subject's arm and resist movement by holding elbow.

    Observer: Palpate pectoralis major and anterior deltoid.

    b. *Subject:* Lie on back on table with arm horizontally extended, palm up. Horizontally adduct the upper extremity to a vertical position, keeping elbow extended.

    Assistant: Resistance may be given at elbow but is not necessary, because gravity furnishes sufficient resistance.

    Observer: Same as in a.

12. **Outward Rotation of Arm.** Shoulder joint: outward rotation; shoulder girdle: possibly adduction and reduction of lateral tilt.

    a. *Subject:* Lying face down on a table with upper arm at shoulder level, resting on table and forearm hanging down off edge of table. Keeping forearm at right angles to upper arm, outward rotate arm at the shoulder joint to limit of motion without allowing upper arm to leave table.

    Assistant: Steady upper arm and resist movement of forearm by holding wrist.

    Observer: Palpate infraspinatus and teres minor.

    b. *Subject:* Sitting erect with upper arm abducted and elbow flexed at right angles with forearm at forward horizontal position. Without moving upper arm, outward rotate at the shoulder joint so that the forearm is in a vertical position (see figure 5.22).

    Assistant: Support upper arm at elbow and give resistance to forearm at wrist.

    Observer: Same as in a.

13. **Inward Rotation of Arm.** Shoulder joint: inward rotation; shoulder girdle: abduction and lateral tilt, and tendency toward elevation.

    a. *Subject:* Same position as in 12a. Inward rotate arm at the shoulder joint.

Assistant: Steady upper arm and resist movement of forearm by holding wrist.
Observer: Palpate teres major and latissimus dorsi.

b. *Subject:* Lie on back on table with upper arm abducted resting on table and forearm raised to vertical position. Inward rotate arm at shoulder joint to the limit of motion.
Assistant: Steady upper arm and resist forearm motion by holding wrist.
Observer: Palpate anterior deltoid and clavicular portion of pectoralis major.

14. **Elevation of Shoulder.**
Subject: In erect position, elevate shoulder girdle, keeping arm muscles relaxed.
Assistant: Resist movement by pressing down on shoulder.
Observer: Palpate trapezius I and II.

15. **Depression of Shoulder.**
a. *Subject:* In erect position with shoulder girdle elevated and elbow flexed, push down with elbow, depress shoulder girdle to normal position.
Assistant: Resist movement by holding hand under elbow.
Observer: Palpate trapezius IV.

b. *Subject:* Take a cross-rest position between two chairs or parallel bars.
Observer: Palpate trapezius IV.

16. **Adduction of Shoulder Girdle** (retraction).
Subject: In erect position with arms abducted, elbows flexed, and fingers resting on shoulders, push elbows backward (horizontally extend at the shoulder joint) keeping the elbows at shoulder level.
Assistant: Stand facing subject and resist movement by pulling elbows forward (horizontally flex at the shoulder joints).
Observer: Palpate middle and lower trapezius (parts III and IV). (This movement is somewhat similar to the one in Lab Experience 10, but here the emphasis is on the shoulder girdle rather than on the arm.)

17. **Abduction of Shoulder Girdle** (protraction).
Subject: In erect position with arm abducted, elbows flexed, and fingers resting on shoulders, horizontally flex at the shoulder joints, attempting to touch the elbows in front of chest.

Assistant: Stand behind subject and resist movement by pulling elbows back (horizontally extend at the shoulder joint).
Observer: Palpate serratus anterior.

Action of the Muscles Other Than the Movers

18. **Stabilization of the Scapula during Forceful Extension of the Arm.**
Subject: In erect position with arm flexed above shoulder level, lower arm against strong resistance.
Assistant: Resist the arm movement by placing hand under the arm just above the subject's elbow.
Observer: Palpate trapezius IV. Explain.

19. **Stabilization of Scapula during Outward Rotation of Humerus.**
Subject: Rotate the arm outward as it hangs at the side.
Observer: Palpate the scapular adductors. Explain.

20. **Rotation of Arm in Abducted Position.**
Subject: With one arm abducted to shoulder level, rotate it first outward, then inward.
Observer: Palpate middle deltoid. Explain its action.

Applications

21. Work in groups of three with the members designated respectively as A, B, and C. Equipment for each group: a volleyball and an empty 12-ounce frozen juice can or another can of approximately same size.

A stands at one end of playing area with left side toward the opposite end.

B stands facing A about two arm lengths away and holds can vertically in right hand with arm flexed and with volleyball balanced on open end of can.

A adjusts distance and swings extended right arm horizontally backward with thumb side up and palm flat. A then swings arm vigorously forward and strikes ball forcefully with palm, attempting to project ball as far as possible.

C observes A's action and writes answers to the following questions without saying them aloud.
a. What is the movement of A's humerus at the shoulder joint in the preparatory movement?

b. Same for the striking movement?

c. What is the position of A's humerus at the moment of impact?

Repeat until each person has taken a turn at being A, B, and C. Report answers to the rest of the group and discuss if not in agreement.

22. Work in partners with one observing while the other performs.

    Starting position: Hang from horizontal bar with palms facing body and with feet hanging clear or, if necessary, with toes just touching floor or bench.

Movement: Chin self with steady pull and hold end position.

Observer: Write joint analysis of (a) starting position of humerus at shoulder joint, and of scapulae; and (b) movement of each. Discuss with partner.

23. Choose a simple motor skill from appendix H. Do a complete anatomical analysis of the shoulder region, following the analysis outline in table 1.2.

REFERENCES AND SELECTED READINGS

Arnheim, D. D., and W. E. Prentice. 1998. *Essentials of athletic training.* 4th ed. St. Louis: McGraw-Hill.

Basmajian, J. V., and C. J. DeLuca. 1985. *Muscles alive.* 5th ed. Baltimore: Williams & Wilkins.

Bigliani, L. U., R. Kelkar, E. L. Flatow, R. G. Pollock, and Y. C. Mow. 1996. Glenohumeral stability: Biomechanical properties of passive and active stabilzers. *Clinical Orthopedics* 330:13–30.

deSousa, O. M., F. Berzin, and A. C. Berardi. 1969. Electromyographic study of the pectoralis major and latissimus dorsi muscles during medial rotation of the arm. *Electromyography* 9:407–16.

Frankel, V. H., and M. B. Nordin. 1989. *Basic biomechanics of the skeletal system.* 2nd ed. Philadelphia: Lea & Febiger.

Logan, G. A., and W. C. McKinney. 1982. *Anatomic kinesiology.* 3rd ed. Dubuque, IA: William C. Brown.

Norkin, C., and P. Levangie. 1992. *Joint structure and function: A comprehensive analysis.* 2nd ed. Philadelphia: F.A. Davis.

Rasch, P. J. 1989. *Kinesiology and applied anatomy.* 7th ed. Philadelphia: Lea & Febiger.

Shevlin, M. G., J. P. Lehmann, and J. A. Lucci. 1969. Electromyographic study of the function of some muscles crossing the glenohumeral joint. *Archives of Physical Medicine and Rehabilitation* 50:264–70.

Smith, E. L. W., L. D. Lehmkuhl, and L. K. Smith. 1996. *Brunnstrom's clinical kinesiology.* 5th ed. Philadelphia: F. A. Davis.

6

THE UPPER EXTREMITY

The Elbow, Forearm, Wrist, and Hand

O U T L I N E

- **The Elbow Joint**
  Structure
  Movements
- **The Radioulnar Joints**
  Structure of Proximal Radioulnar
    Joint
  Structure of Distal Radioulnar Joint
  Movements
- **Muscles of the Elbow
  and Radioulnar Joints**
  Location
  Characteristics and Functions
    of Individual Muscles
- **Muscular Analysis
  of the Fundamental
  Movements of the Forearm**
- **The Wrist and Hand**
  Structure of the Wrist
    (Radiocarpal) Joint
  Movements of the Hand
    at the Wrist Joint
  Structure and Movements
    of the Midcarpal
    and Intercarpal Joints
  Structure of the Carpometacarpal
    and Intermetacarpal Joints
  Movements of the Carpometacarpal
    Joint of the Thumb

Movements of the
  Carpometacarpal and
  Intermetacarpal Joints
  of the Fingers
Structure of the
  Metacarpophalangeal Joints
Movements of the
  Metacarpophalangeal Joints
  of the Four Fingers
Movements of the
  Metacarpophalangeal Joints
  of the Thumb
The Interphalangeal Joints
- **Muscles of the Wrist
  and Hand**
  Location
  Characteristics and Functions
    of Muscles
- **Muscular Analysis
  of the Fundamental
  Movements of the Wrist,
  Fingers, and Thumb**
  The Wrist
  The Fingers
  The Thumb
  The Thumb Metacarpal
  The Thumb Phalanges

■ *Cooperative Actions of the Wrist
and Digits*
    Length of Long Finger Muscles
        Relative to Range of Motion
        in Wrist and Fingers
    Examples of Using the Hands
        for Grasping
■ *Common Injuries of the Forearm,
Elbow, Wrist, and Fingers*
    Fractures of the Forearm

Elbow Dislocation
Elbow Fracture-Dislocation
Sprained or Strained Wrist
Carpal Tunnel Syndrome
Avulsion Fracture
Epicondylitis
■ *Laboratory Experiences*

O B J E C T I V E S

At the conclusion of this chapter, the student should be able to:

1. Name, locate, and describe the structure and ligamentous reinforcements of the articulations of the elbow, forearm, wrist, and hand.
2. Name and demonstrate the movements possible in the joints of the elbow, forearm, wrist, and hand regardless of the starting position.
3. Name and locate the muscles and muscle groups of the elbow, forearm, wrist, and hand, and name their primary actions as agonists, stabilizers, neutralizers, or antagonists.
4. Analyze the fundamental movements of the forearm, hand, and fingers with respect to joint and muscle actions.
5. Describe the common athletic injuries of the forearm, elbow, wrist, and fingers.
6. Perform an anatomical analysis of the elbow, forearm, wrist, and hand in a motor skill.

In much the same way that the shoulder girdle's cooperation with the shoulder joint contributes to the wide range of motion available to
the hand, the cooperative movements of the
elbow, radioulnar, and wrist joints contribute to
the versatility and precision of its movements. Although the hand is intrinsically skillful, its usefulness is greatly impaired when anything interferes
with the motions of the forearm or wrist. Injury to
any one of the joints involved makes this
painfully obvious to the sufferer.

THE ELBOW JOINT

Structure

The elbow is far more complex than the simple
hinge joint that it appears to be. The two bones
of the forearm attach to the humerus in totally
different ways. The humeroulnar joint is indeed
a true hinge joint, but the humeroradial joint is
far from it. It has been classified as an arthrodial
or gliding type of joint, but it is more accurately
described as a restricted ball-and-socket joint.

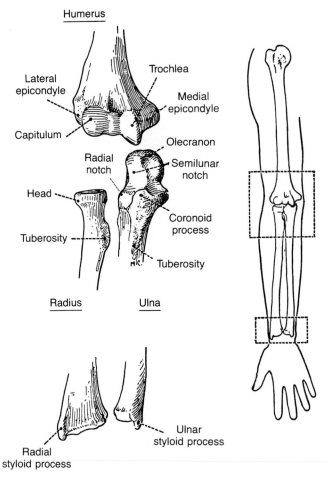

Figure 6.1   The bony structures of the elbow and radioulnar joints, anterior view.

Inspection of the articulating surfaces as depicted in figure 6.1 or of the skeleton itself will help make this clear. The distal end of the humerus presents a spool-like process (trochlea) on the medial side and a spherical knob (capitulum) on the lateral side. The ulna articulates with the humerus by means of a semicircular structure that is cupped around the back and underside of the trochlea. The inner surface of this is known as the semilunar notch. It terminates below and in front in the small coronoid process, and above and in back in the broad olecranon process.

The radius articulates with the humerus by means of a slightly concave, saucerlike disc, which is directly beneath the capitulum when the arm is hanging straight down. In spite of the joint's ball-and-socket structure the radius is unable to abduct or adduct because of the annular ligament that encircles the radial head and binds it to the radial notch of the ulna. Furthermore, because of this and other ligamentous connections with the ulna, the radius is unable to rotate independently (figures 6.2 and 6.3). Hence, the only movements it is free to engage in at the elbow are flexion and extension. For this reason,

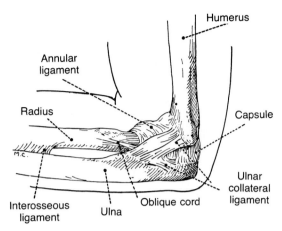

Figure 6.2   Medial aspect of elbow joint showing ligaments.

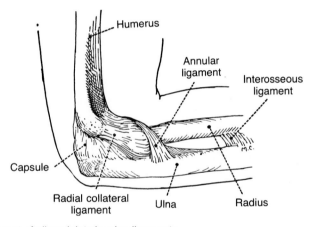

Figure 6.3   Lateral aspect of elbow joint showing ligaments.

one is justified in classifying the elbow joint as a hinge joint.

The two articulations of the elbow joint, as well as the proximal radioulnar articulation, are completely enveloped in a single, extensive capsule. This is lined by synovial membrane, which extends into the proximal radioulnar articulation, covers the olecranon, coronoid, and radial fossae, and lines the annular ligament. The capsule is strengthened by four ligaments: the *anterior, posterior, radial collateral,* and *ulnar collateral.* The last named is the strongest. It is a thick triangular band attached above by its apex to the me-

dial epicondyle of the humerus and below by its base to the medial margins of the coronoid and olecranon processes of the ulna and the intervening ridge.

In the anatomical position, the forearm is abducted in relation to the humerus, an alignment caused by the angle of articulation of the humerus and ulna at the elbow joint. Normally this angle, called the carrying angle, is larger in women than in men. If the forearm were to hang straight down in women as it does in men, it would not clear the female pelvis. Not only is the female's pelvis broader than the male's, her shoulders also are

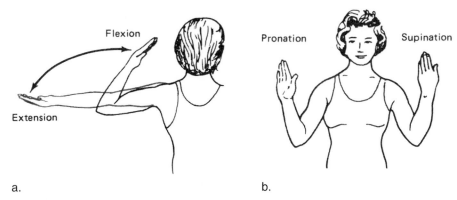

a.   b.

Figure 6.4   Movements of the elbow and radioulnar joints: (a) flexion and extension; (b) right radioulnar joints pronated; left radioulnar joints supinated.

narrower. This exaggerated carrying angle, referred to as cubitus valgus, disappears during elbow flexion or forearm pronation.

Movements
Flexion
From the anatomical position this is a forward-upward movement of the forearm in the sagittal plane (figure 6.4a).

Extension
Return movement from flexion. A few individuals are able to hyperextend the elbow joint. This is probably because of a short olecranon process rather than loose ligaments (figure 6.4a).

THE RADIOULNAR JOINTS

Structure of Proximal Radioulnar Joint
The disc-shaped head of the radius fits against the radial notch of the ulna and is encircled by the annular ligament (see figures 6.1, 6.2, and 6.3). The notch and annular ligament between them form a complete ring within which the radial head rotates. Inasmuch as the superior surface of the radial head articulates with the capitulum of the humerus, rotation must occur here, too, although

strictly speaking, this is not part of the radioulnar joint. The three joints in this region, the humeroulnar, humeroradial, and proximal radioulnar, all share a common capsule.

Structure of Distal Radioulnar Joint
At the distal end of the forearm the radius articulates with the head of the ulna by means of a small notch (see figure 6.1). A triangular fibrocartilaginous disc lies between the head of the ulna and the proximal row of wrist bones (see figure 6.12) and serves to reinforce the joint, as well as to separate it from the wrist. The joint is also strengthened by the *volar radioulnar* and *dorsal radioulnar* ligaments. Both the proximal and distal radioulnar joints are classified as pivot joints.

Movements
Pronation
This is a rotation of the forearm around its longitudinal axis in such a way that the palm turns medially. It corresponds to medial or inward rotation of the humerus.

Supination
This is a rotation of the forearm around its longitudinal axis in such a way that the palm turns lat-

erally. It corresponds to lateral or outward rotation of the humerus. During pronation and supination, the distal end of the radius moves about the ulna, whereas the proximal end of the radius rotates or pivots about its long axis.

Note: When the elbow is in an extended position, pronation of the forearm tends to accompany inward rotation of the upper arm, and supination tends to accompany outward rotation. In the anatomical position of the arm the humerus is rotated outward and the forearm is supinated. The full range of forearm pronation and supination is best seen when the elbow is maintained at a 90-degree angle (see figure 6.4). When the upper arms are at the sides of the body and the forearms are extended forward in the horizontal position, the mid or neutral position relative to pronation and supination is with the thumbs up and the palms facing each other. An excellent way to study what happens to the two forearm bones in these movements is suggested in Laboratory Experience 4.

MUSCLES OF THE ELBOW AND RADIOULNAR JOINTS

Location

The muscles of the elbow and radioulnar joints are listed here according to their positions relative to the joints involved:

Anterior (Elbow Region)
> Biceps brachii
> Brachialis
> Brachioradialis
> Pronator teres

Anterior (Wrist Region)
> Pronator quadratus

Posterior
> Triceps brachii
> Anconeus
> Supinator

Characteristics and Functions of Individual Muscles

Biceps Brachii

This is primarily a muscle of the elbow and radioulnar joints (figure 6.5) but, as noted in the last chapter, it also acts at the shoulder joint. Unless prevented from doing so (by the action of neutralizers or by fixation of the hand when the subject is hanging from a bar), it simultaneously *flexes* and *supinates* the forearm. Studies by Basmajian and others (Basmajian and DeLuca 1985) have shown that the biceps is active during flexion of the supine forearm under all conditions of static and dynamic contraction. In most instances in which the forearm is pronated, however, the biceps shows little activity unless external resistance is applied (figure 6.6). This is because its tendon wraps around the radius and therefore has a poor line of pull. External resistance is also necessary for the biceps to be active in supination of the extended arm. It may be palpated on the anterior surface of the upper arm when the forearm is flexed, especially in the supinated position.

Brachialis

The sole function of this muscle (figure 6.7) is *flexion* of the elbow joint, and it is said to be the unexcelled flexor under all conditions (Basmajian and DeLuca 1985). Because it attaches on the proximal end of the ulna, its line of pull remains the same regardless of whether the forearm is pronated or supinated. It is partially covered by the biceps but can be palpated just lateral to this muscle if the contraction is sufficiently strong, and especially if the forearm is maintained in the pronated position as it is being flexed (see figure 6.6b).

Brachioradialis

In addition to its role as a contributor to elbow *flexion* when the movement is resisted, it has been suggested that this muscle (figure 6.8) may tend to "derotate" the forearm as it flexes. This has not been confirmed by electromyographic research. It has been found, however, that the brachioradialis

Figure 6.5   Biceps muscle of the arm.

neither supinates nor pronates the fully extended forearm unless the movement is strongly resisted. It has also been noted that this muscle is most active in quick movements. It is more active in a semipronated than a supinated forearm position (Basmajian and DeLuca 1985). It may be palpated on the anteroradial aspect of the upper half of the forearm.

Pronator Teres

This is primarily a *pronator* of the forearm (figure 6.8), but it assists in elbow flexion against re-

sistance. The angle of the elbow joint does not influence the pronation activity of this muscle (Basmajian and DeLuca 1985). It is difficult to palpate.

Pronator Quadratus

This muscle's (figure 6.9) sole action is *pronation* of the forearm. EMG experiments have shown that the electrical activity of the pronator quadratus is definitely greater than that of the pronator teres, irrespective of the speed of the movement or the degree of elbow flexion. It is too deep to palpate successfully.

a.

b.

Figure 6.6 Flexion of the forearm: (a) in a position of supination; (b) in a position of pronation. The biceps brachii is less active when the forearm is pronated than when it is supinated.

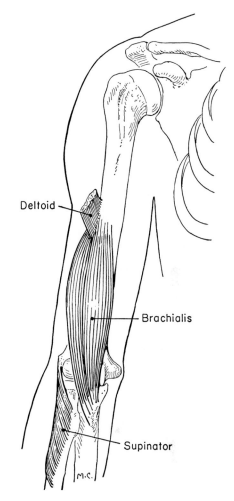

Deltoid

Brachialis

Supinator

M.C.

Figure 6.7 Deep muscles on front of right arm.

Triceps Brachii

Virtually three muscles in one (figures 6.10 and 6.11), the triceps covers the entire posterior surface of the upper arm. Its long head is the only one of the three to cross the shoulder joint. It is a powerful *extensor of the elbow joint* and has two factors in its favor: the number and size of its fibers (p. 50), and a favorable angle of pull

(p. 52). In a comparison of the three heads, it was noted that the medial head appeared to be the principal extensor of the elbow joint, usually accompanied by the lateral head. All three heads participate when there is resistance (Basmajian and DeLuca 1985). The muscle is an easy one to see as well as to palpate.

Anconeus

This muscle, working with the triceps, *extends* the forearm (figure 6.11). This muscle is moderately active during pronation and supination of the

Figure 6.8   Superficial muscles on front of right forearm.

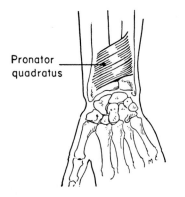

Figure 6.9   Anterior view of distal end of forearm showing pronator quadratus.

forearm, and therefore it is suggested that the anconeus acts as a stabilizer of the elbow joint (Basmajian and DeLuca 1985). The muscle may be palpated on the back of the elbow at the lateral margin of the olecranon process.

Supinator

Although assisted by others, this muscle (see figures 6.7 and 6.10) is the primary one for *supination* under all conditions. Palpation with any degree of success is extremely difficult.

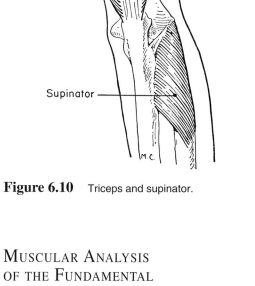

Figure 6.10   Triceps and supinator.

MUSCULAR ANALYSIS OF THE FUNDAMENTAL MOVEMENTS OF THE FOREARM

Flexion

There are three important flexors of the forearm: the brachialis, the brachioradialis, and the biceps—the three Bs. Their relative participation in and contribution to flexion of the forearm have been the subjects of much study. Because elbow flexion may be performed with the forearm pronated, semipronated, or supinated, with or without resistance, slowly or rapidly, with or

against gravity, there have been many variables to study.

Investigators agree that the brachialis serves as a flexor under all conditions, and there is general agreement that the biceps is more active in flexion when the arm is supinated than when it is pronated.

It is now generally accepted that during maximal isometric contractions (1) the biceps is most active electrically when the forearm is supinated and least active when it is pronated; (2) the brachioradialis is most active electrically when the forearm is either in the midposition or

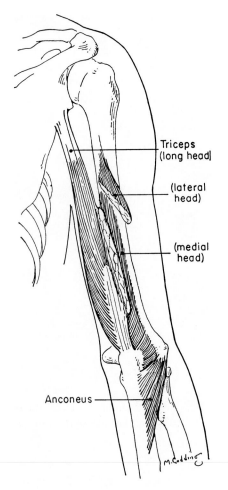

Figure 6.11 Triceps and anconeus.

in supination and least active when the forearm is in extreme pronation or supination; (3) the pronator teres, as a moderate flexor, is most active in a position of pronation; and (4) the isometric force exerted by the elbow flexors during maximal voluntary contractions is greatest when the forearm is supinated or in midposition and least when the forearm is pronated (Basmajian and DeLuca 1985; Sergio and Ostry 1995).

Extension

When not produced by the force of gravity, the forearm is extended at the elbow joint by the triceps and anconeus.

Pronation

Movement of the forearm at the two radioulnar joints. Produced by the combined action of the pronator teres and pronator quadratus.

Supination

Movement of the forearm at the two radioulnar joints. Produced by the supinator and biceps brachii. The two heads of the biceps are not equally active in all supination motions. Brown, Solomon, and Paton (1993) found that activity in each of the heads was related to initial muscle length. The long head of the biceps was found to be more active with a greater muscle length (elbow extension), whereas the short head was more active with a shortened initial muscle length (elbow flexion).

THE WRIST AND HAND

The hand and wrist owe their mobility to their generous supply of joints (figure 6.12). The most proximal of these is the radiocarpal, or wrist, joint. Just beyond this are the two rows of carpal bones, each row consisting of four bones. The carpal joints include the articulations within each of these rows, as well as the articulations between the two rows. The carpometacarpal joints (figure 6.13a) are located at the base of the hand. Closely associated with them are the intermetacarpal joints, those points of contact between the bases of the metacarpal bones of the four fingers. The fingers unite with the hand at the metacarpophalangeal joints. Within the fingers themselves are two sets of interphalangeal joints, the first between the proximal and middle rows of phalanges and the second between the middle and distal rows. The thumb differs from the four fingers in having a more freely movable metacarpal bone and in having only two phalanges instead of three. The metacarpal bone of the thumb is so similar to a phalanx that it might well be described as a cross between a phalanx and a metacarpal (figure 6.13b).

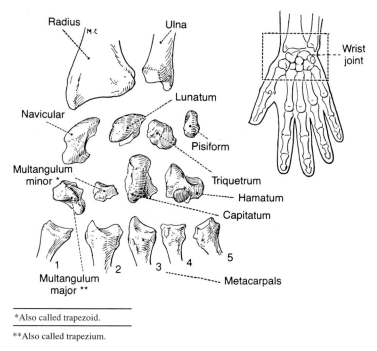

Figure 6.12   Bones of the wrist, anterior view.

Structure of the Wrist (Radiocarpal) Joint

The wrist joint is a condyloid (ovoid) joint formed by the union of the slightly concave, oval-shaped surface of the proximal row of carpal bones (i.e., the scaphoid, lunate, and triquetral bones, but not the pisiform). The distal radioulnar joint is in close proximity to the wrist joint and shares with it the articular disc that lies between the head of the ulna and the triquetral bone of the wrist. However, it is not a part of the wrist joint, because each joint has its own capsule. The capsule of the wrist consists of four ligaments that merge to form a continuous cover for the joint. These are the volar radiocarpal, dorsal radiocarpal, ulnar collateral, and radial collateral (figures 6.14 and 6.15).

Movements of the Hand at the Wrist Joint
Flexion

From the anatomical position (figure 6.16a), this is a forward-upward movement in the sagittal plane, whereby the palmar surface of the hand approaches the anterior surface of the forearm.

Extension

Return movement from flexion.

Hyperextension

A movement in which the dorsal surface of the hand approaches the posterior surface of the forearm—the exact opposite of flexion.

Radial Flexion (Abduction)

From the anatomical position this is a sideward movement in the frontal plane, whereby the hand moves away from the body with the thumb side leading (figure 6.16b). The movement corresponds to abduction of the humerus. This motion is also referred to as radial deviation.

Ulnar Flexion (Adduction)

From the anatomical position this is a sideward movement in the frontal plane, whereby the hand

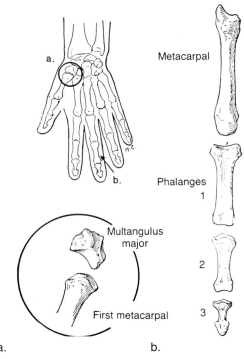

Figure 6.13   Bones of the hand showing selected joint surfaces: (a) carpometacarpal joint of thumb (a saddle joint); (b) metacarpal bone and phalanges of middle finger, anterior view.

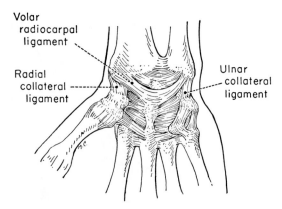

Figure 6.14   Anterior view of right wrist joint showing ligaments.

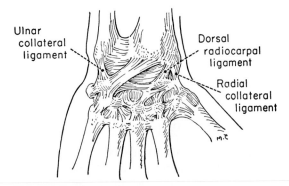

Figure 6.15   Posterior view of right wrist joint showing ligaments.

moves toward the body with the little finger side leading. The movement corresponds to adduction of the humerus. This motion is also referred to as ulnar deviation.

Circumduction

A movement of the hand at the wrist whereby the fingertips describe a circle, and the hand as a whole describes a cone. It consists of flexion, radial flexion, hyperextension, and ulnar flexion occurring in sequence in either this order or the reverse. If there appears to be rotation when one performs this movement, it is taking place in the radioulnar joints, not the wrist joint.

Structure and Movements of the Midcarpal and Intercarpal Joints

These are the joints within the wrist itself. The articulation between the four carpal bones in the proximal row with the four in the distal row is known as the midcarpal articulation. The joints between the adjacent bones within either row are known as the intercarpal joints of the proximal and distal rows, respectively. These joints are all diarthrodial in structure. Within this classification they belong to the nonaxial group and thus permit only a slight gliding motion between the bones. These slight movements, however, add up to a

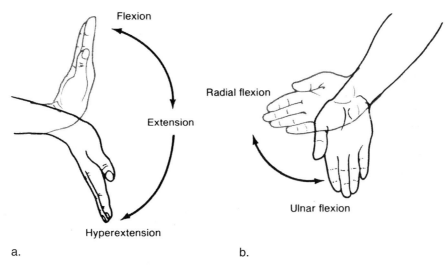

Figure 6.16 Movements of the hand at the wrist joint: (a) flexion, extension, and hyperextension; (b) ulnar and radial flexion.

modified hinge type of movement for the mid-carpal joint as a whole.

A further characteristic of the carpal region is that the bones are shaped and arranged in such a way that the anterior surface is slightly concave from side to side. This provides a protected passageway for the tendons, nerves, and blood vessels supplying the hand. Referred to as the carpal tunnel, this is the site of many pathologies of the hand and wrist. Among the many carpal ligaments, the volar radiocarpal ligament is the strongest. Its fibers radiate from the capitate to the scaphoid, lunate, and triquetral bones on the anterior surface of the wrist.

Structure of the Carpometacarpal and Intermetacarpal Joints (Figures 6.13, 6.17, and 6.18)

The carpometacarpal (trapeziometacarpal) joint of the thumb is a prime example of a saddle joint (see figure 6.13a). It is enclosed in an articular capsule that is stronger in back than in front. The capsule is thick but loose and serves to restrict motion rather than to prevent it. There are no additional ligaments.

The carpometacarpal joints of the four fingers not only are encased in capsules but also are protected by the dorsal, volar, and interosseous carpometacarpal ligaments (figures 6.17 and 6.18). Closely associated with these joints are the intermetacarpal articulations, the joints between the bases of the metacarpal bones of the four fingers. These are irregular joints. They share the capsules of the carpometacarpal joints and are further reinforced by the dorsal, volar, and interosseous basal ligaments and also by the transverse metacarpal ligament, a narrow fibrous band that connects the heads of the four outer metacarpal bones.

Movements of the Carpometacarpal Joint of the Thumb

The names of the movements of the thumb may seem illogical until they are viewed in the context of the resting thumb position, that is, turned on its

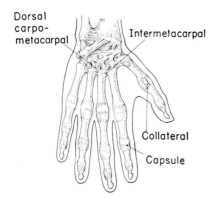

Figure 6.17   Posterior view of ligaments of right hand.

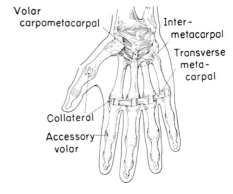

Figure 6.18   Anterior view of ligaments of right hand.

axis so that it faces in a plane perpendicular to the other fingers.

Abduction (Figure 6.19a)

A forward movement of the thumb at right angles to the palm.

Adduction

Return movement from abduction.

Hyperadduction (Figure 6.19b)

A backward movement of the thumb at right angles to the hand.

Extension (Figure 6.19c)

A lateral movement of the thumb away from the index finger, on a level with the palm.

Flexion (Figure 6.19d)

Return movement from extension.

Hyperflexion (Figure 6.19e)

A medially directed movement of the thumb from a position of slight abduction. The thumb slides across the front of the palm.

Circumduction

A movement in which the thumb as a whole describes a cone and the tip of the thumb describes a

circle. It consists of all the movements just described, performed in sequence in either direction.

Opposition (Figure 6.19f)

This movement, which makes it possible to touch the tip of the thumb to the tip of any of the four fingers, is essentially a combination of abduction and hyperflexion and, according to some investigators, slight inward rotation. Others, including the authors, claim that what appears to be inward rotation of the metacarpal is actually a slight medial movement of the greater multangular bone with which the metacarpal articulates. The movements of the metacarpal are accompanied by flexion of the two phalanges, especially the distal. The apparent rotary movement is explained in part by the oblique axis of motion about which abduction and adduction of the thumb occur, and in part by the movement of the greater multangular bone that accompanies flexion of the thumb. The total movement of the thumb in opposition might well be described as a movement of partial circumduction.

Movements of the Carpometacarpal and Intermetacarpal Joints of the Fingers

Largely because of the short ligaments in this region, especially in the case of the second, third, and fourth digits, the motion in both the car-

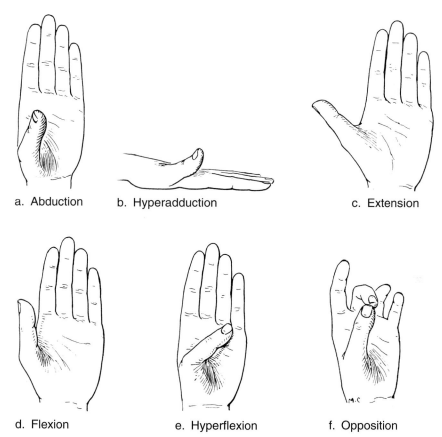

a. Abduction   b. Hyperadduction   c. Extension

d. Flexion   e. Hyperflexion   f. Opposition

Figure 6.19 Movements of the thumb at the carpometacarpal joint.

pometacarpal and intermetacarpal joints is almost nonexistent, being limited to slight gliding. The fifth carpometacarpal joint is slightly more mobile and permits a limited motion of the fifth metacarpal bone, resembling in small degree the motion of the thumb.

Structure of the Metacarpophalangeal
Joints (see Figures 6.13, 6.17, and 6.18)

The joint at the base of the four fingers, uniting the proximal phalanx with the corresponding metacarpal bone, is a condyloid (ovoid) joint. The oval, convex head of the metacarpal fits into the shallow oval fossa at the base of the phalanx. The fossa is deepened slightly by the fibrocartilaginous volar accessory ligament. The joint is encased in a capsule and is protected on each side by strong collateral ligaments.

The metacarpophalangeal joint of the thumb has flatter joint surfaces than do the corresponding joints of the four fingers and has more of the characteristics of a hinge joint. In addition to the articular capsule, it is protected by a collateral ligament on each side and by a dorsal ligament.

Movements of the Metacarpophalangeal Joints of the Four Fingers (Figure 6.20)

Flexion

The anterior surface of the finger approaches the palmar surface of the hand.

Extension

Return movement from flexion. Most individuals are able to achieve slight hyperextension in these joints.

Abduction

For the fourth, fifth, and index fingers this is a lateral movement away from the middle finger. This movement is limited and cannot be performed when the fingers are fully flexed.

Adduction

Return movement from abduction.

Note: In abduction and adduction of the fingers, a different point of reference is used than in abduction and adduction of the hand as a whole. The centerline of the hand—that is, the line passing through the middle finger when the latter is in its normal, extended position—is the reference line for the second, fourth, and fifth digits. Comparable movements of the middle finger are called radial and ulnar flexion.

These lateral finger movements are actually movements of the proximal phalanx, with the action occurring at the metacarpophalangeal joint, but the entire finger moves as a unit since no lateral action is possible at the interphalangeal joints.

Circumduction

The combination of flexion, abduction, extension, and adduction performed in sequence in either direction.

Movements of the Metacarpophalangeal Joints of the Thumb

Flexion

The volar surface of the thumb approaches that of the thenar eminence (base of thumb).

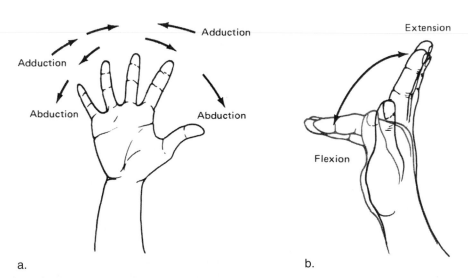

Figure 6.20   Movements of the metacarpophalangeal joints: (a) abduction and adduction; (b) flexion and extension.

Extension

Return movement from flexion. Individuals vary greatly in their ability to hyperextend the thumb at this joint.

The Interphalangeal Joints

These are the joints between the adjacent phalanges of any of the five digits. They are all hinge joints; hence, their only movements are flexion and extension. These correspond to flexion and extension of the first phalanx at the metacarpophalangeal joints. Hyperextension is slight, if present at all. Each joint is enclosed within an articular capsule, which is strengthened in front by an accessory volar ligament and on each side by a strong collateral ligament.

MUSCLES OF THE WRIST AND HAND

Location

The muscles of the wrist, fingers, and thumb are classified according to their location on the forearm or the hand and within each group are listed alphabetically (table 6.1). Of the nineteen muscles of the fingers and thumb, ten are located entirely within the hand and are called intrinsic muscles. Those located outside the hand on the forearm but with tendon attachments on the thumb or fingers are extrinsic muscles.

The wrist flexor muscles originate (proximal attachments) on the medial epicondyle of the humerus or ulna; the wrist extensors have their

TABLE 6.1	Wrist and Hand Muscles
Muscles of the Wrist	
Anterior	**Posterior**
Flexor carpi radialis	Extensor carpi radialis brevis
Flexor carpi ulnaris	Extensor carpi radialis longus
Palmaris longus	Extensor carpi ulnaris
Muscles of the Fingers and Thumb	
On the Forearm (Extrinsic Muscles) (9)	**In the Hand (Intrinsic Muscles) (10)**
Fingers*	Fingers
Extensor digiti minimi	Abductor digiti minimi
Extensor digitorum	Flexor digiti minimi brevis
Extensor indicis	Interossei dorsales manus
Flexor digitorum profundus	Interossei palmaris
Flexor digitorum superficialis	Lumbricales manus
	Opponens digiti minimi
Thumb	Thumb
Abductor pollicis longus	Abductor pollicis brevis
Extensor pollicis brevis	Adductor pollicis
Extensor pollicis longus	Flexor pollicis brevis
Flexor pollicis longus	Opponens pollicis

*To understand the actions of these muscles, it is important to have an exact knowledge of their distal attachments.

proximal attachments on the lateral epicondyle of the humerus. These attachments allow these muscles to remain effective across the wrist joint regardless of the position of the forearm. They also contribute to stabilization of the elbow joint, which contributes further to enhancing effective action of these muscles at the wrist joint. The major disadvantage, as with most multijoint arrangements, is the limiting of the range of motion when there is simultaneous movement across all joints.

Characteristics and Functions of Muscles
Wrist Muscles *(Figures 6.21, 6.22, and 6.23a)*

As one would expect from their location, the *flexor carpi radialis* and *flexor carpi ulnaris* are important flexors of the wrist. The palmaris longus, however, is a weak contributor to wrist flexion and may even be absent in some individuals. The flexor carpi radialis is also active in radial flexion (abduction) and the flexor carpi ulnaris in ulnar flexion. The tendons of these muscles may be readily palpated on the anterior

Figure 6.21   Superficial muscles on front of right forearm.

surface of the wrist (see figure 6.21). The palmaris longus tendon, if present, is clearly visible if the hand is flexed against slight resistance (see figure 6.21). The ulnaris tendon (see figure 6.21) is best identified by its relation to the pisiform bone. It should not be confused with the tendon

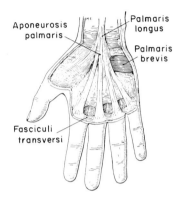

Figure 6.22   Palmar aponeurosis and palmaris muscles of right palm.

lying close on the ulnar side of the palmaris tendon. This is a tendon of the flexor digitorum superficialis, probably the one for the fourth finger (figure 6.24a).

Both *radial extensor* muscles of the wrist are active in extension and radial flexion (abduction), with the *extensor carpi radialis brevis* more active in extension than the *extensor carpi radialis longus.* The *extensor carpi ulnaris* works cooperatively with the extensor carpi radialis muscles in wrist extension and participates in ulnar flexion (adduction) (see figure 6.23).

The three *wrist extensor muscles* may be palpated on the dorsal surface of the forearm when the forearm and hand are resting palm down on a table, the *carpi radialis longus* on the radial side at elbow level and slightly below, the *brevis* slightly below the *longus,* and the *carpi ulnaris* on the ulnar margin of the dorsal surface about midway between the elbow and wrist. The tendon

Figure 6.23   Muscles on back of right forearm: (a) extensor carpi radialis longus and brevis and extensor carpi ulnaris; (b) extensor digitorum and extensor digiti minimi.

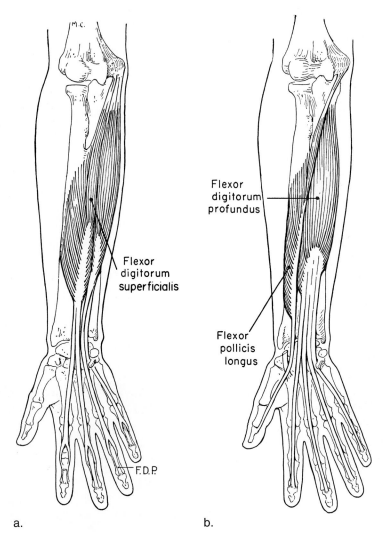

Figure 6.24   Deep muscles on front of right forearm: (a) flexor digitorum superficialis; (b) flexor digitorum profundus and flexor pollicis longus. (F.D.P. = Flexor digitorum profundus.)

of the carpi radialis longus may be palpated on the dorsal surface of the wrist in line with the index finger.

The *flexor carpi radialis* and *extensor carpi radialis longus,* together with the *abductor pollicis longus* of the thumb, team up to produce *radial flexion (abduction)* of the wrist. The *extensor* and *flexor carpi ulnaris* muscles team up similarly to produce *ulnar flexion (adduction).*

Muscles of the Fingers and Thumb
(Figures 6.22 through 6.29)

In most instances, the names of the muscles of the fingers and thumb indicate their chief function. These muscles will therefore not be discussed individually. Some of these muscles, however, have important additional roles, and these should be identified. In addition to being an extensor of the interphalangeal joints, the *extensor digitorum* is

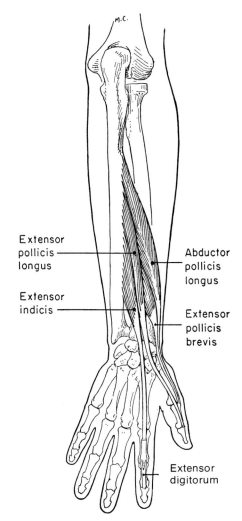

Extensor
pollicis
longus

Extensor
indicis

Abductor
pollicis
longus

Extensor
pollicis
brevis

Extensor
digitorum

Figure 6.25   Posterior muscles of the thumb
and index finger.

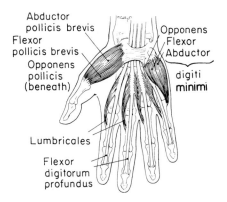

Abductor
pollicis brevis
Flexor
pollicis brevis
Opponens
pollicis
(beneath)

Opponens
Flexor
Abductor

digiti
minimi

Lumbricales

Flexor
digitorum
profundus

Figure 6.26   Anterior view of muscles of right hand.

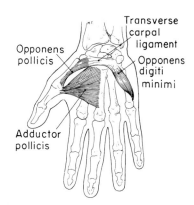

Opponens
pollicis

Transverse
carpal
ligament

Opponens
digiti
minimi

Adductor
pollicis

Figure 6.27   Deep muscles of thumb and fifth
metacarpal.

an important wrist extensor. Similarly, the *flexor
digitorum superficialis* is active in wrist flexion
as well as in flexion at the proximal phalangeal
joints. The *abductor pollicis longus* both abducts
and flexes the metacarpophalangeal joint of the
thumb, and the *abductor pollicis brevis,* together with the *opponens pollicis,* is active in
extension and abduction of the thumb. Both the
flexor and *extensor pollicis longus* are active in
adduction and opposition of the thumb, and the
adductor pollicis participates in opposition and
flexion.

Muscular Analysis of the Fundamental Movements of the Wrist, Fingers, and Thumb

The Wrist

Fundamental movements of the wrist are movements of the hand as a unit. They occur chiefly at
the radiocarpal joint but involve the midcarpal
and intercarpal joints when flexion or hyperextension is carried to the limit of motion.

Flexion

Performed by the flexors carpi radialis, carpi ulnaris, and digitorum superficialis, with possible
help from the palmaris longus, flexor pollicis
longus, and flexor digitorum profundus.

Figure 6.28   Palmar interossei, right hand.

Figure 6.29   Dorsal interossei, right hand.

Extension and Hyperextension

Performed synchronously by the extensors carpi radialis longus, carpi radialis brevis, carpi ulnaris, and extensor digitorum, with possible help from the pollicis longus and extensors indicis and digiti minimi.

Radial Flexion (Abduction)

Performed by the extensors carpi radialis longus and brevis and flexor carpi radialis, with possible help from the abductor pollicis longus and the extensors pollicis longus and brevis.

Ulnar Flexion (Adduction)

Performed by the extensor carpi ulnaris and the flexor carpi ulnaris.

The Fingers

For a better understanding of all the actions of the finger and thumb muscles, they should be studied both on the skeleton (using elastic bands to represent muscles) and on another person. Particular attention should be paid to the relation of each muscle to every joint it crosses, to the muscle's line of pull, and to the leverage involved.

As an aid to recognizing the secondary actions of the muscles, a record of all the joints crossed by all the finger and thumb muscles is included here.

Forearm Muscles of the Fingers

All five of these muscles cross four sets of joints: wrist, carpometacarpal, metacarpophalangeal, and proximal interphalangeal. The extensor digitorum and extensor digiti minimi also cross both the elbow and the distal interphalangeal joint, making a total of six joints crossed. The flexor digitorum superficialis crosses the elbow but not the distal interphalangeal, and both the extensor indicis and flexor digitorum profundus cross the distal interphalangeal joint but not the elbow.

Intrinsic Muscles of the Fingers

Of these six muscles, only the abductor digiti minimi and flexor digiti minimi brevis cross both the carpometacarpal and the metacarpophalangeal joints. The two interossei muscles, dorsales and palmaris, and the lumbricales cross only the metacarpophalangeal joint. The opponens digiti minimi, like the opponens pollicis, crosses only the carpometacarpal joint. The two work together in the cupping action of the palm as well as independently in other opposition movements.

Forearm Muscles of the Thumb

All four of these muscles cross both the wrist and carpometacarpal joints, and all but the abductor pollicis longus also cross the metacarpopha-langeal joint. The extensor and flexor pollicis longus muscles cross the interphalangeal joint as well. The thumb, of course, has no second inter-phalangeal joint.

Intrinsic Muscles of the Thumb

All four of these muscles cross the carpometa-carpal joint, and all but the opponens pollicis cross the metacarpophalangeal joint.

The muscular action of the fingers is given in terms of the movement of each phalanx. Move-ment of the proximal phalanx occurs at the metacarpophalangeal joint, of the middle phalanx at the proximal interphalangeal joint, and of the distal phalanx at the distal interphalangeal joint. For convenience in referring to individual fingers, numbers are assigned as follows: 2 for the index finger, 3 for the middle finger, 4 for the ring fin-ger, and 5 for the little finger.

Flexion

Proximal phalanx Flexed by the lumbricales manus (all fingers), interossei palmaris (palmar interossei) (2,4,5), interossei dorsales manus (2,3,4), flexor digiti minimi brevis (5), and op-ponens digiti minimi (5), with possible help from the flexors digitorum superficialis and pro-fundus.

Middle phalanx Flexed by the flexor digitorum superficialis, which acts on all four fingers and at the same time contributes to flexion of the metacarpal bones.

Distal phalanx Flexed by the flexor digitorum profundus, which also acts on all four fingers and at the same time contributes to flexion of the proximal and middle phalanges.

Extension

Proximal phalanx Extended by the extensor digitorum (all fingers), extensor indicis (2), and extensor digiti minimi (5). The extensor digito-rum is also able to help extend the middle and distal phalanges.

Middle and distal phalanges Extended by the lumbricales manus (all fingers) and interossei dorsales manus (dorsal interossei) (2,3,4). The ab-ductor digiti minimi (5) and the extensor digito-rum (all fingers) are also able to help extend the middle and distal phalanges at the same time that they are extending the proximal phalanx.

Note: When all the fingers flex or extend, the antagonists relax in reciprocal innervation. How-ever, if a single finger moves, the antagonists will contract in an attempt to keep the other fingers still.

Abduction and Adduction

Abduction is brought about by the interossei dor-sales manus (2,4) and abductor digiti minimi (5), and adduction by the interossei palmaris (2,4,5).

Radial and ulnar flexion of the middle finger is performed by the interossei dorsales manus (3).

Opposition

The fifth digit, or little finger, being at the outer margin of the hand, has greater freedom of move-ment than do the other fingers. Through the action of the opponens digiti minimi, the metacarpal bone of this finger can engage in a slight degree of opposition at the carpi metacarpal joint. Together with the thumb, it participates in this movement when the hand is "cupped," as when scooping up water, and also when the tip of the little finger is brought forcibly against the tip of the thumb.

The Thumb

The muscular action of the thumb is given in terms of the movements of the metacarpal bone and the two phalanges, proximal and distal.

The Thumb Metacarpal
Flexion

The metacarpal is flexed and hyperflexed after being slightly abducted by the flexor pollicis bre-vis and the adductor pollicis. The flexor pollicis longus also participates and becomes more domi-nant when the action is full flexion (Basmajian and DeLuca 1985).

Extension

Performed chiefly by the abductor pollicis longus, with help from the opponens pollicis, the abductor pollicis brevis, and the extensors pollicis longus and brevis.

Abduction

Four muscles are responsible for this movement, two from the forearm, the abductor pollicis longus and the extensor pollicis brevis, and two from the thenar eminence, the abductor pollicis brevis and the opponens pollicis. Under some conditions these may be helped by the flexor pollicis brevis.

Adduction

This movement is performed mainly by the adductor pollicis, with some help from the flexor pollicis brevis and, in certain positions, from the extensor pollicis longus.

Opposition

This action is performed mainly by the opponens, but with appreciable help from the flexor pollicis brevis. As opposition is not a single, well-defined movement but varies according to the finger that is being opposed and to the exact position of that finger, the muscles controlling the thumb must adapt to the demands of the situation. This includes the action of the phalanges as well as that of the metacarpal.

The Thumb Phalanges
Flexion

The flexor pollicis longus flexes both of the phalanges. Additional flexors of the proximal phalanx include the flexor pollicis brevis and the adductor pollicis, with help from the abductor pollicis brevis when necessary.

Extension

The extensor pollicis longus extends both of the phalanges. This is joined by the brevis in the extension of the proximal phalanx.

The plane in which flexion and extension of the thumb phalanges occurs is determined by the position of the metacarpal bone of the thumb.

COOPERATIVE ACTIONS OF WRIST AND DIGITS

Length of Long Finger Muscles Relative to Range of Motion in Wrist and Fingers

An interesting characteristic of the long finger muscles is that they do not have sufficient length to permit the full range of motion in the joints of the fingers and wrist at the same time. For instance, one cannot achieve complete flexion of the fingers and wrist simultaneously because the extensor digitorum will not elongate enough to permit it. If maximum *finger* flexion is maintained, the wrist is able to flex only slightly. And, similarly, if maximum *wrist* flexion is maintained, it will be impossible to achieve a real grip with the fingers. They flex incompletely and without appreciable force. Or, if one makes a tight fist and then determines to flex the wrist completely, the individual will soon discover that the fingers loosen their grip and tend to open up in spite of efforts to prevent it. This is not caused by contraction of the finger extensors but by their inability to elongate sufficiently, due to the countercurrent nature of the muscle action of the multiarticular muscles.

The same type of reaction occurs if one attempts to achieve maximum extension of the fingers when the wrist is fully hyperextended. This involuntary movement due to the tension of opposing muscles is known as the tendon or pulley action of multijoint muscles. Because of this arrangement of the muscles, the strongest finger flexion can be obtained when the wrist is held rigid in either a straight or slightly hyperextended position, and the strongest finger extension when the wrist is rigid in either a straight or slightly flexed position. The most powerful wrist action—either flexion or hyperextension—can occur only when the fingers are relaxed. In other words, strong finger action requires a rigid wrist; strong wrist action requires relaxed fingers. The interaction of the wrist and fingers is discussed well by Nordin and Frankel (1989).

Examples of Using the Hands for Grasping

Prehension, or grasping, has been categorized as either a power grip or precision handling. A power grip involves flexion of all fingers, with the role of the thumb being primarily stabilization. The palm is not involved. The interrelationship among the parts depends on the size and shape of the objects being held. There are three basic classifications of the power grip: (1) cylindrical (figure 6.30c), (2) spherical (figure 6.30d and f), and (3) hook (figure 6.30g). Ulnar deviation of the wrist enhances the force of the cylindrical grip. The spherical grip is similar to the

a.

b.

c.

d.   e.   f.   g.

Figure 6.30   Examples of grasps. The muscular involvement depends on the nature of the grasp.

cylindrical grip but with a greater spread of the fingers. The hook grip excludes use of the thumb but sometimes includes use of the palm. Therefore, the hook grip is sometimes categorized as precision handling.

Precision handling involves the use of the thumb and one or two fingers in various positions in order to accommodate a multiplicity of grasping functions. It entails great variability in pressure and fine motor control to manipulate efficiently the various objects.

The muscular involvement also depends on the nature of the grasp. A complex interplay occurs between the extrinsic and intrinsic muscular involvement, which varies with the force and spread of the grasp. Generally speaking, the extrinsic rather than the intrinsic muscles appear to be the major force for compression actions, power gripping, and the gross movements associated with precision gripping. The intrinsic muscles are of greater significance in the refinements of precision movements and the adduction actions that are part of these movements. The wrist extensors are also active during grasping motions, because they stabilize the wrist against the flexion tendencies of those finger flexors that cross the front of the wrist joint (Basmajian and DeLuca 1985).

In sports and gymnastics there is probably less concern with the fine, precise movements of the fingers and thumb than with the grosser movements such as the grasping of balls, striking implements, and suspension apparatus. In general, grasping activities involve flexion of the fingers (usually all three joints), opposition of the thumb metacarpal, and flexion of the phalanges. The degrees of these movements, together with the degree of abduction that may be present in the fingers, depend on the shape and size of the object being grasped, as well as on the purpose of the movement (figure 6.30).

In sport, whether pitching, throwing for distance, or tossing a ball straight upward, the move-

ments of the forearm and hand are of prime importance. The greater the force desired for moving the ball, the greater the contribution of the upper arm, but because this discussion applies only to the forearm and hand, the upper arm is not considered here. Ignoring the finer movements, the essential action of the forearm in both overhand pitching and in throwing for distance is extension; of the wrist, "flexion" from the hyperextended to the extended position (with an abrupt check of the motion when the wrist is straight); and of the fingers, extension.

In a vertical toss, starting with the forearm forward at a slight downward slant—that is, with the elbow at a slightly obtuse angle—the movements are elbow flexion followed by finger extension and wrist flexion from the hyperextended position. The active muscles are mainly the elbow flexors, the wrist flexors in static contraction, and the finger extensors. The reader may find it of interest to analyze the joint and muscle actions in other kinds of throws.

COMMON INJURIES OF THE FOREARM, ELBOW, WRIST, AND FINGERS

Fractures of the Forearm

These are common among children, teenagers, and the elderly and are usually caused either by a direct blow or by falling on a rigidly outstretched arm. It is more usual for both the radius and ulna to break than for either one to break alone, and in the younger age group the fracture of either or both bones is likely to be of the greenstick type.

It is important to immobilize the elbow joint in the treatment of a fractured radius, even though the fracture is close to the wrist. This is because in pronation and supination, as the radial head rotates against both the capitulum of the humerus and the radial notch of the ulna, the broad distal end swings halfway around the ulna. The need for immobilizing the elbow joint in the event of a radial fracture should be apparent to anyone who is conversant with kinesiology.

Elbow Dislocation

The majority of these dislocations consist of the backward displacement of the ulna and radius in relation to the humerus. The most common cause is catching oneself from a fall by taking the weight on the outstretched hand with the elbow in rigid extension or hyperextension. This can be a very serious injury because it is likely to involve blood vessels and nerves.

Elbow Fracture—Dislocation

Elbow dislocations are frequently accompanied by fractures, the most common being a fracture of the medial epicondyle, especially in the middle- to late-adolescent age group in those whose epicondylar epiphyses have not yet closed. These dislocations often occur because of repeated forceful acts such as pitching or serving in tennis.

Sprained or Strained Wrist

This type of wrist injury is very common and, like so many of the other upper extremity injuries, is caused by catching oneself from a fall by thrusting the arm downward and taking the weight on the palm with the hand hyperextended at the wrist and the elbow rigidly extended. Although the injury is usually called a sprain, it is often a strain, since the site of the trouble may be at the tendon attachments rather than at the attachments of the anterior ligaments (Arnheim and Prentice 1998). It may also involve fracture of a carpal bone.

Carpal Tunnel Syndrome

In the wrist, the carpal arch and transverse carpal ligament form the carpal tunnel through which the finger flexors and median nerve pass. Overuse may result in pain caused by nerve compression and numbing of the fingers caused by blood vessel involvement. Carpal tunnel syndrome is a classic example of a repetitive stress injury (RSI). Such injuries are becoming more common as more people spend longer hours working with small hand tools and keyboards. This condition is often treated with rest followed by support and intermittent use. Extreme or very painful conditions may require surgery.

Avulsion Fracture

An avulsion fracture occurs when an external force applied to a finger results in the distal phalanx flexing so sharply that the extensor digitorum tendon pulls off the bit of bone from the base of the phalanx to which it is attached. It occurs at the weakest link in the structure. The probability of occurrence is greatest in youth at the epiphyseal plates and in the elderly, because of osteoporosis.

Epicondylitis

Lateral epicondylitis ("tennis elbow") and medial epicondylitis ("golfers elbow") are further examples of repetitive stress injuries. Although the term epicondylitis implies an inflammatory condition, most such injuries are actually microtraumas or tears in the muscle and soft tissue in the region of the proximal attachment sites of the flexor (medial) or extensor (lateral) muscles of the wrist. Rest, ice, anti-inflammatory drugs and cortizone injections are often prescribed for these conditions. In some cases, pain can be reduced through surgery or counterforce bracing (Field and Savoie 1998; Boyer and Hastings 1999).

Elbow and Forearm: Joint Structure and Function

1. Record the essential information regarding the structure, ligaments, and cartilages of the two articulations of the elbow joint and, likewise, the two radioulnar articulations. Study the movements of these joints both on the skeleton and on the living body, and explain how their structure facilitates or inhibits movement.

2. Using a protractor or goniometer, measure the range of motion on five subjects for the following movements: flexion, pronation, and supination of the forearm.

3. Repeat Laboratory Experience 22 from chapter 5, this time writing the joint analysis of (a) the starting position of the forearm at the elbow and radioulnar joints, and (b) the movement from the starting position to the final pull-up position. Discuss with partner.

4. Assume a handshaking grasp with a skeleton with the elbow flexed and the forearm approximately horizontal. Slowly pronate your forearm and note the movement of the skeleton's forearm. Observe carefully each end of the radius and ulna and describe what happens. Now supinate your forearm as far as possible and carefully observe the radioulnar movements of the skeleton. Note the way the edge of the radial head rotates against the notch of the ulna and the way the superior surface of the radial head revolves against the capitulum of the humerus. At the distal end, note the way the broad articular process of the radius swings around the head of the ulna and the radial shaft crosses over that of the ulna. Note that the ulna itself does not rotate, although it may appear to do so when the elbow is fixed in extension and pronation of the forearm occurs in conjunction with inward rotation of the humerus.

Elbow and Forearm: Muscular Action

Record the results using a format similar to that found in table 1.2.

5. **Flexion**
   Subject: Sit with the entire arm resting on a table. Flex the forearm (a) with palm up (forearm supinated), (b) with thumb up (forearm in neutral position), and (c) with palm down (forearm pronated).
   Assistant: Resist the movement by holding the wrist. Steady the upper arm if necessary.
   Observer: Palpate as many of the forearm flexors as possible. Do you notice any difference in the muscular action in a, b, and c?

6. **Extension**
   a. *Subject:* Lie face down on a table with one arm raised to shoulder level with the upper arm resting on the table, the forearm hanging down. Extend the forearm without moving the upper arm.
      Assistant: Steady the upper arm and resist the forearm at the wrist.
      Observer: Palpate the triceps and anconeus.
   b. *Subject:* On hands and knees, flex and extend the arms at the elbows in a push-up exercise.
      Observer: Palpate the triceps and anconeus.

7. **Supination**
   Subject: Assume a handshaking position with the assistant and supinate the forearm.
   Assistant: Assume the same position with the subject and resist the movement.
   Observer: Palpate and identify the muscles that contract.

8. **Pronation**
   Subject: Assume a handshaking position with the assistant and pronate the forearm.
   Assistant: Assume the same position with the subject and resist the movement.
   Observer: Palpate and identify the muscles that contract. What is their function? Can you palpate the principal movers?

Action of Muscles Other Than Movers

9. **Supination without Flexion**
   Subject: Sit with the arm supported, elbow in a slightly flexed position and relaxed. Supinate the forearm without increasing or decreasing flexion at the elbow.
   Observer: Palpate the triceps. Explain.

10. **Vigorous Flexion of Forearm**
    Subject: Flex forearm vigorously, then check the movement suddenly before completing the full range of motion.

Observer: Palpate the triceps. Does it contract during any part of the movement? Explain.

11. Perform a movement in which the supinator acts as a neutralizer.

Elbow and Forearm: Applications

12. Working with a partner, execute a knee push-up, that is, a push-up from the front lying position, onto the knees instead of the toes, until the elbows are fully extended. Keep the body straight from the knees to the top of the head. Return to the starting position slowly and in good form.
    a. Analyze the joint and muscular action of the elbows in the push-up.
    b. Do the same for the return movement.
    c. What force is responsible for the movement in a? In b?
    d. What is the chief difference in the type of muscular action used in the push-up and in the letdown (return movement)? (See pp. 54–55.)

13. In reading the section on common injuries it may have been noted that several injuries to the forearm, elbow, and wrist are caused by taking the weight on the outstretched hand with the elbow rigidly extended when catching oneself from a fall. The following exercise is designed to accustom one to the practice of giving at the elbow and other upper extremity joints at the moment the hand strikes the ground. If practiced frequently this technique should become a habit.

    Kneel on a gymnasium mat with the knees slightly separated, hips in extension, and body erect. Shift your weight to the side until you lose your balance and fall to a side sitting position with your arm outstretched and your hand reaching to catch your weight. At the moment of contact let your elbow give (i.e., flex) and, if the force is sufficient, roll onto your shoulder and back with knees drawn up. Practice this many times, both to right and left. Experiment with variations.

Wrist and Hand: Joint Structure and Function

14. Record the essential information regarding the structure, ligaments, and cartilages of the radiocarpal, carpometacarpal, metacarpophalangeal, and interphalangeal articulations. Study the movements both on the skeleton and on the living body and explain how the joint structure affects functions. Pay particular attention to the carpometacarpal joint of the thumb.

15. With a protractor or goniometer measure the amount of hyperextension possible at the wrist (a) with the fingers flexed, (b) with fingers extended. Likewise measure the amount of flexion possible at the wrist (a) with the fingers flexed, (b) with the fingers extended. Explain.

Wrist and Hand: Muscular Action

(See procedures for anatomical analysis of movements in chapter 1.) If possible, get someone who plays the piano to serve as a subject.

16. **Flexion at Wrist**
    Subject: Sit with forearm resting on a table with palm up. Flex hand at wrist.
    Assistant: Resist movement by holding palm.
    Observer: Palpate, identify, and explain the action of as many muscles as possible.

17. **Extension and Hyperextension at Wrist**
    Subject: Sit with forearm resting on a table with palm down. Extend hand at wrist.
    Assistant: Resist movement by holding back of hand.
    Observer: Palpate, identify, and explain the action of as many muscles as possible.

18. **Radial Flexion at Wrist**
    Subject: Sit with forearm resting on a table, ulnar side (little finger side of hand) down. Keeping thumb against hand, raise hand from table without moving forearm.
    Assistant: May give slight resistance to hand.
    Observer: Palpate and identify the muscles responsible for radial flexion.

19. **Ulnar Flexion at Wrist**
    Subject: Lie face down or bend forward in such a way that radial side of hand (thumb side) is on supporting surface, with forearm supported and wrist neither flexed nor hyperextended. Keeping little finger against hand, raise hand without moving forearm.
    Assistant: May give slight resistance to hand.
    Observer: Palpate and identify the muscles responsible for ulnar flexion.

20. **Finger Flexion**
    Subject: Sit with forearm resting on a table with palm up. Flex fingers without flexing wrist.

Assistant: Resist movement by hooking own fingers over those of subject.

Observer: Palpate, identify, and explain the action of as many muscles as possible.

21. **Finger Extension**

    Subject: Sit with forearm resting on a table with palm down, fingers curled over edge of table. Extend fingers.

    Assistant: Resist movement by holding hand over subject's fingers.

    Observer: Palpate, identify, and explain the action of as many muscles as possible.

22. **Abduction of Thumb**

    Subject: Place the hand on a table with the palm up and the thumb slightly separated from the index finger. Abduct the thumb at the carpometacarpal joint by raising it vertically upward.

    Assistant: Give slight resistance to the thumb at the proximal phalanx.

    Observer: Palpate the abductor pollicis brevis in the thenar eminence.

23. **Hyperflexion of Thumb in Position of Slight Abduction**

    Subject: Place the hand on a table with the palm up and the thumb slightly raised from the table. Hyperflex the thumb at the carpometacarpal joint.

    Assistant: Give slight resistance to the proximal phalanx of the thumb.

    Observer: Palpate the flexor pollicis brevis in the thenar eminence.

24. **Extension of Thumb**

    Subject: Rest the fully extended hand on its ulnar border with the thumb uppermost. Extend the thumb as far as possible.

Observer: Identify the tendons of the abductor pollicis longus, extensor pollicis longus, and extensor pollicis brevis.

25. **Opposition of Thumb**

    Subject: Press the thumb hard against the tip of the middle finger.

    Observer: Palpate and identify the opponens pollicis and adductor pollicis.

Action of Muscles other than Movers

26. Perform a movement in which the extensor carpi ulnaris and extensor carpi radialis longus and brevis act as neutralizers to prevent flexion at the wrist.

27. Perform a movement in which the extensor carpi ulnaris and flexor carpi ulnaris act as mutual neutralizers.

Hands: Application

28. Inspect the various styles of grasping sport objects in figure 6.30 and analyze a few of these. First identify the joint position of the wrist, fingers, and thumb, and then determine the chief muscular involvement.

Kinesiological Analysis

29. Choose a simple motor skill from appendix H. Do a complete anatomical analysis of the elbow, forearm, wrist, and hand, following the analysis outline in tables 1.1 and 1.2.

REFERENCES AND SELECTED READINGS

Arnheim, D. D., and W. E. Prentice. 1998. *Essentials of athletic training.* 4th ed. St. Louis: McGraw-Hill.

Basmajian, J. V., and J. C. DeLuca. 1985. *Muscles alive.* 5th ed. Baltimore: Williams & Wilkins.

Boyer, M. I., and H. Hastings. 1999. Lateral tennis elbow: "Is there any science out there?" *Journal of Shoulder and Elbow Surgery* 8(5):481–91.

Brown, J. M. M., C. Solomon, and M. Paton. 1993. Further evidence of functional differentiation within biceps brachii. *Electromyography and Clinical Neurophysiology* 33:301–9.

Field, L. D., and F. H. Savoie. 1998. Common elbow injuries in sport. *Sports Medicine* 26(3):193–205.

Goss, C. M., ed. 1980. *Gray's anatomy of the human body.* 36th ed. Philadelphia: Lea & Febiger.

Imaeda, T., K. N. An, and W. P. Cooney. 1992. Functional anatomy and biomechanics of the thumb. *Hand Clinic* 8(1):9–15.

Larson, R. F. 1969. Forearm positioning on maximal elbow-flexor force. *Journal of the American Physical Therapy Association* 49:748–59.

Lee, D. G. 1986. Tennis elbow: A manual therapist's perspective. *Journal of Orthopedic and Sports Physical Therapy* 8:134.

Nordin, M., and V. H. Frankel. 1989. *Basic biomechanics of the musculoskeletal system.* Philadelphia: Lea & Febiger.

Norkin, C., and P. LeVangie. 1992. *Joint structure and function: A comprehensive analysis.* 2nd ed. Philadelphia: F. A. Davis.

Ranney, D. 1995. The hand as a concept: Digital differences and their importance. *Clinical Anatomy* 8:281–87.

Rettig, A. C. 1998. Elbow, forearm, and wrist injuries in the athlete. *Sports Medicine* 25:115–30.

Schaffer, J. P., ed. 1967. *Morris' human anatomy.* 11th ed. New York: Hofner Publishing.

Sergio, L. E., and D. J. Ostry. 1995. Coordination of multiple muscles in two degree of freedom elbow movements. *Experimental Brain Research* 105:123–37.

Stroyan, M., and K. E. Wilk. 1993. The functional anatomy of the elbow complex. *Journal of Sport Physical Therapy* 17:279–88.

THE LOWER EXTREMITY

The Hip Region

OUTLINE

■ *The Pelvic Girdle*
Structure
Movements of the Pelvis
Muscles of the Pelvis
■ *Relationship of the Pelvis
to the Trunk and Lower
Extremities*
Primary Movements of the Pelvis
Secondary Movements
of the Pelvis
■ *The Hip Joint*
Structure
Ligamentous Reinforcements
Movements of the Femur
at the Hip Joint

■ *Muscles of the Hip Joint*
Location
Characteristics and Functions
of Hip Joint Muscles
Muscular Analysis of the
Fundamental Movements
of the Thigh
■ *Common Injuries of the Thigh,
Hip Joint, and Pelvis*
■ *Laboratory Experiences*

OBJECTIVES

At the conclusion of this chapter, the student should be able to:

1. Name, locate, and describe the structure and ligamentous reinforcements of the articulations of the pelvic girdle and hip joint.
2. Name and demonstrate the movements possible in the pelvic girdle and hip joint, regardless of starting position.
3. Name and locate the muscles and muscle groups of the pelvis and hip, and name their primary actions as agonists, stabilizers, neutralizers, or antagonists.
4. Analyze the fundamental movements of the pelvis and thigh with respect to joint and muscle actions.
5. Describe the common athletic injuries of the pelvis, hip, and thigh.
6. Perform an anatomical analysis of the hip region in a motor skill.

The relationship between the pelvic girdle and hip is somewhat similar to that between the shoulder girdle and shoulder joint. Just as the scapula tilts or rotates to put the glenoid fossa in a favorable position for the movements of the humerus, so does the pelvic girdle tilt and rotate to put the acetabulum in a favorable position for the movements of the femur. There are these differences, however. Whereas the left and right sides of the shoulder girdle can move independently, the pelvic girdle can move only as a unit. The difference in depth of socket also limits the movement at the hip joint but is vital to accommodate the weight-bearing function of this joint. Furthermore, whereas the movements of the shoulder girdle take place in its own joints (sternoclavicular and acromioclavicular), the pelvic girdle is dependent on the lumbosacral and other lumbar joints, and the hip joints, for its movements. Hence, an analysis of the movements of the pelvic girdle must always be stated in terms of spinal and hip action.

THE PELVIC GIRDLE

Structure

The pelvis (figure 7.1) is a rigid bony basin that serves as a massive connecting link between the trunk and the lower extremities. Each pelvic bone (os innominatum) is made up of three bones: the ilium, ischium, and pubis. These bones become fused into a single bone by about the time of puberty. The two pelvic bones together form the pelvic girdle. This bony girdle or basin is firmly attached to the sacrum at the sacroiliac articulation, an articulation that is difficult to classify. It presents some of the characteristics of a diarthrodial joint, an articular cavity being present for part of the articulation. It is unlike other diarthrodial joints in one important respect, however. No movement can be voluntarily effected at the sacroiliac joint. Any movement that does occur is involuntary. Just how much motion can occur at the sacroiliac joint is debatable. Some anatomists say that a slight "giving" may occur there as a

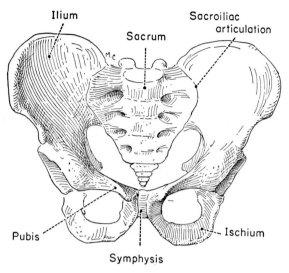

Figure 7.1   Anterior view of pelvis.

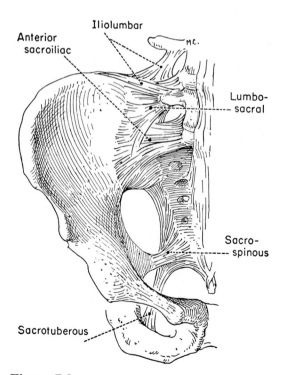

Figure 7.2   Anterior view of sacroiliac articulation showing ligaments.

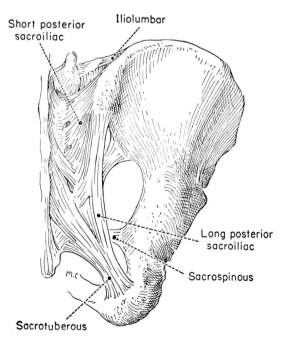

Figure 7.3   Posterior view of sacroiliac articulation showing ligaments.

shock absorption device; others claim that no motion occurs at the joint normally, except in women during pregnancy and parturition, when the ligaments relax to permit a slight spreading of the bones.

The sacrum is firmly bound to the two iliac bones by means of the anterior, posterior, and interosseous sacroiliac ligaments (figures 7.2 and 7.3). It is further reinforced by the iliolumbar, sacrotuberous, and sacrospinous ligaments and by the lower portion of the erector spinae muscle. Because of this firm attachment, the sacrum might well be considered a part of the pelvic girdle. From the point of view of function it is more truly a part of the pelvis than of the spine.

Movements of the Pelvis

Changes in the position of the pelvis are brought about by virtue of the motions of the lumbar spine and the hip joints. Movements in these joints permit the pelvis to tilt forward, backward, and sideward, and to rotate horizontally.

Forward Tilt (Increased Inclination)
(Figure 7.4c)
Movement of the pelvis in the sagittal plane about a frontal-horizontal axis so that the symphysis pubis turns downward and the posterior surface of the sacrum turns upward. To visualize this movement as forward tilt (increased inclination), one might consider the increase in the angle formed by the top of the pubic bone and the horizontal or the increase in deviation of the sacrum and posterior pelvis away from the vertical.

Backward Tilt (Decreased Inclination)
(Figure 7.4b)
A rotation of the pelvis in the sagittal plane about a frontal-horizontal axis so that the symphysis pubis moves forward-upward and the posterior surface of the sacrum turns somewhat downward. This motion is referred to as backward tilt (decreased inclination) because the angle formed by the top of the pubic bone and the horizontal decreases and be-

a.   b.   c.

Figure 7.4   Anteroposterior inclinations of the pelvis: (a) midposition; (b) decreased inclination (backward tilt); (c) increased inclination (forward tilt).

cause there is a decrease in the horizontal inclination of the sacrum and posterior pelvis.

Lateral Tilt *(Figure 7.5a)*
A rotation of the pelvis in the frontal plane about a sagittal-horizontal axis so that one iliac crest is lowered and the other is raised. The tilt is named in terms of the side that moves downward. Thus, in a lateral tilt of the pelvis to the left, the left iliac crest is lowered and the right is raised.

Rotation (Lateral Twist) (Figure 7.5b)
A rotation of the pelvis in the horizontal plane about a vertical (longitudinal) axis. The movement is named in terms of the direction toward which the front of the pelvis turns.

Muscles of the Pelvis

All the muscles that attach to the pelvic bones or to the sacrum serve either to initiate or to control pelvic movements. As one would expect, these

Figure 7.5   Movements of the pelvis: (a) lateral tilt to left; (b) rotation (lateral twist) to right.

are all muscles either of the hip joint or of the lumbar spine, including the lumbosacral junction. The precise combination of movements at these joints depends on whether the pelvic movement is primary or whether it is secondary, supplementing either the spinal movements or those of the hip joint.

Muscles providing the force for primary movements of the pelvis when one is standing with both feet facing forward could be as follows.

Forward Tilt

Hip flexors and lumbosacral spinal extensors.

Backward Tilt

Hip extensors and lumbosacral spinal flexors.

Lateral Tilt to the Right

Left lateral lumbosacral flexors, right hip abductors, and left hip adductors.

Rotation to Right

Left lumbosacral rotators, left hip outward rotators, and right hip inward rotators.

RELATIONSHIP OF THE PELVIS TO THE TRUNK AND LOWER EXTREMITIES

Architecturally, the pelvis is strategically located. Linking the trunk with the lower extremities, it must cooperate with the motion of each yet at the same time contribute to the stability of the total structure. When the body is in the erect standing position, the pelvis receives the weight of the head, trunk, and upper extremities, divides it equally, and transmits it to the two lower extremities. The student will learn how the position of the pelvis is maintained through muscular force couples during the discussion of the biomechanics of rotary motion on pages 345–346. Whenever an individual stands on only one foot, the pelvis automatically adapts itself to this position and transmits the entire weight of the upper part of the body to one of the lower extremities. It requires a fine adjustment to do this in such a way that the balance of the total structure is preserved.

Because the pelvis depends on the joints of the lower spine and those of the hips for its movements, it is not surprising that its motion is sometimes associated with the motion of the trunk or spine, and sometimes with that of the thighs. In such cases the movement of the pelvis may be said to be *secondary* to that of the spine, or of the thighs, as the case may be. In fact, most of its motion belongs in one or the other category. Occasionally, however, the movement seems to be initiated in the pelvis itself, with the spine and thighs cooperating with it. In such an event, the movement of the pelvis might be considered *primary*, and that of the spine and hips secondary. One sees this type of movement when the individual "tucks the hips under" as one would have

Figure 7.6   Lumbar and lumbosacral regions of the spine showing discrepancy in the lower lumbar curve as seen in the vertebral bodies and as seen in the contour of the back. (The sketch is based on an X ray).

to do to change from c to b, or even from c to a, in figure 7.4.

It is not always easy to judge the habitual tilt of the pelvis from the contour of the body. Prominent buttocks, heavy layers of fat, or an unusually convex sacrum can easily mislead the observer. Figure 7.6 shows a sketch based on an X ray that illustrates a type of build in which the contour of the lower back and pelvic region does not correspond to the bony structure. In this illustration the tilt, as judged by the position of the sacrum, is greater than it appears to be from the contour of the lower back. This observation is of importance to those who tend to place emphasis on the position of the pelvis in giving posture instruction.

The joint analyses of the primary and secondary movements of the pelvis are given next.

Primary Movements of the Pelvis

Joint Analysis of the Primary Movements of the Pelvis as Performed from the Fundamental Standing Position

Pelvis	Spinal Joints	Hip Joints
Forward tilt	Hyperextension	Slight flexion
Backward tilt	Slight flexion	Complete extension
Lateral tilt to left	Slights lateral flexion to right	R: Slight adduction L: Slight abduction
Rotation to left (without turning the head or moving the feet)	Rotation right	R: Slight outward rotation L: Slight inward rotation

Secondary Movements of the Pelvis

Joint Analysis of Movements of the Pelvis Secondary to Those of the Spine

Spine	Pelvis
Flexion	Backward tilt
Hyperextension	Forward tilt
Lateral flexion to left	Lateral tilt to left
Rotation to left	Rotation to left

Movements of the Pelvis Secondary to Those of the Lower Extremity

Similar to the relationship between the shoulder girdle and upper extremity, the pelvis moves with the lower extremity to supplement the latter's range of motion for three types of lower extremity movements: (1) movements of both limbs acting in unison, as when swinging them forward or backward in suspension; (2) movements of both limbs acting in opposition, as when walking, running, or doing a flutter kick in swimming; and (3) movements of one limb, as when kicking or when raising one leg to the side. In double-leg swinging the pelvis tilts backward (decreased inclination) when the thigh is flexed at the hip joint, and forward (increased inclination) when

the thigh is raised backward in apparent hyperextension. In opposition movements, when one leg is placed forward and the other backward, the pelvis rotates in the horizontal plane about a vertical axis. This pelvic orientation places the forward-flexed leg in slight outward rotation and the extended rear leg in slight inward rotation at the hip joint. When one thigh is moved sideward in wide abduction, the pelvis tilts laterally, lifting on the side of the abducted leg and lowering on the side of the vertical support leg. Slight abduction of the support leg at the hip joint occurs as a necessary adjustment of the tilted pelvis (figure 7.7). In each of these positions the pelvis positions itself so as to favor the movement of the thighs.

Figure 7.7   Lateral tilt of pelvis secondary to abduction of thigh at hip.

THE HIP JOINT

Structure

The hip joint (figure 7.8), a typical ball-and-socket joint, is formed by the articulation of the spherical head of the femur with the deep cup-shaped acetabulum. The latter, formed by the junction of the three pelvic bones (ilium, ischium, and pubis), is also described as horseshoe shaped because there is a gap (the acetabular notch) at the lower part of the "cup." The entire acetabulum is lined with hyaline cartilage. This is thicker above than below, and the center is filled in with a mass of fatty tissue covered by synovial membrane. A flat rim of fibrocartilage, known as the *acetabular labrum,* is attached by its circumference to the margin of the acetabulum (figure 7.9). It covers the hyaline cartilage, and since it is considerably thicker at the circumference than at the center, it adds to the depth of the acetabulum. Furthermore, being thicker above and behind, it serves to cushion the top and back of the acetabulum against the impact of the femoral head in forceful movements. The head of the femur also

is completely covered with hyaline cartilage, except for a small pit near the center called the *fovea capitis* (see figure 7.8). The cartilage is thicker above and tapers to a thin edge at the perimeter.

Ligamentous Reinforcements

The spherical head, deep socket, and low atmospheric pressure within the joint all lend stability to the hip joint. In addition, several ligaments help limit motion at the hip joint. The *transverse acetabular* ligament is a strong, flat band of fibers continuous with the acetabular labrum, which bridges the acetabular notch and thus completes the acetabular ring.

The *teres femoris* is a flat, narrow triangular band attached by its apex to the fovea capitis near the center of the femoral head, and by its base to the margins of the acetabular ligament (figure 7.10). Its function is to "tie" the head of the femur to the lower part of the acetabulum and thus provide the joint with reinforcement from within.

Outer reinforcement is provided by the three ligaments of the femoral neck, one for each of the

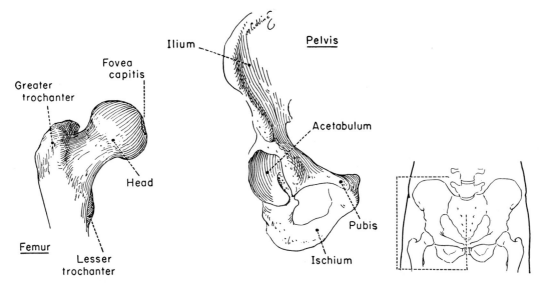

Figure 7.8   Bones of the hip joint.

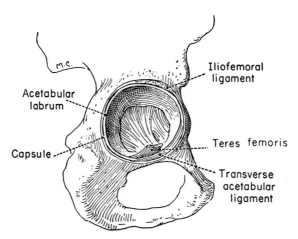

Figure 7.9   Acetabulum of right hip joint.

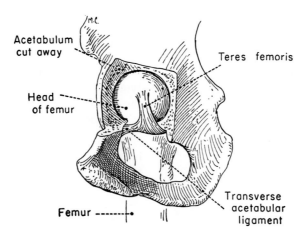

Figure 7.10   Right hip joint from within, looking toward head of femur.

pelvic bones that unite to form the acetabulum (figures 7.11 and 7.12). The *iliofemoral* ligament, called the Y ligament because of its supposed resemblance to an inverted Y, is an extraordinarily strong band of fibers situated at the front of the capsule and intimately blended with it. Because of its position, it serves to check extension and both outward (lateral) and inward (medial) rotation. The *pubofemoral* ligament consists of a narrow band of fibers at the medial anterior and lower portion of the capsule. It prevents excessive abduction and helps check extension and outward rotation. The *ischiofemoral* ligament is a strong triangular ligament at the back of the capsule. It

limits inward rotation and adduction in the flexed position.

Movements of the Femur at the Hip Joint

The movements of the femur (figure 7.13) are similar to those of the humerus but are not quite so free as the latter because of the deeper socket. In studying the movements of the femur, the student should first be aware of the position of the femur in the fundamental standing position. If viewed from the front, it is seen that the shaft is not vertical but slants somewhat medialward. This serves to place the center of the knee joint

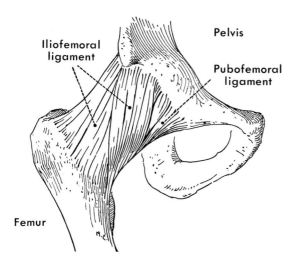

Figure 7.11   Anterior view of right hip joint.

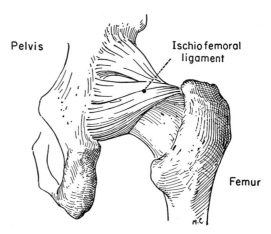

Figure 7.12   Posterior view of right hip joint.

more nearly under the center of motion of the hip joint. Hence, the mechanical axis of the femur—a line connecting the center of the femoral head with the center of the knee joint—is almost vertical (see figure 2.2). The degree of slant of the femoral shaft is related both to the size of the angle between the neck and shaft (angle of inclination) and the width of the pelvis. The angle of inclination decreases with age and the inner spongy or trabecular bone becomes thinner, which makes the femur more susceptible to fracture.

As seen from the side, the shaft bows forward. This characteristic, along with the obtuse neck–shaft angle, provides resistance for the strains and stresses sustained in walking, running, and jumping and for ensuring the proper transmission of weight through the femur to the knee joint. The femur is the longest yet strongest bone of the skeletal system.

Flexion

A forward movement of the femur in the sagittal plane. If the knee is straight, the movement is restricted by the tension of the hamstring muscles. In extreme flexion the pelvis tilts backward to supplement the movement at the hip joint.

Extension

Return movement from flexion.

Hyperextension

A backward movement of the femur in the sagittal plane. This movement is extremely limited. Except in dancers and acrobats, it is possible only when the femur is rotated outward and is probably completely absent in many individuals. The restricting factor is the iliofemoral ligament at the front of the joint. The advantage of this restriction of movement is that it provides a stable joint for weight bearing without the need for strong muscular contraction.

Abduction

A sideward movement of the femur in the frontal plane so that the thigh moves away from the midline of the body. A greater range of movement is possible when the femur is rotated outward. Abduction is limited by the adductor muscles and the pubofemoral ligament.

Adduction

Return movement from abduction. Hyperadduction is possible only when the other leg is moved

Figure 7.13 Movements of the hip joint: (a) flexion, extension, and hyperextension; (b) abduction and adduction; (c) inward and outward rotation; (d) diagonal abduction and adduction.

out of the way. In extreme hyperadduction the teres femoris becomes taut.

Outward (Lateral) Rotation

A rotation of the femur around its longitudinal axis so that the knee is turned outward.

Inward (Medial) Rotation

A rotation of the femur around its longitudinal axis so that the knee is turned inward.

The range of inward and outward rotation is affected by the degree of femoral torsion (twisting of the femur on its long axis so that one end is inwardly rotated with respect to the other). The range of outward rotation usually exceeds that of inward rotation.

Diagonal Adduction

A forward movement of the abducted thigh in a horizontal plane, probably accompanied by reduction of outward rotation.

Diagonal Abduction

A sideward movement of the flexed thigh in a horizontal plane, probably accompanied by outward rotation.

Circumduction

A combination of flexion, abduction, extension, and adduction performed sequentially in either direction.

MUSCLES OF THE HIP JOINT

Location

The muscles acting at the hip joint are listed here according to their position in relation to the joint. They include several muscles that act with equal or greater effectiveness at the knee joint. These are known as the two-joint muscles of the lower extremity. Only their action at the hip joint is considered in this section.

Anterior
Iliopsoas
Pectineus
Rectus femoris
Sartorius
Tensor fasciae latae

Posterior
Biceps femoris
Semimembranosus
Semitendinosus
Gluteus maximus
Six deep outward rotators

Medial
Adductor brevis
Adductor longus
Adductor magnus
Gracilis

Lateral
Gluteus medius
Gluteus minimus

Characteristics and Functions of Hip Joint Muscles

Iliopsoas (Figure 7.14; Also Listed with the Spinal Muscles)

Because the *psoas major, psoas minor,* and *iliacus* muscles share a common distal attachment and act as one muscle at the hip joint, the usual practice of treating them as one muscle is followed here. The muscle is a *strong hip flexor.* Depending on the circumstances, it will either *flex the thigh on the trunk* or it will *flex the trunk as a unit on the thighs* from a supine lying position, or in any position when the movement is performed against resistance. Although some believe it helps stabilize the hip joint in the standing position, others disagree. Results of EMG studies support both views (Basmajian and DeLuca 1985).

The muscle is extremely difficult to palpate. It is impossible to palpate the iliacus, but the *psoas major* may possibly be palpated on slender subjects who are able to keep the abdominal muscles relaxed during testing. Two techniques are suggested:

1. The subject lies on the side, rolled toward the face, and flexes the thigh against slight resistance, without contracting the abdominal muscles. The psoas may be palpated in the groin.

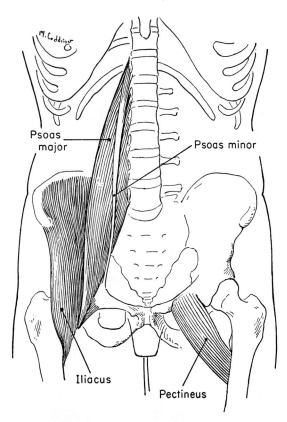

Figure 7.14 Anterior view of pelvic region showing psoas major and minor, iliacus, and pectineus.

2. The subject lies on the back with the lower back arched as much as possible. From this position, one thigh is flexed without contracting the abdominal muscles. An assistant should support the underside of the pelvis and try to keep it from moving. The psoas may be palpated through the abdomen.

Pectineus

This muscle (figure 7.14) is a short, thick, quadrilateral muscle situated lateral and superior to the adductor longus and more or less parallel to it. It *flexes the thigh* and possibly *assists in adduction* when the hip is in a flexed state. Whether it also contributes to outward rotation is debatable. As a flexor it has a good angle of pull that together with its internal structure accounts for its ability

to overcome considerable resistance. It may be palpated at the front of the pubis, just lateral to the adductor longus, but it is difficult to distinguish from the latter muscle.

Rectus Femoris (*Figure 7.15; Also Listed with the Knee Muscles*)

The rectus femoris muscle is the only quadriceps femoris muscle that crosses the hip joint. The muscle *flexes* the thigh and is also active during abduction and lateral rotation. It is a large bipenniform muscle, located superficially on the front of the thigh. It acts on the knee joint as well as the hip and is therefore a two-joint muscle. It shows maximum activity in single joint movements or in the countercurrent actions of hip flexion and knee extension. No activity occurs when the hip flexion is concurrent with knee flexion. It may be palpated as well as seen on the anterior surface of the thigh.

Sartorius (*Figure 7.15; Also Listed with the Knee Muscles*)

This muscle is also a two-joint muscle. Its action on the thigh is *flexion*. It also shows activity in abduction when external resistance is offered, and in outward rotation while sitting.

The sartorius is a long, slender, ribbonlike muscle directed obliquely downward and medialward across the front of the thigh. The sartorius muscle is the longest muscle in the body. It is the most superficial of the anterior thigh muscles and may be readily seen and palpated on slender subjects. On others, it may be palpated at the anterior superior iliac spine. Its name derives from its alleged function of enabling one to sit with the legs "tailor" fashion.

Tensor Fasciae Latae

This muscle (figures 7.15 and 7.18) *flexes and abducts the femur* and *tenses the fascia lata*. It is a small muscle located close in front of and slightly lateral to the hip joint, and it may be palpated about 2 inches anterior to the greater trochanter. Because its pull on the fascia lata is transmitted by

Figure 7.15   Muscles on front of right thigh.

means of the iliotibial tract down to the lateral condyle of the tibia, it helps extend the leg at the knee. Together with the gluteus maximus, which also unites with the fascia lata, it helps stabilize the knee joint in weight-bearing positions. When the lower extremities are fixed, both of these muscles help steady the pelvis and trunk on the thighs.

The Hamstrings *(Figures 7.16 and 7.17; Also Listed with the Knee Muscles)*

The three hamstring muscles—*biceps femoris, semimembranosus,* and *semitendinosus*—are situ-

ated on the back of the thigh, extending from the tuberosity of the ischium down just below the knee joint, with the biceps femoris on the lateral aspect of the posterior surface and the two "semi" muscles on the medial aspect.

The biceps femoris is the lateral hamstring muscle. Only its long head crosses the hip joint. The short head, the only one-joint muscle belonging to the hamstring group, does not cross the hip joint; therefore, it has no part in hip joint movements. The biceps femoris tendon may be palpated on the lateral aspect of the posterior surface of the knee.

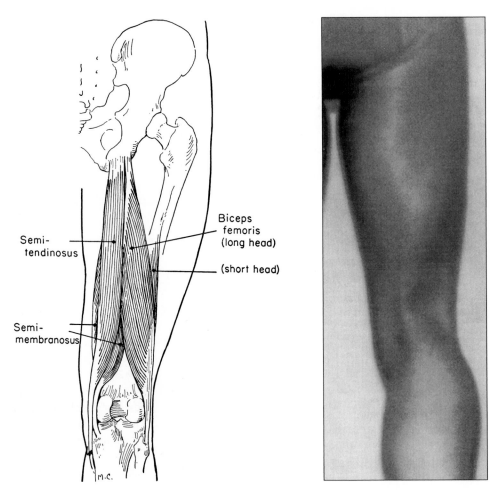

Figure 7.16   Hamstring muscles.

Together the semimembranosus and semi-tendinosus constitute the medial component of the hamstring group. The semimembranosus lies anterior to the semitendinosus and has a shorter, deeper tendon that is extremely difficult to pal-pate. The semitendinosus tendon may easily be palpated on the medial aspect of the posterior sur-face of the knee when the leg is flexed against re-sistance from the prone lying position. It should not be confused with the gracilis tendon, which lies slightly anterior to it. All three muscles *ex-tend the femur* or, if the thighs are bearing weight as in either the standing or long sitting position, they extend the forward flexed trunk as a unit—that is, from the hips. (Spinal action must not be confused with hip action, or vice versa.) The effec-tiveness of the medial hamstrings as extensors of the hip is related to knee joint action. There is maxi-mum activity during hip extension when the knee is either stabilized or flexed simultaneously (Basma-jian and DeLuca 1985). They are inactive, however, during simultaneous hip and knee extension.

Basmajian and DeLuca (1985) report that some investigators found that all three ham-

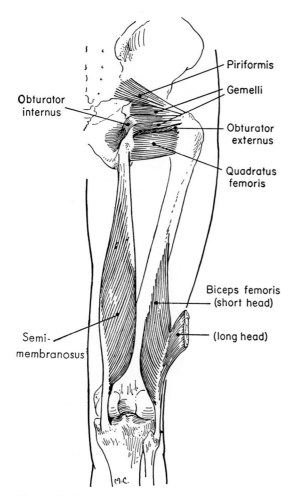

Figure 7.17   Deep posterior muscles of right thigh.

strings, in addition to extending the hip, help stabilize it, except in erect standing. Also, they adduct the femur from the abducted position when the movement is resisted and help rotate the extended femur. The long head of the biceps femoris rotates the femur laterally and the inner hamstrings rotates it medially.

Gluteus Maximus (Figures 7.18, 7.19, and 7.20)

This is the largest and most superficial of the three buttock muscles. It is a potentially *powerful*

hip extensor. It also *rotates the femur outward* when the latter is extended. The *lower portion assists in adduction* from an abducted position if the movement is resisted. The *upper portion abducts* against strong resistance. One can understand these seemingly contradictory functions more readily after studying the relation of the muscle to the hip joint's center of motion as seen from behind. Figure 7.20 shows that roughly one-third of the muscle lies above the center of motion and two-thirds below it. This puts the uppermost fibers in a position for abducting the thigh and the lower fibers in a position for adducting the thigh, whereas the fibers lying directly behind the femoral head are not in position for doing either. The entire muscle may easily be palpated on the posterior surface of the buttock.

The gluteus maximus has been the subject of much EMG study. Contrary to what one might think because of its size and prominence, the gluteus maximus has been shown to be active during the motions named above only when moderate to heavy resistance to the movement exists. And even though it often displays bursts of activity during brief periods of normal and fast walking, its participation is not essential.

The activity of the gluteus maximus in stair climbing has been confirmed in a number of EMG studies. It has also been found to be active in walking up an inclined plane, in extending the femur against resistance, in abducting the femur, especially against resistance and when rotated outward, and in adducting the femur against resistance when in an abducted position. This muscle is also most active during the stance phase of sprint running, as opposed to push-off (Arendt-Nielsen et al. 1991; Jonhagen et al. 1996).

Gluteus maximus activity is also elicited in hyperextension movements of the thigh performed against resistance from the erect standing position, muscle setting, and vigorous hyperextension of the trunk from an erect position. In heavy lifting requiring simultaneous extension of the hips and knees, the gluteus maximus was found to be active during the middle to the last

Figure 7.18   Lateral view of gluteus maximus, tensor fasciae latae, and iliotibial tract.

15 to 20 percent of the movement (Mostardi et al. 1991; Vakos et al. 1994).

The Six Deep Outward Rotators

These six muscles (obturator externus and internus, gemellus superior and inferior, quadratus femoris, and piriformis) (see figure 7.17) form a compact group behind the hip joint. Their fibers run horizontally for the most part. The piriformis, the most superior of the group, is slightly above the joint. The quadratus femoris, the most inferior, is slightly below it. Some of the muscles

have a secondary function such as abduction or adduction, but neither of these functions compares in importance with that of *outward rotation*. They are favorably situated for helping hold the femoral head in the acetabulum.

Adductor Brevis

This muscle (figure 7.21) lies just above the adductor longus and consists of fibers that are almost horizontal when the thigh is in its normal resting or standing position. From this position it both *adducts* and *aids in flexing the femur*. If the

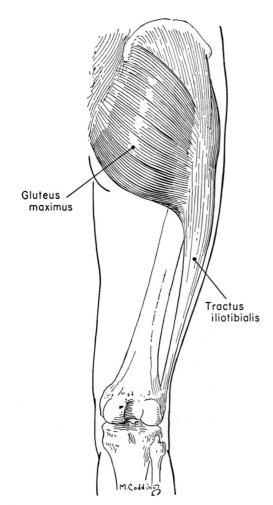

Gluteus
maximus

Tractus
iliotibialis

M.Codding

Figure 7.19   Posterior view of gluteus maximus
and iliotibial tract.

m.c.

Figure 7.20   Diagram showing relation of gluteus
maximus to hip joint.

hip is flexed to a marked degree it combines extension with the adduction, against resistance. It is also active in inward rotation.

Adductor Longus

This muscle (figure 7.21) *adducts* and *flexes the femur*. Steindler (1970) has pointed out that, though it ordinarily helps flex the thigh, when the flexion exceeds about 70 degrees it becomes an extensor as a result of a shift in the relationship between the muscle's line of pull and the joint's

center of motion. In an EMG study made in 1966, de Sousa and Vitti found that this muscle was always active during free adduction and inward rotation (Basmajian and DeLuca 1985). The muscle may be palpated just below its proximal attachment at the medial aspect of the groin.

Adductor Magnus

This muscle (figure 7.21) *extends the thigh as well as adducting it,* and the condyloid or *lowest portion also assists in inward rotation.* De Sousa and Vitti have noted that this muscle was not active during free adduction and extension unless the movement was performed against resistance (Basmajian and DeLuca 1985). Like the other adductors, it was found to be active in inward rotation. The adductor magnus may be palpated on the medial aspect of the middle half of the thigh. The uppermost portion of the muscle—that is, the portion that comes from the pubis—is sometimes treated as a separate muscle called *adductor minimus*.

Gracilis *(Figure 7.21; Also Listed with the Knee Muscles)*

This muscle *adducts* and *flexes the femur*. As the name indicates, it is a slender muscle. Being an

Figure 7.21 Adductor muscles of right thigh.

adductor, it is sometimes called the adductor gracilis and, like the hamstrings, sartorius, and rectus femoris, it is a muscle of the knee as well as the hip joint. EMG studies have shown that it participates in hip flexion only when the knee is extended and that it is most active during the first part of flexion: it also helps rotate the femur medially (inward).

Gluteus Medius

This muscle (figure 7.22a) is essentially an *abductor of the femur*. The *anterior fibers also rotate*

the thigh inward. The muscle may be palpated about 2 or 3 inches above the greater trochanter.

The muscle is an important one in walking and in standing in good posture. When the weight is shifted onto one foot, tension of the gluteus medius and other abductors is an important factor in stabilization of the hip. Lack of such stabilization results in an exaggerated sideward thrust of the supporting hip and a drop of the pelvis on the opposite side (Trendelenburg's sign). Paralysis of this muscle causes a typical limping gait known as the gluteus medius gait. When the weight is

Figure 7.22   Gluteus medius and minimus.

borne on the affected side, the trunk tilts strongly to that side and the opposite hip is thrust into prominence.

Gluteus Minimus

This muscle (figure 7.22b) *rotates inward and abducts*. It is smaller than the gluteus medius and is situated beneath it. Whereas the medius is primarily an abductor and secondarily an inward rotator, the minimus is primarily an inward rotator and secondarily an abductor. The muscles appear to work cooperatively, each one assisting in the other's primary function.

Muscular Analysis of the Fundamental Movements of the Thigh
Flexion

This movement is performed chiefly by the tensor fasciae latae, pectineus (both of these especially during the first half of range), iliopsoas, rectus femoris, and sartorius. The gracilis and adductors longus and brevis assist in flexion in selected positions.

Extension

The three hamstring muscles are the chief hip extensors. The gluteus maximus extends only against resistance. The three adductors also extend against resistance and when the thigh is flexed beyond a 45-degree angle.

Abduction

The chief abductors are the gluteus medius and minimus, the former being the more effective of the two. The sartorius and rectus femoris are active against resistance; the uppermost fibers of the gluteus maximus abduct against resistance during the early part of the movement, and the tensor fasciae latae abducts the thigh when it is extended.

Adduction

The adductor longus is the primary adductor. Other important adductors are the adductors magnus and brevis and the gracilis. The pectineus adducts the flexed thigh, and the lower third of the gluteus maximus assists in the movement when it is performed against resistance. The hamstrings adduct the abducted thigh against resistance.

Outward Rotation

This movement is performed by the six deep outward rotators, biceps femoris, and gluteus maximus.

Inward Rotation

The chief inward rotators are the gluteus medius and minimus, the latter being the more effective of the two. They are assisted by the semimembranosus, semitendinosus, gracilis, and adductor longus. The lower fibers of the adductor magnus rotate the thigh inward when it is extended. Some say that the tensor fasciae latae also helps, but this is debatable.

Diagonal Adduction

Probably performed by the adductors longus and brevis, gracilis, iliopsoas, pectineus, rectus femoris, sartorius, and tensor fasciae latae, and accompanied by the relaxation of the outward rotators.

Diagonal Abduction

Probably performed by the gluteus medius, minimus and upper maximus, and the six deep outward rotators.

COMMON INJURIES OF THE THIGH, HIP JOINT, AND PELVIS

Contusions

Contusions often result from a direct blow to an unprotected or inadequately protected body part. For example, participation in contact sports such as football may result in contusions to the quadriceps muscles due to blows and pinching of the quadriceps muscles between the femur and the external force. Blows to the pelvic area, including the iliac crest, may result in a contusion (hip pointer), muscle strain, or an avulsion fracture, where the muscle pulls away from the iliac crest, taking some bone with it. Landing in a sitting position or a direct blow may cause contusions to the coccyx and/or tuberosity of the ischium. All contusions are very painful, and some may be debilitating, since every movement aggravates the condition. In each case accurate diagnosis is important for proper treatment. When the contusion to a muscle is not treated appropriately, or if the injury occurs repeatedly, myositis ossificans may result.

Myositis Ossificans

This is a condition in which calcification develops following repeated traumas or serious contusions to the muscle. It is likely to occur when the symptoms of muscle injury are so mild that the player insists on continuing to play. The front of the thigh and the brachialis muscle of the upper arm appear to be the most vulnerable area so affected. The frequency with which this condition occurs is caused in large part by poor treatment such as overvigorous massage, manipulation under anesthesia, overstrenuous exercise, and too early return to participation in the activity in which a severe muscle injury has occurred. Myositis ossificans can often be prevented if muscle contusions are given proper treatment (O'Donoghue 1984).

Strains of the Hamstring Muscle Group

A high incidence of hamstring strains occurs among the very active. These tend to happen in running more than in any other activity, especially when a muscular imbalance occurs through fatigue or another condition and when there is a sudden change in direction or speed. A frequent site of the strain is the distal attachment of the biceps femoris muscle on the fibular head. Another common hamstring strain occurs in the pelvic area where the semitendinosus and the long head of the biceps femoris attach to the lower and medial impression on the tuberosity of the ischium. This is usually caused by a forceful movement of the lower extremity involving flexion of the thigh with the knees held in extension. In severe strains there may also be an avulsion fracture, especially if the ossification of the epiphysis is not yet complete.

Hip Conditions

A relatively low incidence of hip joint injuries occurs in athletics. The structure of the joint accounts for the rarity of dislocations, and fractures of the hip joint region are fortunately not a serious threat to athletes. The dangerous age when hip fractures are a real threat is old age, when the bones have lost their toughness, the femoral angle is changed, and the bones become brittle.

LABORATORY EXPERIENCES

Joint Structure and Function

1. Record the essential information regarding the structure, ligaments, and cartilages of the hip joint. Study the movements both on the skeleton and the living body and explain how the joint structure affects the movements.

2. Using a protractor type of goniometer, measure the range of motion in the following joint movements on five different subjects:
   a. Hip flexion, with straight knee
   b. Hip flexion, with flexed knee
   c. Total abduction of both thighs

3. From an erect standing position with the feet together, take a fairly long step forward with the right foot, stopping with weight mostly over the right foot and with the left foot still in place but with the heel raised and the ball of the foot bearing just enough weight to maintain balance. Analyze the joint action that has taken place at each hip joint.

4. Analyze the joint action of each hip joint in each phase of riding a bicycle.

Muscular Action

Identify as many muscles as possible in the following experiments.

5. **Decrease of Pelvic Inclination**
   Subject: Lie on back with knees drawn up and feet resting on floor. Tilt pelvis in such a manner that lumbar spine flexes and therefore flattens.
   Assistant: Kneeling at subject's head and facing subject's feet, place thumbs on the anterior superior iliac spines and fingers under the lower back. Resist movement by pushing iliac spines toward subject's feet.
   Observer: Palpate rectus abdominis and gluteus maximus.

6. **Increase of Pelvic Inclination**
   Subject: In erect standing position, stiffen the knees and push the buttocks as far back as possible.
   Observer: Palpate tensor fasciae latae, sartorius, pectineus, and iliocostalis. Does the adductor longus or gracilis contract?

7. **Lateral Tilt of Pelvis**
   Subject: Stand on one foot on stool with other leg hanging free. Pull free hip up as far as possible.

Assistant: Give slight resistance by holding ankle down.
Observer: Palpate oblique abdominals, iliocostalis, adductor magnus, adductor longus, and gracilis on side of free leg.

8. **Hip Flexion**
   a. *Subject:* Sit on a table with legs hanging over edge. Flex the thigh at the hip joint.
   Assistant: Resist movement slightly by pressing down on knee.
   Observer: Palpate pectineus, tensor fasciae latae, sartorius, rectus femoris, and adductor longus. Does the gracilis contract?
   b. *Subject:* Lie on one side, rolled toward face. Flex thigh of top leg, allowing knee to flex passively.
   Assistant: Resist movement by pushing against knee.
   Observer: Palpate iliopsoas.

9. **Hip Extension**
   a. *Subject:* Stand facing table with trunk flexed forward until it rests on table. Grasp sides of table. Extend one thigh by raising one leg, keeping the knee extended.
   Assistant: Resist movement by pushing down on thigh close to knee. Second time, give resistance at heel.
   Observer: Palpate gluteus maximus, adductor magnus, and hamstrings.
   b. *Subject:* Lie face down on table and extend lower extremity at the hip joint keeping the knee extended.
   Assistant: Resist movement by pushing down on knee.
   Observer: Palpate same muscles as in a.

10. **Hip Abduction**
    Subject: Lie on one side and abduct the top lower extremity at the hip joint.
    Assistant: Resist movement by pushing down on knee.
    Observer: Palpate gluteus maximus, gluteus medius, and tensor fasciae latae.

11. **Hip Adduction**
    Subject: Lie on one side with the top lower extremity abducted; then adduct it.
    Assistant: Resist movement by pressing up against knee.

Note: Unless resistance is applied, the action will be performed by means of the eccentric contraction of the abductors.

Observer: Palpate three adductors and name them.

12. **Outward Rotation of Thigh**

    Subject: Stand on one foot with the other leg flexed at the knee so that the lower leg extends horizontally backward. Rotate the free thigh outward by swinging the foot medially.

    Assistant: Steady subject's knee and resist movement of leg at ankle.

    Observer: Palpate gluteus maximus.

13. **Inward Rotation of Thigh**

    Subject: Stand on one foot with other leg flexed at the knee so that the lower leg extends horizontally backward. Rotate the free thigh inward by swinging the foot laterally.

    Assistant: Steady subject's knee and resist movement of leg at ankle.

    Observer: Palpate gluteus medius, tensor fasciae latae, and lower adductor magnus.

Kinesiological Analysis

14. Choose a simple motor skill from appendix H. Do a complete anatomical analysis of the hip region following the format shown in table 1.2.

REFERENCES AND SELECTED READINGS

Arendt-Nielsen, L., T. Sinkjær, J. Nielsen, and K. Kallesøe. 1991. Electromyographic and kinematic profiles during different gait velocities and inclines. In *Electromyographical kinesiology,* edited by P. A. Anderson, D. J. Hobart, and J. V. Danoff. Amsterdam: Excerpta Medica.

Arnheim, D. D., and W. E. Prentice. 1998. *Essentials of athletic training.* 4th ed. St. Louis: McGraw-Hill.

Basmajian, J. V., and C. J. DeLuca. 1985. *Muscles alive.* 5th ed. Baltimore: Williams & Wilkins.

Duchenne, G. B. 1959. *Physiology of motion,* edited and translated by E. B. Kaplan. Philadelphia: W. B. Saunders.

Fischer, F. J., and S. J. Houtz. 1968. Evaluation of the function of the gluteus maximus muscle. *American Journal of Physical Medicine* 47:182–91.

Goss, C. M., ed. 1980. *Gray's anatomy of the human body.* 36th ed. Philadelphia: Lea & Febiger.

Hamilton, N. 1993. Hip rotator peak torque and hip range of motion in healthy adults. *Clinical Kinesiology* 46(4):2–6.

Jonhagen, S., M. O. Ericson, G. Nemeth, and E. Eriksson. 1996. Amplitude and timing of electromyographic activity during sprint running. *Scandinavian Journal of Medicine and Science in Sports* 6:15–21.

MacConaill, M. A., and J. V. Basmajian. 1969. *Muscles and movements.* Baltimore: Williams & Wilkins.

Merrifield, H. H. 1961. An electromyographic study of the gluteus maximus, the vastus lateralis and the tensor fasciae latae. *Dissertation Abstracts* 21:18–33.

Mostardi, R. A., D. A. Noe, M. L. Jackson, and M. J. Askew. 1991. Electromyographic activity sequencing of selected muscles involved in an isokinetic deadlift. In *Electromyographical kinesiology,* edited by P. A. Anderson, D. J. Hobart, and J. V. Danoff. Amsterdam: Excerpta Medica.

Neuman, D. A., and A. D. Hase. 1994. An electromyographic analysis of the hip abductors during load carriage: Implications for hip joint protection. *The Journal of Orthopaedic and Sports Physical Therapy* 19:296–304.

Nordin, M., and V. H. Frankel. 1989. *Basic biomechanics of the musculoskeletal system.* Philadelphia: Lea & Febiger.

Norkin, C., and P. Levangie. 1992. *Joint structure and function: A comprehensive analysis.* 2nd ed. Philadelphia: F. A. Davis.

O'Donoghue, D. H. 1984. *Treatment of injuries to athletes.* 4th ed. Philadelphia: W. B. Saunders.

Steindler, A. 1970. *Kinesiology of the human body.* Springfield, IL: Charles C Thomas.

Vakos, J. P., A. J. Nitz, A. J. Threkeld, R. Shapiro, and T. Horn. 1994. Electromyographic activity of selected trunk and hip muscles during the squat lift: Effect of varying the lumbar posture. *Spine* 19:687–95.

THE LOWER EXTREMITY

The Knee, Ankle, and Foot

O U T L I N E

- **The Knee Joint**
  Structure
  Menisci
  Ligaments of the Knee
  Movements
- **Muscles of the Knee Joint**
  Location
  Characteristics and Functions
     of Individual Muscles
- **Muscular Analysis**
  of the Fundamental Movements
  of the Leg at the Knee Joint
- **The Ankle and the Foot**
  Structure of the Ankle
  Ligamentous Reinforcement

Structure of the Foot
Movements of the Foot at the
     Ankle, Tarsal, and Toe Joints
- **Muscles of the Ankle and Foot**
  Location
  Characteristics and Functions
     of Individual Muscles
- **Muscular Analysis**
  of the Fundamental
  Movements of the Ankle
  and Foot (Tarsal Joints
  and Toes)
- **Common Injuries of the Leg,**
  Knee, and Ankle
- **Laboratory Experiences**

OBJECTIVES

At the conclusion of this chapter, the student should be able to:

1. Name, locate, and describe the structure and ligamentous reinforcements of the articulations of the knee, ankle, and foot.
2. Name and demonstrate the movements possible in the joints of the knee, ankle, and foot, regardless of starting position.
3. Name and locate the muscles and muscle groups of the knee, ankle,

and foot, and name their primary actions as agonists, stabilizers, neutralizers, or antagonists.
4. Analyze the fundamental movements of the lower leg and foot with respect to joint and muscle actions.
5. Describe the common injuries of the leg, knee, and ankle.
6. Perform an anatomical analysis of the lower extremity in a motor skill.

THE KNEE JOINT

The knee joint is the largest and most complex joint in the human body. It is a masterpiece of anatomical engineering. Placed midway down each supporting column of the body, it is subject to severe stresses and strains in its combined functions of weight bearing and locomotion. To take care of the weight-bearing stresses, it has massive condyles; to facilitate locomotion it has a wide range of motion; to resist the lateral stresses due to the tremendous lever effect of the long femur and tibia, it is reinforced at the sides by strong ligaments; to combat the downward pull of gravity and to meet the demands of such violent locomotor activities as running and jumping, it is provided with powerful musculature. It would be difficult, indeed, to find a mechanism better adapted for meeting the combined requirements of stability and mobility than the knee joint.

Structure

Although the knee is classified as a hinge joint, its bony structure resembles two condyloid or ovoid joints lying side by side, yet not quite parallel (figure 8.1). The lateral flexion permitted in

a single ovoid joint is not possible in the knee joint because of the presence of the second condyle. The two rockerlike condyles of the femur rest on the two slightly concave areas on the top of the tibia's broad head. These articular surfaces of the tibia are separated by a roughened area, called the intercondyloid eminence, which terminates both anteriorly and posteriorly in a slight hollow but rises at the center to form two small tubercles like miniature twin mountain peaks (figure 8.2). During knee extension, the intercondyloid tubercles enter the intercondyloid fossa of the femur. The medial articular surface of the tibia is oval; the lateral is smaller and more nearly round. Each is overlaid by a somewhat crescent-shaped fibrocartilage, known as a semilunar cartilage, or meniscus.

The lower end of the femur terminates in the two rockerlike condyles already mentioned. The lateral condyle is broader and more prominent than the medial. The medial condyle projects downward farther than the lateral. This is evident, however, only when a disarticulated femur is held vertically. In its normal position in the body, the femur slants inward from above. This slant is known as the obliquity of the femoral shaft. Observation of the mounted skeleton will show that

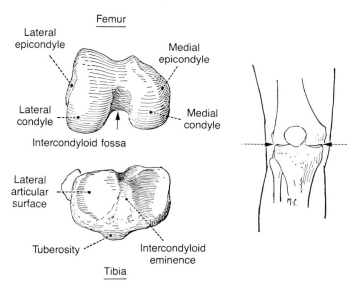

Figure 8.1   Articulating surfaces of knee joint.

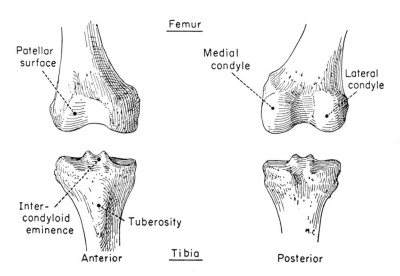

Figure 8.2   Anterior and posterior views of bones of knee joint.

the downward projection of the medial condyle compensates for the obliquity of the femoral shaft.

Another interesting feature of the condyles is that they are not quite parallel. Whereas the lateral condyle lies in the sagittal plane, the medial condyle slants slightly medially from front to back. This is an important factor in the movements of the knee.

Anteriorly, the two condyles are continuous with the smooth, slightly concave surface of the patellar facet for the articulation of the patella. The patella, or kneecap, is a large sesamoid bone located slightly above and in front of the knee

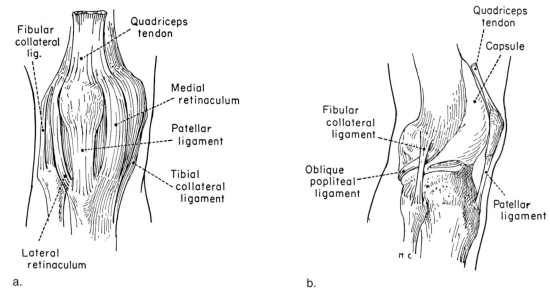

Figure 8.3   (a) Anterior and (b) lateral views of knee joint showing ligaments.

joint. It is held in place by the quadriceps tendon above, by the patellar ligament below, and by the intervening fibers that form a pocket for the patella (figure 8.3).

The articular cavity is enclosed within a loose membranous capsule that lies under the patella and folds around each condyle but excludes the intercondyloid tubercles and cruciate ligaments. It is supplemented by expansions from the fascia lata, iliotibial tract, and various tendons. The oblique popliteal ligament covers the posterior surface of the joint completely, shielding the cruciate ligaments and other structures not enclosed within the capsule.

The synovial membrane of the knee joint is the most extensive of any in the body. It folds in and around the joint in a manner far too complicated to attempt to describe here. There are numerous bursae in the vicinity of the knee joint. The largest and most important of these bursae are the prepatellar, infrapatellar, and suprapatellar bursae.

Menisci

The menisci (figure 8.4) are circular rims of fibrocartilage situated on the articular surfaces of the head of the tibia. They are relatively thick at their peripheral borders but taper to a thin edge at their inner circumferences. Thus they deepen the articular facets of the tibia and, at the same time, serve in a shock-absorbing capacity. The inner edges are free, but the peripheral borders are attached loosely to the rim of the head of the tibia by fibers from the inner surface of the capsule.

The lateral meniscus forms an incomplete circle, conforming closely to the nearly round articular facet. Its anterior and posterior horns, which almost meet at the center of the joint, are attached to the intercondyloid eminence.

The medial cartilage is shaped like a large letter C, broader toward the rear than in front. Its anterior horn tapers off to a thin strand attached to the anterior intercondyloid fossa. It is not as freely movable as the lateral cartilage because of its secure anchorage to the medial (tibial) collateral ligament at the medial side of the knee and the semimembranosus muscle posteriorly. Largely because of these points of attachment, the medial cartilage is more frequently injured than the lateral.

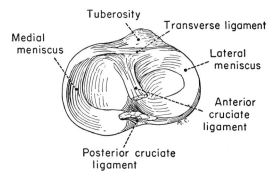

Figure 8.4   The menisci of the knee joint.

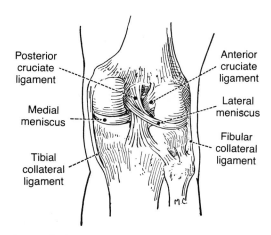

Figure 8.5   Posterior view of knee joint showing cruciate ligaments.

Ligaments of the Knee*
Patellar Ligament (Figure 8.3)

This is a strong, flat ligament connecting the lower margin of the patella with the tuberosity of the tibia. Passing over the front of the patella, the superficial fibers are continuations of the central fibers of the quadriceps femoris tendon.

Medial (Tibial) Collateral Ligament
(Figures 8.3a and 8.5)

This is a broad, flat, membranous band on the medial side of the joint. It is attached above to the medial epicondyle of the femur below the adductor tubercle and below to the medial condyle of the tibia. It is firmly attached to the medial meniscus. This fact should be noted because of its significance in knee injuries. It serves to check extension and to prevent motion laterally.

Lateral (Fibular) Collateral Ligament
(Figures 8.3 and 8.5)

This is a strong, rounded cord, attached above to the back of the lateral epicondyle of the femur and below to the lateral surface of the head of the fibula. It serves to check extension and to prevent motion medially.

Oblique Popliteal Ligament (Figure 8.3b)

This is a broad, flat ligament, covering the back of the knee joint. It is attached above to the upper margin of the intercondyloid fossa and posterior surface of the femur and below to the posterior margin of the head of the tibia. Medially it blends with the tendon of the semimembranosus muscle, and laterally with the lateral head of the gastrocnemius. It too protects against hyperextension.

The Cruciate Ligaments (Figure 8.5)

These are two strong, cordlike ligaments situated within the knee joint, although not enclosed within the joint capsule. They are called cruciate because they cross each other. They are further designated anterior and posterior, according to their attachments to the tibia. They serve to check certain movements at the knee joint. They limit extension and prevent rotation in the extended position. They also check the forward and backward sliding of the femur on the tibia, thus safeguarding the anteroposterior stability of the knee.

Anterior cruciate ligament (Figure 8.5)   This passes upward and backward from the anterior intercondyloid fossa of the tibia to the back part of the medial surface of the lateral condyle of the femur.

*Detailed descriptions of individual ligaments are included here because of their importance to a good understanding of the complex injuries experienced by this joint.

Posterior cruciate ligament *(Figure 8.5)*   This is a shorter and stronger ligament than the anterior. It passes upward and forward from the posterior intercondyloid fossa of the tibia to the lateral and front part of the medial condyle of the femur.

Transverse Ligament (Figure 8.4)

This is a short, slender, cordlike ligament, connecting the anterior convex margin of the lateral meniscus to the anterior end of the medial meniscus.

The Iliotibial Tract (Figures 7.18 and 7.19)

The iliotibial tract is said to act like a tense ligament that connects the iliac crest with the lateral femoral condyle and the lateral tubercle of the tibia. At the knee joint the tract serves as a stabilizing ligament between the lateral condyle of the femur and the tibia.

Movements

The movements that occur at the knee joint are primarily flexion and extension. A slight amount of rotation can take place when the knee is in the flexed position and the foot is not supporting the weight or during the initial stages of flexion and the final stages of extension (figure 8.6).

Flexion and Extension

The movements of flexion and extension at the knee are not as simple as those of a true hinge joint. This can be demonstrated in the classroom by holding a disarticulated femur and tibia together in a position of extension and then, holding the tibia stationary, flexing the femur on the tibia as though the individual were assuming a squat or sitting position. If no other adjustment is made, the femoral condyles will roll back completely off

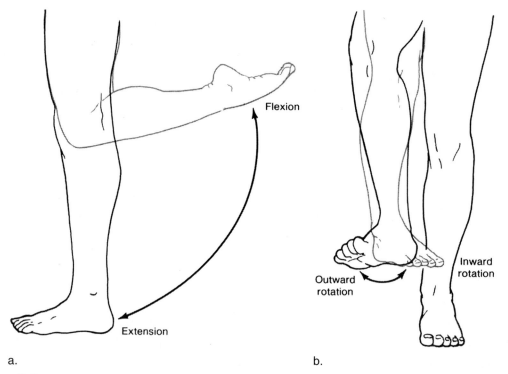

a.   b.

Figure 8.6   Movements of the knee joint: (a) flexion and extension; (b) inward and outward rotation (in flexed, non-weight-bearing position).

the top of the tibia. What prevents this from happening in real life is the fact that, as the condyles roll backward, they simultaneously glide forward and thus remain in contact with the menisci throughout each phase of the movement. In addition, the anterior cruciate becomes taut and prevents further backward translation. Conversely, when the femur extends on the tibia, the forward roll of the femoral condyles is accompanied by both a backward glide and the pull of the posterior cruciate to help prevent forward dislocation.

Because the femoral condyles are not quite parallel and the medial condyle is slightly longer, a slight degree of rotation occurs during the initial phase of flexion and the final phase of extension. This can be seen readily on the living subject who stands with the knees slightly flexed and then extends them completely. The patellae turn slightly medialward, indicating slight inward rotation of the thighs. Because of the inequality of the two condyles, the medial condyle continues to roll forward after the lateral condyle has ceased its movement. The inward rotation of the femur that accompanies the completion of extension is commonly known as the "locking" or "screw home" mechanism of the knees. In persons who tend to hyperextend their knees habitually, the rotation is more pronounced.

When the leg is flexed or extended in a non-weight-bearing position, the tibia rotates on the femur, instead of vice versa. The final phase of extension is accompanied by slight outward rotation of the tibia. At the beginning of flexion the tibia rotates inward until the midposition is attained.

The rotation that occurs in the final stage of extension and the initial phase of flexion is an inherent part of these movements and should not be confused with the voluntary rotation that can be performed when the leg is not bearing weight and the knee is in a flexed position.

Inward and Outward Rotation in the Flexed Position

In spite of the fact that the knee joint is classified as a hinge joint, its condylar structure accommodates movement other than just flexion and extension under certain conditions. When the leg has

been flexed at the knee, the collateral ligaments become slack and it is possible to rotate the leg on the thigh through a total range of about 50 degrees. This can occur, however, only when the leg is not bearing the body weight. It is impossible, for instance, to rotate either the leg or the thigh in this manner when the body is in a stooping position. A good way to demonstrate rotation of the tibia is to sit on a chair with the heel resting lightly on the floor. In this position, with the knee and thigh held motionless, the foot should be turned first in and then out. The action will be that of inward and outward rotation of the tibia. The movement taking place within the foot itself should be discounted. Taut collateral and cruciate ligaments prevent rotation when the leg is extended at the knee, either in a weight-bearing or non-weight-bearing position (Goss 1980). Inward or outward movements of the foot in the extended position are due to rotation at the hip joint.

MUSCLES OF THE KNEE JOINT

Location

The muscles acting on the knee joint are classified as anterior or posterior according to the relation of their distal tendons to the transverse axis of the joint.

Anterior	Posterior
Quadriceps femoris group	Hamstring group
Rectus femoris	Biceps femoris
Vastus intermedius	Semimembranosus
Vastus lateralis	Semitendinosus
Vastus medialis	Sartorius
	Gracilis
	Popliteus
	Gastrocnemius

Characteristics and Functions of Individual Muscles

Quadriceps Femoris Group

This group (figures 8.3, 8.7, and 8.8) consists of the rectus femoris and the vasti: vastus intermedius,

Figure 8.7   Front of thigh showing rectus femoris and sartorius muscles.

vastus lateralis, and vastus medialis. Of these, only the rectus femoris, the most superficial of the four, crosses the hip joint. The vastus intermedius lies posterior to the rectus and is completely covered by it. The distal portions of the four muscles unite to form a single broad, flat tendon that attaches to the base of the patella, the base being the upper border. In some texts this is given as the distal attachment of the quadriceps group, with no further explanation. If this ended the matter, one would wonder how muscles that did not cross the knee joint could extend it. Obviously, the patellar ligament connecting the patella with the tuberosity of

the tibia is a vital part of the quadriceps femoris. Actually, the patella is a sesamoid bone encased within the quadriceps tendon, with the patellar ligament being but a continuation of this and the tibial tuberosity the true distal point of attachment. All four muscles extend the leg at the knee joint and function as a unit in doing so.

The vastus lateralis and vastus medialis, with their fibers converging toward the patella, act with the vastus intermedius and rectus femoris, with their longitudinal approach, to steady the knee joint in weight-bearing positions and to maintain a balanced tension on the patella. There

Figure 8.8   Front of thigh showing three vasti muscles and the gracilis.

is very little activity from these muscles, however, in relaxed standing. Because the three vasti are one-joint muscles they are *powerful knee extensors,* regardless of the position of the hip joint. Their greatest activity is during the last part of knee extension. The vastus medialis is the most active of the three throughout the greatest range of knee extension. Its lower portion is also important in preventing lateral dislocation of the patella. When the knee is fully extended, static contraction of the quadriceps serves to pull up or "set" the patella, a mild exercise used in rehabilitation of the injured knee. This pull on the patella

is not directly vertical but is at an angle to the femur. The pull angle of the quadriceps is commonly referred to as the Q angle. This angle is measured as shown in figure 8.9, at the intersection of lines drawn from the center of the patella to the anterior superior iliac spine and from the tibial tuberosity to the center of the patella. Normal Q angles range from 8 degrees to 17 degrees, usually slightly higher in females than in males. Large Q angles have been associated with increased incidence of patellofemoral problems, as a result of the increasingly off-center pull (Woodland and Francis 1992).

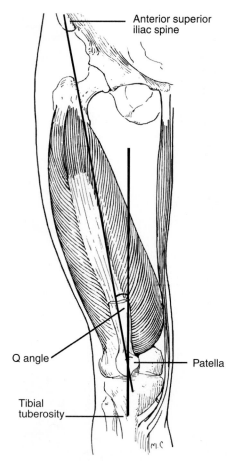

Anterior superior iliac spine

Q angle

Patella

Tibial tuberosity

Figure 8.9   Q angle.

The two-joint *rectus femoris* (also listed with the hip muscles) is of bipenniform structure with all except the lowest fibers slanting obliquely downward and sideward from the central tendon and the lowest fibers being approximately vertical (see figure 8.7). The upper three-quarters of the muscle consists of the muscle fibers, with the last quarter, down to the base of the patella, being the muscle's distal tendon. The entire muscle contracts regardless of whether it is producing movement at the hip joint or knee joint. It is most effective at the knee joint when the hip joint is extended. The muscle may be palpated on the central-anterior surface of the thigh.

The majority of the *vastus lateralis* fibers slant downward and medialward to the tendon. The muscle may be palpated on the anterolateral aspect of the thigh, lateral to the rectus femoris.

Most of the fibers of the *vastus medialis* slant downward and lateralward to the tendon, with the lowest ones almost horizontal in direction. If the lateralis and medialis were looked upon as one muscle, it would be considered to be of bipenniform construction, with the fibers slanting in direct opposition to those of the rectus femoris. The fleshy part of both the medialis and lateralis extends down almost to the level of the base of the patella. The vastus medialis may be palpated on the anteromedial aspect of the lower third of the thigh, medial to the rectus femoris.

Hamstring Group

(Also listed with the hip muscles.) The hamstrings (figures 8.10 and 8.11), so named from their large, cordlike tendons behind the knee joint, consist of the biceps femoris, semimembranosus, and semitendinosus muscles. Although the biceps femoris constitutes the lateral hamstring, its long head lies approximately along the midline of the posterior aspect of the thigh, as far down as the popliteal space. The long head comes from the tuberosity of the ischium, and the short head originates from the linea aspera on the posterior surface of the thigh. The two join at the distal tendon close to the lateral condyle of the femur, not far above the tendon's attachment to the head of the fibula. It is an important *flexor of the knee*. When the knee is flexed and not bearing weight, the biceps femoris can rotate the lower leg outward. Its tendon may be palpated behind the knee on its lateral aspect. The long head is fusiform in construction; the short head is penniform.

The *semimembranosus* and *semitendinosus* constitute the medial hamstrings. The former lies deeper than the latter and attaches higher on the tibia. The semitendinosus is attached to the medial surface of the tibia, below the head, just below the attachment of the gracilis and behind that of the sartorius. Like the biceps femoris, they

Figure 8.10   Hamstring muscles.

flex the knee joint. Unlike the biceps femoris, the semimembranosus and semitendinosus medially rotate the unweighted and flexed tibia. The semitendinosus may be palpated on the medial aspect of the posterior surface of the knee. The tendon of the semimembranosus is almost impossible to palpate successfully because it is shorter than its partner and is partially covered by the latter, as well as by the gracilis tendon.

Nearly everyone is familiar with the limiting effect of the hamstrings. Many experience difficulty in touching the toes with the fingers without bending the knees and in sitting erect on the floor with the legs extended straight forward because the hamstrings are frequently not long enough to permit such extreme stretching at the hips and knees simultaneously.

Sartorius

(Also listed with the hip muscles.) This is a long, slender, ribbonlike muscle (see figure 8.7) superficially located and directed obliquely downward and medialward across the front of the thigh. On its way to its distal attachment, it curves around behind the bulge of the medial condyles in such a way that its line of pull is posterior to the axis of

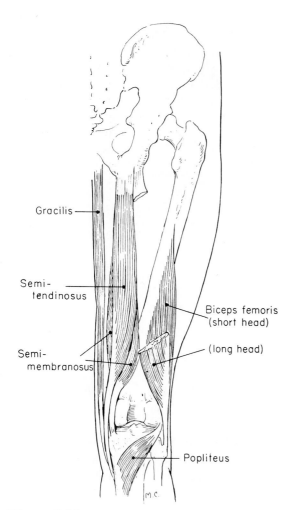

Figure 8.11   Posterior muscles of thigh and knee.

the knee joint. Thus, in spite of the fact that at least two-thirds of the muscle, including both its proximal and distal attachments, lies on the anterior aspect of the lower extremity, its action at the knee joint is generally *flexion,* not extension. It also assists in inward rotation of the tibia when the leg is flexed at the knee and *is not bearing weight.* The line of pull of the sartorius is determined by the direction of its distal tendon, between the latter's point of contact with the medial condyle of the tibia and its attachment to the upper anteromedial surface of the tibial shaft, al-

most as far forward as the anterior crest. It may be palpated at the anterior superior iliac spine, as well as along its entire length, where it is clearly visible on a thin, well-muscled subject.

Gracilis

(Also listed with the hip muscles.) This is a long, slender muscle (see figures 8.8 and 8.11) situated on the medial aspect of the thigh. Its action at the knee joint is *flexion.* It also is slightly active in *inward rotation of the tibia when the knee is in a flexed position and the foot is not bearing weight.* It may be palpated on the medial aspect of the posterior surface of the knee, anterior to the semitendinosus tendon but close to it.

Popliteus

This muscle (see figure 8.11) *rotates the tibia inward* and *helps flex the knee.* In structure and function it resembles the pronator teres muscle of the elbow. In a subject who is standing, it "unlocks" the knee joint preliminary to flexion. It also helps protect and stabilize the knee joint from forward dislocation of the femur when a squatting position is assumed and maintained. During walking, it is active throughout most of the weight-bearing phase (Basmajian and DeLuca 1985).

Gastrocnemius

(Also listed with the ankle muscles.) This large calf muscle (see figure 8.23), although primarily a muscle of the ankle joint, has an important function at the knee joint. It is in a position to help *flex* the knee and does so when the leg is not bearing weight. It also functions at the knee as a *posterior ligament* to protect the joint in movements involving violent extension, as in running and jumping.

When the foot is fixed in weight bearing, *the gastrocnemius can help maintain knee extension.* It does this when the hip and knee are in strong extension and when plantar flexion of the ankle is inhibited, such as when the line of gravity passes in front of the knee and ankle joints. Under these circumstances the gastrocnemius is able to pull back and down on the femoral condyles, thus contributing to knee extension. Its activity in "relaxed standing at ease" was found in three-fourths of subjects tested barefooted. The wearing of high heels increased the frequency of subjects whose muscles were active. The muscle is easy to palpate, including both the muscle belly in the calf and the tendon behind the ankle.

MUSCULAR ANALYSIS OF THE FUNDAMENTAL MOVEMENTS OF THE LEG AT THE KNEE JOINT

Flexion

The knee joint has five important flexors, namely the three hamstring muscles (biceps femoris, semimembranosus, and semitendinosus), the sartorius, and the gracilis; the latter is especially important during the early part of flexion, provided that the hip is not flexing simultaneously. Two additional muscles that help with flexion are the popliteus and gastrocnemius.

It should be remembered that when the weight is borne by the feet and the knees are allowed to flex, as in stooping, the knee flexors are not responsible for the movement. The flexion is produced by the force of gravity and is controlled by the extensor muscles that are contracting eccentrically, that is, in lengthening contraction.

The three adductors have also been shown to be active in most children during flexion and extension of the knee with or without external resistance. They were also active under the same conditions in most adults during knee flexion, but activity of these muscles during extension occurred only when resistance was applied (Basmajian and DeLuca 1985).

Extension

This action is performed by the four muscles that make up the quadriceps femoris group: the rectus femoris, the vastus intermedius, the vastus lateralis, and the vastus medialis.

Muscles sometimes act in surprising ways. A good example of this is the action of the gastrocnemius at the knee when the weight is on the foot. When the weight is not on the foot, the gastrocnemius is an assistant flexor of the knee. Its primary function is extension (plantar flexion) of the ankle joint. When the foot is bearing weight, flexion of the leg at the knee cannot take place unless the ankle is dorsiflexing at the same time. If this dorsiflexion is prevented, the weight-bearing knee is unable to flex. Under these circumstances the gastrocnemius contracts in what might be called the reverse direction; that is, it acts on its proximal attachments and pulls backward and downward on the femoral condyles, and with the foot fixed this contributes to knee extension. Because of such reversals, it is not desirable for a student to memorize muscular actions. The circumstances under which the movement is performed are of vital importance.

Outward Rotation of the Tibia

This action is performed by the biceps femoris. It can occur only when the knee is flexed in a non-weight-bearing situation.

Inward Rotation of the Tibia

This action is performed chiefly by the semimembranosus, semitendinosus, and popliteus, with possible help from the gracilis and sartorius. As with outward rotation, it can occur only when the knee is flexed and the foot is not bearing weight.

THE ANKLE AND THE FOOT

The foot has two functions of great importance: support and propulsion. In studying the structure of the foot, one should keep these functions in mind, because only by seeing the foot in terms of the combined static and dynamic demands made upon it can one fully appreciate its intricate mechanism.

The foot is united with the leg at the ankle joint. Within the foot itself are the seven tarsal bones. Two of the joints in this region are of sufficient importance to the kinesiologist to merit special attention. These are the subtalar and midtarsal joints, the latter including the talonavicular and calcaneocuboid articulations. The movements within the foot occur mainly at these two joints.

The structure of the ankle, tarsal joints, and toes will be described separately, but the muscles of these three regions will be discussed together, because many of them act on more than one joint.

Structure of the Ankle

The ankle (talocrural) joint (figures 8.12, 8.13, and 8.14) is a hinge joint. It is formed by the articulation of the talus (astragalus) with the malleoli of the tibia and the fibula. The malleolus of the fibula lies more posterior and extends more distally than that of the tibia. The malleoli of the tibia and fibula, bound together by the transverse tibiofibular ligament, the anterior and posterior ligaments of the lateral malleolus, and the interossei, constitute a mortise into which the upper, rounded portion of the talus fits. The transverse tibiofibular ligament secures the lateral and medial malleoli and the back surface of the talus. The ankle joint is surrounded by a thin, membra-

nous capsule that is thicker on the medial side of the joint. In the back it is a thin mesh of membranous tissue and is not continuous, as are most capsules. It is reinforced by several strong ligaments.

Ligamentous Reinforcement

The medial side of the ankle joint is protected by five strong ligamentous bands (see figure 8.13), four of them connecting the medial malleolus of the tibia with the posterior tarsal bones, the calcaneus, talus, and navicular. These four ligaments are known collectively as the deltoid ligament. Individually they are the calcaneotibial, the anterior talotibial, the tibionavicular, and the posterior talotibial ligaments. The fifth band (plantar calcaneonavicular) provides a horizontal connection between the navicular bone and the sustentaculum tali projection on the medial aspect of the calcaneus. It is also known as the spring ligament.

The lateral side of the ankle is reinforced (see figure 8.14) by three ligaments collectively called the lateral collateral ligament. These connect the lateral malleolus with the upper lateral aspect of the calcaneus and with anterior and posterior portions of the talus. The components of the lateral

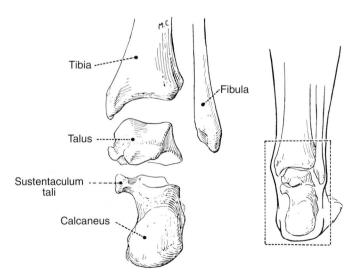

Figure 8.12   Bones of ankle and subtalar joints, posterior view.

collateral ligament are named the calcaneofibular, anterior and posterior talofibular ligaments, respectively. The lateral ligaments are weaker than the medial ligaments, and the anterior talofibular ligament is the weakest of all. Inspection of figures 8.13 and 8.14 gives one the impression that the lateral side of the ankle is less protected than the medial. These facts help explain the high incidence of lateral ankle sprains.

Structure of the Foot

The foot as a whole (figures 8.15 and 8.16) is usually described as an elastic arched structure, the keystone of the arch being the talus. This

bone has several marks of distinction. Aside from being the connecting link between the foot and the leg, it is distinguished by having no muscles attached to it and by receiving and transmitting the weight of the entire body (with the exception of the foot itself), a function that requires great strength and firm support.

The foot has two arches, a longitudinal and a transverse. The longitudinal arch extends from the heel to the heads of the five metatarsals. It is sometimes described as being made up of an inner and an outer component. The outer component includes the calcaneus, cuboid, and fourth and fifth metatarsals (figure 8.16a). The inner component consists of the calcaneus, talus, navicular, three

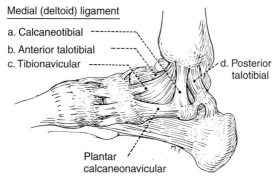

Figure 8.13   Medial ligaments of ankle joint.

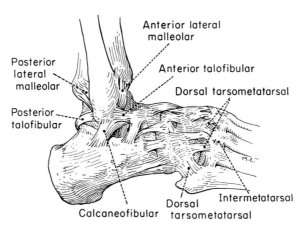

Figure 8.14   Lateral ligaments of ankle joint.

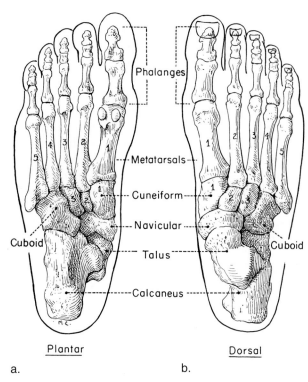

Figure 8.15   Bones of the foot: plantar and dorsal views.

cuneiforms, and the three medial metatarsals (figure 8.16b). The outer component has a nearly flat contour and lacks mobility; hence, it is better adapted to the function of support. The inner component, with its greater flexibility and its curving arch, is adapted to the function of shock absorption, so important in all forms of locomotion. Contrary to popular opinion, the height of the longitudinal arch is not indicative of the strength of the arch. Thus, a low arch is not necessarily a weak one, *provided it is not associated with a pronated (i.e., abducted and everted) foot.*

The transverse arch is the side-to-side concavity on the underside of the foot formed by the anterior tarsal bones and the metatarsals. The anterior boundary of this arch under the metatarsal heads is known as the metatarsal arch. There is some disagreement as to whether this should be called an arch, since it flattens completely when bearing weight. The metatarsal arch exists, therefore, only in non-weight-bearing situations.

The toes, especially the large and powerful "big toes," are largely responsible for propulsion. They provide the push-off at the end of the step. Their use in locomotion is directly proportional to the vigor and speed of the walk or run.

The strength and elasticity of the foot, which is comprised of twenty-six bones, are due largely to the ligaments that bind the bones together and to the muscles that work to preserve the balance of the foot. Thus, both ligaments and muscles share the responsibility for maintaining the integrity of the feet.

Subtalar Joint (Talocalcaneal)

This is the joint (figure 8.17) between the underside of the talus and the upper and anterior aspects of the calcaneus, or heel, bone. It is reinforced by

Figure 8.16   Bones of the foot: lateral and medial views.

Figure 8.17   Ligaments of tarsal joints.

four small talocalcaneal ligaments. A fifth ligament, the *plantar calcaneonavicular,* is probably
the most important of all. It is a broad, thick ligament that connects the sustentaculum tali projection of the calcaneus with the underside of the
navicular bone. It passes under the talus and aids
in supporting it. It is actually part of the subtalar
joint, because it contains a fibrocartilaginous
facet that is lined with synovial membrane. This
is commonly called the *spring ligament* because
of the yellow elastic fibers that give it its elasticity. The importance of this ligament can be readily understood when one remembers that the talus
receives the weight of the entire body. The shock-
absorbing function of this elastic support is obvious. It is probably equally obvious that excessive
prolonged pressure on this ligament through im-
proper use of the feet will cause it to stretch permanently and thus result in a lowered arch.

Unfortunately, figure 8.17b gives a somewhat misleading picture of this ligament. Although it looks like a cord-shaped ligament on the
medial aspect of the ankle, the part that shows in
the picture is actually just the medial border of a
broad ligament that extends beneath the head of
the talus, like a taut hammock.

Midtarsal Joint (Transverse Tarsal; Chopart's Joint)

The midtarsal joint consists of two articulations,
the lateral one being the calcaneocuboid joint and
the medial one the talonavicular. Viewed from
above, the continuous line of articulation—the
talonavicular and calcaneocuboid—forms a somewhat shallow letter S (figures 8.15b and 8.18). The
talonavicular joint is a modified ball-and-socket
joint and permits somewhat restricted movements
about three axes. The calcaneocuboid joint is nonaxial and permits only slight gliding motions.
These seem to be supplementary or secondary to
the freer motions of the talonavicular joint. Several
ligaments reinforce these joints, but the ones that
give the most support are the *long and short plantar (calcaneocuboid) ligaments.* These are both
wide, thick ligaments of great strength.

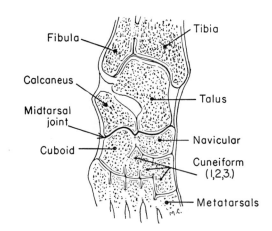

Figure 8.18   Oblique section of tarsal bones
showing midtarsal joint.

Tarsometatarsal Joints

These joints (figures 8.15 and 8.19) are nonaxial, with the possible exception of the great toe
joint, which looks slightly like a saddle joint.
The movements are of a gliding nature that resembles a restricted form of flexion, extension,
abduction, and adduction.

Intermetatarsal Joints

These joints (see figures 8.14 and 8.19) include
two sets of side-by-side articulations, those between the bases and those between the heads of the
metatarsal bones. They are all nonaxial joints. The
articulations between the heads of the metatarsal
bones are an important part of the metatarsal arch.
The total result of the movements occurring there
is a spreading or flattening of the arch when the
weight is on it and a return to its plantar concavity
when the weight is taken off it.

Metatarsophalangeal Joints

These joints (see figures 8.15 and 8.19) may best
be described as a modified form of condyloid
joint. The joint of the great toe differs from the
others in that it is larger and has two sesamoid
bones beneath it.

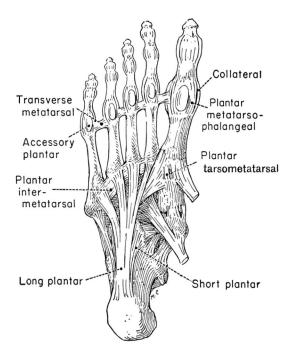

Figure 8.19   Plantar ligaments of foot.

Labels on figure:
Transverse metatarsal
Accessory plantar
Plantar inter- metatarsal
Long plantar
Collateral
Plantar metatarso- phalangeal
Plantar tarsometatarsal
Short plantar

Interphalangeal Joints

As is true of the fingers, these are all hinge joints (see figures 8.15 and 8.19).

Movements of the Foot at the Ankle, Tarsal, and Toe Joints

Ankle Joint

The movements of the ankle joint occur about an axis that is usually described as frontal-horizontal but is actually slightly oblique, as evidenced by the slightly posterior position of the lateral malleolus relative to the medial. This is of minor significance, but it explains the tendency of the foot to turn out when it is fully dorsiflexed and to turn in when fully plantar flexed (figure 8.20).

Dorsiflexion (flexion)   A forward upward movement of the foot in the sagittal plane, so that the dorsal surface of the foot approaches the anterior surface of the leg.

Plantar flexion (extension)   A forward downward movement of the foot in the sagittal plane, so that the dorsal surface of the foot moves away from the anterior surface of the leg.

Tarsal Joints

The movements that take place at the *midtarsal, subtalar,* and other *tarsal* joints occur together and are usually closely related to the ankle joint movements. Except for the talonavicular joint, which belongs to the ball-and-socket category, they are all nonaxial joints and therefore permit only slight gliding movements (figure 8.20).

Dorsiflexion   Slight decrease in convexity of dorsal surface and in concavity of plantar surface of tarsal region. Accompanies dorsiflexion of ankle.

Plantar flexion   Increase in convexity of dorsal surface and in concavity of plantar surface of tarsal region. Accompanies plantar flexion of ankle.

Inversion and adduction (supination)   A lifting of the medial border of the arch combined with a medial bending of the front of the foot.

Eversion and abduction (pronation)   A slight raising of the lateral border of the foot combined with a slight lateral bending of the front of the foot.

Tarsometatarsal and Intermetatarsal Joints

These joints have a slight gliding motion. The first metatarsal bone has a slightly greater degree of motion at these joints than do the other metatarsals because of the absence of any ligament between its base and the base of the second metatarsal.

Metatarsophalangeal Joints

Flexion, extension, and limited abduction and adduction.

Figure 8.20 Movements of the foot at the ankle and tarsal joints: (a) dorsiflexion and plantar flexion; (b) supination and pronation (tarsal joint only).

Interphalangeal Joints

Flexion and extension; also hyperextension, especially of the great toe.

MUSCLES OF THE ANKLE AND FOOT

Location

Eleven of the twenty-two muscles of the ankle and foot are intrinsic, that is, they are located entirely within the foot. The other eleven are extrinsic; they have distal tendon attachments on the foot but are otherwise located outside it (table 8.1). A twelveth extrinsic muscle, the plantaris, has been omitted because it is a vestige often absent in human beings. When present it assists the ankle extensor muscles.

Characteristics and Functions of Individual Muscles

Tibialis Anterior

This muscle (figure 8.21a) lies along the full length of the anterior surface of the tibia from the lateral condyle down to the medial aspect of the tarsometatarsal region. Approximately one-half to two-thirds of the way down the leg it becomes tendinous. The tendon passes in front of the medial malleolus on its way to the first cuneiform. The muscle *dorsiflexes the ankle and foot,* and *supinates (inverts and adducts) the tarsal joints* when the foot is dorsiflexed. In EMG studies it was found that one-half the subjects in free standing had activity in the tibialis anterior that went away when the subjects leaned forward (Basmajian and DeLuca 1985). The muscle may be palpated on the anterior surface of the leg just lateral to the tibia.

TABLE 8.1	Ankle and Foot Muscles
Extrinsic Muscles	**Intrinsic Muscles**
Anterior Aspect of Leg	Extensor digitorum brevis
Tibialis anterior	Flexor digitorum brevis
Extensor digitorum longus	Quadratus plantae
Extensor hallucis longus	Lumbricales
Peroneus tertius	Abductor hallucis
Lateral Aspect of Leg	Flexor hallucis brevis
Peroneus longus	Adductor hallucis
Peroneus brevis	Abductor digiti minimi
Posterior Aspect of Leg	Flexor digiti minimi brevis
Gastrocnemius	Dorsal interossei
Soleus	Plantar interossei
Tibialis posterior	
Flexor digitorum longus	
Flexor hallucis longus	

Extensor Digitorum Longus

This muscle (figures 8.21b and 8.22) *extends the four lesser toes.* It also *dorsiflexes both the ankle and the tarsal joints* and *helps evert and abduct the latter.* It is a penniform muscle, situated lateral to the tibialis anterior muscle in the upper part of the leg and lateral to the extensor hallucis longus in the lower part. Just in front of the ankle joint the tendon divides into four tendons, one for each of the lesser toes. The muscle may be palpated on the anterior surface of the ankle and the dorsal surface of the foot, lateral to the tendon of the extensor hallucis longus.

Extensor Hallucis Longus

This muscle (see figure 8.21a) *extends and hyperextends the great toe.* It also *dorsiflexes the ankle and the tarsal joints.* Like the preceding muscle, it is penniform in structure. Its upper portion lies beneath the tibialis anterior and extensor digitorum longus, but about halfway down the leg the tendon emerges between these two muscles, thus becoming superficial. After it reaches the ankle the tendon slants medially across the dorsal surface of the foot to the top of the great toe. It may be palpated on the dorsal surface of the foot and great toe.

Peroneus Tertius

This muscle (see figure 8.22) *dorsiflexes and pronates (everts and abducts) the tarsal joints* and *dorsiflexes the ankle.* It is a small muscle that lies lateral to the extensor digitorum longus, sometimes described as the fifth tendon of the latter muscle. It may be palpated on the dorsal surface of the foot close to the base of the fifth metatarsal.

Peroneus Longus

This muscle (see figure 8.22) *plantar flexes, everts, and abducts the tarsal joints,* and *plantar flexes the ankle.* It also is most active during the propulsive phase of walking. It is situated superficially on the lateral aspect of the leg with its distal tendon passing behind the lateral malleolus and proceeding forward and downward to the margin of the foot, where it passes behind the tuberosity of the fifth metatarsal. At this point it turns under the foot, passes through the peroneal groove of the cuboid, and slants forward

Figure 8.21   Anterior muscles of the leg.

across the plantar surface of the foot to its attachment at the base of the first metatarsal and first cuneiform, not far from the attachment of the tibialis anterior. The muscle belly may be palpated on the lateral surface of the lower half of the leg and just above and behind the lateral malleolus.

Peroneus Brevis

This muscle (see figures 8.21a and 8.22) *plantar flexes and everts and abducts the tarsal joints* and

helps plantar flex the ankle. It is a penniform muscle, lying beneath the peroneus longus on the lower half of the lateral aspect of the leg. Its tendon passes behind the lateral malleolus immediately anterior to the tendon of longus and continues forward just above the longus tendon to its attachment on the tuberosity of the fifth metatarsal, below the attachment of the peroneus tertius. It may be palpated on the lateral margin of the foot, just posterior to the base of the fifth metatarsal.

Figure 8.22   Lateral muscles of the leg. (P.B. = peroneus brevis; P.L. = peroneus longus)

Gastrocnemius

(Also listed with the knee muscles.) This is a powerful fast-twitch fiber muscle (figure 8.23) for *plantar flexing the foot at the ankle joint.* It is the most superficial muscle on the back of the leg and can be seen as two bulges in the upper part of the calf when it is well developed. Its two heads, together with the soleus, constitute the triceps surae. The lateral and medial portions of the muscle remain distinct from each other as far down as the middle of the back of the leg. Then they fuse to form the broad tendon of Achilles.

The most familiar function of this muscle is to *enable one to rise on the toes.* Many anatomists have thought that it acted only when the movement was resisted, but an EMG investigation by Sheffield and coworkers revealed that it was active in unresisted *plantar flexion* in subjects lying in the supine position (Basmajian and DeLuca 1985). It has also been shown to be active in most individuals during normal relaxed standing. The muscle has a large angle of pull, approximately 90 degrees when the foot is in its fundamental position. Its internal structure

Figure 8.23   Gastrocnemius.

and its leverage combine to make it an exceedingly powerful muscle. In a 1967 EMG study, Herman and Bragin concluded that its most important role was plantar flexing in large contractions and in the rapid development of tension (Basmajian and DeLuca 1985). It may be palpated in the calf of the leg and on the back of the ankle.

Soleus

Like the gastrocnemius, this muscle (figure 8.24) *plantar flexes the foot at the ankle joint.* It lies beneath the gastrocnemius, except along the lateral aspect of the lower half of the calf where a portion of it lies lateral to the upper part of the calcaneal tendon. Its fibers are inserted into the calcaneal tendon in a bipenniform manner. It is predominantly comprised of slow-twitch fibers. In an EMG study of the leg muscles, when the subjects balanced on one foot, the soleus was consistently more active than the gastrocnemius. In another study the soleus was most active in minimal contractions and when the foot was in a dorsiflexed position. This seems to imply that it was especially active in the reduction of dorsiflexion. Campbell and coworkers, using fine wire

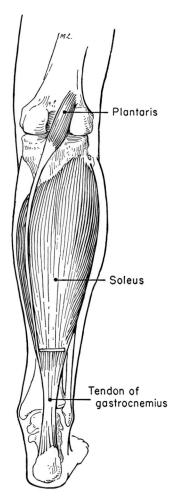

Figure 8.24   Posterior muscles of the leg, middle layer.

Figure 8.25   Tibialis posterior. (P.L. = peroneus longus; T.P. = tibialis posterior.)

electrodes, have shown that the medial part of the soleus is a strong dynamic and static plantar flexor, whereas the lateral part is primarily a stabilizer (Basmajian and DeLuca 1985). The muscle may be palpated slightly lateral to and below the lateral bulge of the gastrocnemius.

Tibialis Posterior

This muscle (figure 8.25) *plantar flexes the tarsal joints and helps plantar flex the ankle.* It participates in *supination (inversion and adduction)* when the foot is plantar flexed. It is the deepest

muscle on the back of the leg. The main part of the muscle covers the intermuscular septum between the tibia and the fibula. In the lower front of the leg its tendon slants across the medial side of the ankle, passes behind the medial malleolus and above the sustentaculum tali, and then turns under the foot around the medial margin of the navicular bone to insert into its underside. The muscle is penniform in structure. Because of its direction of pull and its numerous attachments on the plantar surface of the tarsal bones, an important function of this muscle appears to be maintenance of the

Flexor digitorum
longus

F.H.L.

F.D.L

P.L.

Figure 8.26   Flexor digitorum longus and flexor
hallucis longus; (F.H.L. = flexor hallucis longus; F.D.L. =
flexor digitorum longus; P.L. = peroneus longus.)

longitudinal arch in a reserve capacity such as is
needed in a weak foot.

Flexor Digitorum Longus

This muscle (figure 8.26) *flexes the four lesser
toes, plantar flexes and helps invert and adduct
the tarsal joints, and helps plantar flex the ankle.*
It is situated on the medial side of the back of the
leg behind the tibia. Penniform in structure, its
distal tendon passes behind the medial malleolus
between the tendons of the tibialis posterior and

flexor hallucis longus. Beneath the tarsal bones it
divides into four tendons that go to the distal phalanx of each of the four lesser toes.

Flexor Hallucis Longus

This muscle (figure 8.26) *flexes the great toe,
plantar flexes and helps invert and adduct the
tarsal joints, and helps plantar flex the ankle.* It is
situated on the lateral side of the back of the leg,
behind the fibula and the lateral portion of the
tibia. The fibers unite with the distal tendon in a
penniform manner. The tendon crosses behind the
ankle to the medial side, passes behind and beneath the sustentaculum tali, and runs forward
under the medial margin of the foot to the distal
phalanx of the great toe. It is the most posterior of
the three tendons that pass behind the medial
malleolus. One of its important functions is to
provide the push-off in walking, running, and
jumping. It may be palpated on the medial border
of the calcaneal tendon close to the calcaneus.

Intrinsic Muscles of the Foot

These muscles (figures 8.27, 8.28, and 8.29) will
be treated as a group rather than individually.
There are eleven of these small muscles or muscle groups. All but one, the extensor digitorum
brevis, are on the plantar surface and are usually
described as being arranged in four layers. The
dorsal interossei muscles, although included in
the deepest layer, are situated between the
metatarsal bones rather than on either surface (see
figure 8.21b). The extensor digitorum brevis,
which includes the hallucis although the latter is
sometimes described as a separate muscle, is situated on the dorsal surface of the foot (see figure 8.21a). With the exception of the *lumbricales*
and the *quadratus plantae,* which help flex the
lesser toes, the names of these muscles indicate
their functions. As one might expect, these intrinsic muscles are much more highly developed in
primitive people than in people who habitually
wear shoes.

Various research investigations have shown
that the intrinsic muscles act as a functional unit,

Figure 8.27   Plantar muscles of the foot, superficial layer.

Figure 8.28   Plantar muscles of the foot, middle layer.

Figure 8.29   Plantar muscles of the foot, deep layer.

have a significant role in stabilization of the foot during propulsion, and tend to show more activity in feet that are habitually pronated. They do not show activity during relaxed standing in either normal or pronated feet and are not active in the normal *static* support of the longitudinal arches. They do, however, show definite activity in voluntary attempts to increase the height of the arches. They are also definitely active in the movement of rising on the toes.

Plantar Fascia

On the plantar surface of the foot the muscles are covered by fascia (figure 8.30), divided into medial, central, and lateral portions. The central portion, known as the plantar aponeurosis, is particularly strong and fibrous. It extends under the whole length of the foot, connecting the tuberosity of the calcaneus with the bases of the proximal phalanges of the five toes. This is an exceedingly strong band that serves as an effective binding rod for the longitudinal arch.

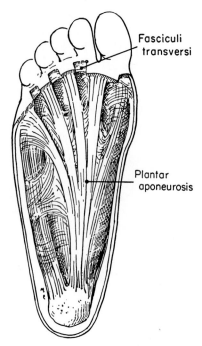

Figure 8.30   Plantar fascia of the foot (superficial).

MUSCULAR ANALYSIS OF THE FUNDAMENTAL MOVEMENTS OF THE ANKLE AND FOOT (TARSAL JOINTS AND TOES)

The Ankle
Dorsiflexion

Performed by the tibialis anterior, peroneus tertius, extensor digitorum longus, and extensor hallucis longus.

Plantar Flexion

Performed by the gastrocnemius, soleus, and peroneus longus, with possible help from the tibialis posterior, peroneus brevis, flexor digitorum longus, and flexor hallucis longus.

The Tarsal Joints
Dorsiflexion

The same as for dorsiflexion of the ankle.

Plantar Flexion

Performed by the tibialis posterior, flexor digitorum longus, flexor hallucis longus, and peroneus longus and brevis.

Supination (Inversion and Adduction)
(Figure 8.31b)

Performed by the tibialis anterior (when the foot is dorsiflexed) and tibialis posterior (when the foot is plantar flexed), with possible help from the flexor digitorum longus and flexor hallucis longus (Basmajian and DeLuca 1985).

Pronation (Eversion and Abduction)
(Figure 8.31a)

Performed by the peroneus longus, brevis, and tertius, with possible help from the extensor digitorum longus.

The Toes (Exclusive of the Intrinsic Muscles)
Flexion

Performed by the flexor digitorum longus and flexor hallucis longus.

Extension

Performed by the extensor digitorum longus and extensor hallucis longus.

Maintenance of the Arches

Many investigators have studied the structure of the arches and the role of muscles in maintaining them. Some have stated that the arch is supported by muscle contraction alone, whereas others have concluded that the arches are supported exclusively by passive structures, bones, and ligaments or the combination of muscular contraction and passive structures.

a.   b.

Figure 8.31   The feet and legs in weight-bearing position: (a) in eversion and abduction; (b) in inversion and adduction.

In 1963 Basmajian and Stecko investigated the activity of six muscles (tibialis anterior, tibialis posterior, peroneus longus, flexor hallucis longus, abductor hallucis, and flexor digitorum brevis) during static standing under various load conditions. Using twenty young men as subjects, they found that the subjects could support loads of 100 to 200 pounds, standing on one foot without any evidence of muscular action, and that with loads of 400 pounds some muscles became active but many still remained inactive. They concluded from these findings that the arches' first line of defense is ligamentous and that the muscles constitute a dynamic reserve, which is called into action reflexively when the load is excessive (Basmajian and DeLuca 1985).

In a strong foot, muscle activity is involved for balance, adjusting the foot when encountering uneven surfaces, during locomotion, and when incurring other stresses such as standing on tiptoes.

In a weak foot, such as with flat feet, muscles play a greater role. However, it has been demonstrated consistently that bones and ligaments are the primary structures for maintaining the arches.

COMMON INJURIES OF THE LEG, KNEE, AND ANKLE

The Leg
Skin Bruises (Contusions)

These injuries are very common because of the exposed position of the tibia and its lack of protection. A direct blow may cause an injury that varies in severity all the way from a simple bruise to a severe traumatic tibial periostitis, a condition in which the periosteum may be seriously damaged. Unlike the femur, the tibia has no anterior muscles to cushion it against sharp blows. It is important, therefore, to make every effort to protect the bone by the use of shin guards or other forms of padding in activities where there is a high risk of shin bruising.

Shin Splints

This condition is usually associated with overuse and produces symptoms of tenderness and pain on the medial surface of the tibia. The onset is gradual and the condition may be due to repeated tiny tears where the tibialis posterior or anterior attaches to the tibia or to tears or sprains in the interosseous membrane. Softer surfaces and supporting the arches may be helpful in relieving the symptoms, but rest is often necessary for recovery.

Leg Fracture

The most common leg fracture experienced in athletics is that of the fibula, a fracture that tends to occur in the lower two-thirds of the leg. A fibular fracture is not usually of serious consequence, provided it is not accompanied by damage to the ankle joint, the condition of greatest concern being rupture of the tibiofibular ligament. A complicating condition that is likely to accompany this is displacement of the bones, owing to the forceful pull of antagonistic muscles. If this results in instability of the ankle joint, the consequences can be extremely serious, causing a permanent disability (Arnheim and Prentice 1998).

The Knee

Vulnerability of the Knee Joint

There can be no question as to the vulnerability of the knee. It is probably the most susceptible to injury of any of the joints in the body. Two factors appear to be responsible for this: its complicated structure and its position midway between the hip and the sole of the foot. Superficially, it looks like a hinge joint, but its action combines the movements of a hinge with the gliding of an irregular joint. Furthermore, when it is flexed it is capable of a slight degree of medial and lateral rotation. Several writers have called attention to the strains and stresses to which the knee is subject and have emphasized the need to be aware of these forces

for knee function. Additionally, misalignments that cause the unequal or off-center transmission of forces through the knee joint are predisposing factors contributing to knee injuries. Common examples of these conditions are knock-knees (genu valgum) and bowlegs (genu varum). In knock-knees (genu valgum) the knees are closer to the midline of the body than is normal. In the standing position the knees are closer together than the feet, so that when the feet are placed side by side, the knees are either pressed together or are slightly overlapping with one behind the other. Mechanically, the condition means that the weight-bearing line of the lower extremity passes lateral to the center of the knee joint. This puts the medial ligament (tibial collateral) under increased tension and subjects the lateral meniscus to increased pressure and friction. Such a joint is an unstable one. Not only is it more prone to injury than a well-aligned joint, but in all weight-bearing positions postural strains are constantly present. The condition of bowlegs (genu varum) is just the reverse of knock-knees, with the additional complication of the long bones themselves being curved laterally.

Contusion

This condition occurs frequently among athletes and can be caused either by a fall or by a blow against the front or side of the knee. The problem presented by a contusion of the knee is that it often masks a more serious injury, such as ligament damage. Therefore, if there is uncertainty, this injury should be treated as the more serious injury to prevent further deterioration.

Collateral Ligament Sprain

This is doubtless one of the most, if not *the most,* frequently reported knee injury, at least in the world of sports (Arnheim and Prentice 1998). To understand the reason for this, a thorough knowledge of the structure of the joint is essential (pp. 182–186 and figure 8.32). Although classified as a hinge joint, it is by no means a typical one like the interphalangeal finger joints, for instance. In flexion and in the return from flexion, a

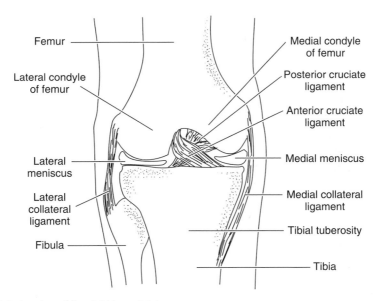

Figure 8.32   Anterior view of the right knee joint.

From D. D. Arnheim, *Modern Principles of Athletic Training,* 7th ed., p. 567. Copyright © 1989 Mosby College Publishing, St. Louis. Reprinted by permission.

certain amount of gliding occurs. When the knee is flexed it is capable of a slight amount of voluntary rotation. When it receives a blow from the side or when it is subjected to severe wrenching in the weight-bearing position, it can easily be forced beyond its normal range of rotary motion. Furthermore, although abduction and adduction are not normal knee motions—that is, one cannot voluntarily perform them—the leg can be passively abducted or adducted by an outside force. A slight degree of this probably does no harm, but a severe lateral blow or violent wrenching is likely to tear the ligament on the opposite side.

Because the knee is protected medially, the majority of knee sprains are caused by a blow from the lateral side toward the medial side or by a severe medialward twist (Arnheim and Prentice 1998). This means that the leg has been violently adducted and medially rotated at the knee joint. The stress is primarily on the ligaments on the inner side of the knee. If the force is great enough to be transmitted to the deep layer of the tibial collateral ligament, it is likely to affect the medial meniscus, which is attached to the ligament. Injuries to the lateral side are much less common. Cruciate ligament sprain and rupture are often encountered when forces cause the tibia to move forward or backward.

Strengthening of the muscles that cross the knee joint is an important part of the rehabilitation of injured knee joints. The muscles and their tendons help stabilize the joint and provide support that may be compromised because of the damaged ligaments. Moreover, it is important to maintain the strength of these muscles for their stabilizing role in sustaining the integrity of the joint and preventing injuries to it.

Deep Knee Bending

Squatting, or deep knee bending, is a movement that is used in many ways, both in daily life activities and in sports and other physical education activities. It is used by the baseball catcher as the ready-to-catch position. It is also used as a starting position for running races, for executing various stunts, as an exercise for physical fitness or training, and for landing after jumping down from a height. In the home, on the street, and almost anywhere it is used for picking up objects from the floor or ground. Whether performed slowly or quickly, the basic muscular pattern is the same. In downward movement, the hip and knee joints are flexing and the ankle joints are dorsiflexing. The joint movements are *caused* by the force of gravity; they are *controlled* by the muscles that normally cause the opposite movements but that, for this purpose, are engaged in *eccentric contraction.* In the return movement— that is, the return to the erect standing position— the same muscles are working but this time in *concentric contraction.*

The demands placed on the muscles and ligaments of the knee joint during deep squats are severe. These factors should be considered when contemplating the assignment of exercises involving repeated full squats or long-held squat positions. A much safer alternative would be a half-squat exercise.

Chondromalacia

Chondromalacia of the patella most often occurs among young adults and affects the cartilage on the articulating surface of the patella. The etiology of this degenerating disease is unknown, but it is conjectured that an incongruence between the patella and the femur may contribute to this disease. Common symptoms include pain upon movement, swelling, and a grating sensation. Treatment includes isometric exercise, wearing a band (brace) for support, and limiting certain activities.

Osgood-Schlatter Disease

Osgood-Schlatter disease, affecting adolescents, is caused by repeated usage of the knee extensors, resulting in a tearing or avulsion at the epiphysis of the tibial tuberosity, the point for attachment of the patellar tendon. Symptoms include swelling, hemorrhage, and pain when running, jumping, or kneeling. Treatment includes

ice therapy, rest, and subsequent isometric strengthening exercises.

The Ankle

Of all the injuries to which the lower extremity is prone, those affecting the ankle joint have the highest incidence. One reason for this is thought to be the arrangement of the muscles. The long tendons cross the ankle in a way that makes for lack of bulkiness and for good leverage but contributes little to stabilization (Arnheim and Prentice 1998). Consequently, this joint is unusually susceptible to strains, sprains, dislocations, and fractures.

Strains

A strain is a muscle injury. This includes the muscle tendon and the connective tissue by means of which the muscle is attached to the bone. Landing from jumping exposes the tendons of the ankle and foot muscles to the danger of strain. The impact of landing may force the ankle joints beyond their normal range of motion. This gives the Achilles tendon a sudden wrench that may cause tearing, either at the point of the tendon's attachment to the bone or at the junction between the tendon and the muscle belly. This is potentially a very debilitating injury requiring expert treatment.

The distal tendons of both the anterior and posterior tibial muscles are also subject to strain. The aftereffects of each of these can be quite troublesome, because they are both inverters (supinators) of the foot, in addition to which the posterior tibial helps support the longitudinal arch in weak feet or under exceptional stress.

Sprains

A sprained ankle is all too familiar. It results from a sudden wrench or twist and is usually associated with forced inversion of the foot with the lateral ligaments being stretched or torn and sometimes ruptured or pulled off of the bone. The affected ligaments are any of those on the lateral aspect of the ankle—the calcaneofibular, anterior talofibular, and posterior talofibular. The interosseous talocalcaneal ligament, although not strictly an ankle ligament, may also be affected.

Fractures

Ankle fractures are usually caused by a sudden wrenching or twisting, the same factors that cause sprains but, whereas sprains are the result of excessive inversion of the foot, fractures result from excessive eversion. The majority of ankle fractures occur to the malleoli, especially the lateral malleolus. In the more serious fractures some dislocation as the result of a separation between the tibia and fibula is also likely, with a consequent widening of the socket or mortise. Prompt and adequate treatment to restore the joint integrity is all important if permanent damage is to be avoided.

LABORATORY EXPERIENCES

Knee Joint: Joint Structure and Function

1. Record the essential information regarding the structure, ligaments, and cartilages of the knee joint. Study the movements both on the skeleton and on the living body and explain how the joint structure affects movements.

Muscular Action

Identify as many muscles as possible in the following experiments.

2. **Flexion at Knee**
   Subject: Lie face down and flex leg at knee by raising foot.
   Assistant: Steady subject's thigh and resist movement by pushing down on ankle.
   Observer: Palpate biceps femoris, semitendinosus, gracilis, sartorius, and gastrocnemius.

3. **Extension at Knee**
   a. *Subject:* Rise from a squat position.
      Observer: Palpate quadriceps femoris.
   b. *Subject:* Sit on table with legs hanging over edge. Extend leg.
      Assistant: Steady subject's thigh and resist movement by holding ankle down.
      Observer: Palpate quadriceps femoris.

4. **Outward Rotation of Leg with Knee in Flexed Position**
   Subject: Sit on table with legs hanging over edge. Rotate foot laterally as far as possible without moving thigh.

   Assistant: Steady subject's thigh and give slight resistance by holding foot.
   Observer: Palpate biceps femoris.

5. **Inward Rotation of Leg with Knee in Flexed Position**
   Subject: Sit on table with legs hanging over edge. Rotate foot medially as far as possible without moving thigh.
   Assistant: Steady subject's thigh and give slight resistance by holding foot.
   Observer: Palpate semitendinosus, gracilis, and sartorius.

Ankle and Foot: Joint Structure and Function

6. Record the essential information regarding the structure, ligaments, and cartilages of the ankle, subtalar, and midtarsal joints. Study the movements of these joints both on the skeleton and on the living body and explain how the joint structures affect the movements.

7. Using a goniometer, compare the total range of plantar and dorsiflexion of the ankle in a group of five or more subjects (a) with extension at the knee, and (b) with flexion at the knee.

8. Make a similar comparison between two groups, one consisting of three to five varsity-level swimmers and the other of the same number of recreational swimmers, or make a similar comparison between ballet and nonballet dancers.

Ankle and Foot: Muscular Action

Identify as many muscles as possible in the following experiments.

9. **Plantar Flexion**

   Subject: Perform each of the following actions:
   a. Stand and rise on the toes. b. Hold one foot off the floor and extend it vigorously.
   Observer: Compare the muscular action of the leg in a and b.

10. **Dorsiflexion**

    Subject: Sit on a table with the legs straight and with the feet over the edge. Dorsiflex one foot as far as possible.
    Assistant: Resist the movement by holding the foot.
    Observer: Identify the tibialis anterior, peroneus tertius, extensor digitorum longus, and extensor hallucis longus.

11. **Pronation (Eversion and Abduction)**

    Subject: In same starting position as in Laboratory Experience 10, pronate one foot without extending it.
    Assistant: Steady the leg at the ankle and resist the movement by holding one foot.
    Observer: Identify the muscles that contract.

12. **Supination (Inversion and Adduction)**

    Subject: In same position as in Laboratory Experience 10, supinate one foot as far as possible.
    Assistant: Steady the leg at the ankle and resist the movement by holding the foot.
    Observer: Identify the muscles that contract.

Kinesiological Analysis

13. Choose a simple motor skill from appendix H. Do a complete anatomical analysis of the lower extremity following the analysis outline in table 1.2.

REFERENCES AND SELECTED READINGS

Aagaard, P., E. B. Simonsen, S. P. Magnusson, B. Larson, and P. Dyhre-Poulsen. 1998. A new concept for isokinetic hamstring:quadriceps muscle strength ratio. *American Journal of Sports Medicine* 26:231–37.

Arnheim, D. D., and W. E. Prentice, 1998. *Essentials of athletic training.* 4th ed. St. Louis: McGraw-Hill.

Basmajian, J. V., and J. C. DeLuca. 1985. *Muscles alive.* 5th ed. Baltimore: Williams & Wilkins.

Cavanagh, P. R., E. Morag, A. J. M. Boulton, M. J. Young, K. T. Deffner, and S. E. Pammer. 1997. The relationship of static foot structure to dynamic foot function. *Journal of Biomechanics* 30:243–50.

Cicotti, M. G., R. K. Keran, J. Perry, and M. Pink. 1994. An electromyographic analysis of the knee during functional activities. 1. The normal profile. *American Journal of Sports Medicine* 22:645–50.

Cox, A. J. 1990. Biomechanics of the patello-femoral joint. *Clinical Biomechanics* 5:123–30.

Goss, C. M., ed. 1980. *Gray's anatomy of the human body.* 36th ed. Philadelphia: Lea & Febiger.

Hamilton, N., and H. Deutsch. 1994. Quadriceps muscle group activity related to hip angle and load. *Clinical Kinesiology* 48:55–60.

Nordin, M., and V. H. Frankel. 1989. *Basic biomechanics of the musculoskeletal system.* Philadelphia: Lea & Febiger.

Norkin, C., and P. Levangie. 1986. *Joint structure and function: A comprehensive analysis.* Philadelphia: F.A. Davis.

Stefanyshyn, D. J., and B. N. Nigg. 1997. Mechanical energy contribution of the metatarsophalangeal joint to running and sprinting. *Journal of Biomechanics* 30:1081–85.

Woodland, L. H., and R. S. Francis. 1992. Parameters and comparisons of the quadriceps angle of college-aged men and women in the supine and standing positions. *The American Journal of Sports Medicine* 20:208–11.

C H A P T E R

9

THE SPINAL COLUMN AND THORAX

O U T L I N E

■ *Structure and Articulations of the Spinal Column*
Articulations of the Vertebral Bodies
Ligamentous Reinforcement
Articulations of the Vertebral Arches
Atlanto-Occipital Articulation
Atlantoaxial Articulation
■ *Movements of the Spine as a Whole*
Individual Movements
Summary of Spinal Movements
Regional Classification of Spinal Movements
Summary of Factors Influencing Stability and Mobility of the Spine
■ *Muscles Operating the Spinal Column*
Location
Characteristics and Functions of Individual Spinal Muscles

■ *Muscular Analysis of the Fundamental Movements of the Head and Spine*
Cervical Spine and Atlanto-Occipital Joint
Thoracic and Lumbar Spine
■ *Structure and Articulations of the Thorax*
■ *Movements of the Thorax*
Enlargement of the Thorax in Inhalation
Phases of Respiration
■ *Muscles of Respiration*
Characteristics of Individual Muscles with Primary Function in Respiration
Characteristics of Individual Muscles with Secondary Function in Respiration
■ *Muscular Analysis of Respiration*
■ *Common Injuries of the Neck, Back, and Thorax*
■ *Laboratory Experiences*

215

OBJECTIVES

At the conclusion of this chapter, the student should be able to:

1. Name, locate, and describe the structures and ligamentous reinforcements of the articulations of the spinal column and thorax.
2. Name and demonstrate the movements possible in joints of the spinal column and thorax, regardless of starting position.
3. Name and locate the muscles and muscle groups of the spinal column and thorax and name their primary actions as agonists, stabilizers, neutralizers, or antagonists.
4. Analyze the fundamental movements of the spinal column and thorax with respect to joint and muscle actions.
5. Describe the common injuries of the spinal column and thorax.
6. Perform an anatomical analysis of the movements of the spinal column in a motor skill.

STRUCTURE AND ARTICULATIONS OF THE SPINAL COLUMN

If you were faced with the problem of devising a single mechanism that would simultaneously (1) give stability to a collapsible cylinder, (2) permit movement in all directions and yet always return to the fundamental starting position, (3) support three structures of considerable weight (a globe, a yoke, and a cage), (4) provide attachment for numerous flexible bands and elastic cords, (5) transmit a gradually increasing weight to a rigid basinlike foundation, (6) act as a shock absorber for cushioning jolts and jars, and (7) encase and protect a cord of extreme delicacy, you would be staggered by the immensity of the task. Yet the spinal column fulfills all these requirements with amazing efficiency. It is at the same time an organ of stability and mobility, of support and protection, and of resistance and adaptation. It is an instrument of great precision, yet of robust structure. Its architecture and the manner in which it performs its many functions are worthy of careful study. From the kinesiological point of view, we are interested in the spine chiefly as a mechanism for maintaining erect posture and for permitting movement of the head, neck, and trunk.

To understand these functions of the spine, it is necessary to have a clear picture, first of the spinal column as a whole and second of the distinguishing characteristics of the different regions. The spinal column, consisting of seven cervical, twelve thoracic, and five lumbar vertebrae, the sacrum (five fused sacral vertebrae), and the coccyx (three to five fused vertebrae), presents four curves as seen from the side (figure 9.1). At birth, the vertebral column is convex backward. The thoracic and sacrococcygeal curves remain convex to the rear and are considered primary curves. The cervical and lumbar curves reverse direction of the curvature during infancy and early childhood and are referred to as secondary curves. The curvature at the cervical region develops when the infant raises its head; the lumbar region develops its anterior convexity when the infant assumes an upright posture and begins to walk. The curves are a response to gravity and continue to develop through puberty.

An exaggerated curve in the thoracic region is referred to as a kyphosis, and one in the lumbar

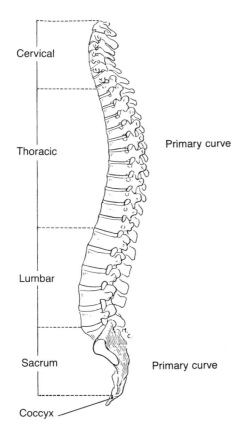

Cervical

Thoracic

Primary curve

Lumbar

Sacrum

Primary curve

Coccyx

Figure 9.1 Lateral view of the spinal column showing anteroposterior curves.

There are two sets of interspinal articulations, those between the vertebral bodies and those between the vertebral arches. The latter are in pairs, with one on either side of each vertebra. The articulations of the first two vertebrae are atypical and will be described separately.

Such a close relationship exists between the structure of the spinal column and the movements that take place in its different regions that the student will find it well worth the effort to acquire a thorough grasp of the structure, particularly of the joints, before proceeding to the movements. If possible, both a skeleton and a strung set of vertebrae should be referred to frequently while studying spinal structure.

Articulations of the Vertebral Bodies

These joints (figure 9.2) are classified as synchondroses or cartilaginous joints. The bodies of the vertebrae are united by means of fibrocartilages, otherwise known as intervertebral discs. These correspond to the surfaces of the adjacent vertebral bodies, except in the cervical region, where they are smaller from side to side. They adhere to the hyaline cartilage both above and below, with no articular cavity in this type of joint. In thickness they are fairly uniform in the thoracic region, but in the cervical and lumbar regions they are thicker in front than in back. Altogether, they constitute one-fourth the length of the spinal column. Each disc consists of two parts, an outer fibrous rim and an inner pulpy nucleus known as the nucleus pulposus. This is a ball of firmly compressed elastic material, a little like the center of a golf ball. It constitutes a center of motion and permits compression in any direction, as well as torsion. The intervertebral discs are also important as shock absorbers, resisting compressive forces.

The discs consist of a large percentage (80 to 90 percent) of water. With advancing age, this fluid is absorbed and the discs shrink and become brittle. This change is noticeable in the reduced height and a significant increase in disc problems in older people.

region is referred to as a lordosis. Kyphotic curves have a backward convexity. Lordotic curves have a forward convex curve. A lateral deviation of the spine is called a scoliosis. Any significant deviation from the expected gradual curves as well as misalignments among the vertebrae may seriously affect an individual's movement capabilities or predispose a person to injury.

From the first cervical to the fifth lumbar vertebra, the vertebral bodies become increasingly larger. This is an important factor in fulfilling the weight-bearing role of the spine. The vertebral bodies decrease in size from the first sacral through the coccygeal region. The sacral vertebrae complete the pelvic girdle, which transmits the weight of the head and trunk onto both femoral heads.

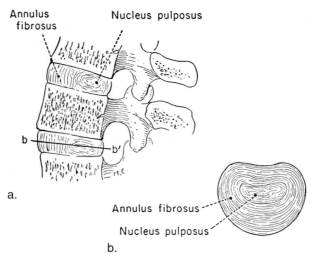

Figure 9.2   (a) Sagittal section of lumbar vertebrae and intervertebral fibrocartilages. (b) Transverse section of intervertebral fibrocartilage, through b-b′.

Ligamentous Reinforcement

The joints of the spinal column are reinforced by several ligaments (figures 9.3 and 9.4). The vertebral bodies are held together by two long ligaments, one in front and one in back. The anterior longitudinal ligament starts as a narrow band and widens as it descends from the occipital bone to the sacrum. The posterior longitudinal ligament, descending from the occipital bone to the coccyx, is relatively narrow throughout but has lateral expansions opposite each intervertebral fibrocartilage. Both ligaments are stronger in the thoracic region than in either the cervical or the lumbar region (table 9.1).

Articulations of the Vertebral Arches

The articulations (figure 9.5) between the facets of the vertebral arches are nonaxial diarthrodial joints. Each of these joints has an articular cavity and is enclosed within a capsule. A slight amount of gliding motion is permitted. The resultant movement of each vertebra is determined largely by the direction in which the articular facets face. The cervical spine appears to be somewhat of an exception, however. The facets in this region slant at about a 45 degree angle, lying halfway between the horizontal and the frontal planes (figure 9.6a). Such a slant would seem to favor rotation and lateral flexion and to be unfavorable to flexion and hyperextension. Yet these latter movements occur as freely as does lateral flexion, whereas rotation from the second cervical vertebra down can be rated as only moderate. In the thoracic region they lie slightly more in the frontal and less in the horizontal plane than do the cervical articulations, and they have a slight inward and outward slant (figure 9.6b). The upper facets face backward, slightly upward, and lateralward; the lower facets face forward, slightly downward, and medialward. They are adapted equally well to rotation and to lateral bending. In the lumbar region, except at the lumbosacral articulation, the articular facets lie more nearly in the sagittal plane (figure 9.6c). The upper facets face inward and slightly backward; the lower facets face outward and slightly forward. Furthermore, the upper facets present slightly concave surfaces and the lower facets convex. By this arrangement of the facets, the lumbar vertebrae are virtually locked

Figure 9.3   Anterior longitudinal ligament of the spine: (a) anterior view; (b) sagittal section of vertebrae showing lateral view of ligament.

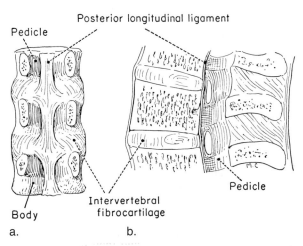

Figure 9.4   Posterior longitudinal ligament of spine: (a) frontal section of vertebrae showing posterior view of ligament; (b) sagittal section of vertebrae showing lateral view of ligament.

against rotation. The slight amount of rotation that does occur is made possible by the looseness of the capsules. At the lumbosacral articulation the facets lie somewhat more in the frontal plane than is true of the other lumbar joints.

The ligaments reinforcing these joints may be identified in figure 9.7. The ligamenta flava and the interspinous and supraspinous ligaments are all thickest and strongest in the lumbar region. There remain two rather thin ligaments, the inter-

transverse, connecting the transverse processes of adjacent vertebrae, and the ligamentum nuchae, which is the continuation of the supraspinous ligament in the cervical region (see table 9.1).

Atlanto-Occipital Articulation

This is the articulation (figure 9.8) between the head and the neck. It consists of a pair of joints, one on each side. Each condyle of the occipital

TABLE 9.1	Ligaments of the Vertebral Column	
Ligaments	**Function**	**Region**
Anterior longitudinal	Limits extension. Reinforces anterior portion of annulus fibrosus.	Axis to sacrum well developed in lumbar and thoracic
Anterior atlantoaxial (continuation of anterior longitudinal ligament)	Limits extension.	Axis and atlas
Posterior longitudinal	Limits flexion. Reinforces posterior portion of annulus fibrosus.	Axis to sacrum
Ligamentum flavum	Limits flexion, especially in lumbar area.	Axis to sacrum
Ligamentum nuchae (continuation of the supraspinous ligaments)	Limits flexion.	Cervical region
Supraspinous Posterior atlantoaxial (continuation of ligamentum flavum)	Limits flexion. Limits flexion.	Thoracic and lumbar Atlas and axis
Tectorial membrane (continuation of posterior longitudinal ligament)	Limits flexion.	Axis to occipital bone
Interspinous	Limits flexion.	Primarily lumbar
Intertransverse	Limits lateral flexion.	Primarily lumbar
Alar	Limits rotation of head to same side and lateral flexion to opposite side.	Axis to skull

From: C. Norkin and P. Levangie, *Joint Structure and Function: A Comprehensive Analysis,* p. 128. Copyright © 1983 F. A. Davis, Philadelphia. Reprinted by permission.

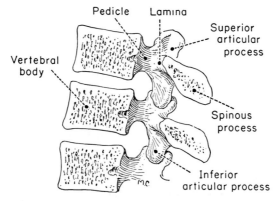

Figure 9.5 Sagittal section of vertebrae showing articulations of the vertebral arches.

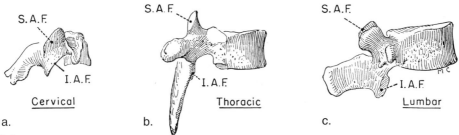

Figure 9.6 Articular facets of vertebrae: (a) cervical; (b) thoracic; (c) lumbar. (S.A.F. = Superior articular facet. I.A.F. = Inferior articular facet.)

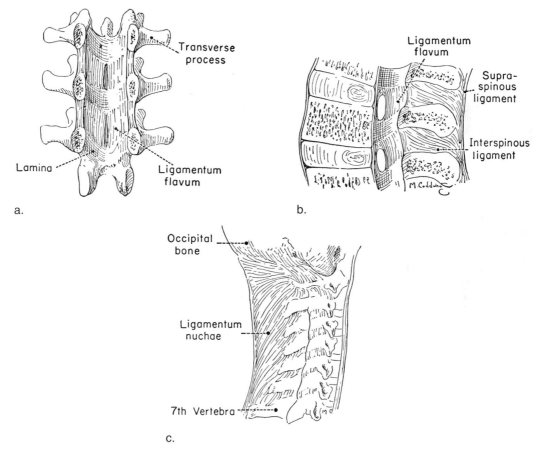

Figure 9.7 Ligaments of vertebral articulations: (a) frontal section of three lumbar vertebrae showing anterior view of vertebral arches and ligamentum flavum; (b) sagittal view of lumbar vertebrae showing ligaments of vertebral arches; (c) side view of cervical spine showing ligamentum nuchae.

bone of the skull articulates with the corresponding superior articular fossa of the first vertebra, known as the atlas. Each articulation by itself belongs to the condyloid (ovoid) classification, but the movement that occurs in the two joints together is more like that of a hinge joint. The rigid relationship between the two joints results in a restriction of the lateral motion that would normally

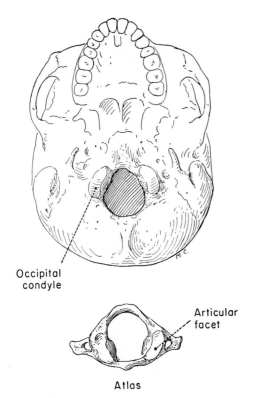

Occipital
condyle

Articular
facet

Atlas

Figure 9.8   Bones forming atlanto-occipital
articulation.

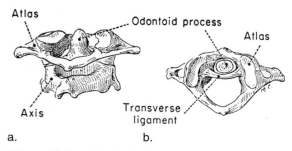

a.   b.

Figure 9.9   Atlantoaxial articulation: (a) posterior
view; (b) superior view.

occur in an ovoid joint. The movements that take place at the atlanto-occipital articulation are chiefly flexion and extension, with a slight amount of lateral flexion (figure 9.10a and b). Combining these four motions results in limited circumduction. There is no rotation.

Atlantoaxial Articulation

This is a perfect example of a pivot joint—a joint whose sole function is rotation (figure 9.9). The toothlike peg (odontoid process, or dens) that projects upward from the second cervical vertebra, otherwise known as the axis, or epistropheus, fits into the ring formed by the inner surface of the anterior arch of atlas and the transverse ligament that bridges across the tips of the arch. Because no rotation occurs at the atlanto-occipital joint, rotation of atlas on axis will carry the head

with it; thus the movement occurring at the atlantoaxial joint contributes to the movement of the head on the trunk (figure 9.10c).

MOVEMENTS OF THE SPINE AS A WHOLE

Individual Movements

The movements of the spinal column, which resemble those of a ball-and-socket joint, are described as follows.

Flexion

This is a forward-downward bending in the sagittal plane about a frontal-horizontal axis (figure 9.11a). It involves a compression of the anterior parts of the intervertebral discs and a gliding motion of the articular processes. It occurs more freely in the cervical, upper thoracic, and lumbar regions. The cervical curve may be reduced to a straight line and the lumbar curve, in flexible individuals, may be reversed. The greatest anteroposterior motion in the lumbar spine usually occurs between the fifth lumbar vertebra and the sacrum.

Extension and Hyperextension

Extension is the return movement from flexion (figure 9.11b). Hyperextension is a backward-downward movement in the sagittal plane. It occurs most freely in the cervical and lumbar regions, and particularly at the lumbosacral junction. In the thoracic region, hyperextension is

Figure 9.10   Movements of the head and neck: (a) flexion, extension, and hyperextension; (b) lateral flexion; (c) rotation.

limited by the overlapping of the spinous processes.

Lateral Flexion

This is a sideward bending in the frontal plane about a sagittal-horizontal axis (figure 9.11c). It is freest in the cervical region and quite free in the lumbar region and at the thoracolumbar junction, but it is limited in the thoracic region by the pres-ence of the ribs. Each rib (except the 1st, 10th, 11th, and 12th) articulates with two adjacent ver-tebrae and the intervening disc, and each rib (ex-cept the 11th and 12th) articulates with the trans-verse process of the lower of the two vertebrae (figure 9.12). Thus the ribs serve as splints, re-stricting lateral flexion of the thoracic spine to a marked degree. It is amazing that any motion can take place there at all.

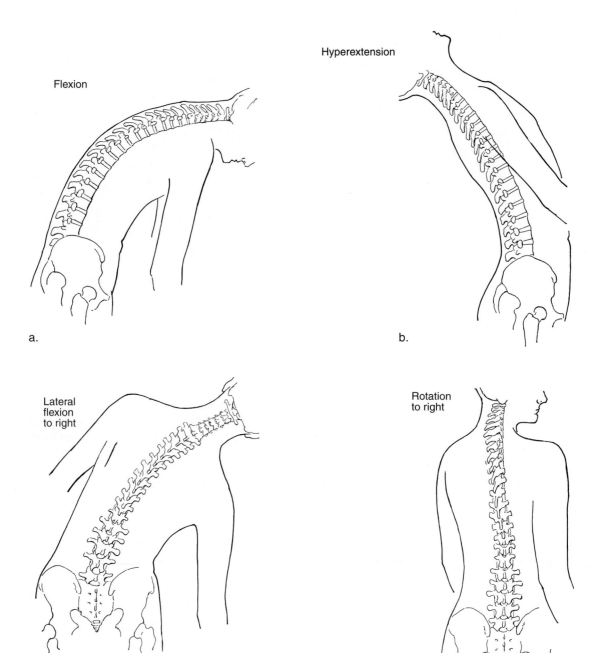

Figure 9.11   Movements of the spinal column.

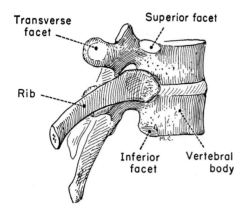

Figure 9.12 Articulation of a rib with two adjacent vertebrae.

For several reasons—the slant of the articular processes, the presence of the anteroposterior curves of the spine, and muscular and ligamentous tensions—lateral flexion is always accompanied by a certain amount of torsion. When lateral flexion is performed from the erect position, the maximum movement occurs in the lumbar region and at the thoracolumbar junction, with only slight involvement of the lower thoracic spine. (The cervical spine is excluded from this discussion.) The torsion occurs in the same part of the spine and consists in a turning of the vertebral bodies toward the side of the lateral flexion. Thus, if the spine bends to the right (forming a curve concave to the right), the vertebral bodies of the lumbar and lower thoracic vertebrae turn slightly to the right, with the spinous processes, therefore, turning to the left.

If the lateral flexion is performed from a position of hyperextension, and the hyperextension is maintained throughout the movement, the lateral flexion moves lower in the spine, occurring almost entirely below the eleventh thoracic vertebra. The torsion occurs in this same region and in the same manner that it does when the lateral flexion is performed from the erect position. The position of hyperextension seems to lock the thoracic spine against lateral movements.

If the lateral flexion is performed from a position of forward flexion, the movement occurs higher in the spine than ordinarily, the greatest deviation being at the level of the eighth thoracic

vertebra. The torsion in this case reverses itself. Thus, in a side bend to the right, the vertebral bodies turn to the left and the spinous processes to the right. This reversal is not inconsistent. It is directly related to the anteroposterior curves of the spine. In the first two examples—that is, when the lateral flexion is performed either from the erect or from the hyperextended position—most of the movement takes place in the lower part of the spine, the part that is concave to the rear. The rotation that accompanies the side bend in these two cases is called concave side rotation because the bodies turn in the direction of the concave, or inner, side of the laterally curved spine. When the side bend is performed from the flexed position, most of the movement takes place in the thoracic spine, the region that is convex to the rear. The rotation that accompanies the lateral flexion in this case is called convex side rotation because the vertebral bodies turn in the direction of the convex, or outer, side of the laterally curved spine.

Rotation

This is a rotary movement of the spine in the horizontal plane about a vertical (longitudinal) axis (see figure 9.11d). Spinal rotation is named by the way the front of the upper spine turns with reference to the lower part. Thus, a turning of the head and shoulders to the right constitutes rotation to the right. A turning of the legs and pelvis to the left, without turning the upper part of the body, also constitutes rotation of the spine to the right since the anatomical relationships are the same as in the former example. The movement of rotation is most free in the cervical region, with 90 percent of the movement being attributed to the atlantoaxial joint. It is next most free in the thoracic region and at the thoracolumbar junction. Owing to the interlocking of the articular processes, it is extremely limited in the lumbar region, there being only about 5 degrees of rotation to each side. In the cervical region there is no rotation between the atlas and the skull, but free rotation at the pivot joint between atlas and axis. Whenever rotation occurs in the spine, it is accompanied by a slight amount of unavoidable lateral flexion to the same side.

When performed from the erect position, rotation of the spine (below the seventh cervical vertebra) occurs almost entirely in the thoracic region. When performed from the position of hyperextension, the movement shifts lower in the spine, occurring in the vicinity of the thoracolumbar junction. When performed from the flexed position, the rotation is higher than usual, occurring in the upper thoracic spine. Regardless of the position in which the rotation is performed—whether erect, flexed, or hyperextended—the slight lateral flexion that accompanies it is always to the same side as the rotation. Thus if the spine rotates to the left, it flexes slightly to the left. This movement is very slight, however, and can scarcely be detected.

Circumduction

This is a circular movement of the upper trunk on the lower, a combination of flexion, lateral flexion, and hyperextension, but not including rotation.

Summary of Spinal Movements

Flexion; extension; hyperextension
> Free in all three regions
> Cervical and thoracic curves may be reduced to straight lines
> Limited hyperextension in thoracic region due to downward orientation of spinous processes
> Lumbar curve may be reversed in flexible subjects

Lateral flexion
> Free in cervical and lumbar regions
> Limited in thoracic region by rib attachments
> Accompanied by torsion

Rotation
> Freest at top of spine, least free at bottom
> Limited in lumbar region due to superior and inferior articular surfaces oriented in sagittal plane
> Accompanied by slight lateral flexion

Circumduction
> Sequential combination of flexion, lateral flexion, and hyperextension

Regional Classification of Spinal Movements

Atlanto-occipital joint
> Flexion and extension
> Hyperextension
> Slight lateral flexion

Atlantoaxial joint
> Rotation

Remaining cervical joints
> Free flexion and extension
> Free hyperextension
> Free lateral flexion
> Free rotation

Thoracic region
> Moderate flexion
> Slight hyperextension (inhibited by spinous processes)
> Moderate lateral flexion (inhibited by ribs)
> Free rotation

Lumbar region
> Moderate to free flexion and extension
> Free hyperextension
> Free lateral flexion
> Slight rotation (inhibited by orientation of articular surfaces)

Summary of Factors Influencing Stability and Mobility of the Spine

Before considering the muscular analysis of the spinal movements it is advisable to review some of the special characteristics that contribute to the spine's stability and modify its mobility in one way or another.

Pressure and Tension Stresses

The tendency of the compressed intervertebral discs to push the vertebrae apart, combined with the tendency of the ligaments to press them together, is an important factor in the stability of the spinal column. Throughout life the discs are the main shock-absorbing mechanisms in the vertebral column.

Anteroposterior Curves

The alternating anteroposterior curves of the spinal column influence the nature and the degree of movements that occur in the different regions. Individual variations from the so-called normal curves cause variations in the movement patterns. The anteroposterior curves are said to serve as a safeguard against the development of abnormal lateral curves (curvature of the spine, scoliosis).

Relative Thickness and Shape of the Intervertebral Discs

There is a direct relationship between the thickness of the discs and the degree of movement permitted, with greater freedom of motion where the discs are thick.

Thickness and Strength of the Ligaments

These differ in the different regions and have a corresponding influence on the motions permitted in each region (see table 9.1).

Direction and Obliquity of the Articular Facets

These are characteristic for each region and play an important part in determining the type of motion permitted in each.

Size and Obliquity of the Spinous Processes

These overlap like shingles in the thoracic region, hence limiting hyperextension. In the lumbar region they are horizontal and, although they are wide, they do not restrict motion.

Articulations of the Ribs with the Vertebrae

These limit lateral flexion in the thoracic region.

MUSCLES OPERATING THE SPINAL COLUMN

Location

The muscles responsible for the movements of the spine, with the exception of two groups, have at least one attachment on the spinal column or the skull. The exceptions are the abdominal and the hyoid muscles. Both groups are superficially located on the front of the body. Nevertheless, both groups, the abdominal muscles in particular, are effective movers or stabilizers of the spine. The muscles are listed according to aspect and region.

Anterior Aspect

Cervical Region

    Prevertebral muscles (longus capitis and colli, rectus capitis anterior, and lateralis)

    Hyoid muscles (suprahyoids and infrahyoids)

Thoracic and Lumbar Regions

    Abdominal muscles

        Obliquus externus abdominis

        Obliquus internus abdominis

        Rectus abdominis

        Transversus abdominis

Posterior Aspect

Cervical Region Only

    Splenius capitis and cervicis

    Suboccipitals (rectus capitis posterior major and minor, obliquus capitis superior and inferior)

Cervical, Thoracic, and Lumbar Regions

    Erector spinae (iliocostalis, longissimus, and spinalis)

    Deep posterior spinal muscles (multifidi, rotatores, interspinales, intertransversarii, and levatores costarum)

    Semispinalis thoracis, cervicis, and capitis

Lateral Aspect

Cervical Region

 Scalenus anterior, posterior, and medius (commonly called the three scalenes)

 Sternocleidomastoid

 Levator scapulae

Lumbar Region

 Quadratus lumborum

 Psoas major

Characteristics and Functions of Individual Spinal Muscles

Anterior Aspect

Prevertebral Muscles   As figure 9.13 shows, the longus colli and capitis extend vertically up the front of the vertebrae, the colli from the upper three thoracic to the first cervical (atlas) and the capitis from the lower cervical to the occipital bone. The rectus capitis muscles pass obliquely upward from the atlas to the skull, the anterior slanting medially and the lateralis laterally. With the exception of the longus colli, these muscles flex the head and neck when the left and right muscles act together. Acting separately, they flex the head and neck laterally or rotate it to the opposite side. The longus colli acts only on the neck and is active in resisted forward flexion, resisted lateral flexion, and rotation to the same side. It also stabilizes the neck during coughing, talking, and swallowing.

Hyoid muscles   Also called the strap muscles, these are small anterior muscles in the cervical region (figure 9.14). There are four suprahyoids and four infrahyoids. Together they flex the head and neck. They are primarily muscles of some phase of swallowing, but they contract in cervical flexion whenever the movement is performed against resistance. By neutralizing one another's pull on the hyoid bone their action is transferred to the head and thence to the cervical spine. They may be palpated just below the jaw bone.

Abdominal Muscles

Obliquus externus abdominis   The fibers of this muscle (figure 9.15) run diagonally upward

Figure 9.13   Prevertebral muscles of cervical spine (anterior view).

and outward from the lower part of the abdomen, the two muscles together forming an incomplete letter V, as seen from the front. When both sides contract they flex the thoracic and lumbar spine against gravity or other resistance. When only one side contracts in combination with other anterior, lateral, and posterior muscles on the same side, it *flexes the spine laterally*. When it combines with other spinal rotators, it rotates the spine to the opposite side—that is, the right muscle *rotates the spine to the left*.

Investigators have found that external obliques show the greatest activity in movements performed from the supine position such as forward and/or lateral flexion. Both of the obliques have been found to increase activity in order to stabilize the spine in response to applied loads or to support lower-limb motion. In addition the external and internal obliques working together were found to show activity during a Valsalva maneuver (holding the breath while contracting the abdominal muscles forcefully). The external oblique may be palpated at the side of the abdomen.

Obliquus internus abdominis   This muscle (figure 9.16) lies beneath (i.e., deeper than) the external oblique. Its fibers fan out from the crest of the ilium, most of them passing diagonally

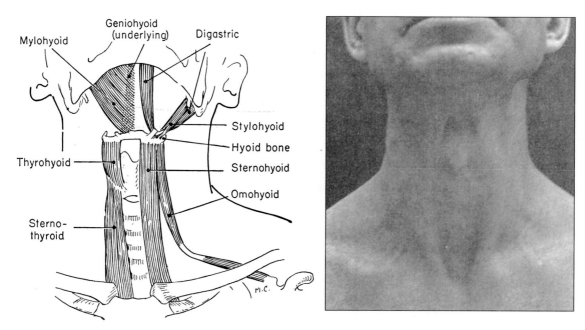

Figure 9.14   Hyoid muscles (anterior view).

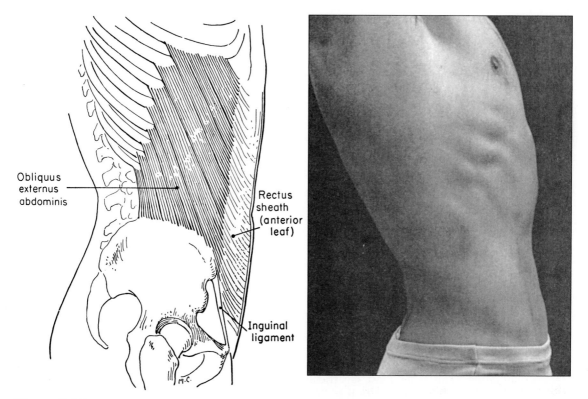

Figure 9.15   External oblique abdominal muscle (obliquus externus abdominis).

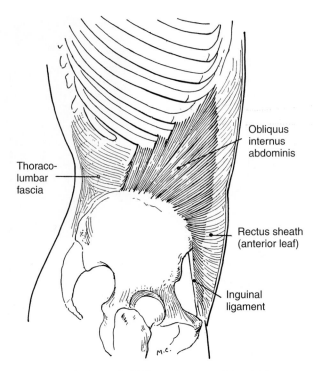

Figure 9.16   Internal oblique abdominal muscle (obliquus internus abdominis).

forward and upward toward the rib cartilages and sternum, some horizontally forward toward the linea alba, and some diagonally forward and downward toward the crest of the pubis. Of the three abdominal muscles acting on the spine, this one is most active in rotation. EMG experiments have also shown it to have marked activity in leaning backward and in decreasing the pelvic tilt from the supine position during leg raising and lowering (hip flexion/extension), although these functions may vary with individuals (Shields and Heiss 1997). In summary, the internal oblique *flexes the lumbar and thoracic spine, flexes the spine laterally, and rotates the spine to the same side*. It may be palpated at the side of the abdomen, below the external oblique. It may also be palpated through the external oblique when the latter is relaxed, as in rotation.

Rectus abdominis   This is the most superficial of the abdominal muscles (figure 9.17). It is situ-

ated on the anterior surface of the abdomen on either side of the linea alba. It is a long, flat band of muscle fibers extending longitudinally between the pubis and the lower part of the chest. At three different levels transverse fibrous bands known as tendinous inscriptions cross the muscle fibers. The muscle is enclosed within a sheath formed by the aponeuroses of the other muscles making up the abdominal wall. The upper rectus was found to be more active in exercises involving the upper part of the body, such as spine flexion from the supine position. The lower rectus was found to be more active in moments involving a decrease of pelvic tilt, such as in the supine position bending the knees and lifting them toward the face until the fifth lumbar vertebra is raised approximately 5 inches above the supporting surface (Sarti et al. 1996). In brief, the rectus abdominis *flexes the lumbar and thoracic spine*, and *one side working alone helps flex the spine laterally*. The muscle may be palpated on the front of the abdomen

Figure 9.17   Rectus abdominis.

about 2 or 3 inches from the midline, from the pubis to the sternum.

Transversus abdominis   This muscle (figure 9.18) is made up of a broad sheet of fibers that run horizontally from the thoracolumbar fascia and cartilages of the lower ribs forward to the linea alba. Unlike the other abdominal muscles, it is not a mover of the spinal column; its pull is inward against the abdominal viscera, and hence it is a strong muscle of exhalation and expulsion. It does, however, help *stabilize the trunk* when acts requiring great effort are performed and may be primarily responsible for the maintenance of intra-abdominal pressure during lifting.

The Abdominal Muscles as Spinal Flexors
The rectus abdominis and the external and internal obliques work together to flex the lumbar and thoracic spine. They play a small part, however, in flexing the spine from an erect position. This movement is produced by the force of gravity and controlled by the extensors in eccentric contraction. The only circumstance that would necessitate continued contraction of the abdominal muscles would be if the spine were being flexed against resistance, such as would occur if a person were lifting a weight by pulling down on a pulley rope and supplementing arm strength by flexing the spine instead of by the more efficient method of bending the knees and using the body weight.

The abdominal muscles are markedly active when the spine is being flexed from a supine position, especially at the beginning of this movement before the hips start to flex. Their activity is increased if a weight is held against the chest or on top of the head. (Obviously, the head and

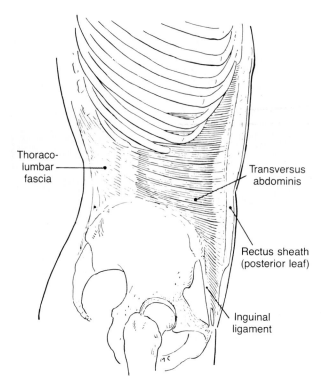

Figure 9.18   Transversus abdominis.

neck flexors are also working hard.) Once the hips start to flex, the abdominal muscles play a double role—namely, as movers in flexing the spine and as stabilizers of the pelvis against the pull of the hip flexors. When a straight spine sit-up is performed, the abdominal muscles do not act as movers at all. In this exercise, the trunk as a whole is flexing at the hip joints on the lower extremities. As the hip flexors are attached to the movable pelvis, the latter needs to be stabilized against their pull, and this is done by means of the static contraction of the abdominal muscles. If the latter are not strong enough to prevent the tilting of the pelvis, the abdominal action then becomes an involuntary eccentric or lengthening contraction. If the student is thoroughly familiar with the attachments of the abdominal muscles, he or she will know that they cannot be movers

in this exercise because they *do not cross the hip joints.*

The abdominal wall   The abdominal wall consists of the four abdominal muscles. Together, these muscles form a strong anterior support for the abdominal viscera. They are subject to considerable stress from the pressure of the latter against their inner surface. The more stretched they become, as in the case of a protruding abdomen, the more heavily the organs rest upon the abdominal wall, subjecting it to direct gravitational stress. Thus a vicious circle is set in motion. The pressure against the lower abdominal wall stretches it still more, causing its protrusion to increase and subjecting it to ever-increasing gravitational stress. As is so often the case, correction of this postural fault is much more diffi-

Figure 9.19   Posterior and lateral muscles of cervical spine.

cult than its prevention. A strong abdominal wall
is greatly to be desired.

Posterior Aspect

Splenius capitis and cervicis   These two muscles consist of bands of parallel fibers, slanting
outward as they ascend from their centrally located lower attachments to their more laterally located upper attachments. The capitis is much
broader than the cervicis. Figure 9.19 clearly
shows the left cervicis and the right capitis muscles. The viewer should try to visualize both muscles on both sides. When the left and right sides
contract together, they serve to *extend and hyperextend the head and neck.* They also help support
the head in erect posture. One side contracting
alone can *flex the head and neck laterally and
also rotate them to the same side.* The muscles
may be palpated on the back of the neck just lateral to the trapezius and posterior to the sternocleidomastoid above the levator scapulae, especially if the head is extended against resistance in

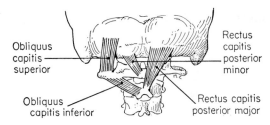

Figure 9.20   Suboccipital muscles (posterior view).

the prone position and the shoulders are kept relaxed. It is difficult to identify them, however.

Suboccipital group   This is a group of four
short muscles (figure 9.20) situated at the back of
the lower skull (occipital bone) and upper two
vertebrae (atlas and axis). It includes the obliquus
capitis superior and inferior, and the rectus capitis
posterior major and minor. Acting together on
both sides, this group extends and hyperextends
the head. When one side acts alone it *flexes the
head laterally or rotates it to the same side.*

Erector spinae   The muscle (figure 9.21) commences as a large mass in the lumbosacral region but soon divides into three branches.

The *iliocostalis* branch consists of lumbar, thoracic, and cervical portions that are named *lumborum, thoracis, and cervicis,* respectively. It receives an additional tendon of origin from each rib throughout the thoracic region and gives off small slips to insert into the ribs in the thoracic region and into the transverse processes of the vertebrae in the cervical region.

The *longissimus* branch consists of three distinct portions that, in fact, appear to be three separate muscles (figure 9.21). *Longissimus thoracis* is a broad band lying against the angles of the ribs, *longissimus cervicis* is narrower and lies slightly closer to the spine, connecting the transverse processes of the upper thoracic vertebrae with those of the lower cervical vertebrae, and *longissimus capitis* is a thin strand that lies against the vertebrae for its lower two-thirds and then slants outward and upward to the mastoid process of the temporal bone.

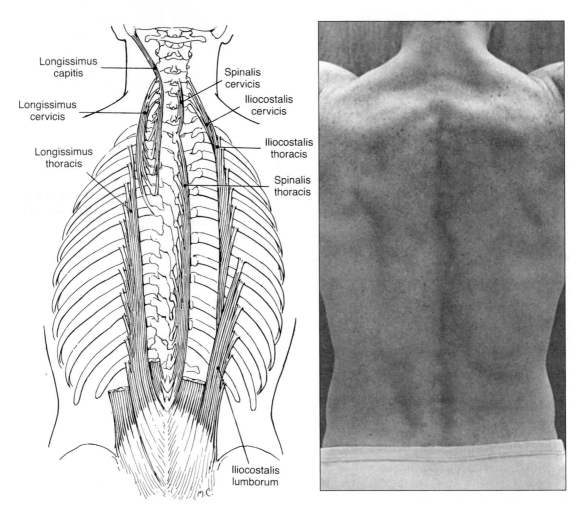

Figure 9.21   The erector spinae.

The *spinalis* branch lies against the vertebrae and is attached by separate slips to the spinous processes. It is of significance in the thoracic region only.

Electromyographic studies have shown that the erector spinae contributes little to the maintenance of erect posture unless a deliberate effort is made to extend the thoracic spine more completely or unless the weight is carried forward over the balls of the feet, in which case some static contraction of the muscle is required. In ordinary standing the level of activity is quite low (Basmajian and DeLuca 1985).

In forward flexion from the standing position, the erector spinae undergoes eccentric contraction until the weight of the trunk is supported by the ligaments. When the trunk returns from this position the muscle contracts concentrically until the body is again erect and balanced (Basmajian and DeLuca 1985). However, many times the lumbar region of this muscle does not become active to initiate the return from full flexion and often there are moments when this muscle is quiet during continued extension.

Dolan, Mannion, and Adams (1994), among others, have found that from 16 percent to 31 percent of force generated in extension can be explained by "passive" tissues. These passive elements may include intervertebral discs, ligaments, the series elastic component of muscle, or other structures. Pauly (1966) found that in almost all vigorous exercises performed from the standing position, the most active part of the erector spinae was the spinalis and the least active was the iliocostalis lumborum. The muscle engages most forcefully in its functions of extension, hyperextension, and lateral flexion when these movements are performed against gravity or other resistance. Hyperextension from the prone lying position is considered the best exercise for strengthening the erector spinae (Pauly 1966).

In brief, when the two sides of the muscle contract with equal force, the erector spinae *extends the head and spine* (assuming that all of its branches are contracting). When one side contracts alone, especially in conjunction with lateral and anterior muscles of the same side, it causes lateral flexion. And when one side alone contracts in a certain precise combination with lateral and anterior muscles—some on the same side, some on the opposite side—it rotates the head and spine to its own side. The lumbar and lower thoracic portions of the muscle may be palpated in the two broad ridges on either side of the spine.

Deep posterior spinal muscles   This group (figure 9.22) includes the multifidi, rotatores, interspinales, intertransversarii, and levatores costarum. The latter is primarily a muscle of the thorax but is included here as a possible assistant in extension and lateral flexion. These muscles consist of small slips, in most cases inserting into the vertebrae immediately above their lower attachments. Some of the fibers run vertically, and some slant medially as they ascend. The former are best developed in the cervical and lumbar regions where their action is that of extension. The latter are best developed in the thoracic region where they either extend or rotate. It has been suggested that the muscles in this group are responsible for localized movements. It seems likely that they also help stabilize the spine. In brief, acting symmetrically they *extend and hyperextend the spine* and acting asymmetrically they *rotate the spine to the opposite side and assist in lateral flexion.*

Semispinalis thoracis, cervicis, and capitis   These muscles (figure 9.23) lie close to the vertebrae beneath the erector spinae. The thoracis and cervicis portions consist of small bundles of fibers that slant medially as they ascend to the spinous processes several vertebrae above. The lower portion of the semispinalis capitis—that is, the portion starting from the upper thoracic vertebrae—has a slight medial slant, but the bundles in the cervical region attaching to the occipital bone are vertical. Like the muscles in the preceding group they extend and hyperextend the thoracic and cervical spine when both sides contract

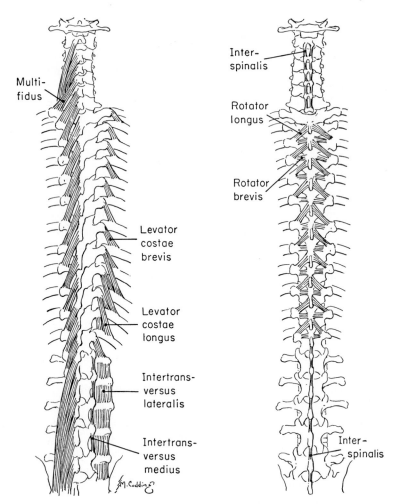

Figure 9.22   Deep posterior muscles of the spine including part of the transversospinalis (multifidus, rotators, and semispinalis).

together, and when only one side contracts they cause *lateral flexion and rotation to the opposite side.*

Transversospinalis   This is not a different muscle from those already listed but represents a different organization of the deep muscles of the back. Some texts use this term for the three spinal muscles whose fibers slant medially as they ascend, namely the *semispinalis, multifidi, and rotatores* (see figures 9.22 and 9.23).

Thoracolumbar fascia   Although not a muscle, the thoracolumbar fascia (see figure 9.18) is described here because of its importance to the deep muscles of the spine and erector spinae. It binds these muscles together, holding them close to the skeletal structure and separating them from the more superficial muscles of the back. In the lumbar region it curves around the lateral margin of the erector spinae and folds in front of it to attach to the tips of the transverse processes of the vertebrae and to the intertransverse ligaments. Its lat-

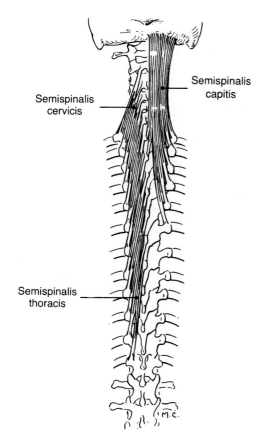

Figure 9.23   Semispinalis (posterior view), including part of the transversospinalis (multifidus and rotators).

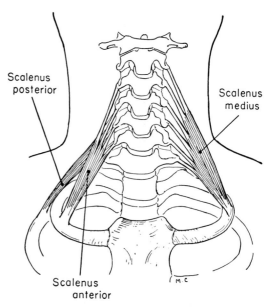

Figure 9.24   The scalenes: anterior, posterior, and medius (anterior view).

eral portion provides attachment for the transverse abdominis (see figure 9.18), and its posterior portion blends with the aponeurosis of the latissimus dorsi (see figure 5.14).

Lateral Aspect

Scalenus anterior, posterior, and medius   The three scalenes (figure 9.24) run diagonally upward from the sides of the two upper ribs to the transverse processes of the cervical vertebrae. Acting together, they flex the cervical spine and, acting on one side at a time, they *flex the neck laterally.* They also serve to elevate the upper ribs in forced inspiration. They may be palpated on the side of the neck between the sternocleidomastoid

and the upper trapezius but are difficult to identify (Basmajian and DeLuca 1985).

Sternocleidomastoid   This muscle (figure 9.25) arises from two heads, one from the top of the sternum and the other from the top of the clavicle about 2 inches lateral to the first. They unite to attach to bones of the skull close below and behind the ear. Acting together, they flex the head and neck. Acting on one side at a time, they flex the head and neck laterally; they also rotate them to the opposite side (see figure 9.27a). They may be easily palpated, as well as seen, on the side of the neck from just under the ear to the front of the neck on either side of the sternoclavicular joint.

Levator scapulae (see figure 9.19)   (Also listed with the muscles of the shoulder girdle.) When one scapula is fixed, the muscle on that side will help flex the cervical spine laterally. If both muscles contract at the same time when both scapulae are fixed, they neutralize each other without effecting

Figure 9.25 Sternocleidomastoid muscle.

any movement. This action may possibly help stabilize the neck, especially when the body is in the prone position, supported on "all fours."

Quadratus lumborum This flat muscle (figure 9.26) is situated behind the abdominal cavity at the side of the lumbar spine. It extends from the crest of the ilium to the lowest rib and has slips branching medially to attach to the tips of the transverse processes of the upper four lumbar vertebrae. Acting bilaterally, it is credited with stabilizing the pelvis and lumbar spine. Acting unilaterally, it flexes the lumbar spine to the same side (lateral flexion). In a 1972 EMG study, Waters and Morris (in Basmajian and DeLuca) found that together with other posterior spinal muscles, as well as with the abdominal muscles, it contracted regularly in each cycle of walking. According to the electromyogram reproduced in *Muscles Alive* (Basmajian and DeLuca 1985), its action appears to coincide with the moment of heel contact. The muscle may be palpated on a thin, muscular subject just lateral to the erector spinae in the lumbar region.

Psoas (Also listed with the muscles of the hip.) Like the quadratus lumborum, the psoas (see figure 7.14) is situated at the back of the abdominal cavity. Together, these two form the posterior abdominal wall. Although the psoas is primarily a muscle of the hip joint, its action on the lower spine and pelvis is of interest. Because the psoas major muscle at its promixal end attaches to the sides of the bodies to the front and lower borders of the transverse processes of all the lumbar vertebrae, it has been thought to be a mover of the lumbar portion of the spinal column.

Although there appear to be diverse opinions regarding such muscular actions, it seems likely that the differences are not of great importance. Frequently, when there is lack of agreement regarding movement, one may safely assume that the true function of the muscular contraction, with reference to the joints in question, is more likely to be stabilization or balance than purposeful movement. In their edition of *Brunnstrom's Clinical Kinesiology,* Lemkuhl and Smith (1983) described this type of action with unusual clarity. They liken the muscles that are situated near the

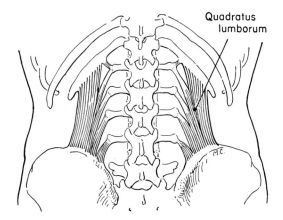

Figure 9.26   Quadratus lumborum (posterior view).

spinal column (erector spinae, psoas major, and so on) to guy ropes supporting an upright pole. When the pole starts to tip, the tension of the ropes on the opposite side increases. In like manner, if a person starts to lean backward, possibly to favor weak posterior muscles, the muscles on the front of the spine spring into action. Thus, it would appear that the most important role of the psoas is *stabilization or balancing of the spine* in response to other forces acting on the latter. In addition, unilateral contraction contributes to *lateral flexion* of the lumbar spine.

MUSCULAR ANALYSIS OF THE FUNDAMENTAL MOVEMENTS OF THE HEAD AND SPINE

In general, the muscles situated anterior to the spine flex it, those posterior to it extend it, and those lateral to it, when acting on one side only, either flex it laterally or rotate it, depending on the requirements of the intended movement. *Because of the effect of gravity, however, the anterior muscles fulfill their function as flexors most successfully when the body is supine, the posterior muscles as extensors when the body is prone, and the lateral muscles as lateral flexors when the body is resting on the side.* These facts should

be kept in mind when one is analyzing the muscular actions of the fundamental movements.

Cervical Spine and Atlanto-Occipital Joint
Flexion
This movement is performed chiefly by the sternocleidomastoid, the three scalenes, and the prevertebral muscles. The supra- and infrahyoid muscles, whose chief function is to move the hyoid bone up or down in movements related to swallowing and vocalizing, give added force to cervical flexion when they contract together and movements of the mouth are prevented.

Extension and Hyperextension
Many muscles contribute to these movements: the splenius capitis and cervicis, the capitis and cervicis portions of the erector spinae, semispinalis, deep posterior spinal muscles, and the suboccipitalis. When the left and right sides of trapezius I contract together, they also help extend the head and neck.

Lateral Flexion
This movement is performed by the simultaneous contraction of the extensors and flexors of the same side. Specifically, the chief lateral flexors include the capitis and cervicis portions of the splenius, erector spinae, semispinalis, three scalenes, and sternocleidomastoid. The suboccipitals, cervical portions of the deep posterior spinal muscles, and levator scapulae are in a position to aid in lateral flexion when they are needed.

Rotation
The sternocleidomastoid and deep posterior spinal muscles rotate the head and neck to the opposite side and the splenius, erector spinae, and occipitals rotate them to the same side (figure 9.27).

Thoracic and Lumbar Spine

The muscles that produce motion in the trunk are arranged in such a way that their effectiveness depends heavily on their distance from the vertebral

Rt. sterno-
cleidomastoid

a.

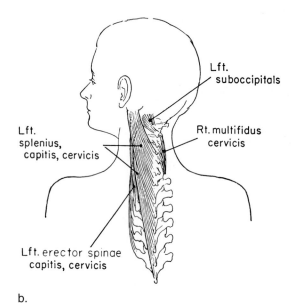

Lft.
suboccipitals

Lft.
splenius,
capitis, cervicis

Rt. multifidus
cervicis

Lft. erector spinae
capitis, cervicis

b.

Figure 9.27   Muscles that contract to rotate the head and neck to the left.

column. Both the relative size of the trunk muscles and their arrangement in the body play a role in producing trunk motion and in the etiology of injuries to the vertebral areas. Figure 9.28 shows both the relative sizes and the locations of the various muscles of this region.

Flexion

This movement is performed by the three abdominal muscles: the rectus abdominis and external

and internal obliques. As an aid to their effective action the pelvis must often be stabilized by the hip flexors, especially when the movement is performed from the supine position.

Extension and Hyperextension

The thoracic and lumbar portions of the erector spinae and the semispinalis thoracis are the chief extensors, but the deep posterior spinal muscles also have a significant role. When hyperextension

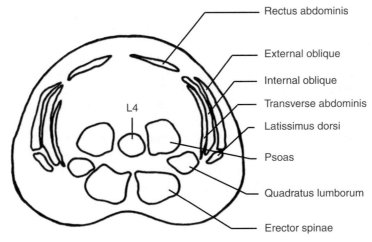

Figure 9.28   Relative positions of the trunk muscles as shown by magnetic resonance imaging.

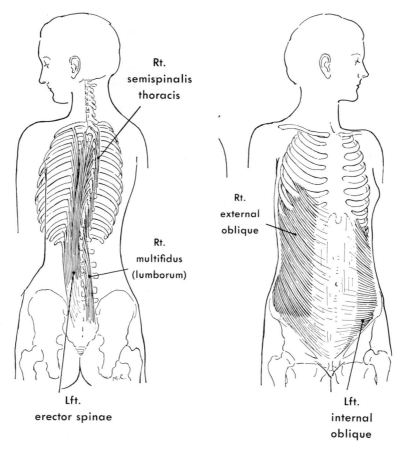

Figure 9.29   Muscles that contract to rotate the trunk to the left.

is performed from the prone lying position, the erector spinae is particularly active.

Lateral Flexion

Many muscles are active in this movement—the erector spinae, internal and external oblique abdominals, and quadratus lumborum in particular, with the semispinalis thoracis, rectus abdominis, deep posterior spinal muscles, psoas, and latissimus dorsi supplying additional force if needed. When the trunk is flexed to the right from a sidelying position on the left, the working muscles are those on the right side of the trunk.

Rotation

Rotation to the left (figure 9.29) is effected by the left internal oblique abdominal muscle and the thoracic and lumbar portions of the left erector spinae, especially the iliocostalis thoracis branch, the right external oblique abdominal muscle, semispinalis thoracis, multifidus, and other deep posterior spinal muscles.

STRUCTURE AND ARTICULATIONS OF THE THORAX

The thorax is a bony cartilaginous cage with an inverted V-shaped opening in front beneath the sternum (figure 9.30). It is formed mainly by the ribs and their cartilages but also includes the sternum, which constitutes the anterior base of attachment for the ribs, and the thoracic portion of the spine, which provides the posterior base of attachment. The upper seven ribs whose cartilages articulate directly with the sternum are called true ribs and the remaining five, false ribs. This is a misleading term, the only difference being that the latter do not articulate with the sternum. In each case the cartilages of the eighth, ninth, and tenth ribs unite with the cartilage above; the eleventh and twelfth ribs, known as the "floating ribs," have no anterior attachment but end anteriorly in cartilaginous tips.

The angle formed by the margins of the lower rib cartilages at the front of the chest is known as the subcostal angle. This is characteristically wider in individuals of stocky build than in those of slender build. The thorax is wider from side to side than it is from front to back and slightly flattened in front. An infant or young child has a more "barrel-shaped" chest than does an adult—that is, a thorax whose anteroposterior diameter more nearly approaches its transverse diameter than is the case in an adult.

Before studying the articulations and the movements of the thorax, the student should review the ribs by observing them on a skeleton, noting especially their shape and the way in which they twist. If no skeleton is available, he or she should look carefully at pictures of the ribs, such as those shown in figure 9.31.

All but the lowest two ribs articulate anteriorly with the sternum, either directly or indirectly, and all articulate posteriorly with the vertebrae. More specifically, with the exception of the first, tenth, eleventh, and twelfth ribs, the head of each rib articulates with two adjacent vertebrae, thus spanning the disc between (figure 9.32). The first, tenth, eleventh, and twelfth ribs articulate with a single vertebra. Except in the case of the last two ribs, each rib has an additional vertebral articulation between the tubercle of the rib and the adjacent transverse process of the vertebra (figure 9.33). All of these articulations are nonaxial, diarthrodial joints and permit only a slight gliding action.

There are four groups of sternocostal articulations: (1) the sternocostal joints between the costal cartilages and the sternum; (2) the joints between each rib and its cartilage, known as the costochondral joints; (3) the joints between one costal cartilage and another, called the interchondral joints; and (4) the two intersternal joints, one between the manubrium and body of the sternum, the other between the body and the xiphoid process (figure 9.34).

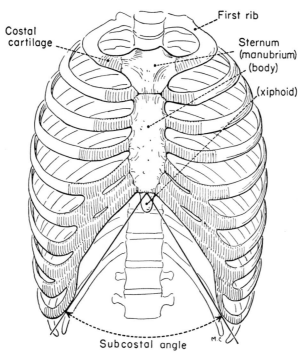

Figure 9.30   Anterior view of thorax.

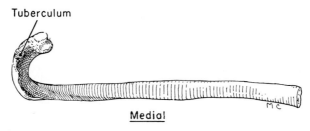

Figure 9.31   Rib: (a) posterior view; (b) medial view.

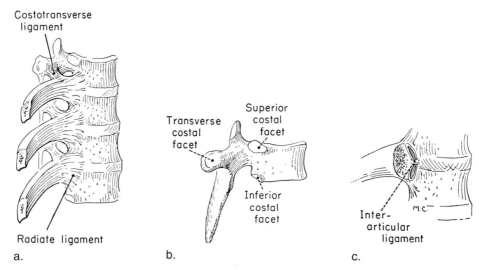

Figure 9.32   Anterior and lateral views of costovertebral articulations.

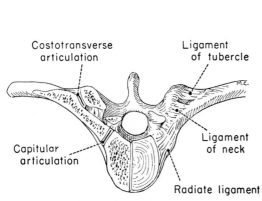

Figure 9.33   Superior view of costovertebral articulations.

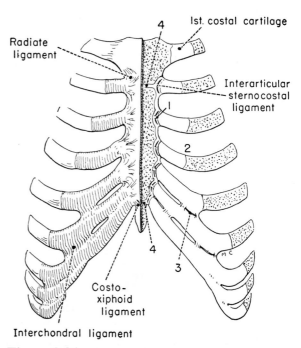

Figure 9.34   Sternocostal articulations (1 = sternocostal; 2 = costochondral; 3 = interchondral; 4 = intersternal).

MOVEMENTS OF THE THORAX

Because most of the ribs are attached both posteriorly and anteriorly, their movement is extremely limited. In the thoracic expansion associated with inhalation, the anterior ends of the ribs are elevated in a flexion type of movement. This is accompanied by a slight eversion in which the lower margin of the central portion of the rib turns upward and lateralward, the inner surface being made to face somewhat downward. As the anterior ends of the upper ribs move upward, they also push forward, carrying the sternum forward and upward with them. In the case of the lower ribs the anterior ends move laterally, thus "opening" the chest and widening the subcostal angle.

Although expansion of the thorax is ordinarily associated with inhalation for the purpose of providing the body with oxygen, there is another purpose: Whenever one exerts maximal muscular effort of short duration, a deep breath is taken and held while exerting the effort. This action stabilizes the ribs and sternum and thus provides firm anchorage for the upper extremity and trunk muscles that are used in forceful lifting, pushing, and pulling.

Enlargement of the Thorax in Inhalation

In inhalation the thorax is enlarged in three diameters: transverse, anteroposterior, and vertical.

Increase in the Transverse Diameter

This effect (figure 9.35) results from the elevation and eversion of the lateral portion of the ribs. The shape and twist of the ribs together with their anterior and posterior attachments are responsible for what has so aptly been called their "bucket handle inspiratory movement." The elevation of the lower ribs is accompanied by a lateral movement of their anterior ends. This widening of the lower thorax increases the power of the diaphragm by putting it on a stretch.

Increase in the Anteroposterior Diameter

This effect (figure 9.35) is produced by the elevation of the anterior ends of the obliquely placed ribs and of the body of the sternum, the latter being caused by the rib movement. The elevation of the anterior ends of the ribs causes the ribs to assume a more horizontal position and results in a straightening of the costal cartilages. The movements of the thorax in the anteroposterior and transverse diameters are inseparable. The expansion in both

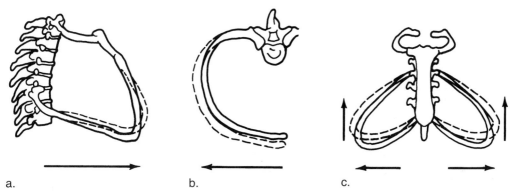

a.   b.   c.

Figure 9.35   Expansion of thorax during inhalation: (a) lateral view; (b) superior view; (c) anterior view.

directions when the ribs are elevated is the inevitable result of their shape and of the oblique direction of their axes in motion.

Increase in the Vertical Diameter

This effect is brought about primarily by the depression of the central tendon of the diaphragm, but elevation of the upper two ribs makes a slight contribution. In forced inspiration the thoracic spine may extend to its limit, and this also contributes to a further increase in the vertical diameter.

Phases of Respiration

Based on their conclusions on their own findings as well as on those of several other investigators, Basmajian and DeLuca (1985) recognize four phases of respiration. In brief, these are as follows.

Preinspiration

This is a brief static phase that precedes the intake of air.

Inspiration

This phase is characterized by expansion of the thorax and the taking in of air.

Pre-expiration

This is a brief static phase that follows inspiration and precedes expiration.

Expiration

This phase is characterized by an outflow of air accompanying a decrease in thoracic volume.

MUSCLES OF RESPIRATION

The muscles associated with respiration may be divided into two groups. The first group consists of the muscles of the thorax and includes those muscles associated with the ribs whose primary function is respiration. The second group consists of those muscles of the spine and shoulder girdle whose functions in respiration, although important, are not their primary functions. Because only their activity in respiration is described here, the reader is directed to other sections of the text for additional information on the muscles included in this latter group.

Muscles with Primary Function of Respiration

> Diaphragm
>
> Intercostales, externi and interni
>
> Levatores costarum
>
> Serratus posterior inferior
>
> Serratus posterior superior
>
> Transversus thoracis

Muscles with Secondary Function of Respiration

> Abdominals
>
> Erector spinae
>
> Extensors of cervical and thoracic spine
>
> Pectoralis major and minor
>
> Quadratus lumborum
>
> Scalenes, anterior, posterior, and medius
>
> Sternocleidomastoid
>
> Trapezius I and II

Characteristics of Individual Muscles with Primary Function in Respiration

Diaphragm

This muscle (figure 9.36) is a dome-shaped sheet that separates the thoracic and abdominal cavities from each other. Its contraction causes depression of its central tendon, and this increases the vertical dimension of the thorax. It also has a tendency to lift the lower ribs, but this appears to be resisted by the quadratus lumborum and iliocostalis lumborum. As the diaphragm moves downward it presses against the abdominal organs which, in turn, push forward against the relaxed abdominal wall. By increasing the intra-abdominal pressure, these actions help in defecation, vomiting, and other forms of expulsion. Although primarily a muscle of inspiration, a number of EMG studies

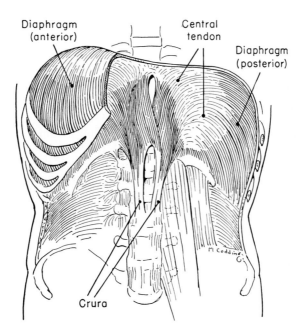

Figure 9.36   The diaphragm.

have revealed the presence of electrical activity in the diaphragm during both the pre-expiratory and expiratory phases (Basmajian and DeLuca 1985). It was suggested that this continuation of activity in the expiratory phase might be a braking action that serves the purpose of resisting or slowing down the elastic recoil of the lungs. This appears to imply that the contraction is eccentric or lengthening in nature, much like the action of the knee and hip extensors in resisting gravitational force in a slow, deep knee bend. The finding that the diaphragm did not show any activity in forced expiration seems to bear this out. Two other findings were also revealed by EMG studies: (1) that all portions of the diaphragm contract simultaneously, a positive indication that the muscle functions as a unit, and (2) that the diaphragm is unquestionably the chief muscle of inspiration (Basmajian and DeLuca 1985).

Intercostales, Externi and Interni

These muscles (figure 9.37) are two layers of similar sets of muscles, each set consisting of

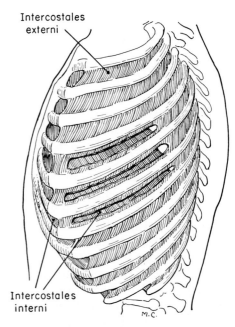

Figure 9.37   The intercostal muscles.

short parallel fibers that connect adjacent ribs. The fibers of the outer set slant downward and forward from one rib to the rib below, and those of the inner set slant in the reverse direction, that is, downward and backward. An interesting point is that the slant of each set is similar to the slant of the corresponding oblique abdominal muscle. Both sets extend posteriorly as far as the angles of the ribs. In front, the external layer extends only as far forward as the costal cartilages, whereas the internal extends to the sternum. Hence the anterior portion of the internal intercostals is not covered by the external layer.

These muscles have long been regarded as important respiratory muscles, second only to the diaphragm, but for many years there has been a lack of agreement concerning their specific functions. Some investigators have claimed that both sets elevate the ribs, some that one set elevates and the other depresses, and some that both the external intercostals and the anterior (uncovered) portion of the internal layer elevate, and the remainder of the internal depresses. Even electromyographic research has not settled the question of functions. One reason may be that, as refinements are made in techniques, investigators do not want to repeat the old methods, thus making comparisons invalid. If several research teams could agree on using the same techniques under similar conditions, the findings of one or more studies might confirm those of others.

In the past, it has been assumed that if a muscle is active during a certain phase of breathing it is making a direct contribution to the movement characteristic of that phase. For instance, if a muscle that attaches to the ribs, as do the intercostals, were to contract during the inspiratory phase, it would be assumed that it was helping expand the thorax. Jones and associates (Basmajian and DeLuca 1985), however, have suggested a theory concerning the intercostals that deserves serious consideration. Their group noted that both sets of intercostals were constantly active during quiet breathing but showed no rhythmic fluctuation as one would expect if they were causing the

rhythmic movements of the thorax. They explained this observation by suggesting that the function of the intercostals was to supply the tension needed to keep the ribs at a constant distance from each other and to increase the intrathoracic pressure.

At the risk of putting too much emphasis on the findings from a single study, the results of Taylor's EMG investigation of the intercostal muscles, in which he used very fine needle electrodes, are briefly reported here (Basmajian and DeLuca 1985).

External Intercostals
A. No action at all in quiet breathing.
B. Where two layers of muscles are present (i.e., both external and internal), the external acts in inspiration only. (In the light of the first notion it is assumed that this means in deep or forced inspiration.)

Internal Intercostals
A. Where two layers of muscles are present, the internal acts during expiration only. This was noted in the lower lateral part of the thorax during quiet expiration.
B. In the cartilaginous region in front where the internal is not covered by the external, electrical activity was noted during inspiration.

Most recently, studies have shown that the first two internal intercostals are always active in quiet inspiration, with the remainder of the intercostals being recruited from top to bottom in vigorous inspiration. During normal expiration, intercostal muscle usage is deactivated in the reverse order, that is, from bottom to top. During vigorous expiration, all the intercostal muscles are active (Basmajian and DeLuca 1985).

Levatores Costarum
These little muscles (figure 9.38), slanting down and slightly outward from the tip of the transverse process of each vertebra to the rib below, with additional bands in the case of the seventh, eighth,

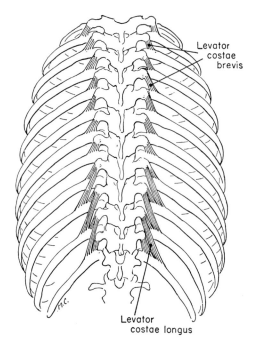

Figure 9.38   Levatores costarum (levator costae).

Figure 9.39   Serratus posterior superior and inferior.

ninth, and tenth vertebrae passing to the second rib below, are in a position to exert a lifting effect on the ribs but have poor leverage for this as their attachments to the ribs are quite close to the costovertebral joints. In spite of this, it is assumed that they help elevate the ribs during inspiration.

Serratus Posterior Inferior

Like four chevrons, these broad bands (figure 9.39) connect the lower borders of the lowest four ribs with the spinous processes and ligaments of lower vertebrae (lower two thoracic and upper two or three lumbar). They are assumed to *depress the four ribs and to stabilize* them against the pull of the diaphragm. They are too deep to palpate or to test electromyographically by present techniques.

Serratus Posterior Superior

Like four steeply slanted, inverted chevrons, these bands (figure 9.39) connect the upper borders of the second, third, fourth, and fifth ribs with the spinous processes and ligaments of the lower two or three cervical and the upper two thoracic vertebrae. They are assumed to help *elevate the four ribs* and in so doing to *expand the upper thorax.* Like the inferior, this muscle is too deep to palpate or to check by present EMG means.

Transversus Thoracis

This muscle (figure 9.40) connects the lower half of the inner surface of the sternum and adjoining

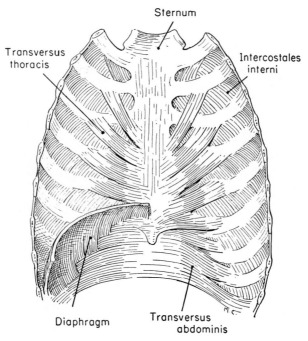

Figure 9.40   Posterior (inner) view of anterior wall of thorax.

costal cartilages with the lower borders and inner surfaces of the costal cartilages of the second, third, fourth, fifth, and sixth ribs. It consists of flat bands that radiate upward and outward from the inner surface of the sternum to the ribs, the lowest fibers being continuous with those of the transversus abdominis.

Characteristics of Individual Muscles with Secondary Function in Respiration
Abdominals

The abdominals (see figures 9.15, 9.16, and 9.17) are considered to be the most important muscles for expiration, yet they do not become active until the expiration is forced. Normal quiet breathing is considered passive, and very little muscular activity occurs during it. The transversus abdominis, in that order, the internal and the external obliques, have been found to be the most important muscles of forced expiration (Abe et al. 1996; Cress-

well, Grundstrom, and Thorstensson 1992). It was also noted that they do not initiate expiration but help complete it. Although the rectus also contracts in expiration, it was found to be of little importance as compared with the other abdominals. Vigorous contraction of the abdominals is present in all expiratory actions such as coughing, sneezing, straining, or vomiting.

Erector Spinae

This extensive muscle (see figure 9.21) of the back serves to *stabilize the spine and pelvis* against the pull of the abdominal muscles. By resisting the tendency of the latter to flex the spine, it forces them to concentrate their activity on abdominal compression.

Extensors of Cervical and Thoracic Spine

These muscles (see figures 9.22 and 9.23) *stabilize the head and neck* against the pull of the scalenes and the sternocleidomastoid.

Pectoralis Major and Minor

A few investigators have reported activity of the pectoralis major (see figures 5.4 and 5.11) in deep inspiration but have not made it clear what function the muscle is performing. It seems reasonable to assume that when an individual holds the arms vertically upward or is suspended by the hands, the pectoralis major would help elevate the sternum and upper six ribs. The pectoralis minor is likewise in a position to lift the third, fourth, and fifth ribs when the thoracic spine is extended and the scapulae are stabilized.

Quadratus Lumborum

An EMG study conducted in 1965 by Boyd and coworkers confirms the assumption that this muscle (see figure 9.26) anchors the last rib against the pull of the diaphragm, which would otherwise tend to lift it and, in so doing, lose some of the force for depressing its central tendon (Basmajian and DeLuca 1985).

Scalenes, Anterior, Posterior, and Medius

These three muscles (see figure 9.24) are assuming greater importance as respiratory muscles as the result of EMG research. They connect the transverse processes of the cervical vertebrae with the first two ribs. They were formerly thought to be primarily lateral flexors of the neck and secondarily accessory or stabilizing muscles of respiration, their function being to anchor the first two ribs for the intercostals. Results of two investigations more than ten years apart give strong evidence of the scalenes' role as true respiratory muscles in quiet inspiration as well as in forced (Basmajian and DeLuca 1985). These muscles may be palpated on the side of the neck between the sternocleidomastoid and upper trapezius muscles.

Sternocleidomastoid

As an accessory muscle of respiration, this muscle (see figure 9.25) showed marked electrical activity in forced inspiration. It helps elevate the sternum and clavicle. In vigorous inspiration the head is usually held firmly erect, and, instead of flexing the head and neck, the sternocleidomastoid has a slight lifting effect on the sternum and sternal end of each clavicle. It may be palpated on the side of the neck just below the ear and on the front of the neck at the junction of the clavicle and sternum.

Trapezius I and II

In reviewing EMG studies of the trapezius, Basmajian and DeLuca (1985) were unable to find confirmation of Duchenne's inclusion of this muscle (see figure 5.6) as an accessory in respiration. It is included here as a possible stabilizer of the shoulder girdle against the downward pull of the pectoralis minor. As yet, this theory has not been confirmed.

MUSCULAR ANALYSIS OF RESPIRATION

On the whole, EMG studies have tended to reinforce the muscular analysis of respiration as presented in older kinesiology texts, but there have been some unexpected revelations. The student who is interested in pursuing this subject is advised to read Basmajian and DeLuca's (1985) excellent summaries of EMG investigations before examining the original reports of individual studies.

Inspiration

The action of the diaphragm accounts for about one-third of the air exchanged in normal breathing. Action in the scalenes and the intercostals (especially the external) also occurs in quiet inspiration. With forced inspiration, these major muscles of inspiration, as well as the sternocleidomastoid, serratus posterior superior, levatores costarum, quadratus lumborum, erector spinae, and pectoralis major and minor, are active.

Expiration

Quiet expiration is generally considered to be a passive act. However, some activity has been recorded in the intercostals, serratus posterior muscles, diaphragm, and quadratus lumborum. The major muscles of forced expiration are the transversus abdominis and oblique abdominals. The erector spinae are active as stabilizers against the pull of the abdominals. Other participants include the transversus thoracic and intercostals. The diaphragm has been found to be quiet during vigorous expiration.

COMMON INJURIES OF THE NECK, BACK, AND THORAX

Neck Injuries

Although these fortunately are not common except in severe falls, blows, or accidents, they are of prime concern. If there is the slightest suspicion of serious injury, it is literally of vital importance that the individual not be moved at all until after having been examined by a physician, and then only under the physician's close supervision. *The danger of death or paralysis from the neck down cannot be overemphasized.*

Contusions of the Spine

These injuries are undoubtedly much more common among athletes than among nonathletes. The muscles involved are usually those on either side of the spinous processes. Ordinarily the contusion is not serious, but it may cause a hematoma. Another possible complication is painful stiffness, which may last for several days. Muscle spasm often occurs in the more severe contusions of the lower back.

Back Strains and Sprains

Strains (injuries to muscles) and sprains (injuries to ligaments) are both common injuries, largely because there are so many muscles and ligaments in the region of the spine. In the early stages of these injuries it is often difficult to distinguish between them. The strain is usually the result of either a violent contraction, a movement in more

than one plane, or poor posture. A sprain may be caused by the same kind of movements that cause a strain, but in sprains the damage is a tearing of the ligaments.

An acute back strain that is not given proper treatment is likely to develop into a chronic strain and become a perpetual problem. This is usually more common in the lower back than in the upper. Prevention of back strain and sprain is of major concern in the planning of conditioning and rehabilitation programs.

Fractures of Transverse Process of Lumbar Vertebra

These injuries occur quite frequently in sports, either from a severe blow or from a violent muscular contraction. In either case, the damage to the muscle and soft tissue will be treated. The damage to the bone itself will not be dangerous except for pain. This is understandable when one reviews the attachments of the back muscles, especially those of the semispinalis muscle and the deep posterior muscles of the spine.

Herniated Disc

The conditions that cause a herniated disc, namely the compression of two adjacent vertebrae with such magnitude that the annulus fibrosus is ruptured, are often brought about by repeated heavy lifting with the body in poor alignment. If this has happened to an athlete, however, participation in athletics is unwise until the rupture can be repaired. Otherwise the nucleus pulposus is likely to protrude through the break in the disc and press on the spinal cord or a spinal nerve. The area most likely to be affected is the lumbar spine, especially between the fourth and fifth lumbar vertebrae. This condition can be, but does not have to be, painful.

Rib Fractures

These injuries are fairly common in contact sports like football and wrestling, or in traumatic blows to the chest. The usual causes are either direct blows or forceful compressions. Sudden, violent, muscular contraction may also be a cause. In most fracture injuries, two or more ribs are likely to be involved. A fracture should be suspected if breathing is accompanied by severe pain. A possible serious complication of rib fractures is damage to the soft tissues when the broken ends of the bone are pushed inward (Arnheim and Prentice 1998).

Whiplash

A whiplash is a cervical sprain resulting from a violent motion. In a whiplash injury the neck is violently moved through an S-curve, with the upper portion of the cervical spine undergoing flexion while the lower portion of the cervical region is hyperextending or fixed. The pain often occurs one day after the injury and involves muscle strains and tears to ligaments. It may also include a herniated disc in the cervical region.

Low Back Pain

Nonspecific low back pain has become a frequent complaint, accounting for more missed work days than any other form of injury. Low back pain can arise from poor posture, inefficient lifting, repetitive stress, or other factors. Pain may range in severity from mildly annoying to producing serious functional impairment. Frequently treatment for low back pain involves exercises to reduce forward pelvic tilt or to strengthen abdominal muscles.

LABORATORY EXPERIENCES

Joint Structure

1. Study the bones of the spinal column. Classify the structure for each of the following joints, including the articulations of both the bodies and the arches. Explain how the structure of each joint affects its function.
   a. Atlanto-occipital
   b. Atlantoaxial
   c. A middle cervical joint
   d. The joint between the seventh cervical and the first thoracic vertebrae
   e. A middle thoracic joint
   f. The joint between the twelfth thoracic and the first lumbar vertebrae
   g. A middle lumbar joint
   h. The lumbosacral joint

Joint Action

2. Have a subject sit tailor fashion on a table and flex the spine as completely as possible. Observe the shape of the spine as seen from the side. Compare the three regions of the spine as to forward flexibility.

3. Have a subject sit astride a chair, facing its back, and hyperextend the spine as completely as possible. Observe the shape of the spine, as in 2.

4. Have a subject sit astride a bench and laterally flex the spine as far as possible, first to one side and then to the other. Observe from the rear.

5. Have a subject sit astride a bench with the hands at the neck, then rotate the trunk as far as possible, first to one side, then to the other. Observe and compare the regions of the spine as to rotating ability.

6. Observe flexion, hyperextension, lateral flexion, and rotation of the spine in several subjects, preferably subjects representing different body builds, and note individual differences.

7. Have a subject lie face down on a table with the legs and pelvis supported on the table, the trunk extending forward beyond the table, and the hands clasped behind the neck.
   a. Have the subject flex the spine laterally. Compare the thoracic and lumbar regions. Note the torsion accompanying the lateral flexion.
   b. Have the subject flex the spine and then flex it laterally. Observe as in a.
   c. Have the subject hyperextend the spine (with someone helping support the elbows) and then flex laterally. Observe as in a.
   d. Have the subject rotate the trunk to one side as far as possible. Compare the thoracic and

lumbar regions. Is any lateral flexion apparent in the spine?

  e. Have the subject flex the spine and then rotate it. Observe as in a.

  f. Have the subject hyperextend the spine and then rotate it. Observe as in d.

8. **Movement of the Thorax in Respiration**
Subject: Breathe naturally for a while, then as deeply as possible.
Observer: (a) Place the hands on the sides of the thorax and note the movement in the lateral diameter. (b) Place one hand on the ribs at the subcostal angle (just below the sternum) and the other hand against the back at the same level. Note the movement in the anteroposterior diameter. (c) Place the fingers on the sternum. Can you detect any movement in normal respiration? In deep respiration?

Muscular Action

The purpose of these exercises is not to test the strength of the muscles but to enable the observer to study the action of the muscles in simple movements of the body. The procedure, therefore, is quite different from that followed by the physical therapist in testing muscle strength. It is suggested that students work in groups of three: one acting as the subject, one as an assistant helping support or steady the stationary part of the body and giving resistance to the moving part, and one palpating the muscles and recording the results. The procedures in appendix C may be used for this purpose. They may also be used for the analysis of other movements.

9. **Flexion of the Neck**
  a. *Subject:* Lie on the back and lift the head, bringing the chin toward the chest.
    Observer: Palpate and identify as many of the contracting muscles as possible.
  b. *Subject:* Lie on the back and lift the head, leading with the chin.
    Observer: Compare the action of the sternocleidomastoid in b with its action in a.

10. **Extension and Hyperextension of the Neck**
  a. *Subject:* Lie face down on a table with the head over the edge. Raise the head as far as possible, hyperextending both the head and the neck.
    Assistant: May resist the movement if stronger muscular action is desired.

Observer: Palpate and identify as many of the contracting muscles as possible.

  b. *Subject:* Lie face down on a table with the head over the edge. Raise the head as far as possible with the chin tucked in.
    Assistant: Resist the retraction of the chin.
    Observer: Compare the muscular action in b with that in a.

11. **Lateral Flexion of the Head and Neck**
Subject: Lie on one side and raise the head toward the shoulder without turning the head or tensing the shoulder.
Assistant: Give slight resistance at the temple.
Observer: Palpate and identify as many muscles as possible.

12. **Rotation of the Head and Neck**
Subject: Sit erect and rotate the head to the left as far as possible.
Assistant: Give fairly strong resistance to the side of the jaw.
Observer: Palpate the sternocleidomastoids. Which one contracts?

13. **Flexion of the Thoracic and Lumbar Spine**
Subject: Lie on the back with the arms folded across the chest. Flex the head, shoulders, and upper back from the table, keeping the chin in. There is no need to come to a sitting position, since this is intended as a movement of spinal, not hip, flexion.
Assistant: Hold the thighs down.
Observer: Palpate the rectus abdominis and the external oblique abdominal muscle.

14. **Extension and Hyperextension of the Thoracic and Lumbar Spine**
Subject: Lie face down with the hands on the hips. Hyperextend the head and trunk as far as possible.
Assistant: Hold the feet down.
Observer: Palpate the erector spinae and the gluteus maximus. What is the function of the latter muscle in this movement?

15. **Lateral Flexion of the Thoracic and Lumbar Spine**
Subject: Lie on one side with the bottom arm placed across the chest and the hand resting on the opposite shoulder, and with the hand of the top arm resting on the hip. Laterally flex the trunk.
Assistant: Hold the legs down. If necessary, help the subject by pulling at the elbow.

Observer: Palpate the rectus abdominis, external oblique abdominal muscle, erector spinae, and latissimus dorsi.

16. **Rotation of the Thoracic and Lumbar Spine**
    Subject: Sit astride a bench with the hands placed behind the neck. Rotate to one side as far as possible without leaving the bench.
    Assistant: Resist the movement by grasping the subject's arms close to the shoulders and pushing (or pulling) in the opposite direction.
    Observer: Palpate as many of the spinal and abdominal muscles as possible. Disregard the muscles of the scapula and arm.

17. **Muscular Action in Forced Inhalation**
    a. *Subject:* Inhale through a small rubber tube, pinching it slightly in order to furnish resistance.
       Observer: Note the action of the sternocleidomastoid, cervical and thoracic extensors, and upper trapezius. Can any other muscular action be detected? If so, explain.
    b. *Subject:* Run in place or around the room until short of breath. Hang from a horizontal bar.
       Observer: Can you detect any action of the pectoralis major accompanying inhalation? (By stabilizing the arms, the hanging position causes the pectoralis major to act on the ribs.)

18. **Muscular Action in Vigorous Exhalation**
    Subject: Blow through a small rubber tube, pinching it slightly or holding a finger loosely over the end or blow into a spirometer, flarimeter, or toy balloon.

Observer: Note the action of the abdominal muscles and the erector spinae. Explain.

Action of the Muscles other than the Movers

19. **Sit-Up**
    Subject: Lie on the back and come to a sitting position, keeping the spine as rigid as possible.
    Assistant: Hold the feet down.
    Observer: Palpate the abdominal muscles, erector spinae, and sternocleidomastoid. Explain the function of each.

20. **Double Leg Lowering**
    Subject: Lie on the back. Raise both legs, then slowly lower them half way.
    Observer: Palpate the abdominal muscles and erector spinae. Explain the function of each.

21. **Trunk Flexion**
    Subject: Stand with the feet slightly separated. Flex forward from the hips, keeping the back flat.
    Observer: Palpate the erector spinae. Explain its function.

22. **Push-Up**
    Subject: Assume a front-leaning rest position on the hands and toes with the body straight. Let the arm flex at the elbows until the chest almost touches the floor, then push up again, keeping the body straight the entire time. Do not let the body sag or hump.
    Observer: Palpate the abdominal muscles. Explain their function.

Kinesiological Analysis

23. Choose a simple motor skill from appendix H. Do a complete anatomical analysis of the motions of the spinal column following the analysis outline in table 1.2.

REFERENCES AND SELECTED READINGS

Abe, T., N. Kusuhara, N. Yoshimura, T. Tomita, and P. A. Easton. 1996. Differential respiratory activity of four abdominal muscles in humans. *Journal of Applied Physiology* 80:1379–89.

Arnheim, D. D., and W. E. Prentice. 1998. *Essentials of athletic training.* 4th ed. St. Louis: McGraw-Hill.

Basmajian, J. V., and J. C. DeLuca. 1985. *Muscles alive.* 5th ed. Baltimore: Williams & Wilkins.

Campbell, E. J. M. 1952. An electromyographic study of the role of the abdominal muscles in breathing. *Journal of Physiology* 177:222–33.

Cresswell, A. G., H. Grundstrom, and A. Thorstensson. 1992. Observations on intra-abdominal pressure and patterns of abdominal intramuscular activity in man. *Acta Physiologica Scandinavia* 144:409–18.

De Troyer, A., M. Estenne, V. Ninane, D. Van Gansbeke, and M. Gorini. 1990. Transverse abdominis muscle function in humans. *Journal of Applied Physiology* 68:1010–16.

Dolan, P., A. F. Mannion, and M. A. Adams. 1994. Passive tissues help the back muscles to generate extensor moments during lifting. *Journal of Biomechanics* 27:1077–85.

Hodges, P. W., and C. A. Richardson. 1997. Contraction of the abdominal muscles associated with movement of the lower limb. *Physical Therapy* 77:132–42.

Jones, D. S., and J. E. Pauly. 1957. Further electromyographic studies on muscles of costal respiration in man. *Anatomy Record* 128:733–46.

Kumar, S., Y. Narayan, and M. Zedka. 1996. An electromyographic study of unresisted trunk rotation with normal velocity among healthy subjects. *Spine* 21:1500–12.

Kumar, S., M. Zedka, and Y. Narayan. 1999. EMG power spectra of trunk muscles during graded maximal voluntary isometric contraction in flexion-rotation and extension-rotation. *European Journal of Applied Physiology* 80:527–41.

Lemkuhl, L. D., and L. K. Smith. 1983. *Brunnstrom's clinical kinesiology.* 4th ed. Philadelphia: F. A. Davis.

Loney, P. L., and P. W. Stratford. 1999. The prevalence of low back pain in adults: A methodological review of the literature. *Physical Therapy* 79:384–95.

Norkin, C., and P. Levangie. 1983. *Joint structure and function: A comprehensive analysis.* Philadelphia: F. A. Davis.

Pauly, J. E. 1966. An electromyographic analysis of certain movements and exercises. I. Some deep muscles of the back. *Anatomy Record* 155:223–34.

Sarti, M. A., M. Monfort, M. A. Fuster, L. A. Villaplana. 1996. Muscle activity in upper and lower rectus abdominus during abdominal exercises. *Archives of Physical Medicine and Rehabilitation* 77:1293–97.

Shields, R. K., and D. G. Heiss. 1997. An electromyographic comparison of abdominal muscle synergies in the curl and double straight leg lowering exercises with control of the pelvic position. *Spine* 22:1873–79.

Fundamentals of Biomechanics

Introduction to Part II

As seen by the kinesiologist, the human body is a highly complex machine constructed of living tissue. As such it is subject to the laws and principles of mechanics as well as those of biology. The principles of mechanics are directly applicable both to the movements of the human body and to the implements it handles. Principles of balance and equilibrium, motion, and the application of forces apply equally to people in motion as they do to rockets and wheels, gears and missiles. A study of the fundamental principles of mechanics as they apply to movement skills will aid the teacher, therapist, and coach in the analysis of skills for the intelligent evaluation of technique and correction of error. Applications in research can lead to the determination of the relative merits of existing techniques as well as to the development of techniques yet unknown.

Interest in mechanical analysis and study as part of physical education was due in large measure to the influence of three pioneers. C. H. McCloy, from the University of Iowa, toured the country in the late 1930s and 1940s giving lectures with demonstrations showing specific ways in which performance could be improved by the application of appropriate mechanical principles. He was the first to develop a course in the mechanical analysis of motor skills. Pioneer efforts in cinematographic analysis by Ruth Glassow at the University of Wisconsin also contributed to interest in the application of the fundamental principles of mechanics and physics to sports skills among physical educators in the United States. During this same period Thomas Cureton, whose undergraduate degree was in electrical engineering, taught mechanics of sports and physical activities at Springfield College. His research and writing at this time concentrated on the applications of physics to physical education and on the principles of cinematographic analysis (Atwater 1980). During the 1950s and early 1960s, research on the mechanics of sports activities increased in scope and variety as others became involved and as methodology and equipment

improved, but it was in the late 1960s and early 1970s that a lively interest in the mechanical analysis of humans in motion emerged. Graduate programs designed to prepare specialists in the mechanics of human motion appeared, and the results of vastly improved research methodology, technology, and instrumentation became apparent in a growing body of literature. There was a new area of study that many have named biomechanics of sport and others have called mechanical kinesiology.

In the branch of science called biomechanics, the principles and methods of mechanics are applied to the structure and function of biological systems (Atwater 1980). Because biology is concerned with all living things, biomechanics is a very broad branch of science, and the biomechanics of sport is only one of the applied areas in which applications are made of the same common core of knowledge and fundamental research found in physics, mathematics, anatomy, and physiology. Other fields of applied biomechanics include industrial engineering and ergonomics, physical rehabilitation, medicine and biomedical physics, and aerospace science.

Of the fields of applied biomechanics the biomechanics of sport, dance, and physical education are the least advanced, but increased availability and use of advanced technology in the form of computers and electronic recording devices have resulted in research and study that formerly was almost prohibitive because of the agonizing amount of time they consumed. Additional impetus has also been supplied through the founding in 1973 of the International Society of Biomechanics (ISB) and, in 1977, the American Society of Biomechanics (ASB). The influence of these societies in stimulating study and disseminating knowledge through international meetings has done much to advance knowledge in this fascinating field of applied biomechanics, the biomechanics of sport and physical education.

Part II introduces the student to some elementary concepts necessary for understanding the biomechanics of sport and physical education. Chapter 10 presents mechanical concepts and terminology basic to the study of mechanics as an aspect of kinesiology. The need to understand basic mathematical concepts in order to use appropriate formulas and understand basic principles is also set forth in this chapter. The level of mathematics needed for this and subsequent chapters is relatively elementary and, with the aid of the examples given and the mathematics review in appendix E, the average kinesiology student should have no difficulty. Under no circumstances, however, should the student become so involved with juggling numbers in this part that the sight of the forest is lost for the trees.

Part II continues with a chapter on the fundamentals of motion description, with particular emphasis placed on an understanding of projectiles and "free flight." Specific applications are made to sport and physical education activities. A similar approach is followed in subsequent chapters on the conditions of linear motion, the conditions of rotary motion, and the center of gravity and stability. Each chapter concludes with a variety of problems and exercises designed to help the student understand the direct application of principles of mechanics to the execution of skills in sport and physical education.

Throughout Part II the student is encouraged to think in terms of applying newly gained knowledge of the biomechanical aspects of motion to the analysis of familiar motor skills. Using the analysis outline presented in table 1.1, each new mechanical concept should be applied to an evaluation of a motor skill. Such practice in using knowledge for analysis will help build a strong foundation for the growing practitioner in human movement analysis.

References

Atwater, A. E. 1980. Kinesiology/biomechanics: Perspectives and trends. *Research Quarterly for Exercise and Sport* 51:193–218.

Nelson, R. C. 1971. Biomechanics of sport: An overview. In *Selected topics in biomechanics,* edited by J. M. Cooper, 31–37. Chicago: The Athletic Institute.

Wartenweiler, J. 1979. The manifold implications of biomechanics. In *Biomechanics IV,* edited by R. C. Nelson and C. A. Morehouse, 11–14. Baltimore: University Park Press.

Internet Resources

A number of sites on the World Wide Web may be of interest to the student studying the mechanical aspects of kinesiology. Among those that might be most helpful are the following:

http://www.usfca.edu/ess/resourcepage.htm
This is a good starting point with links to many courses and tutorials.

http://www.iupui.edu/~rbahamon/trigpg1.html
Review of trigonometry.

http://www.physics.uoguelph.ca/tutorials/tutorials.html
Physics tutorials including algebra, conversions, trigonometry, vectors, torque, and free-body diagrams.

http://www.celos.psu.edu/kinematics/
A 3-D kinematics tutorial that is fairly advanced. There is a good section (aplet) on 2-D vectors.

http://www.iago.stfx.ca/people/edemont/Courses/375/assignments/mainpage.html
Interactive physics simulations online. This page requires a browser plug-in.

http://www.bsu.edu/classes/kwon/PEP294
Online labs from a course at Ball State University.

http://www.osu.orst.edu/instruct/exss.323
Biomechanics homework problems for practice.

http://www.nyu.edu/classes/mcdonough/biomech2.htm
Sets of biomechanics problems with answers from a physical therapy point of view.

http://www.silver.neep.wisc.edu/~lakes
Downloadable biomechanics laboratory problems—fairly advanced.

http://www.exploratorium.edu/sports/index.html
Interesting short articles on science (including mechanics) applied to sport.

*Note: All Internet sites are transient by nature and may cease to be active without warning. New sites are continually being activated.

TERMINOLOGY AND MEASUREMENT IN BIOMECHANICS

O U T L I N E

■ *Introduction to Terminology*
Mechanics
Biomechanics
■ *Quantities in Biomechanics*
The Language of Science
Units of Measurement
Scalar and Vector Quantities
■ *Vector Analysis*
Vector Representation
Combination of Vectors
Resolution of Vectors
Location of Vectors in Space
Graphic Resolution and
    Combination of Vectors
Trigonometric Resolution and
    Combination of Vectors
Value of Vector Analysis
■ *Laboratory Experiences*

O B J E C T I V E S

At the conclusion of this chapter, the student should be able to:

1. Define the terms mechanics and biomechanics, and differentiate between them.
2. Define the terms kinematics, kinetics, statics, and dynamics, and state how each relates to the structure of biomechanics study.
3. Convert the units of measurement employed in the study of biomechanics from the U.S. system to the metric system, and vice versa.
4. Describe the nature of scalar and vector quantities, and identify such quantities as one or the other.
5. Demonstrate the use of the graphic method for the combination and resolution of two-dimensional vectors.

6. Demonstrate the use of the trigonometric method for the combination and resolution of two-dimensional vectors.

7. Identify the scalar and vector quantities represented in individual motor skills and describe the vector quantities using vector diagrams.

INTRODUCTION TO TERMINOLOGY

As it is presently constituted, kinesiology is an area of study concerned with the musculoskeletal analysis of human motion and the study of mechanical principles and laws as they relate to the study of human motion. Students of human motion capable of accurately analyzing the musculoskeletal actions occurring in the execution of a movement are well on their way toward knowing what is happening during that movement. Those who have taken the further step of acquiring a working knowledge of how human motion is governed by physical laws and principles have added an additional dimension to their understanding of how and why the motion occurs as it does. Together, all this information provides a scientific foundation upon which to make appropriate decisions concerning the safest, most effective, and most efficient execution of any movement pattern. It is only through such study that definitive answers may be found concerning the "best" way for an individual to perform a skill and the reasons *why* the method selected is indeed the best. In sport, for example, the record-breaking "form" of one athlete may or may not be appropriate for another of different body build and size. In fact, although they break records, top performers' techniques may include actions that, if eliminated, would result in even greater performance. Unless subjected to scientific scrutiny, discrimination between the success factors and deterrent factors may be confused or not even identified.

Mechanics

Where *forces* and *motion* are concerned, the area of scientific study that provides accurate answers to what is happening, why it is happening, and to what extent it is happening is called *mechanics*. It is that branch of physics concerned with the effect that **forces** have on bodies and the motion produced by those forces. The study of mechanics is engaged in by those people whose occupations or professions require an understanding of force, matter, space, and time. Engineers, to a large extent, are involved with the application of mechanics. Navigation, astronomy, space, and communications experts all study mechanics. The same is true of individuals concerned with the study of human motion and the forces causing it. The laws and principles used to explain the motion of planets or the strength of buildings and bridges apply equally to humans. *All* motion, including motions of the human body and its parts, is the result of the application of forces and is subject to the laws and principles that govern force and motion.

Biomechanics

When the study of mechanics is limited to living structures, especially the human body, it is called *biomechanics.* **Biomechanics** is an interdisciplinary science based on many of the fundamental disciplines found in the physical and life sciences. Generally, biomechanics is considered to be that aspect of the science concerned with the basic laws governing the effect forces have on the state of rest or motion of animals or humans, whereas the applied areas of biomechanics deal with solving practical problems. Anatomists, orthopedists, space engineers, industrial engineers, biomedical engineers, physical therapists, physical educators, dancers, and coaches all have an interest in biomechanics and in applying its principles to the improvement of human movement. Professional applications may differ, but the same basic laws of biomechanics provide a common foundation for all. In this context the part of biomechanics that applies to sport, dance, and physical education may be considered to be that part of kinesiology that involves the mechanics of human motion.

Statics and Dynamics

The study of biomechanics is divided into two areas, **statics** and **dynamics.** *Statics* covers situations in which all forces acting on a body are balanced, and the body is in equilibrium. A body in a static situation would exhibit either no motion or a constant, unchanging motion. With a knowledge of the principles of statics, one may have a better understanding of levers and a greater ability to solve problems such as locating the body's center of gravity or center of buoyancy.

The branch of biomechanics dealing with bodies subject to *unbalance* is called *dynamics.* The principles of dynamics explain circumstances in which an excess of force in one direction or a turning force causes an object to change speed or direction. In this situation an object might move from a static position to one of motion or might undergo some change in the motion state. Principles of work, energy, and accelerated motion are included in the study of dynamics.

Kinematics and Kinetics

The terms **kinematics** and **kinetics** are also part of the vocabulary of the study of mechanics. Kine-

matics has been referred to as the geometry of motion. It describes the motion of bodies in terms of time, displacement, velocity, and acceleration. The motion occurring may be in a straight line (linear kinematics) or rotating about a fixed point (angular kinematics). Kinematics is concerned only with the analytical and mathematical descriptions of all kinds of motion and *not* with the forces that cause the motion. The branch of mechanics that considers the *forces* that produce or change motion is called *kinetics.* The most complex of biomechanics studies, it is the area least developed in physical education and physical therapy, and of most challenge to research today. Linear kinetics is concerned with the causes of linear motion, and angular kinetics deals with the forces that cause angular motion.

QUANTITIES IN BIOMECHANICS

The Language of Science

In the study of human motion, as in the study of any science, careful measurement and the use of mathematics are essential for the classification of facts and the systematizing of knowledge. Mathematics is the language of science. It enables us to express relationships quantitatively rather than merely descriptively. It provides objective evidence of the superiority of one technique over another and thus forms the basis for developing effective measures for improving both the safety and the effectiveness of performance. Furthermore, it makes possible continuing advancement of knowledge through research. Had it not been for the use of mathematics, the contributions of great scientists like Archimedes, Galileo, and Newton would not have been possible.

In the biomechanical aspects of kinesiology, as in all mechanics, the depth of understanding of the principles and laws that apply to it is greatly increased through experimental and mathematical evidence. Hence, it is to the kinesiologist's advantage to become conversant with appropriate mathematical concepts and techniques. The mathematics needed for the quantitative treatment of the simple mechanics discussed in this text is not difficult. It consists of elementary algebra and right triangle trigonometry. A review of these essential mathematical concepts is presented in appendix E.

Units of Measurement

The units of measurement employed in the study of biomechanics are expressed in terms of space, time, and mass. Currently in the United States, there are two systems of unit measurement for these quantities, the U.S. system and the metric system. Although the metric system is currently used in research and literature, a comparison of equivalent values is helpful. Table 10.1 presents some common units used in biomechanics study and their U.S. and metric equivalents.

Length

In the metric or decimal system, all units differ in size by a multiple of 10. In ascending order, linear units are millimeters, centimeters, meters, and kilometers. In the U.S. system the basic unit of length is the foot. Other possible units are inches, yards, and miles.

Area or Volume

In the metric system, square centimeters or square meters are used for area, and cubic centimeters, liters, or cubic meters are used for volume. In the U.S. system, area units are square inches or feet, and cubic inches, cubic feet, quarts, or gallons denote volume.

Mass and Force (Weight)

Mass is the quantity of matter a body contains. The **weight** of a body depends on its quantity of matter and the strength of the gravitational attraction acting on it. The measure of gravitational *force* is called weight. The mass of an object will not change even if taken to the moon, but its weight will. The kilogram, equal to the mass of a liter of water, is the unit of mass in the metric system. The unit of force (weight) is the newton (N), and for most of the United States a mass of

TABLE 10.1	Comparions of U.S. and Metric Systems of Measurement		
Unit	Metric System	U.S.	Equivalents
Length	centimeter (cm)	inch (in)	1 in = 2.54 cm
	meter (m) = 100 cm	foot (ft)	1 cm = 0.3937 in
	kilometer (km) = 1000 m	mile (mi) = 5280 ft	1 ft = 0.305 m
			1 m = 3.28 ft
			1 mi = 1.609 km
			1 km = 0.621 mi
Area	square meter (100 cm^2)	square foot (144 in^2)	1 in^2 = 6.45 cm^2
			1 cm^2 = 0.155 in^2
Volume	cubic cm (cm^3)	cubic in (in^3)	1 qt = 0.946 liter
	liter (1000 cm^3)	quart (57.75 in^3)	1 liter = 1.06 qt
			1 in^3 = 16.39 cm^3
			1 cm^3 = 0.06 in^3
Mass	kilogram (kg)	slug (32 lb)	1 kg = 0.068 slug
			1 slug = 14.6 kg
Force (weight)	newton (0.102 kg)	pound (lb)	1 lb = 0.454 kg
			1 kg 2.21 lb
			1 N = 0.225 lb
Time	second	second	

1 kilogram weighs approximately 9.80 newtons. In the U.S. system the pound is the basic unit of force (weight). The mass unit is the slug (from the English word for sluggish). A mass of 1 slug weighs approximately 32 pounds for the gravitational pull present at the latitude and longitude of most of the United States.

Time

The basic unit of time for both systems of measurement is the second.

Scalar and Vector Quantities

Quantities that are used in the description of motion may be classified as either scalar or vector in nature.

Scalar quantities are single quantities. They possess only size or amount. This size or amount is referred to as magnitude and completely describes the scalar quantity. The units of measure described in the previous section are primarily scalar quantities because they are described only by magnitude. Examples of scalar quantities would be such things as a speed of 8 kilometers per hour, a temperature of 70 degrees, an area of 2 square kilometers, a mass of 10 kilograms, or a height of 2 meters.

There are also double quantities that cannot be described by magnitude alone. These double quantities are called **vector** quantities. A vector quantity is described by both magnitude and direction. Examples of vector quantities would be a velocity of 8 kilometers per hour in a northwest direction, 10 newtons of force applied at a 30-degree angle, a displacement of 100 meters from the starting point. The importance of clearly designating vector quantities can be seen if the direction component of the double quantity is altered. For instance, if two people on opposite sides of a door push with equal magnitudes (amounts) of force, the door will not move. If, on the other hand, they both push on the same side of the door, thus changing the *direction* of one of the forces, the result will be very different. The nature of the movement of the door depends on both the *amount* and *direction* of the force. Force, therefore, is a vector quantity. If the individual who ran 8 kilometers runs 8 more kilometers, the total distance run will be 16 kilometers. However, if the runner goes 8 kilometers in one direction, reverses, and runs back to the starting point, the change in position, or **displacement,** is zero. The runner is 0 kilometers from the starting point. Displacement, then, is also a vector quantity possessing both magnitude and direction. Numerous quantities in biomechanics are vector quantities. In addition to force, displacement, and velocity already mentioned, some other examples are momentum, acceleration, friction, work, and power. Vector quantities exist whenever *direction* and *amount* are inherent characteristics of the quantities.

VECTOR ANALYSIS

Vector Representation

A vector is represented by an arrow whose length is proportional to the magnitude of the vector. The direction in which the arrow points indicates the direction of the vector quantity. Figure 10.1 shows examples of arrows indicating the vector quantities of force, displacement, and velocity.

Vector quantities are equal if magnitude and direction are the same for each vector. Although all of the following vectors are of the same length (magnitude), only two are equal vector quantities. They are the two that also have the same direction (d and f).

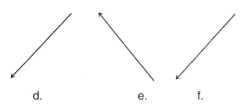

a.   b.   c.   d.   e.   f.

a. Displacement

b. Force   c. Velocity

Figure 10.1   Examples of vector amounts represented by arrows: (a) displacement; (b) force; (c) velocity.

Combination of Vectors

Vectors may be combined by addition, subtraction, or multiplication. They are added by joining the head of one with the tail of the next while accounting for magnitude and direction. The combination results in a new vector called the **resultant.** The resultant vector is represented by the distance between the last head and the first tail. Figure 10.2 shows examples of vectors that have been combined by addition. Note that the head of the re-

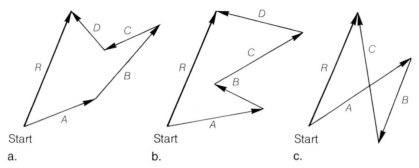

Start   Start   Start

a.   b.   c.

Figure 10.2 Vectors are added by joining the head of one with the tail of the next. The same resultant vector *R,* in examples (a), (b), and (c), may be obtained from the combination of dissimilar components.

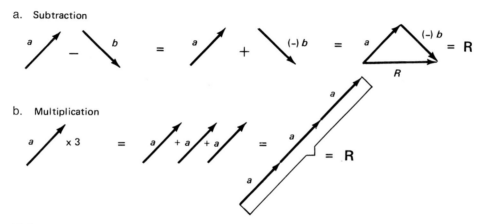

Figure 10.3 Vectors may be combined by subtraction or multiplication.

sultant *R* meets the *head* of the last component vector. These drawings also show that very different component vectors may produce the same resultant.

The subtraction of vectors is done by changing the sign of one vector (multiply by −1) and then adding as before (figure 10.3a). The multiplication of a vector by a number changes its magnitude only, not its direction (figure 10.3b).

Resolution of Vectors

As just explained, the combination of two or more vectors results in a new vector. Con-

versely, any vector may be broken down or resolved into two component vectors acting at right angles to each other. The vector in figure 10.1c represents the velocity with which the shot was put. Should one wish to know how much of that velocity was in a horizontal direction and how much in a vertical direction, the vector must be resolved into horizontal and vertical components. In figure 10.4, *A* and *B* are the vertical and horizontal *components* of resultant *R.* The vector addition of these components once again would result in the resultant vector *R.* The arrows over *A, B,* and *R* indicate that they are vector quantities.

Figure 10.4   A resultant vector may be resolved or broken down into two component vectors acting at right angles to each other. The velocity vector *R* has a horizontal component *B* and a vertical component *A*.

Location of Vectors in Space

In describing motion it is helpful to have a frame of reference within which one can locate a position in space or change in position. It is possible to locate an object in three dimensions, but to simplify understanding, the description that follows is limited to motion in two dimensions, that is, one plane.

The position of a point *P* can be located using either *rectangular* coordinates or *polar* coordinates. In the two-dimensional rectangular coordinate system, the plane is divided into four quadrants by two perpendicular intersecting lines. The horizontal line is the *x* axis and the vertical line is the *y* axis. Values along either axis are

measured from the point of intersection of the two axes where *x* and *y* are both equal to zero (0, 0). The location of point *P* is represented by two numbers, the first equal to the number of *x* units and the second to the number of *y* units away from the intersection or origin. In figure 10.5, the rectangular coordinates for point *P* are *(x, y)* in a and (13, 5) in b. In this latter example, point *P* is at the head of vector *R* and, the location of the vector tail is at the origin, this vector's location in space is established. The tail is at (0, 0), and the head is at (13, 5).

Point *P* may also be described using polar coordinates. These consist of the distance *(r)* of point *P* from the origin and the angle (θ) that the line *r* makes with the *x* axis. The polar coordinates for point *P* in figure 10.5c are *(r, θ)*. If *P* is the vector head, *r* equals the vector's magnitude, and θ is equal to its direction. In polar terms the vector's description is *(r, θ)*.

In these coordinate systems, degrees are customarily measured in a counterclockwise direction. Also, by convention, *x* values to the right of the *y* axis are positive (+) and those to the left are negative (−). The *y* values above the *x* axis are positive and those below are negative. Point *A* in figure 10.6 has *(x, y)* coordinates of (4.3, 2.5) and *(r, θ)* coordinates of (5, 30°). The *(x, y)* coordinates for point *B* are (−1.5, −3) and the polar coordinates are (3.4, 240°).

Graphic Resolution and Combination of Vectors

Within this frame of reference, quantities encountered in the study of biomechanics may be portrayed and handled graphically. Consider a jumper who takes off with a velocity of 9.6 meters per second (m/sec) at an angle of 18 degrees. Because the takeoff velocity has both magnitude and direction, it is a vector quantity and may be *resolved* into its components. By selecting a linear unit of measurement to represent a unit of velocity, such as 1 cm to represent 1 meter per second of velocity, and by constructing a line of the

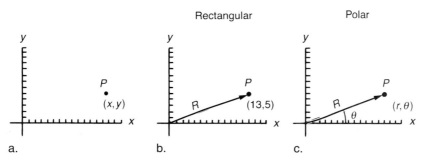

Figure 10.5   A point in space may be located in two dimensions using an *x* and *y* axis as a frame of reference. In (a) point *P* is *x* units from the *y* axis and *y* units from the *x* axis. In (b) point *P* is 13*x* units from the *y* axis and 5*y* units from the *x* axis. In (c) point *P* is *r* units from the *x, y* intersection and θ degrees from the *x* axis.

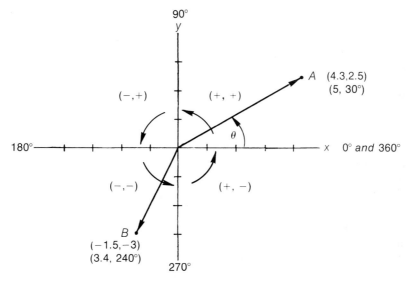

Figure 10.6   Coordinate quadrants. Values of *x* and *y* are positive in the upper right quadrant and negative in the lower left. And *x* is negative in the upper left and *y* is negative in the lower right.

appropriate length at an angle of 18 degrees to the *x* axis, one can determine the horizontal and vertical components of velocity for that jump. This is done by constructing a right triangle in which the hypotenuse is the vector, representing the total velocity of the jump, the vertical side is the vertical velocity, and the horizontal side is the horizontal velocity (figure 10.7). The horizontal and vertical velocity components are determined by

carefully measuring the lengths of the respective sides of the triangle and converting those amounts to velocity values by using the conversion factor. In this illustration, the conversion factor selected was 1 cm = 1 m/sec. The values obtained from measuring the lengths of the sides and applying the conversion factor were 5.2 m/sec of horizontal velocity component and 1.7 m/sec of vertical velocity.

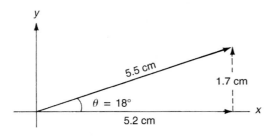

Given
Velocity of jump = 5.5 m/sec
Angle of takeoff = 18°

Solution
Let 1 cm = 1 m/sec

Then: Velocity of jump = 5.5 cm
Horizontal velocity x = 5.2 cm = 5.2 m/sec
Vertical velocity y = 1.7 cm = 1.7 m/sec

Figure 10.7 Graphic method of vector resolution. The horizontal and vertical velocity components of the broad jump with an initial velocity of 5.5 m/sec at a direction of 18 degrees are determined by drawing vector components to scale.

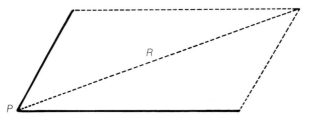

Figure 10.8 A "parallelogram of forces" used for determining the composite effect of two forces applied to the same point.

The *combination* of vectors to determine the resultant vector may also be obtained graphically by the construction of a parallelogram, the sides of which are linear representations of the two vectors. The first step is to mark a point *P* on a piece of paper. This represents the point at which the two vectors are applied. From this point two vector lines are drawn to scale, with the correct angle between them—that is, the same angle that actually exists between the two vectors. By using these two lines as two sides, a parallelogram is constructed with the addition of two more lines to form the other two sides (figure 10.8). The diagonal is then drawn from the point of application *P* to the opposite corner. This diagonal represents both in magnitude and direction the composite effect of the two separate vectors. It is the resultant vector R.

When one wishes to determine the resultant of *three* or more vectors acting at one point, a similar procedure is followed. First, the resultant of two of the vectors is found. A second parallelogram is then constructed using the third vector as one side and the resultant of the first two vec-

tors as the second side. The resultant vector of this second parallelogram is the resultant of all three vectors (figure 10.9).

Another graphic method combines the vectors by adding them head to tail. Suppose muscle *J* has a force of 1000 newtons and is pulling on bone E–F at an angle of 10 degrees, and muscle *K* has a force of 800 newtons and is pulling at an angle of 40 degrees (figure 10.10a). The composite effect of these two muscles may be described in terms of the amount of force and the direction or angle of pull of that composite force. Again a linear unit of measure is selected to represent a unit of force, and the vectors are placed in reference to the *x, y* axes so that the tail of the force vector for muscle *K* is added to the head of the force vector for muscle *J* (figure 10.10b). The scale used in this example is 1 cm = 400 N. The resultant vector was drawn connecting the tail of *J* with the head of *K*. Its length represents the resultant force of the two muscles. The force in newtons was obtained by multiplying the vector length by the conversion factor, 1 cm = 400 N. The direction of the result-

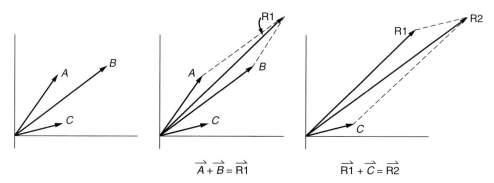

$$\overrightarrow{A} + \overrightarrow{B} = \overrightarrow{R1} \qquad \overrightarrow{R1} + \overrightarrow{C} = \overrightarrow{R2}$$

Figure 10.9   Parallelogram method used for determining the composite effect of three or more forces applied to the same point. R_1 is resultant of combined forces A and B. R_2 is resultant of combined forces R_1 and C. Thus A + B + C = R_2.

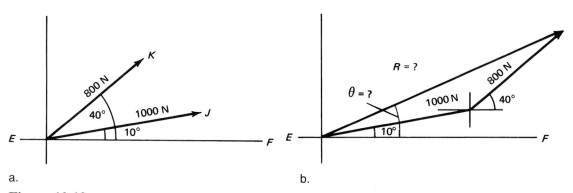

a.   b.

Figure 10.10   Combination of vectors using graphic method. Vector J is added to vector K taking into account magnitude and direction. Resultant R is drawn by connecting the tail of J to the head of K. When measured with a ruler, R equals 7 cm, which according to the scale is equivalent to 1750 N. The resultant angle θ, when measured with a protractor, is 23.5°.

ant force is indicated by the angle between the x axis and the resultant (measured with a protractor). Careful use of a protractor and ruler produced an R of 4.4 cm, which is equivalent to 1760 newtons pulling in a direction of 23.5 degrees. Like the parallelogram technique, this method is not limited to two vectors. Any number of vectors may be combined in this fashion.

Trigonometric Resolution and Combination of Vectors

Although the graphic method has value for portraying the situation, it does have serious draw-backs when it comes to calculating results. Accuracy is difficult to control in the drawing and measuring process, and the procedure is slow and unwieldy. A more accurate and efficient approach makes use of trigonometric relationships for both combining and resolving vectors.

Any vector may be resolved into horizontal and vertical components if the trigonometric relationships of a right triangle are employed. Let us use the previous example of the jumper whose velocity at takeoff was 9.6 m/sec in the direction of 18 degrees with the horizontal (see figure 10.7). To find the horizontal velocity (V_x) and vertical velocity (V_y) at takeoff a right triangle is constructed.

With the takeoff velocity (R) as the hypotenuse of the triangle, the vertical and horizontal components of velocity become the vertical and horizontal sides of the triangle (figure 10.11). To obtain the values of V_x and V_y the sine and cosine functions are used as shown in figure 10.11. The horizontal velocity of the jump V_x turns out to be 9.1 m/sec and the vertical velocity V_y is 3.0 m/sec.

The combination of vectors is also possible with the use of right triangle trigonometric relationships. If two vectors are applied at right angles to each other, the solution should appear rea-

sonably obvious because it is the reverse of the example just explained. If a baseball is thrown with a vertical velocity of 15 m/sec and a horizontal velocity of 26 m/sec, the velocity of the throw and the angle of release may be determined as shown in figure 10.12. The resultant velocity— that is, the velocity of the throw—is 30 m/sec and the angle of projection is 30 degrees.

If more than two vectors are involved or if they are not at right angles to each other as shown in previous examples, the resultant may be obtained by determining the x and y components for

Given: $R = 9.6$ m/sec

              $\theta = 18°$

To find: Value of V_y

              $\sin \theta = \dfrac{opp}{hyp} = \dfrac{V_y}{R}$

              $V_y = \sin 18° \times 9.6 = .3090 \times 9.6$

              $\boxed{V_y = 3.0 \text{ m/sec}}$

To find: Value of V_x

              $\cos \theta = \dfrac{adj}{hyp} = \dfrac{V_x}{R}$

              $V_x = \cos 18° \times 9.6 = .9511 \times 9.6$

              $\boxed{V_x = 9.1 \text{ m/sec}}$

Figure 10.11   Resolution of a vector using the trigonometric method. Horizontal and vertical components are determined by using cosine and sine functions.

Given: $V_y = 15$ m/sec
        $V_x = 26$ m/sec

Find: R and θ

Solution: $R^2 = V_y^2 + V_x^2$

$R^2 = 15^2 + 26^2 = 901$

$\boxed{R^2 = \sqrt{901} = 30 \text{ m/sec}}$

$\theta = \arctan \dfrac{V_y}{V_x}$

$\theta = \arctan \dfrac{15}{26}$

$\boxed{\theta = 30°}$

Figure 10.12   Trigonometric solution to combination of two vectors applied at right angles.

each individual vector and then summing these individual components to obtain the x and y components of the resultant. Once the x and y components are known, the magnitude and direction of R may be obtained. Let us consider the problem treated graphically in figure 10.10, in which we were interested in determining the composite force of the two muscles and the resultant direction or angle of pull. To solve this problem trigonometrically, the horizontal and vertical components for each muscle must first be determined, as shown here:

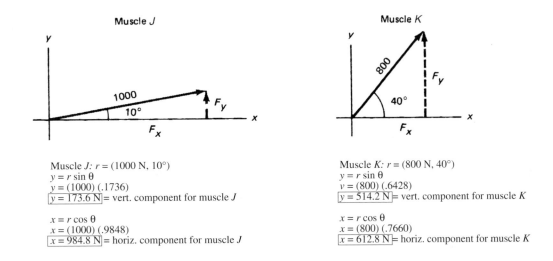

Muscle J: $r = (1000$ N, $10°)$
$y = r \sin \theta$
$y = (1000) (.1736)$
$\boxed{y = 173.6 \text{ N}}$ = vert. component for muscle J

$x = r \cos \theta$
$x = (1000) (.9848)$
$\boxed{x = 984.8 \text{ N}}$ = horiz. component for muscle J

Muscle K: $r = (800$ N, $40°)$
$y = r \sin \theta$
$v = (800) (.6428)$
$\boxed{y = 514.2 \text{ N}}$ = vert. component for muscle K

$x = r \cos \theta$
$x = (800) (.7660)$
$\boxed{x = 612.8 \text{ N}}$ = horiz. component for muscle K

Next, to obtain the y component of the resultant effect of the *two* muscles, the y values for muscles J and K are summed ($\Sigma y = 173.6 + 514.2$; $\Sigma y = 687.8$ N). Similarly, the x component for R is the sum of the x values for J and K ($\Sigma x = 984.8 + 612.8$; $\Sigma x = 1597.6$ N).

As we have seen before, a knowledge of the horizontal (x) and vertical (y) components makes it possible to determine the resultant vector. A triangle is formed and the unknown parts are found. Figure 10.13 presents the solution once the x and y values for muscles J and K have each been

Given: $\Sigma y = 687.8$ N
            $\Sigma x = 1597.6$ N
Find: θ and r

Solution: $\theta = \arctan \dfrac{\Sigma y}{\Sigma x}$

$\theta = \arctan \dfrac{687.8}{1597.6} = .4305$

$\boxed{\theta = 23.3°}$

$R = \dfrac{687.8}{\sin 23.3°} = \dfrac{687.8}{.3955}$

$\boxed{R = 1739 \text{ N}}$

Figure 10.13   Trigonometric combination of summed vectors. The sum of all x components becomes the horizontal vector component; the sum of all y components becomes the vertical vector component. R and θ are determined by combining Σx and Σy.

summed. The summed F_y and F_x values form the two sides of the triangle and the unknown resultant force is the hypotenuse. Using the tangent relationship between the two sides, the resultant angle of pull of the two muscles was calculated to be 23.3 degrees. With this additional information, the composite or resultant force of 1739 newtons was found using the $\sin \theta$ = opposite/hypotenuse relationship.

In the explanation of coordinate systems it was shown that values of x and y may be negative and that values of θ may exceed 90 degrees (see figure 10.6). An example of a problem with these additional factors is that of the hiker who plots the stated course and then must determine the resultant displacement at the completion of the course:

A hiker walks the following course: 2000 meters at 30 degrees, 1000 meters at 100 degrees, and 500 meters at 225 degrees. What is her resultant displacement? The solution is presented in figure 10.14.

Value of Vector Analysis

The ability to handle variables of motion and force as vector or scalar quantities should improve one's understanding of motion and the forces causing it. The effect that a muscle's angle of pull has on the force available for moving a limb is better understood when it is subjected to vector analysis. Similar study of the direction and force of projectiles improves one's understanding of the effect of gravity, angle of release, and force of release upon the flight of a projectile. The effect of several muscles exerting their combined forces on a single bone is also clarified when treated quantitatively as the combination of vector quantities to obtain a *resultant*. Indeed, the effect that a change in any variable may produce becomes much more apparent. Without the use of a vector relationship, it would be difficult if not impossible to describe motion and forces in meaningful, quantitative terms.

Resolution of Individual Vectors:

For 2000 m at 30°:

x = 2000 m cos 30° y = 2000 m sin 30°
x = 2000 m × .866 y = 2000 m × .500
x = 1732 m y = 1000 m

For 1000 m at 100°:

θ = 100° − 90° θ = 10°
x = −1000 m sin 10° y = 1000 m cos 10°
x = −1000 m × .174 y = 1000 m × .985
x = −174 m y = 985 m

For 500 m at 225°:

θ = 225° − 180° θ = 45°
x = −500 m cos 45° y = −500 m sin 45°
x = −500 m × .707 y = −500 m × .707
x = −353.5 m y = −353.5 m

x = 1732 + (−174) + (−353.5) = 1204.5 m
y = 1000 + 985 + (−353.5) = 1631.5 m

$R = \sqrt{x^2 + y^2} = \sqrt{1204.5^2 + 1631.5^2} = \boxed{2028 \text{ m}}$

$\theta = \arctan \dfrac{y}{x} = \dfrac{1631.5}{1204.5} = 1.354 \quad \boxed{\theta = 53.6}$

Figure 10.14   Combination of vectors involving negative values of x and y and values of θ larger than 90 degrees.

LABORATORY EXPERIENCES

1. Define the following key terms:
   Statics
   Dynamics
   Kinematics
   Kinetics
   Scalar
   Vector
   Component vector

2. Express the following units in metric terms:
   a. A force of 25 pounds
   b. A mass of 5 slugs
   c. A distance of 11 inches
   d. A velocity of 20 feet per second
   e. A volume of 3 quarts

3. Determine the distance between each set of points (scale: 1 unit = 10 cm).
   a. (2, 3); (5, 7)
   b. (1, 2); (3, 3)
   c. (1.5, 3.0); (6, 6)
   d. (0, 0); (6.2, 3.6)

4. Find the x and y component for each of the following vectors:
   a. 45 m/sec at 25°
   b. 85 N at 135°
   c. 118 kg at 310°
   d. 25 m/sec^2 at 210°

5. A basketball official runs 20 meters along the sideline in one direction, reverses, and runs 8 meters. What is the distance run? What is the displacement? Draw a vector diagram.

6. The muscular force of a muscle is 650 N and the muscle is pulling on the bone at an angle of 15 degrees. What are the vertical and horizontal components of this force?

7. At the moment of release, a baseball has a horizontal velocity component of 25 meters per second and a vertical velocity component of 14 meters per second. At what angle was it released, and what was its initial velocity in the direction of the throw in m/sec? In ft/sec?

8. A child is being pulled in a sled by a person holding a rope that has an angle of 20 degrees with the horizontal. The total force being used to move the sled at a constant forward speed is 110 N. How much of the force is horizontal? Vertical?

9. An orienteer runs the following course: 1000 meters at 45°, 1500 meters at 120°, 500 meters at 190°.
   a. Draw the course to scale accurately.
   b. Determine the resultant displacement graphically.
   c. Determine the resultant displacement trigonometrically.
   d. Explain any differences you have between your graphic and trigonometric results.
   e. Express the orienteer's position at the end of the course in terms of rectangular coordinates; polar coordinates.

10. A football lineman charges an opponent with a force of 175 pounds in the direction of 310 degrees. The opponent charges back with a force of 185 pounds in the direction of 90 degrees. What is the resultant force and in what direction will it act?

11. Referring to figures 2.2 and 7.21, make a tracing of the femur and adductor longus muscle. Draw a straight line to represent the mechanical axis of the femur and another to represent the muscle's line of pull.
    a. Using a protractor, determine the angle of pull of the muscle (angle formed by muscle's line of pull and mechanical axis of bone).
    b. Assuming a total muscle force of 900 N, calculate the force components.

12. Muscle A has a force of 450 N and is pulling on a bone at an angle of 15 degrees. Muscle B has a force of 600 N and is pulling on the same bone at the same spot but at an angle of 30 degrees. Muscle C has a force of 325 N and is pulling at the same spot with an angle of pull of 10 degrees. What is the composite effect of these muscles in terms of amount of force and direction?

13. Name as many vector and scalar quantities you can think of that are part of the games of football, tennis, or golf.

14. Choose one of the following sports:
    Volleyball
    Soccer
    Field hockey
    a. For that sport make a list of the individual motor skills represented and classify each skill

according to the classification model presented in chapter 1 (p. 6).
b. Name the underlying mechanics objective for each skill identified (chapter 1, p. 13).

c. Identify the scalar and vector quantities that are a part of each skill identified. For each skill, draw and label a vector diagram for *one* of the vector quantities named.

REFERENCES AND SELECTED READINGS

Atwater, A. E. 1980. Kinesiology/biomechanics: Perspectives and trends. *Research Quarterly for Exercise and Sport* 51:193–218.

Groves, R., and D. N. Camione. 1983. *Concepts in kinesiology.* 2nd ed. Philadelphia: Saunders College Publishing.

Hamill, J., and K. M. Knutzen. 1995. *Biomechanical basis of human movement.* Baltimore: Wiiliams & Wilkins.

Hay, J. G. 1993. *The biomechanics of sports techniques.* 4th ed. Englewood Cliffs, NJ: Prentice Hall.

Rodgers, M. M., and P. Cavanagh. 1984. Glossary of biomechanical terms, concepts, and units. *Physical Therapy* 64:1887–1901.

Tözeren, A. 2000. *Human body dynamics: Classical mechanics and human movement.* New York: Springer.

THE DESCRIPTION OF HUMAN MOTION

O U T L I N E

- **Motion**
  Relative Motion
  Cause of Motion
  Kinds of Motion
  Kinds of Motion Experienced
      by the Body
  Factors That Determine the Kind
      of Motion
  Factors Modifying Motion
- **Kinematic Description of Motion**
  Linear Kinematics
  Angular Kinematics
- **Laboratory Experiences**

O B J E C T I V E S

At the conclusion of this chapter, the student should be able to:

1. Name the kinds of motion experienced by the human body, and describe the factors that cause and modify motion.

2. Name and properly use the terms that describe linear and rotary motion: position, displacement, distance, speed, velocity, and acceleration.

3. Explain the interrelationships that exist among displacement, velocity, and acceleration, and use the knowledge of these interrelationships to describe and analyze human motion.

4. Describe the behavior of projectiles, and explain how angle, speed, and height of projection affect that behavior.

5. Describe the relationship between linear and rotary movement, and explain the significance of this relationship to human motion.

6. Identify the critical kinematic components that would be used to fully describe the skillful performance of a selected motor task.

MOTION

If we are to understand the movements of the human musculoskeletal system and the objects put into motion by this system, we need first to turn our thoughts to the concepts of motion itself. What is motion? What determines the kind of motion that will result when an object or a part of the human body is made to move? How is motion described in mechanical terms? How do these generalities about motion apply to movements of the musculoskeletal system? Indeed, how does one know that motion is occurring?

Relative Motion

Motion is the act or process of changing place or position with respect to some reference object. Whether a body is at rest or in motion depends totally on the reference. When a person is walking down the street or riding a bicycle or serving a tennis ball, it seems obvious that movement is involved. Less obvious is the motion status of the sleeping passenger in a smoothly flying plane or of an automobile parked at a curb. If the earth is the reference point, all but the parked car are in motion relative to the earth, and even the parked car is in motion if the reference point is the sun. On the other hand, if the bicycle is the reference point, the person riding it is at rest relative to the bicycle, and the sleeping passenger is at rest with respect to anything in the plane. The relative motion of each is defined in relation to the specific reference object or point. It is possible, therefore, to be at rest and in motion at the same time relative to different reference points. The sleeping passenger is at rest relative to the plane and in motion relative to the earth. The relative motion of two bodies depends entirely on their relative velocities through space. Two joggers running at 8 km/hr in the same direction are at rest with respect to each other. However, if one jogs at 8 km/hr and the other at 10 km/hr, the slower jogger would be considered to be at rest with respect to the faster but the faster would be in mo-

tion both with respect to the slower runner and to the earth.

Cause of Motion

It is difficult to think of motion without visualizing a specific object in the act of moving. If we did not actually see how it changed from a stationary condition to a moving one, we might wonder what caused it to be set in motion. Did someone pull on it, or push against it, or perhaps blow on it or even attract it with a magnet? What are these assumed causes of motion? Without exception, each cause of motion is a form of force. Force is the instigator of movement. If we see an object in motion, we know that it is moving because a force has acted on it. We know, too, that the force must have been sufficiently great to overcome the object's inertia, or resistance to motion, for unless a force is greater than the resistance offered by the object it cannot produce motion. We can push against a stone wall all day without moving it so much as 1 millimeter, but a bulldozer can knock the wall down at the first impact. The magnitude of the force relative to the *magnitude of the resistance* is the determining factor in causing an object to move.

Kinds of Motion

What are the ways in which an object may move? The hand moves in an arc when the forearm turns at the elbow joint and the neighboring joints are held motionless. A hockey puck may slide across the ice without turning. On the other hand, it may revolve as it slides. A figure skater spins in place. Arrows, balls, and jumpers move through the air in an arc known as a parabola. As we note the different ways in which objects move, we are impressed with the almost limitless variety in the patterns of movement. Objects move in straight paths and in curved paths; they roll, slide, and fall; they bounce; they swing back and forth like a pendulum; they rotate about a center, either partially or completely; and they frequently rotate at the same time that they move as a whole from one place to another. Although the variety of ways in which objects move appears to be almost limitless, careful consideration of these ways reveals that there are, in actuality, only two major classifications of movement patterns. These are translatory, or linear, and rotary, or angular. Either an object moves in its entirety from one place to another or it turns about a center of motion. Sometimes it does both simultaneously.

Translatory Movement

This kind of movement is termed translatory because the object is translated as a whole from one location to another. Translatory movement is commonly called linear motion and is further classified as rectilinear or curvilinear. *Rectilinear motion* is the straight-line progression of an object as a whole with all its parts moving the same distance in the same direction at a uniform rate of speed. The child on the sled in figure 11.1, a water skier pulled by a boat, or a bowling ball moving in a straight path are examples of rectilinear motion.

Curvilinear motion refers to all curved translatory movement; that is, the object moves in a curved pathway. The paths of a ball or any other projectile in flight, the wrist during the force phase in bowling (figure 11.2), or a skier in a sweeping turn are all examples of curvilinear motion.

Figure 11.1   An example of rectilinear motion.

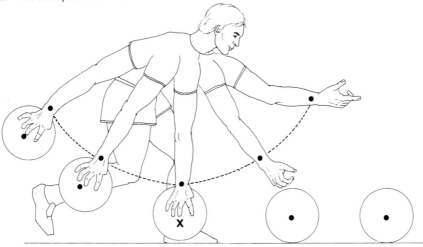

Figure 11.2   The wrist follows a curvilinear path during the delivery of a bowling ball. (Drawn from motion picture film tracing.)

A special form of curvilinear motion, which on the surface does not appear to be translatory, is that called *circular motion*. This type of motion occurs when an object moves along the circumference of a circle, that is, a curved path of constant radius. The logic for calling this type of motion linear relates to the fact that it occurs when an unbalanced force acts on a moving body to keep it in a circle. If that unbalanced force stops acting on the object and the object is free to move, it will move in a linear path tangent to the direction in which it is moving at the moment of release. A classic example is an object tied to the end of a string and swung in circles around the head. When the object is released it will fly off in a straight line. The hammer in the hammer throw follows a circular path until it is released, at which time it flies along a curvilinear path until it lands. The path of a ball held in the hand as the arm moves around in windmill fashion is another example of circular motion. If the ball is released during the motion, it will fly off at a tangent and continue in a straight line until gravity forces it into a curved path. Other examples of bodies in circular motion are the gondola on a moving Ferris wheel or the knot on the ring of a spinning lariat.

Rotary, or Angular, Motion

This kind of motion is typical of levers and of wheels and axles. Rotary, or angular, motion occurs when any object acting as a radius moves about a fixed point. The distance traveled may be a small arc or a complete circle and is measured as an angle, in degrees. Most human body segment motions are angular movements in which the body part moves in an arc about a fixed point. The axial joints of the skeleton act as fixed points for rotary motion in the segments. The arm engages in rotary motion when it moves in windmill fashion about a fixed point or axis in the shoulder. The head's motion in the act of indicating "no," the lower leg in kicking a ball, or the hand and forearm in turning a doorknob are all examples of rotary, or angular, motion. In each instance the moving body segment may be likened to the radius of a circle. The arm moving in windmill fashion and the lower leg and foot in kicking are the radii (figure 11.3). In

Figure 11.3   Example of angular motion. The lower leg rotates about an axis in the knee joint. Similarly, the thigh engages in rotary motion moving about an axis in the hip joint. (Drawn from motion picture film tracing.)

the "no" action of the head and in the doorknob being turned by the forearm and hand, the radius is perpendicular to the long axis running vertically through the middle of the head and lengthwise through the middle of the forearm and hand, respectively. These movements are not to be confused with circular motion. Circular motion describes the motion of any point on the radius, whereas angular motion is descriptive of the motion of the entire radius. When a ball is held in the hand as the arm moves in a windmill fashion, the ball is moving with circular motion, while the arm acts as a radius moving with angular motion about the fixed point of the shoulder.

Other Movement Patterns

Reciprocating motion denotes repetitive movement. The use of the term is ordinarily limited to repetitive translatory movements, as illustrated by a bouncing ball or the repeated blows of a ham-

a.   b.

Figure 11.4   General motion: linear motion of one part of the body (the hand) resulting from angular motion of several segments of the body. (a) Just before lunge (thrust). (b) At completion of lunge.

mer, but technically it includes all kinds. The term oscillation refers specifically to repetitive movements in an arc. Familiar examples of this type of movement are seen in the pendulum, metronome, and playground swing.

Often an object displays a combination of rotary and translatory movement. This is sometimes referred to as general motion. The bicycle, automobile, and train move linearly as the result of the rotary movements of their wheels. Likewise, people, as they walk or run down the street, experience translatory motion because of the angular movement of their body segments. The angular motions of several segments of the body are frequently coordinated in such a way that a single related segment will move linearly. This is true in throwing darts, in shot putting, and in a lunge in fencing (figure 11.4). Because of the angular motions of the forearm and upper arm, the hand travels linearly and thus is able to impart linear force to the dart, to the shot prior to the release, and to the foil.

Kinds of Motion Experienced by the Body

The human body experiences all kinds of motion. Because most of the joints are axial, the body segments must undergo primarily angular motion (figure 11.5). A slight amount of translatory motion is seen in the gliding movements of the plane

or irregular joints but these movements are negligible in themselves. They occur chiefly in the carpal and tarsal joint and in the joints of the vertebral arches in conjunction with angular movements in neighboring axial joints.

The body as a whole experiences rectilinear movement when it is acted on by the force of gravity, as in coasting down a hill (figure 11.1) or in a free fall (figure 11.6), and likewise when acted on by an external force, as in water skiing (figure 11.7). It experiences general motion in forward and backward rolls on the ground and in somersaults in the air, and rotary motion in twirling on ice skates. It experiences curvilinear translatory motion in diving and jumping, and it experiences reciprocating motion when swinging back and forth on a swing or a bar.

Factors That Determine the Kind of Motion

Thus far we have considered the cause of motion and the various kinds of motion on the basis of movement patterns or paths. Now we must turn to another question. What determines the kind of motion that will result when an object is made to move? The best way for the student to discover the answer is to produce each kind of motion and then analyze what was done to obtain the desired kind of motion.

Figure 11.5   An example of movement of the body caused by the body's own muscular activity. Movements of individual body segments are primarily angular. (Drawn from motion picture film tracing.)

To make an object move linearly, we discover that it must be free to move and that either we must apply force uniformly against one entire side of the object or we must apply it directly in line with the object's center of gravity. The object will move in a straight line provided it does not meet an obstacle or resistance of some sort. If its edge hits against another object or encounters a rough spot, the moving object will turn about its point of contact with the interfering obstacle. If we attempt to push a tall cabinet across a supporting surface that provides excessive friction, such as a cement floor, the cabinet will tip, even though we place our hands exactly in line with the cabinet's center of gravity and push in a horizontal direction. To move it linearly it will be necessary to apply the push lower than the cabinet's center of gravity to compensate for the friction.

If one part of an object is "fixed," rotary motion will occur when sufficient force is applied on any portion of the object that is free to move. A lever undergoes rotary motion because, by definition, some portion of it remains in place. If it is desired to move an object in the manner of a lever it is necessary to provide a "fulcrum" or an axis and to apply force to the object at some point other than at the fulcrum. Thus, if rotary motion of a freely movable object is desired, it is necessary to apply force to it "off center" or to provide an "off center" resistance that will interfere with the motion of part of the object.

Reciprocating motion is caused by a uniform repetition of opposing force applications, and the oscillation of a pendulum is produced by repeated applications of gravitational force to a suspended object that is free to move back and forth and that is in any position other than its resting position.

In summary, the kind of motion that will be displayed by a moving object depends primarily on the kind of motion permitted in that particular kind of object. If it is a lever, it is permitted only

Figure 11.7   An example of movement of the body caused by an external force.

Figure 11.6   Landing from a vertical jump. An example of linear movement of the body caused by the force of gravity. (Drawn from motion picture film tracing.)

angular motion; if it is a pendulum, oscillatory motion; and so on. If it is a freely movable object, it is permitted either translatory or rotary motion, depending on the circumstances. These circumstances include the point at which force is applied with reference to the object's center of gravity, the environmental pathways of movement available to the object, and the presence or absence of additional external factors that modify the motion.

Factors Modifying Motion

Motion is usually modified by a number of external factors, such as friction, air resistance, and water resistance. Whether these factors are a help

or a hindrance depends on the circumstances and the nature of the motion. The same factor may facilitate one form of motion, yet hinder another. For instance, friction is a great help to the runner because maximum effort may be exerted without danger of slipping; yet, on the other hand, friction hinders the rolling of a ball, as in field hockey, golf, and croquet. Again, wind or air resistance is indispensable to the sailboat's motion, but unless it is a tailwind, it impedes the runner. Likewise, water resistance is essential for propulsion of the body by means of swimming strokes and of boats through the use of oars and paddles, yet at the same time it hinders the progress of both the swimmer and the boat, especially if these present a broad surface to the water. For this reason, swimmers keep the body level, and designers plan streamlined boats. One of the major problems in movement is to learn how to take advantage of these modifying factors when they contribute to the movement in question and, on the other hand, how to minimize them when they are detrimental to the movement. A more detailed discussion of forces influencing motion is presented in the chapters on the conditions of linear and rotary motion.

The motion of the segments of the body is also modified by anatomical factors. These include friction in the joints (minimized by synovial fluid), tension of antagonistic muscles, tension of ligaments and fasciae, anomalies of bone and joint structure, atmospheric pressure within the joint capsule, and the presence of interfering soft tissues. Except for the limitations because of fat or muscle bulk, these modifying factors are classified as internal resistance.

KINEMATIC DESCRIPTION OF MOTION

Motion has been defined as the act or process of changing place or position with respect to some reference point. Thus, to talk about motion, a starting point must be identified. Once this is done the resultant motion, regardless of whether it is translatory or rotary, may be characterized according to the distance and direction away from the starting point, the speed of the movement, and any change in speed that may occur. This kind of motion study is called kinematics. Motion is described in terms of displacement, velocity, and acceleration with no consideration of or reference to the forces that cause or modify the motion. Linear kinematics is concerned with translatory motion and angular kinematics with rotary motion.

Linear Kinematics
Distance and Displacement

The distance an object is removed from a reference point is called its displacement. Displacement does not indicate how far the object travels in going from point A to point C. It only indicates the final change of position. A person who walks north for 3 kilometers to point B and then east for 4 kilometers to point C has walked a distance of 7 kilometers, but the displacement with respect to the starting point is only 5 kilometers (figure 11.8). Similarly, a basketball player who runs up and down the court several times has traveled a considerable distance, but the displacement with respect to one of the end lines may be zero. Or

consider the poor golfer who, blinded by the late afternoon sun, hits the ball so erratically and frequently that the route to the green, 450 yards away, crosses and recrosses the fairway many times. Regardless of the zigzag path to the green and the many changes of direction needed to get there, the ball's displacement is the straight-line distance from the tee to the green.

Displacement is a vector quantity having both magnitude and direction. It is not enough to indicate only the amount of positional change. That alone would be *distance,* a scalar quantity. The direction of the vector must also be defined. When the golfer finally reaches the green, the displacement from the hole to green is 450 yards west. And the walker's displacement in figure 11.8 is 5 km, in a northeast direction.

Speed and Velocity

Speed and *velocity* are two words that are frequently used to describe how fast an object is moving. These terms are often used interchangeably, but in fact there is a significant difference. Speed is related to distance and velocity to displacement. Speed tells how fast an object is moving—that is, the distance an object will travel in a given time—but it tells nothing about the direction of movement.

$$\text{Average speed} = \frac{\text{distance traveled}}{\text{time}} \text{ or} = \frac{\mathbf{d}}{\mathbf{t}}$$

Examples of speed measurements are a car traveling at 7 km/hr, the wind blowing at 60 mph, a ball thrown with a speed of 30 m/sec, or a sprinter running at 10 m/sec.

Velocity, on the other hand, involves direction as well as speed. Speed is a scalar quantity; whereas velocity is a vector quantity. In many activities this difference is of no concern, but in others it is of extreme importance. The speed of a football player carrying the ball may be impressive, but if not directed toward the opponent's goal, it is not providing yardage for a first down. Although the speed may be great, the velocity in the desired direction may indeed be zero. Veloc-

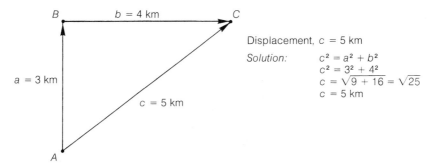

Displacement, c = 5 km

Solution: $c^2 = a^2 + b^2$
$c^2 = 3^2 + 4^2$
$c = \sqrt{9 + 16} = \sqrt{25}$
$c = 5$ km

Figure 11.8   Displacement is the resultant distance an object is removed from its starting point.

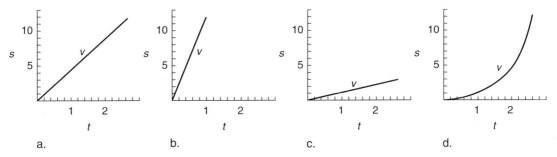

a.   b.   c.   d.

Figure 11.9   Examples of displacement-time graphs for uniform and nonuniform motion. The velocity in (a), (b), and (c) is constant.

ity is speed in a given direction. It is the amount of displacement per given unit of time. This is the same as saying that velocity is the rate of displacement, or

$$\text{Average velocity} = \frac{\text{displacement}}{\text{time}} \text{ or } = \frac{\mathbf{s}}{\mathbf{t}}$$

In the diagrams in figure 11.9, displacement values (s) are represented on the y axis and the time values (t) are on the x axis. If displacement values are plotted to correspond with their time values, the line formed by connecting these plotted values represents the rate of displacement or velocity (v). When the rate of displacement does not change—that is, when the distance and direction traveled is the same for each equal time period— the velocity is constant, and the velocity line on the diagram is a straight line. In figures 11.9a, b, and c the velocity is constant, but in figure 11.9d the curved line indicates that the rate of displace-

ment changes, and therefore the velocity is not constant. When there is greater displacement per unit of time, the velocity increases, as does the slope of the velocity line in the diagram. Figure 11.9b shows the fastest velocity and c the slowest. In d, the displacement starts at a slow rate and then increases. If a, b, c, and d represent runners on a straight track, a, b, and c would each be running at a constant but different velocity, with b's velocity the fastest and c's the slowest. Runner d starts out at a slow velocity but increases the rate of displacement until the resultant velocity is the fastest of all four.

Where velocity is constant, as in a, b, and c, the motion is said to be uniform. When the amount of displacement per unit of time varies, nonuniform motion occurs. Uniform motion is not a common characteristic of human motion, because most human movements are likely to have many variations in the rate of displacement.

When the velocity of human motion is given, it is usually an average velocity that tells only the total displacement occurring in a stated period of time. Although a long-distance runner who ran the Boston marathon, a distance of 26 miles, 385 yards, in 2.5 hours had an average velocity of 10.4 mph, it is doubtful that the velocity was uniformly 10.4 mph through the run. If one were to record the time at which the runner passed frequent and equally spaced distance points along the route, a displacement-time graph could be prepared to show the variations in the runner's speed at various points in the course of the race. This kind of information can be quite useful in helping a coach or participant analyze the performance and strategy of the race, and plan changes where needed. The narrower the distance intervals used, the greater is the possibility that critical variations in speed will become apparent. The use of cinematography permits a similar analysis of brief and fast events. The distance and time data necessary for graphing and analyzing the motion patterns are obtained indirectly from the film record.

In equation form, average velocity is

$$\bar{v} = \frac{s}{t}$$

The symbol $\bar{v}$ represents displacement, and t represents time. The average velocity of a tennis ball served 19 meters in 0.35 seconds is 19 divided by 0.35, or 54.3 m/sec in the direction of the service court.

Acceleration

When velocity changes, its rate of change is called **acceleration.** A sprint runner has an initial velocity of 0 m/sec. When the gun signals the beginning of a race, the sprinter's velocity begins to change by increasing. The rate of change in velocity is acceleration. Acceleration may be positive or negative. An increase is considered positive, and a decrease such as slowing down at the end of the race is negative. Negative acceleration is also called deceleration.

In equation form, acceleration is expressed as

$$\bar{a} = \frac{v - u}{t}$$

where $\bar{a}$ represents average acceleration, v is the final velocity, and u is the initial velocity. In other words, acceleration is any change in velocity divided by the time interval over which that change occurred.

In the example of the sprint runner, a graph of the sprinter's velocity throughout the race can be used to illustrate acceleration (figure 11.10). As the sprinter is waiting in the starting blocks, the velocity is zero. In section a of the race, the sprinter changes from a velocity of 0 to a velocity of 9 m/sec after the first 5.6 seconds. Because this is an increase in velocity, this is positive acceleration. The acceleration for this phase of the race, the rate of change in velocity, equals the difference between the final velocity (9 m/sec) and the initial velocity (0 m/sec) divided by the time interval (5.6 sec), or 1.8 m/sec^2. In section b of the race the velocity does not change but remains at a constant 9 m/sec. Because there is no change in velocity, the acceleration for this phase would be zero. To prove this, we use the equation

$$\bar{a} = \frac{v - u}{t} = \frac{9 \text{m/sec}}{9 - 5/\text{sec}} = \frac{0}{4/\text{sec}} = 0$$

In section c the sprinter increases velocity again just before the finish. In this phase the acceleration is not constant, so calculating an average velocity would not produce a true representation of the changes in velocity that are occurring. It is more accurate to calculate several instantaneous accelerations to plot a curve. By visually examining the curve, it can be seen that the acceleration at the beginning of this short phase is greater than the acceleration at the end of the phase. Section d of the race starts as the sprinter crosses the finish line. At this point the velocity is 10 m/sec. The sprinter now decreases velocity to come to a stop (0 m/sec) after the race. This slowing down represents negative acceleration, or deceleration.

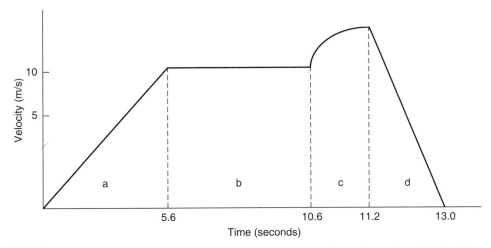

Figure 11.10 An acceleration curve showing a constant acceleration (uniform change in velocity) in (a), zero acceleration (no change in velocity) in (b), varying acceleration in (c), and constant deceleration (uniform slowing) in (d).

Because velocity is always displacement divided by time and acceleration is velocity divided by time, acceleration is really displacement divided by time divided by time, and the units for measurement must reflect this. The time unit must appear twice in acceleration units. The logic for this is apparent when the units of m/sec are used for velocity in the equation for average acceleration:

$$\bar{a} = \frac{\left(\dfrac{\text{final m}}{\text{sec}} - \dfrac{\text{initial m}}{\text{sec}}\right)}{\text{sec}}$$

After the subtraction is completed this equation becomes

$$\bar{a} = \frac{\dfrac{m}{\text{sec}}}{\text{sec}}$$

or, as commonly written, m/sec/sec or m/sec^2. Thus, the average acceleration of the runner in the example is 1.6 m/sec^2.

One usually thinks of acceleration in terms of a change in the amount of distance covered in equal units of time. Acceleration also occurs when, although the speed remains constant, there is a change in direction. The example given for

figure 11.10b is that of a runner keeping a steady pace on a straight track with no acceleration. If the runner, still running at the same speed, shifts to a circular track, acceleration occurs because of the change in direction, and the velocity-time graph would look more like figure 11.10c.

Uniformly Accelerated Motion

When the acceleration rate is constant, the velocity change is the same during equal time periods. Under these conditions motion is said to be uniformly accelerated. This type of acceleration does not occur with great frequency, because the change in velocity of bodies in motion is usually irregular and complicated. However, one common type of uniform acceleration is important in sport and physical education, the acceleration of freely falling bodies.

Neglecting air resistance, objects allowed to fall freely will speed up or accelerate at a uniform rate owing to the acceleration of gravity. Conversely, objects projected upward will be slowed at a uniform rate that is also due to the acceleration of gravity. The value for the acceleration of gravity changes with different locations on the earth's surface, but for most of the United States this value can be considered to be 32 ft/sec^2 or 9.80 m/sec^2.

Regardless of its size or density, a falling object will be acted on by gravity so that its velocity will increase 9.8 m/sec each second it is in the air. A dropped ball starting out with a velocity of 0 m/sec will have a velocity of 9.8 m/sec at the end of 1 second, 19.6 m/sec at the end of 2 seconds, 29.4 m/sec at the end of 3 seconds, and so on. A second ball weighing twice as much will fall with exactly the same acceleration. It too will have a velocity of 29.4 m/sec at the end of 3 seconds. Of course, this example does not consider the resistance or friction of air, which can be appreciable. The lighter the object, the more it is affected. After an initial acceleration, light objects such as feathers or snowflakes may stop accelerating entirely and fall at a constant rate. Consider, for instance, the difference between the behavior of a badminton shuttle and a golf ball when dropped from a height.

The denser and heavier the free-falling object, the less air friction affects it, especially if the distance of the fall is not too great. Even heavy objects, such as sky divers falling from great distances, eventually reach a downward speed large enough to create an opposing air resistance equal to the accelerating force of gravity. When this happens, the diver no longer speeds up but continues to fall at a steady speed. This speed is called terminal velocity and amounts to approximately 120 mph (53 m/sec) for a falling sky diver. With the parachute open, the diver's velocity decreases to 12 mph steady velocity.

Laws of uniformly accelerated motion In spite of the reality of air resistance, much can be learned about the nature of free-falling bodies and uniform acceleration through a knowledge of the laws of uniformly accelerated motion. Because the acceleration of gravity is constant, the distance traveled by a freely falling body, as well as its downward velocity, can be determined for any point in time by application of these laws. Expressed in equation form, they are

$$v = u + at$$
$$s = ut + \tfrac{1}{2}at^2$$
$$v^2 = u^2 + 2as$$

Galileo's experiments with inclined planes enabled him to work out these equations. They apply to any type of linear motion in which acceleration is uniform. Their specific application to the effect of gravity on freely falling objects is presented in table 11.1. If the initial velocity (u) is zero, as it is when an object is allowed to fall freely from a stationary position, the equations may be simplified:

$$v = at$$
$$s = \tfrac{1}{2}at^2$$
$$v^2 = 2as$$

The student may also discover that some authors, when applying these equations specifically to gravity, replace a, the symbol for acceleration, with the symbol g.

The time an object takes to rise to the highest point of its trajectory is equal to the time an object takes to fall to its starting point. Similarly, the release speed and landing speed are the same. Other than the fact that the directions are reversed, the upward flight is a mirror image of the downward flight. Proof that the release velocity and landing velocity are equal in amount but opposite in direction can be shown mathematically by substitution of values in the motion equations. Following vector conventions, velocities upward are positive and those downward are negative. Thus the acceleration of gravity is treated as a negative value.

Example Assuming that a ball is thrown upward so that it reaches a height of 5 meters before starting to fall, what is its initial velocity as it leaves the hand? What is its final velocity as it lands in the hand?

Upward Throw Velocity
Given: $v = 0$
$a = -9.80$ m/s^2
$s = 5$
Find: $u = ?$

Downward Landing Velocity
Given: $u = 0$
$a = -9.80$ m/s^2
$s = 5$
Find: $v = ?$

Solution Using eq. (11.3) $v^2 = u^2 + 2as$

$v^2 = u^2 + 2as$	$v^2 = u^2 + 2as$
$u^2 = v^2 - 2as$	$v^2 = 0 - (2 \times 9.8 \times 5)$
$u^2 = 0 + (2 \times 9.8 \times 5)$	$v^2 = -98.0$
$u^2 = 98.0$	$v = -\sqrt{98}$
$u = \sqrt{98.0}$	
$u = 9.90$ m/sec	$v = -9.90$ m/sec

TABLE 11.1	Effect of Gravity on a Freely Falling Object

	Time	Distance Traveled $s = ut + \frac{1}{2}at^2$	Final Velocity $v = u + at$	Average Velocity $\bar{v} = \dfrac{u + v}{2}$
U.S.	1 sec	16 ft	32 ft/sec	16 ft/sec
$a = 32$ ft/sec^2	2 sec	64 ft	64 ft/sec	32 ft/sec
	3 sec	144 ft	96 ft/sec	48 ft/sec
	4 sec	256 ft	128 ft/sec	64 ft/sec
	5 sec	400 ft	160 ft/sec	80 ft/sec
Metric	1 sec	4.9 m	9.8 m/sec	4.9 m/sec
$a = 9.80$ m/sec^2	2 sec	19.6 m	19.6 m/sec	9.8 m/sec
	3 sec	44.1 m	29.4 m/sec	14.7 m/sec
	4 sec	78.4 m	39.2 m/sec	19.6 m/sec
	5 sec	122.5 m	49 m/sec	24.5 m/sec

Projectiles

An object that has been given an initial velocity and then allowed to move in free fall under the influence of gravity is a projectile. Balls that are thrown, kicked, or hit; javelins; bullets or missiles; jumpers, divers, and gymnasts while in the air are all examples of projectiles.

An object or a body is projected into the air for any of several reasons. In the case of the diver or the gymnast, the purpose of the projection is to gain maximum time in the air, or time of flight. The longer the *time of flight* the athlete can produce, the greater the number of acrobatic moves that can be performed. In other activities, a decreased time of flight may serve to deceive or avoid an opponent, as in the volleyball spike, or a smash in tennis, or an onside kick in football. Projectiles may also be released for the purpose of producing *maximum horizontal displacement.*

The long jumper, the discus thrower, the shot-putter, and the batter in baseball are all examples of projection of an object for distance. Maximum displacement may also be in the vertical direction. Projections for maximum vertical displacement include such activities as the high jump and the pole vault. Projection of a body or an object for *maximum accuracy* is the purpose of actions such as shooting in basketball or soccer, passing, archery, or golf. When accuracy is the primary concern, a compromise often must be made between horizontal displacement and time in the air.

Once released, projectiles follow a predictable path. If air resistance is ignored because it is considered negligible, this path will be a parabola. The characteristic parabolic path of a projectile is the result of the constant downward force of gravity. This means that gravity will decelerate any upward motion at a

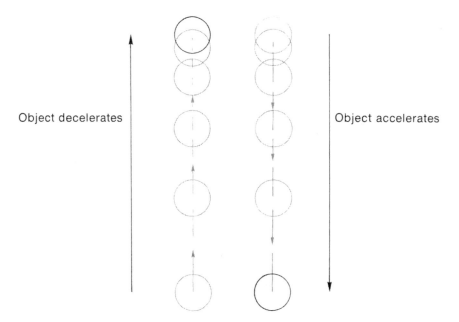

Object decelerates

Object accelerates

Figure 11.11   Objects projected upward are decelerated by the downward force of gravity at the same rate as those allowed to fall downward are accelerated. Both objects will cover the same distance in the same time. (Drawn from motion picture film tracing.)

rate of 9.8 m/sec² or will accelerate any downward motion at the same rate (figure 11.11). All objects in free fall have the same downward acceleration whether they start from a resting position with a drop or fall or have been given some initial velocity.

Two forces then, are acting on a projectile: the projecting force and gravity. The projecting force is a vector quantity that may act at any desired angle, depending on the purpose of the projection. The application of the projecting force produces an initial velocity in the object at some angle of projection. Because this initial release velocity is a vector quantity, it can be resolved into two component velocities, one vertical and one horizontal. The vertical component of velocity, being a vector parallel to gravity, will be directly affected by gravity. The horizontal component will not. Gravity is also a vector force that

always acts in a vertical, downward direction. This downward force of gravity acts completely independently of any horizontal component of the projecting force (figure 11.12).

If an object or a body is projected with only a horizontal velocity, then gravity, as the second force, will still act to cause that object to fall. If one object falls freely from rest at the same time that another is projected horizontally from the same height, both objects will hit the ground at the same time. However, they will hit in different places. The dropped object will land immediately below the point of release, whereas the projected object will land some distance away. Gravity has acted on both objects equally, giving them equal vertical velocities in the downward direction, so they will fall at the same rate and land at the same time. The difference in landing points is the result of the horizontal velocity possessed by the pro-

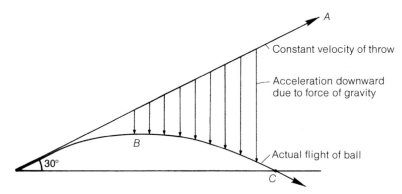

Figure 11.12 Effect of gravity on the flight of a projectile.

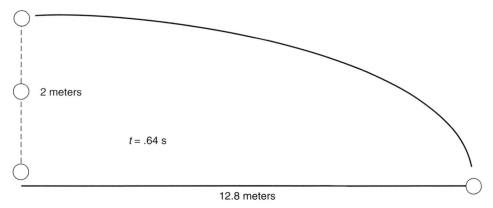

Figure 11.13 A horizontally projected object and a free-falling object released from the same height will land at the same time but in different places.

jected object. In the time it took both objects to fall, the horizontal velocity of the projected object carried that object some distance from the point of release. This distance can be calculated using the velocity equation

$$V = s/t \qquad \text{or} \qquad s = V * t$$

If, for instance, these two objects were balls released at a height of 2 meters, they would take .64 seconds to fall to the ground. If one was projected horizontally with a velocity of 20 m/sec, it would strike the ground at a distance of 12.8 meters from the release point ($s = 20$ m/sec $*$ .64 sec) (figure 11.13).

To change the time an object is in the air, the velocity produced by projection must have some vertical component. This may be an upward component, opposing gravity, or a downward component being added to gravity. The time an object is in the air may also be varied by altering the height of release. If the balls in the previous examples were released from a height of 3 meters, both balls would be in the air for .78 seconds. Using the velocity equation again, it can be determined that the horizontally projected ball would now travel 15.6 meters from the point of release ($s = 20$ m/sec $*$ .78 sec $= 15.6$ meters).

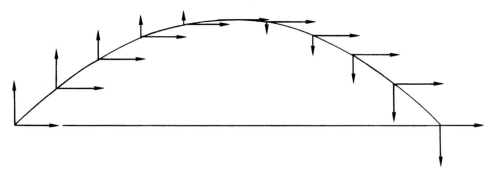

Figure 11.14   Magnitude of horizontal and vertical velocities during projectile flight.

An object that is projected with only upward velocity will be decelerated by gravity until it reaches a velocity of zero. At this point, it will start to drop back toward the release point, accelerating as it falls. When the object reaches the release point, it will possess the same velocity it was given at release. The time required to reach the highest point will be equal to the time it takes to fall back to the height from which it was released.

More often than not, objects put into flight will be projected in some direction other than exactly vertical or horizontal. A projectile of this type has both horizontal and vertical components of the initial velocity vector. Again, these two component velocities are considered independently. The horizontal component of velocity remains constant following release (if air resistance is neglected), as no force is available to change this velocity. The vertical component of velocity will be subject to the uniform acceleration of gravity. When the object is projected with some upward angle, gravity will act to decelerate the object to zero vertical velocity and then accelerate the object again as it falls downward. During this period of vertical deceleration and acceleration, the object is also undergoing constant horizontal motion. This combination of these two independent factors produces the parabolic flight path of the projectile as portrayed in figure 11.14.

The horizontal distance an object will travel in space depends on both its horizontal velocity and the length of time the object is in the air, or time of flight. The time of flight depends on the maximum height reached by the object, and that, in turn, is governed by the vertical velocity imparted to the object at release. Thus the horizontal distance an object will travel depends on both the horizontal and vertical components of velocity. As will be remembered from the earlier discussion of vectors, the magnitudes of these two components will be determined by the magnitude of the initial projection velocity vector and by the angle that indicates the direction of this vector, referred to as the angle of projection. With this in mind, it can be seen that a projectile with a low angle of projection will have a relatively high horizontal velocity in relation to the vertical velocity. The low vertical velocity does little to resist the pull of gravity, which therefore requires very little time to decelerate the object to a vertical velocity of zero and start the drop back down. In this instance, vertical distance is low, and therefore time of flight is short, allowing little time for horizontal travel. On the other hand, if the angle of projection is large, it takes longer for the object to decelerate to zero velocity, allowing a much longer time of flight. In this instance, however, there is little horizontal velocity, so little distance can be covered in the time available. Thus it would seem that the optimum angle of projection would be a 45-degree angle, with equal magnitudes for the horizontal and vertical components. In fact, the actual optimal angle of projection depends on several factors, including purpose

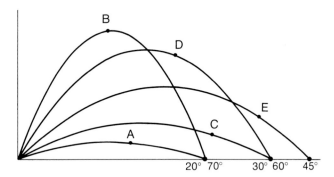

Figure 11.15   The angle of projection influences the horizontal and vertical distance covered by a projectile. Complementary angles of projection produce the same horizontal displacement.

of the projection. A 45-degree angle of projection will maximize horizontal distance only if release height and landing height are the same. In this case, the object will approach the landing at approximately the same angle as that at which it was projected (figure 11.15).

If an object is projected from above the ground, as in many throwing events, a lower angle of projection may produce optimum results. This is because the object thrown will have a somewhat increased time of flight as it covers the extra distance between the height of release and the ground as it falls. With this increased time of flight, a slightly reduced vertical velocity and a slightly increased horizontal velocity will usually be optimal. The greater the difference between release height and landing height, the lower the angle of projection needs to be. If initial velocity can be increased, the optimum angle can also be increased back toward a 45-degree angle. From this discussion, then, it can be concluded that *speed of release, angle of projection,* and *height of release* are the three factors that control the range of a projectile.

Angular Kinematics

Angular kinematics is very similar to linear kinematics because it is also concerned with displacement, velocity, and acceleration. The im-

portant difference is that the displacement, velocity, and acceleration are related to rotary rather than to linear motion, and although the equations used to show the relationships among these quantities are quite similar to those used in linear motion, the units used to describe them are different (table 11.2).

Angular Displacement

The human skeleton is made up of a system of levers that by definition are rigid bars that rotate about fixed points when force is applied. When any object acting as a rigid bar moves in an arc about an axis, the movement is called rotary, or angular, motion. An attempt to describe angular motion in linear units presents real problems. As an object moves in an arc, the linear displacement of particles spaced along that lever varies. Particles near the axis have a displacement in inches, meters, feet, or centimeters that is less than those farther away. For example, in the underarm throw pattern, the hand moves through a greater distance than the wrist and the wrist a greater distance than the elbow. Rotary motion needs rotary units to describe it. As might be expected, these units relate to the units of a circle and the fact that the circumference of a circle C is equal to $2\pi r$, where r is the radius and π is a constant value of 3.1416.

There are three interchangeable rotary, or angular, units of displacement: degrees, revolutions,

TABLE 11.2	Relationships Between Rotary and Linear Motion	
	Linear	**Rotary**
SYMBOLS		
Displacement	s	θ
Velocity	$v, u, \bar{v}$	$\omega_v, \omega_u, \bar{\omega}$
Acceleration	$a, \bar{a}$	$\alpha, \bar{\alpha}$
Time	t	t
EQUATION		
Displacement	$s = u + \frac{1}{2}at^2$	$\theta = \omega_u + \frac{1}{2}\alpha t^2$
Velocity	$v = u + at$	$\omega_v = \omega_u + \alpha t$
	$v^2 = u^2 + 2as$	$\omega_v^2 = \omega_u^2 + 2\alpha\theta$
Acceleration	$\alpha = \dfrac{v - u}{t}$	$\alpha = \dfrac{\omega_1 - \omega_u}{t}$
LINEAR AND ANGULAR CONVERSIONS		
Displacement	$s = \theta r$	$\theta = \dfrac{s}{r}$
Velocity	$\bar{v} = \bar{\omega}r$	$\bar{\omega} = \dfrac{v}{r}$
Acceleration	$a = \alpha r$	$\alpha = \dfrac{a}{r}$

and radians. One radian is the same as 57.3 degrees, and one full revolution is the same as 360 degrees or 2 *p* radians of displacement. The word revolution is not stated, but it is understood when we say that a diver executed a 1 1/2 somersault tuck. The dive could also be described as a tuck somersault of 540 (360 + 180) degrees or 3 *p* radians. Degrees are used most frequently in the measurement of angles, but radians, the term favored by engineers and physicists, are the units most often required in equations of angular motion. The symbol for angular displacement is the Greek letter θ (theta).*

Angular Velocity

The rate of rotary displacement is called angular velocity, symbolized as ω (omega). Angular velocity is equal to the angle through which the radius turns divided by the time it takes for the displacement:

$$\bar{\omega} = \frac{\theta}{t}$$

It is expressed as degrees/second, radians/second, or revolutions/second. A softball pitcher who moves the arm through an arc of 140 degrees in 0.1 second has an average angular velocity of 1400 degrees per second. This could also be expressed as 3.88 revolutions per second or 24.43 radians per second. This velocity is called average velocity because film studies of pitchers show that the angular displacement during the execution of the skill is not uniform, and a velocity such as this represents the average velocity over the time span through which the displacement is measured. As with linear movements, most angular human movements are likely to be variable and not uniform. The longer the time span through which the displacement is measured, the more variability is averaged. Thus, if one is interested in the velocity at a

*For a review of the geometry of circles and an additional explanation of degrees, radians, and revolutions, see appendix E, Part 5.

Figure 11.16 Variations in the angular displacement of a golf club over equal time intervals during the execution of a golf drive. (Drawn from motion picture film tracing.)

specific instant in a skill, the displacement must be measured over an extremely small time span.

Figure 11.16 shows the variations in displacement during the execution of a golf drive. Each displacement between images occurs over the same time period (approximately .0067 seconds), so greater spacing between images indicates greater angular displacement over the same time or greater velocity. When the total angular displacement of the golf club was measured from the beginning of the downswing to the point of contact with the ball and divided by the time it took for the swing, the average velocity of the club was 2148 degrees/second (37.5 rad/sec). The "instant" velocity at a, however, was 1432 degrees/sec, and at b it was 2864 degrees/sec. Illustrations such as this, which

show a motion as it occurs over very small spans of time, are produced with high-speed film or video. This golfer was filmed at a rate of approximately 150 frames per second, or .0067 seconds per picture.

Angular Acceleration

In the discussion of linear velocity, a change in velocity was called acceleration. The same is true for changes in angular velocity. Angular acceleration α (alpha) is the rate of change of angular velocity and is expressed in equation form as

$$\alpha = \frac{\omega_v - \omega_u}{t}$$

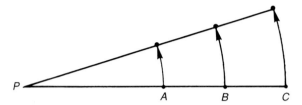

Figure 11.17   Lever *PA* > *PB* > *PC*. Although the angular displacement for all three levers is the same, the linear displacement at the end of the longer levers is greater than that at the end of the shorter levers.

where ω_v is final velocity, ω_u is initial velocity, and *t* is time. If, in figure 11.16, the angular velocity is 25 rad/sec at a and 50 rad/sec at b and the time lapse between a and b is .11 seconds, the angular acceleration between a and b is 241 rad/sec/sec. This value for a, indicating that the velocity increased 241 radians per second each second, would be true, of course, only if the velocity increased at a uniform rate. Otherwise this value has to be considered as an average of accelerations that may have been higher or lower during the time period studied.

Relationship Between Linear and Angular Motion

The description of angular motion in terms of displacement, velocity, and acceleration can tell us a great deal about human movements, but nothing in such a description accounts for or shows the effect of the length of the radius on the outcomes of the movements. We know that, all other things being equal, a baseball hit in the middle of a bat will not go as far as one hit at the end, that a ball hit by a tennis racket will travel farther than a ball hit with the hand, and that a golf driver will cause a struck ball to travel farther than a nine iron. In each instance, greater force is imparted to the struck object because the radius of the striking implement (distance between axis and point of contact) is longer and greater linear velocity is generated at its end.

As can be seen in figure 11.17, lever *PA* is shorter than lever *PB,* and lever *PB* is shorter than lever *PC.* If all three levers move through the same angular distance in the same amount of time, it is apparent that point *C* traveled farther in a curvilinear manner than either point *A* or point *B.* This curvilinear distance is difficult to measure but may be easily calculated if the angular displacement (θ) and the length of the radius (*r*) are known. The equation that expresses the relationship between angular and linear displacement is $s = \theta r$. Because the linear displacement of point *C* took the same amount of time as the displacements of points *A* and *B*, point *C* moved with a greater linear velocity than either of the other two points. Point *B* had a smaller linear velocity than point *C* but a larger linear velocity than point *A.* All three levers have the same *angular velocity,* but linear velocity of the circular motion at the end of each lever is proportional to the length of the lever. An object moved at the end of a long radius will have a greater linear velocity than one moved at the end of a short radius, *if the angular velocity is kept constant. The longer the radius, the greater is the linear velocity of a point at the end of that radius.* Thus it is to the advantage of a performer to use as long a lever as possible to impart linear velocity to an object if the long lever length does not cause too great a sacrifice in angular velocity. The longer the lever, the more effort it takes

Figure 11.18   Increasing the length of the radius decreases the angular velocity when the linear velocity remains constant.

to swing it. Therefore, the optimum length of the lever for a person depends on the individual's ability to maintain angular velocity. A child who cannot handle the weight of a long radius is better off with a shortened implement that can be controlled and swung rapidly, whereas a strong adult profits by using a longer radius.

If the reverse occurs—that is, if the linear velocity is kept constant—an increase in radius will result in a decrease in angular velocity. Once an object is engaged in rotary motion, the linear velocity at the end of the radius stays the same because of the conservation of momentum. The radius of rotation for a pike somersault dive is longer than that for a tuck somersault, and the radius for a layout somersault is longer than that for a pike somersault. If one starts a dive in an open position and then tucks tightly, the radius of rotation decreases but, because the linear velocity does not change, the angular velocity increases. The same situation occurs when a figure skater rotates slowly about a vertical axis with arms and one leg out to the side and brings the arms and leg close to the axis. The radius decreases and the angular velocity increases. To slow down, the skater again reaches out with arms and leg. Figure 11.18 shows the effect of shortening the radius while maintaining a constant linear velocity at the end of the radius. *Shortening the radius will increase the angular velocity, and lengthening it*

will decrease the angular velocity. Points *a* and *b* on radii *A* and *B* have moved through the same linear distance, but the angular displacement for *A* is greater than that for *B*. If the displacements of *a* and *b* each take place in the same amount of time, the linear velocities will be equal, but the angular velocity for *A* will be greater than that for *B*.

The relationship that exists between the angular velocity of an object moving in a rotary fashion and the linear velocity at the end of its radius is expressed by the equation

$$\bar{v} = \omega r$$

To use any of the equations relating linear and angular motion, the angular measures must be expressed in radians. If the angle is expressed in degrees, it can be converted to radians simply by dividing by 57.3.

Either form of the equation shows the direct proportionality that exists between linear velocity and the radius. For any given angular velocity, the linear velocity is proportional to the radius. If the radius doubles, the linear velocity does likewise. And for any given linear velocity, the angular velocity is inversely proportional to the radius. If the radius doubles, the angular velocity decreases by half. To achieve higher linear velocities at the end of levers, the motions must be done with longer levers or higher angular velocities (figure 11.19).

Figure 11.19   Long levers and high angular velocities result in high linear velocities at the ends of the levers. Thus the tennis racket, an extension of a long body lever, is able to impart high linear velocity to the ball.

LABORATORY EXPERIENCES

1. Define the following key terms:

Linear motion	Velocity
Angular or rotary motion	Acceleration
Distance	Gravity
Speed	Projectile
Displacement	

2. Choose one of the following activities:

   Running long jump
   Basketball jump shot
   Softball pitching

   Identify the critical linear and angular kinematic elements of the selected skill. Explain how each of these elements contributes to successful performance.

3. An Olympic skater who participated in the men's speed-skating events had the following times: 1500 m in 2 min 2.96 sec; 5000 m in 7 min 23.61 sec; and 10,000 m in 15 min 1.35 sec. What was his average speed for each of these events?

4. Using the concept of acceleration, explain how a swimmer can have a better time for a 100-m race in a 25-m pool than in a 100-m pool.

5. How much time will a batter have to decide to swing at a pitch and still hit it under these circumstances?
   a. The pitcher throws the ball at 80 mph.
   b. The distance from the ball release to the plate is 56 ft.
   c. It takes the batter .30 second to get the bat to the desired contact point.

6. With the help of several classmates, prepare a displacement-time graph and a velocity-time graph for your performance on the 50– or 100–meter dash. Class members should be spaced at 5–meter intervals along your running path, each with a stopwatch. On the signal for you to go, each timer will start the watch and stop it when you pass that timer's position. Prepare a table with the following data for each run:
   a. Distance intervals
   b. Times recorded at each interval
   c. Times over each 5–yard interval (subtract adjacent times)
   d. Average velocity over each 5-meter interval

$$v = \frac{s}{t} = \frac{15}{t_2 - t_1}$$

For each set of data, prepare a displacement-time graph and a velocity-time graph for the whole run. Describe your run in terms of displacement, velocity, and acceleration. Compare your graphs with those of other members of the group, and note any differences.

7. An arrow shot straight up into the air reached a height of 75 m. With what velocity did it leave the bow? How long was the arrow in the air?

8. Place one coin near the edge of a table and another on the end of a ruler (as shown in the following diagram). While pressing the center of the ruler to the table with an index finger strike one end of it in the direction indicated so that both coins land on the ground. Diagram the path of each. Which hits the floor first? Explain.

Figure 11.20

9. Throw a ball so that it is projected vertically upward. Catch it at the same height it was released. Have a partner measure the time the ball is in the air—that is, from the time of release to the time the ball lands in your hand. Determine the velocity of the ball at the moment of release and the distance the ball traveled before it started its descent. Graph the flight of the ball on a piece of graph paper.

10. While walking along at a constant speed project a ball vertically into the air. If you continue to walk without changing your speed or direction, where will the ball land? Explain. Draw a diagram of the ball's flight indicating the forces acting on it.

11. Assume that you are able to throw a ball with a velocity of 24 m/sec and at an angle of 45 degrees with the horizontal. If it is caught at the same height from the ground at which it was released, neglecting air resistance, how far will it go? How long will it be in flight? Repeat with a 30–degree angle of release. How would these values change if the landing height were lowered?

12. Using figure 11.3, determine the angular velocity of the lower leg at the knee joint at the beginning of the force phase and at the moment of foot contact with the ball. The time between each stick figure tracing is .0156 second. What is the linear velocity at the ankle at the moment of contact if the lower leg is 35 centimeters (knee joint to ankle joint)?

References and Selected Readings

Adrian, M. J., and J. M. Cooper. 1994. *The biomechanics of human movement.* 2nd ed. Indianapolis: Benchmark Press.

Hay, J. G. 1993. *The biomechanics of sports techniques.* 4th ed. Englewood Cliffs, NJ: Prentice Hall.

Kreighbaum, E., and K. M. Barthels. 1990. *Biomechanics.* 3rd ed. New York: Macmillan.

Pate, R. R., B. McClenaghan, and R. Rotella. 1984. *Scientific foundations of coaching.* Philadelphia: Saunders College Publishing.

Tözeren, A. 2000. *Human body dynamics: Classical mechanics and human movement.* New York: Springer.

Winter, D. A. 1990. *Biomechanics of human movement.* 2nd ed. New York: Wiley.

Zatsiorsky, V. M. 1998. *Kinematics of human motion.* Champaign. IL: Human Kinetics.

THE CONDITIONS OF LINEAR MOTION

OUTLINE

- **The Nature of Force**
  Aspects of Force
  Resolution of Forces
  Composite Effects of Two
    or More Forces
- **Newton's Laws of Motion**
  Law of Inertia
  Law of Acceleration
  Law of Reaction
- **Forces That Modify Motion**
  Weight
  Contact Forces
  Elasticity and Rebound
  Fluid Forces
- **Free-Body Diagrams**
- **Work, Power, and Energy**
  Work
  Energy
- **The Analysis of Linear Motion**
- **Laboratory Experiences**

OBJECTIVES

At the conclusion of this chapter, the student should be able to:

1. Name, define, and use the following terms properly as they apply to linear motion: force, inertia, mass, weight, momentum, and impulse.

2. Explain what is meant by the terms magnitude, direction, and point of application of force, and use these terms properly as they apply to internal and external forces.

3. Explain the effect of specified changes in the magnitude, direction, and point of application of force on the motion state of a body.

4. Define and give examples of the terms linear forces, concurrent forces, and parallel forces.

5. Determine the magnitude, direction, and point of application of muscle forces in hypothetical situations in which specific muscles are considered in isolation.

6. State Newton's laws as they apply to linear motion.
7. Explain the cause and effect relationship between the forces responsible for linear motion and the objects experiencing the motion.
8. Name and define the basic external forces responsible for modifying motion: weight, normal reaction, friction, elasticity, buoyancy, drag, and lift.
9. Draw and analyze simple two-dimensional free-body diagrams in which all applicable external forces are properly accounted for.
10. Explain the work–energy relationship as it applies to a body experiencing linear motion.
11. Define and use properly the terms work, power, kinetic energy, and potential energy.
12. Using the concepts that govern linear motion, perform a mechanical analysis of a selected motor skill.

THE NATURE OF FORCE

Objects start moving when they are pushed or pulled, that is, when some type of force acts on them. Forces produce motion, stop motion, and prevent motion. They may increase speed, decrease speed, or cause objects to change direction. They may push or pull to cause motion or produce a net effect so that bodies remain stationary. *Force is defined as that which pushes or pulls through direct mechanical contact or through the force of gravity to alter the motion of an object.* It is the effect that one body has on another. The identification of forces that act to produce motion of the body or of an object is an important element of a kinesiological analysis.

The action of a force may be internal or external. Internal forces are defined as forces exerted by bodies on other bodies within a defined system, whereas external forces are those exerted by bodies within an arbitrarily specified system on bodies outside the specified system. Internal forces cause differences in body shape, and external forces cause displacement of the body. In kinesiology, the system under consideration is the human body. Internal forces are therefore usually classified as muscle forces that act on the various structures of the body, and external forces are those outside the body. The best-known external force is weight, or gravitational force. Wind or water resistance forces, friction, or forces due to other objects acting on the body are also external forces.

Aspects of Force

Force is a vector quantity. Force possesses both magnitude and direction, as do all vector quantities. Force also has an exact point of application on the object. To describe a force fully, all three of these characteristics must be identified and taken into account. A change in any one of them alters the nature of the motion. Applying a force of insufficient magnitude, for instance, might produce no motion. A weight lifter trying to lift a 250 N barbell with 150 N of force would be unsuccessful. If the force applied by the weight lifter were increased to 260 N, the barbell would move if the force were applied in the proper direction and at the proper point of application. If the direction of the force is downward, the barbell will not be lifted upward. If the force is applied to only one end of the barbell, the bar will rotate rather than move upward in a linear manner. To successfully lift the 250 N barbell, the lifter must apply a force greater than 250 N in an *upward direction,* through the center of gravity of the barbell.

Magnitude, direction, and point of application as they relate to both external and internal forces are explained in the following sections.

Magnitude

The amount or size of the force that is being applied makes up the magnitude of the force vector. The basic unit of force in the U.S. system is the pound, and in the metric system it is the newton. In the weight-lifting example just used, the magnitude of the muscle force used in the first unsuccessful attempt was 150 N. The force being exerted by the barbell had a magnitude of 250 N. This 250 N force was the result of the pull of gravity acting on the mass of the barbell. This force is commonly referred to as weight. Weight can be expressed as mass times the acceleration due to gravity, or

$$w = mg$$

When one holds a ball in the hand, the pull of gravity is felt as the weight of the ball. The ball stays in the hand as long as an equal and opposite force acting between the hand and the ball balances the downward gravitational force. In this example the equal and opposite force is muscular. When the opposing force is removed, the ball drops and gravity's pull is apparent in the downward motion of the ball. The weight of the ball is the magnitude of the force of gravity acting on the ball.

The magnitude of muscular force is in direct proportion to the number and size of the fibers in the muscle that is contracting. If muscles contracted individually, it would be a relatively easy matter to measure the force exerted by each one in a given movement. Because they normally act in groups, however, their force or strength is measured collectively. It is customary to measure maximum muscular strength by performing a simple movement against the resistance of a dy-

namometer, spring balance, or similar instrument. The instrument thus serves as the resistance to an anatomical lever whose force is provided by a group of muscles that act as a functional team to produce the movement of the lever. Among the muscle groups that are frequently measured by this method are the finger flexors (grip strength), elbow flexors, and knee extensors.

The magnitudes of external forces other than gravity depend on other factors. Most of these external forces will be discussed in more detail later in this text.

Point of Application

The point of application of a force is that point at which the force is applied to an object. Where gravity is concerned this point is always through the center of gravity of an object. For practical purposes it may be assumed that the point of application of muscular force is the center of the muscle's attachment to the bony lever. This usually corresponds to the muscle's insertion or distal attachment. Technically, however, it is the point of intersection between the line of force and the mechanical axis of the bone or segment serving as the anatomical lever. This axis does not necessarily pass lengthwise through the shaft of the bony lever. If the bone bends or if the articulating process projects at an angle from the shaft, the greater part of the axis may lie completely outside the shaft, as in the case of the femur (see figure 2.2). *The mechanical axis of a bone or segment is a straight line that connects the midpoint of the joint at one end with the midpoint of the joint at the other end or, in the case of a terminal segment, with its distal end.*

Direction

The direction of a force is along its action line. Because the force of gravity pulls all objects toward the earth's center, the direction of gravitational forces is vertically downward. The force of gravity acting on an object would be represented as a downward-directed vector starting at the center of gravity of the object.

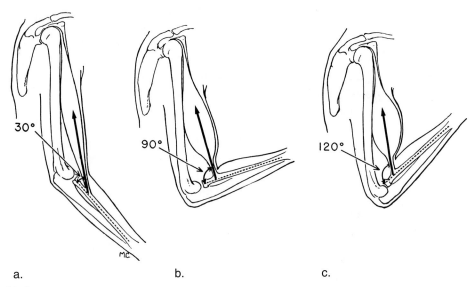

Figure 12.1 Angles of muscle pull: (a) an angle less than 45 degrees; (b) an angle of 90 degrees; (c) and angle greater than 90 degrees.

The direction of a muscular force vector is in the direction of the muscle line of pull. This direction is identified by the muscle angle of pull, which is defined as the angle between the line of pull and that portion of the mechanical axis of bone that lies between the point of application of the muscle force and the joint, which acts as the fulcrum (figure 12.1).

Resolution of Forces

Because force has the qualities of both magnitude and direction, it is a vector quantity. Graphically, the magnitude of the force is represented by the length of the vector line. The point of application of the force is the point where the force vector starts. The vector line represents the line of force, and the arrowhead indicates the direction of the force application (figure 12.2).

Angle of Pull

As with any vector, a force may be resolved into a vertical and a horizontal component, and the relative size of these component vectors depends on the angle at which the force is applied. Where

muscles are involved, the size of a muscle's angle of pull changes with every degree of joint motion, and consequently so do the sizes of the horizontal and vertical components. These changes have a direct bearing on the effectiveness of the muscle's pulling force in moving the bony lever. The larger the angle between 0 degrees and 90 degrees, the greater the vertical component and the less the horizontal component (see figure 12.1).

The vertical component of muscle pull is always perpendicular to the lever and is called the rotary component. It is that part of the force that moves the lever. The horizontal component is parallel to the lever and is the nonrotary component. It does not contribute to the lever's movement. The angle of pull of most muscles in the resting position is less than a right angle, and it usually remains so throughout the movement (see figure 12.1a). This means that the nonrotary component of force is directed toward the fulcrum, which gives it a stabilizing effect. By pulling the bone lengthwise toward the joint, it helps maintain the integrity of the joint. Under most circumstances, therefore, muscular force has two simultaneous functions—movement and stabilization.

Figure 12.2   Graphic representation of a force vector. The magnitude of the force is the vector line, A; the point of application is the beginning of the vector, B; and the direction of the vector is represented by the arrowhead and the angle θ.

In the latter capacity it supplements the ligaments, an excellent example of the body's efficiency, because muscles perform this stabilizing function only during the period when the segment is moving, at which time the integrity of the joint may be threatened.

Occasionally the angle of pull becomes greater than a right angle, which means that the nonrotary component of force is directed away from the fulcrum and is therefore a dislocating component. This does not happen in many instances, however, and, when it does, the muscle is close to the limit of its shortening range and is therefore not exerting much force (see figure 12.1c).

When the angle of pull is 90 degrees, the force is completely rotary. When it is 45 degrees the rotary and stabilizing (nonrotary) components are equal. Because the angle of pull usually remains less than 45 degrees, more of the muscle's force serves to stabilize the joint than to move the lever. In fact, there are some muscles whose angles of pull are always so small that their contributions to motion would seem to be negligible. This appears to be true of the coracobrachialis and the subclavius muscles. It is interesting to note that the upper extremity is frequently called upon to perform violent, powerful movements, as well as to support the body weight in suspension. The joints that bear the brunt of this violence and strain are the shoulder and sternoclavicular joints.

They might well become dislocated more easily than they do, were it not for the coracobrachialis and the subclavius muscles, which pull the bones lengthwise toward their proximal joints and thus serve to stabilize these joints.

The effect the angle of pull has upon the rotary force of a muscle for a given angle is demonstrated in the following problem. The solution clearly shows an increase in rotary force with each increase in angle size.

Example

Muscle *M* exerts a force of 100 N at insertion and is pulling at an angle of 30 degrees. How much of its force is rotary? Stabilizing? How do these values change when the angle of pull is 10 degrees? 75 degrees? (See figure 12.3).

Solution

Angle of pull of 30°:

Construct a right triangle where $\sin 30° = \dfrac{A}{100}$.

Rotary component equals $100 \times \sin 30° = 50$ N.
Stabilizing component equals $100 \times \cos 30° = 86.6$ N.

Angle of pull of 10°:

Construct a right triangle where $\sin 10° = \dfrac{A}{100}$.

Rotary component *A* equals $100 \times \sin 10° = 17.36$ N.
Stabilizing component *B* equals $100 \times \cos 10° = 98.48$ N.

Angle of pull of 75°:

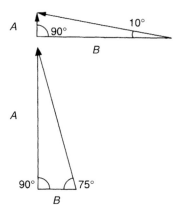

Construct a right triangle where $\sin 75° = \dfrac{A}{100}$.

Rotary component equals $100 \times \sin 75° = 96.59$ N.
Stabilizing component equals $100 \times \cos 75° = 25.88$ N.

Anatomical Pulley

The small angle of pull that most muscles have when in their normal resting position has already been noted. Were it not for anatomical devices that serve as fixed single pulleys, some muscles would probably be unable to effect any move-

ment whatsoever. The anatomical pulley serves the same purpose as the mechanical fixed single pulley, that of changing the direction of force by changing the angle of pull of the muscle providing the force.

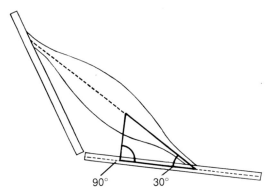

Figure 12.3   Method of constructing a right triangle for the purpose of determining the components of muscular force by the trigonometric method. Note that the hypotenuse coincides with a portion of the muscle's line of pull, and the side adjacent coincides with the mechanical axis of the bone into which the muscle is inserted.

Figure 12.4   The medial condyles at the knee joint serving as a pulley to increase the angle of pull of the gracilis tendon.

This increase in muscle angle of pull acts to increase the rotary component of the muscle force. For instance, the angle of pull of the gracilis is increased by means of the bulging medial condyles both above and below the knee joint over which the tendon passes before it attaches to the tibia (figure 12.4). The patella serves the same purpose for the quadriceps by increasing its angle of pull as it crosses the front of the knee (figure 12.5). A pulley changing the angle of pull so that it changes the nature of the movement is illustrated by the peroneus longus muscle, which, by passing behind the lateral malleolus before it turns under the foot to attach to the first cuneiform and base of the first metatarsal bone, plantar flexes the foot at the ankle (figure 12.6). If it passed in front of the malleolus, its angle of pull would be shifted in front of the ankle joint, and this would cause it to dorsiflex the foot. In this example the lateral malleolus serves as the "fixed pulley."

Resolution of External Force

The resolution of a single external force vector into component force vectors acting at right angles to each other is accomplished in the same

Figure 12.5   By increasing the angle of pull the patella increases the rotary force component of the quadriceps femoris.

From M. Williams and H. R. Lissner, *Biomechanics of Human Motion.* Copyright © 1962 W. B. Saunders, Orlando, FL. Reprinted by permission.

Figure 12.6 The lateral malleolus serving as a pulley for the peroneus longus tendon.

Figure 12.7 The diagonal pushing force (R) consists of a horizontal and a vertical component. Only the horizontal component (X) serves to overcome the table's resistance to being moved. The vertical component (Y) adds to the resistance. (Drawn from a photograph.)

manner as that explained for muscular forces and would be used when the force is applied at an oblique angle. If, instead of giving a piece of furniture a horizontal push, one pushes it by standing close to it with the arms held at a forward-downward slant, only part of the force will push

the table forward (figure 12.7). The force is applied to the table at an oblique angle and thus has both a vertical and a horizontal component. Whether or not the table moves forward depends on the amount of the total force applied in the horizontal direction. If sufficient, only the horizontal component of force will overcome the table's resistance to move. The downward component merely pushes the table against the floor and increases the friction between the floor and the table. The closer one can come to applying all the available force in the desired direction of movement, the more efficient will be the action. Another example of this principle is demonstrated in pulling actions. If a child's sled or wagon is drawn by too short a rope, there will be a relatively large lifting component and a small forward pulling component. Because the purpose is to pull the wagon horizontally, it is more efficient to use a long rope because this gives a relatively greater horizontal or pulling component.

Composite Effects of Two or More Forces

Frequently two or more forces are applied to the same object. A canoe may be acted on by both the wind and the paddler. One force tends to send the canoe north and the other east. While in flight a punted ball's path is the result of the force imparted to it by the kicker, the downward force of gravity, and the force of the wind, if any. In the body it is rarely, if ever, the case that an individual muscle acts by itself. For example, at least four muscles may act in flexion of the forearm, and more than five contribute to flexion of the leg at the knee joint. The effect that composite forces have on the human body to cause or modify motion may be classified according to their direction and application as linear, concurrent, or parallel.

Linear Forces

Forces applied in the same direction along the same action line are called linear forces. If a horizontal push is applied to a piece of furniture and the push is applied in line with the object's center of gravity, the object will move forward in a horizontal direction, if, of course, there is no additional conflicting force or resistance. If another force is applied to the furniture in line with and in the same direction as the first force, the resultant of the two forces has a value equal to the sum of the two forces ($a + b = c$).

Similarly, if the forces act in opposite directions, the resultant still equals the algebraic sum of the two forces ($a + (- b) = c$). This might be the case in a tug of war.

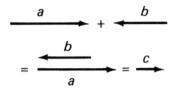

Examples of more than one force applied at the same point and acting in identical directions in the body are rare. Possibly there are two such examples: the gastrocnemius and the soleus acting at the ankle joint, and the psoas and the iliacus acting at the hip joint. In each of these examples, the two muscles have a common tendon for their distal attachments.

Concurrent Forces

Forces acting at the same point of application but at different angles are called concurrent forces. Several football players opposing each other in a blocking situation furnish opposing forces that may be considered as acting at one point (figure 12.8). The resultant outcome of the blocking is found using the method known as the combination of vectors described in chapter 10. This method assumes a common point of application. Although this situation is common externally, it is not true of the majority of muscles that act on the same bone. Very few muscles have a common point of attachment. Nevertheless, the principle of finding the composite effect of two or more forces, with respect to magnitude and direction, is as true for forces acting on body segments as for forces acting on external objects. The important thing to remember is that the resultant magnitude of two or more concurrent forces is not their arithmetic sum, and the resultant direction of two concurrent forces is not halfway between them unless the two forces are of equal magnitude. The *resultant of two or more concurrent forces depends on both*

Figure 12.8   Opposing forces acting at one point but at different angles are called concurrent forces.

the magnitude of each force and the angle of application—that is, the direction of each force. The techniques of vector resolution and combination must be used when doing force calculations.

Parallel Forces

In addition to linear forces, in which all forces occur along the same action line, and concurrent forces, in which forces acting at different angles are applied at the same point, another situation exists in which forces not in the same action line but *parallel* to each other act at different points on a body. The two students in figure 12.9 are carrying a weight between them. Each one exerts an upward force on an end while the weight exerts a downward force between them. There are three parallel forces here, two in one direction and the third in an opposite direction. All three forces are acting on the same object but at different points.

Another example of this situation is that of holding a 10-N weight in the hand when the forearm is flexed so that the angle of pull of the biceps is 90 degrees. The force of gravity may be represented as acting at two different points to push the forearm and the weight down while the

Figure 12.9   Example of parallel forces. The box exerts a downward force while both carriers exert parallel forces upward.

force of the biceps acting in the opposite direction at another point pulls the forearm up. All three forces are parallel to each other but act at different points (figure 12.10).

The effect parallel forces have on the object they act on depends on the magnitude, direc-

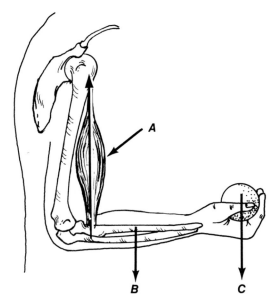

Figure 12.10 Example of parallel forces in equilibrium. The force of the biceps (*A*) balances the opposite force of gravity acting on the forearm at its center of gravity (*B*) and on the weight held in the hand (*C*).

tion, and application point of each force. Parallel forces may act in the same or opposite directions. They may be balanced and cause no motion, or they may cause linear or rotary motion. When parallel forces act on an object, their relationship to the object's fixed axis or to its center of gravity, if it can move freely, determines the resultant action. In the case of the weight held at opposite ends by two students, the weight will remain balanced and motionless if all the forces about the center of gravity are balanced. The weight will move upward in a linear fashion if the students exert equal parallel forces upward that are greater than the downward force of the weight, and they will move in a rotary fashion about their center of gravity if the students exert equal and opposite parallel forces. Other examples of parallel forces are shown in figure 12.11.

NEWTON'S LAWS OF MOTION

The fact that motion is related to force in a precise manner was observed by Sir Isaac Newton in the seventeenth century. He formulated three laws of motion that explain why objects move as they do. Although all of these laws cannot be proved on earth, even in ideal experimental situations, they are accepted as universal truths to explain the effects of force.

Law of Inertia

Newton's first law of motion states that **a body continues in its state of rest or of uniform motion unless an unbalanced force acts on it.** This Law of Inertia means that an object at rest remains at rest, and one in motion will continue at a constant speed in a straight line unless acted on by a force. In effect, the law identifies the conditions under which there is no external force. The fact that objects at rest need a force to move them seems obvious, but the need for force to slow or stop an object in motion is not always as apparent. We have all seen moving objects come to rest of their own accord, or what seems to be their own accord, but, in fact, other forces in the form of friction or air resistance caused the change in velocity. The tendency for a body to stay in motion for long periods of time is possible to observe more clearly in laboratory conditions where the effects of friction and air resistance can be minimized. Nevertheless, numerous examples of Newton's first law can still be observed in sport and everyday experiences. Base runners in baseball know that it takes force to change velocity suddenly to avoid overrunning a base. Skiers continue into space if they traverse a hill or mogul at high speed (figure 12.12). And nearly everyone at sometime or another has experienced the frightening situation of continuing to move forward when the vehicle in which one is riding stops suddenly.

The property of an object that causes it to remain in its state of either rest or motion is called

a.

b.

c.

Figure 12.11   Example of parallel forces producing (a) linear motion, (b) rotary motion, and (c) no motion. (a and c drawn from motion picture film tracing; b drawn from photograph.)

Figure 12.12   An example of Newton's first law of motion.

inertia. Because of inertia, force is needed to change the velocity of an object. The amount of force needed to alter the object's velocity is directly related to the amount of inertia it has. The measure of inertia in a body is its mass, that is, the quantity of matter it possesses. The greater the mass of an object, the greater its inertia. A bowling ball obviously has greater inertia than does a volleyball. A tennis racket has greater inertia than a badminton racket, and a textbook more than a magazine.

Law of Acceleration

Newton's second law of motion, the Law of Acceleration, concerns acceleration and momentum, and it tells how the quantities of force, mass, and acceleration are related and how to measure force when it exists. The law states that **the acceleration of an object is directly proportional to the force causing it, is in the same direction as the force, and is inversely proportional to the mass of the object.** It is quite easy to show that change in velocity (acceleration) of an object is proportional to the force and in the direction of the

force. The velocity of a pitched ball reflects the force with which it is thrown, and it moves in the direction of the line of force at the moment of release. Similarly, it takes less braking force to stop a baseball moving at 5 meters per second than it does to stop a pitch of 50 meters per second. In both instances, the change in velocity is directly proportional to the amount of force and is in the direction of the force. The mass of the ball is a measure of its inertia, and the greater the inertia, the more force it takes to change the object's velocity. Thus, a bowling ball requires more force to put it in motion than a playground ball, and the same is true for stopping it. Acceleration is inversely proportional to mass.

Newton's second law may be expressed in equation form as

$$F = ma$$

For this to be possible, the force unit is the pound when acceleration is in feet/second/second and mass is in slugs. When acceleration is in meters/second/second and mass is in kilograms, force is expressed in newtons (see table 10.1).

With this equation it is possible to determine the force needed to produce a given linear acceleration of a body if the weight of the body is known. Because we know that $m = \dfrac{w}{g}$, the equation for force, $F = ma$, can be written as $F = \dfrac{w}{g} \times a$, the force needed to accelerate a 300-N object 2 m/sec^2 is 61N, or $\left(\dfrac{300}{9.8 \text{ m / sec}^2} \times 2\text{m / sec}^2 \right)$.

Impulse

The Law of Acceleration dictates that when sufficient force is applied to a mass, an acceleration will occur according to the equation

$$F = ma$$

Because acceleration is the rate of change in velocity, this equation can be rewritten as

$$F = \frac{m(v - u)}{t}$$

substituting $(v - u/t)$ for a. Multiplying both sides by time produces a new equation:

$$Ft = m(v - u)$$

In other words, the product of a force and the time over which this force acts will produce a change in the velocity of the mass. This product of force and time is called **impulse.** From the impulse equation, $Ft = m(v - u)$, it should be apparent that the force required to produce a given change of velocity in a given time period is proportional to the mass. It is also easy to see that as any change in velocity of an object of a given mass increases, so must the impulse increase proportionately. Conversely, if either force or time is increased, the velocity of the mass must also increase. Doubling either the force or the time over which a force is applied will double the velocity change.

The importance of creating as large an impulse as possible is evident in the skillful execution of many sports techniques. A baseball pitcher uses a form that allows the longest time over which to apply the force to the ball before releasing it. This same long windup is seen in the technique used by hammer throwers, discus throwers, and shot-putters. In each instance the performer accelerates the object to be thrown as much as possible by generating as much force as strength permits and by using body segment adjustments that increase the time over which the force can be applied (figure 12.13).

The impulse relationship also shows that force cannot be generated to cause a change in velocity unless time is available over which the force is applied. This helps explain the value of the follow-through in throwing, kicking, and striking movements. Although the follow-through does not affect the flight of the object once the object has left the throwing or striking implement, it does help ensure that the missile will stay in contact with the implement that is imparting force to it for as long as possible. The ball is actually carried along by the foot, golf club, or tennis racket, and the longer the time the force of the implement can be applied to the ball, the greater will be the change in velocity in the ball.

Momentum

The impulse equation is also written as

$$Ft = mv - mu$$

Figure 12.13   Example of impulse generation. (Drawn from motion picture film tracing.)

The product of mass and velocity (*mv* or *mu*) is momentum, and any change in momentum is equal to the impulse that produces it. Momentum is a quantity of motion that may be increased or decreased by increasing or decreasing either the mass or the velocity. The shot-putter who is able to push the shot with a greater speed than the opponent will cause the shot to have greater momentum at the moment of release. And, even though the mass is less, a small child may topple an adult if the child's faster speed is sufficient to produce a larger momentum than the person the child collides with. Similarly, heavier bowling balls released with the same speed as lighter balls have greater momentum, and a heavier tennis racket will strike a tennis ball with greater momentum and cause a greater change in momentum in the tennis ball than will a lighter racket.

An increase in momentum occurs when the force is applied in the direction of the motion. Force applied in the opposite direction produces a slowing down or decrease in momentum. This is what happens when one catches a fast ball or lands from a jump or a fall. In both instances relatively large momentums are reduced to zero and large impulses occur. The momentum of the ball is large because of its large velocity, and the momentum of the person falling is great because of a large mass. Looking again at the impulse equation, $Ft = mv - mu$, it can be seen that a short stopping time will require a large stopping force and that an increase in stopping time will reduce the amount of stopping force needed to change the momentum of the object to zero. This is why it is necessary to increase the stopping time by "giving" when catching the ball or when landing from a jump or fall. Without the "give" the impulse will not be enough, the momentum will not decrease to zero, and the ball will not be caught, or the momentum will reach zero but the force will be so great that injury in the form of damaged bones, joints, and soft tissue may result. A 20-N force falling for 5 seconds has the same impulse as a 100-N force falling for 1 second.

Law of Reaction

Newton's third law of motion considers the way forces act against each other. A book lying on a table (figure 12.14) exerts a downward force on the table, and because the book is stationary, another equal and opposite force must be acting on the book. Newton's first law states that unbalanced forces produce motion. Because we have no motion here, we must have a balanced force system. The downward force of the book on the

Figure 12.14   Equal and opposite reactions. *H* = *S* (forces of hand and bag) and *B* = *T* (book and table).
From M. Williams and H. R. Lissner, *Biomechanics of Human Motion.* Copyright © 1962 W. B. Saunders, Orlando, FL. Reprinted by permission.

Figure 12.15 To accelerate forward, a walker must push backward. Notice how the front part of the footprint in the sand is more deeply depressed than the rear.

table is balanced by an upward force of the table on the book. The same is true when a person walks across a floor. The feet push back against the floor with the same magnitude as the floor pushes forward against the feet. Without the forward push of the floor against the feet, forward progress would not be possible. Notice how the front part of the foot in the footprint in figure 12.15 makes a deeper impression than the heel. To accelerate forward, the walker has to push backward. For this reason, runners push against starting blocks at the beginning of a race so that a strong forward reaction push can be received from the blocks. In each of these instances, forces of equal magnitude are exerted in opposite directions. One force is called the action force and the other is the reaction force.

Newton's Law of Reaction states that **for every action there is an equal and opposite reaction.** Whenever one body exerts a force on a second body, the second body exerts an equal and opposite force on the first.

In locomotion on the surface of the earth (ground or floor), this reaction force is referred to as *ground reaction force.* The ground reaction force vector is equal in magnitude and opposite in direction to the force vector that is being applied to the ground. In walking, as the foot pushes

down and back against the ground, the ground pushes up and forward against the foot. Notice how the front part of the footprint in figure 12.15 makes a deeper impression in the front than the heel does in the back. Notice also how the sand had to be compressed by the walker before it was solid enough to produce an equal and opposite reaction. This is one reason that walking on soft sand or snow is more difficult than walking on a firm surface.

Although ground reaction force is necessary for locomotion, such forces do place stress on the body. It sometimes becomes necessary to minimize ground reaction force to prevent injury. A pole vaulter, for example, uses ground reaction force in the run and the takeoff but needs to minimize the ground reaction force at landing. The use of a landing pit or crash pad allows the vaulter to alter momentum by increasing the time over which velocity is reduced. In the impulse equation, $Ft = m(v - u)$, if time (t) is increased, force (F) must decrease. A decrease in the force component of impulse is a decrease in the action force. On the Law of Reaction, a decrease in the action force will produce an equal and opposite decrease in the ground reaction force.

Action and reaction show up in countless other ways when objects are in motion. When a boat is rowed, the oars exert a force against the water and the water pushes against the oars with an equal and opposite reaction, causing the boat to be pushed forward as the force is transferred from the oar to the boat through the oarlock. The force of a volleyball can be felt pushing back against the hand as it is served with a forward force. A similar force is observed when a gun is shot or an arrow is released from a bow. The recoil of the gun or bow is due to the reaction force of the bullet or arrow to the action force of the gun or bow.

Conservation of Momentum

When an object is set in motion by a force, the momentum (mv) of the object is changed. Because the force that causes this change in momentum must have an equal and opposite force, another equal and opposite momentum change must occur in the object producing the reactive force. The time the objects are in contact with each other would also be equal, and therefore the impulses (Ft) would be equal. This means that $m_1v_1 - m_1u_1 = m_2v_2 - m_2u_2$. This principle is summarized in the Law of Conservation of Momentum, which states that **in any system where forces act on each other the momentum is constant.** Thus, if an impact or action between objects occurs, the momentums before impact must equal the momentums after the impact, provided, of course, that no momentum is lost through friction or other forces. The momentum of a golf ball changes from zero to a larger quantity after it is struck by a club (figure 12.16). Neglecting air resistance and friction, the momentum of the club will also change so that the momentum of ball and club after impact will equal the momentum of ball and club before impact.

This is proved by using the impulse equation

$$m_bv_b - m_bu_b = m_cv_c - m_cu_c$$

where the subscript b refers to the ball and the subscript c to the club. Rearranged, this equation becomes

$$m_bu_b - m_cu_c = m_bv_b - m_cv_c$$

That is, the combined momentums before impact equal the combined momentums after impact. Momentum is conserved; none is lost.

The conservation of momentum may be easily apparent in some instances, whereas in others it is harder to visualize. When one steps out of a canoe onto a dock, the canoe is pushed back by the passenger as the passenger is pushed forward by the canoe. The change in momentum of the canoe backward ($m_1v_1 - m_1u_1$) will equal the change in momentum of the passenger forward ($m_2v_2 - m_2u_2$). Here the action–reaction relationship is evident in the movements of both the canoe and the person. But if the same person steps off an ocean liner, the change in momentum of the ship is imperceptible, yet it will still equal the change in momentum of the passenger. Because the mass

Figure 12.16 Momentum of club and ball before impact equals momentum of club and ball after impact. (Drawn from motion picture film tracing.)

of the ship is so great, its velocity is not apparent. In both instances, the change in the mass–velocity product of the passenger equals the change in the mass–velocity product of the boat (canoe or ship), and momentum is conserved. Incidentally, if the passenger disembarking from the canoe does not account for the backward acceleration of the canoe, the step toward the dock may be a wet one.

Summation of Forces

The forces generated by the muscle structure of the body may be summated from one segment to another. In generating momentum, these forces, applied over a period of time, are used to build momentum, which is then transferred from segment to segment. In a typical throwing pattern, for instance, force is first generated in the muscles of the lower extremity as the legs extend to push against the ground. The momentum generated is transferred to the trunk, where the application of further muscular force acts to increase momentum, primarily through an increase in velocity. This momentum is then transferred to the upper arm. The great decrease in mass when moving from trunk to upper arm produces an increase in velocity, in accord with the momentum equation (*mv*) and the fact that momentum within a system must be conserved. If the muscles of the rotator cuff contract to provide further impulse, velocity will increase further. This sequential transfer of momentum continues with mass decreasing and velocity increasing until momentum is finally transferred to the thrown ball.

FORCES THAT MODIFY MOTION

In addition to the forces that produce motion, a number of forces act to modify motion in some manner. These modifying forces must be considered when studying the kinetics of linear motion. When the kinesiological analysis model presented in chapter 1 is applied to a motor skill, the forces that modify motion must be included in any discussion of the nature of the forces involved. Six of these forces are commonly categorized as follows:

1. **Weight**
2. **Contact forces**
    a. Normal reaction
    b. Friction
3. **Fluid forces**
    a. Buoyancy
    b. Drag
    c. Lift

For purposes of discussion in this chapter, an additional category of elasticity and rebound has been added.

Weight

In what came to be known as the Law of Gravitation, Newton (remember the apple) was the first to point out that all bodies are attracted to each other in direct proportion to their masses and in inverse proportion to the square of the distance between them. The amount of this attraction be-

tween bodies on earth is negligible except for the attraction between the earth itself and the bodies on it. Because of the earth's huge mass, this attraction is quite noticeable. The force is called gravity, and it is measured as the weight of the body applied through the center of gravity of the body and directed toward the earth's axis (figure 12.17). The closer a body is to the earth's center, the greater is the gravitational pull and, therefore, the more it weighs. When the body moves far enough away from the earth's center, such as to the moon, the decrease in the gravitational pull is apparent, as in the ease of giant leaps made by astronauts. The mass of the body is the same as on earth, but the weight has decreased in proportion to the gravitational pull. The relation between weight, mass, and gravity is represented in equation form as $W = mg$. The force of weight must be considered in all motion analyses.

Figure 12.17 Gravitational force is measured as the weight of the body applied through the center of gravity of the body and directed toward the center of the earth.

Contact Forces
Normal Reaction

As Newton's third law states, for every action there is an equal and opposite reaction. That is, the forces acting between two bodies are equal and acting in opposite directions. This implies that forces always exist in pairs. A child hanging from a bar pulls down on the bar as the bar pulls up on the child. In the same way, the bar pushes down on the supports as the supports push up on the bar. A diver pushes down on the board and the board pushes back, or a jumper pushes off the ground and the ground pushes back (figure 12.18). Every time there is a push, there has to be a push back. Without the reactive force there would be no motion.

Figure 12.18   Example of normal reactive force. As the jumper pushes down on the ground, the ground pushes back. (Drawn from motion picture film tracing.)

Friction

Friction is the force that opposes efforts to slide or roll one body over another. Without friction it would be impossible to walk or run or do much of any kind of moving. On the other hand, friction increases the difficulty of moving objects about with its deterrent effect. There are numerous examples in which we attempt to *increase* friction for more effective performance. The use of rubber-soled shoes on hardwood floors or wet decks, spikes on golf shoes, and rubber knobs on hiking boots improve friction with the supporting surface. Chalk on the gymnast's hands, on work gloves, and on cloth grips on tennis rackets are all used to decrease slippage. Even the surfaces of balls are designed to increase friction through irregularities such as the fuzz on the tennis ball or the dimples on a golf ball. Attempts to decrease friction are also evident in physical activity. The sole of one of a bowler's shoes is made to have little friction so that it can slide more easily in the approach. Sharp ice skates apply pressure on the ice and cause slight melting, thus making it easier for the skates to move across the ice. Ice covered with a slight film of water is more slippery than colder, drier ice. Skis are waxed, bicycles are greased, and roller skates have ball bearings, each for the purpose of minimizing the retardant effect of friction.

The amount of friction between one surface and another depends on the nature of the surfaces and the forces pressing them together. Generally speaking, smooth surfaces have less friction than rough surfaces. The area of surfaces in contact with each other does not affect friction. A footlocker pulled along on one end would take as much force to pull as one on its side. An empty footlocker, however, would take less force than one full of books. **Friction is proportional to the force pressing two surfaces together.**

The force of friction acts parallel to the surfaces that are sliding over each other and opposite to the direction of motion. In figure 12.19 the book is pressing down on the table with a force W equal to its weight. The reactive force of the table T pushes up against the book. The force

Figure 12.19 The coefficient of friction is the ratio between the force needed to overcome the friction P to the force holding the surfaces together W.

needed to put the book in motion is P. The force resisting the motion F is the force due to friction. F equals in magnitude the force P attempting to move the book. The ratio of the force needed to overcome the friction P to the force holding the surface together W is called the coefficient of friction μ (mu).

$$\mu = \frac{P}{W}$$

This coefficient indicates the starting friction ratio for these two surfaces. It is an experimentally determined value that depends on the nature of the contact surfaces. Mu (μ) is a constant for any two given surfaces. The larger the coefficient, the more the surfaces cling together. The smaller the coefficient, the easier it is for the two surfaces to begin sliding over each other. A coefficient of 0.0 would indicate completely frictionless surfaces. The equation also shows that the coefficient of friction is totally dependent on the force holding the surfaces together (W) and the force needed to slide one surface over the other (P). The coefficient will decrease as P decreases.

Friction is overcome by changing either the nature of the two surfaces or the force. If one attempts to push an object forward with a force directed diagonally downward, the force holding the surfaces together is increased and so is the friction. Consequently, the effort needed to move the object increases proportionately. On the other hand, a force directed diagonally forward-upward would decrease the force holding the surfaces together, diminish the friction, and make the moving task somewhat easier.

Starting friction, the friction that resists the start of motion, is greater than sliding friction, the friction that resists continued motion. It takes less force to keep something sliding than it does to start it sliding. At low speeds friction usually decreases as speed increases, but at extremely rapid speeds friction increases proportionately until the heat it generates causes the sliding surfaces to disintegrate. Whereas sliding friction is less than starting friction, rolling friction is much less than sliding friction. The movement of heavier objects is much easier when they are put up on wheels. As with sliding friction, rolling friction varies with the nature of the surfaces and the magnitude of the force pushing the two surfaces together. Smooth, hard surfaces roll or are rolled upon more easily than soft, irregular surfaces. Field hockey players, soccer players, and golfers know this and must adjust their games to varying surfaces. Obviously, the rolling friction over thick, high, wet grass will be greater than that over a hard, dry, closely cropped surface. Similarly, bicycles, wheelchairs, and skates are much easier to use on smooth, hard pavement than on soft surfaces.

The coefficient of friction between two objects may also be found by placing one object on the second and tilting the second until the first starts to slide. The tangent of the angle of the second object with the horizontal is the coefficient of friction (figure 12.20). Bunn (1972) cited an interesting application of the use of μ with respect to the gripping power of basketball shoes. The amount of lean a player may safely take is equal to the angle θ that the player makes with the vertical, whose tangent $= \dfrac{P}{W}$. P is the amount of horizontal force needed to cause the feet to start sliding horizontally and W is the weight of the player (figure 12.21). Shoes allowing a greater lean would certainly afford their wearers an advantage in the game. For this information to be of

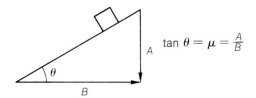

$$\tan \theta = \mu = \frac{A}{B}$$

Figure 12.20   An inclined plane may be used to determine the coefficient of friction μ between two surfaces.

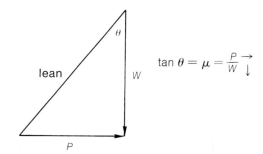

$$\tan \theta = \mu = \frac{P}{W} \; \substack{\rightarrow \\ \downarrow}$$

Figure 12.21   The amount of lean a basketball player can safely assume depends on the friction between the floor and his shoes.

use to shoe manufacturers, however, a standard type of floor surface would have to be determined.

Elasticity and Rebound

Objects that rebound from each other do so in a fairly predictable manner. The nature of a rebound is governed by the elasticity, mass, and velocity of the rebounding surfaces, the friction between the surfaces, and the angle with which one object contacts the second.

Any time two or more objects come into contact with each other, some distortion or deformation occurs. Whether or not the distortion is permanent depends on the elasticity of the interacting objects. Elasticity is the ability of an object to resist distorting influences and to return to its original size and shape when the distorting forces are removed. The force that acts on an object to distort it is called *stress*. The distortion that occurs is called *strain* and is proportional to the stress causing it. Stress may take the form of tension, as in the stretching of a spring; compression, as in the squeezing of a tennis ball (figure 12.22); bending, such as the bending of a fencing foil; or torsion, as in the twisting of the spring. In all cases the object tends to resume its original shape when the stress is removed. If the stress is too large, the elastic limit of the object is exceeded and permanent distortion occurs.

Coefficient of Elasticity

Substances vary in their resistance to distorting forces and in their ability to regain their original shapes after being deformed. One usually thinks of a material such as rubber as being highly elastic, because it yields easily to a distorting force and returns to its original shape. Actually, substances that are hard to distort and return perfectly to their original shapes are more elastic. Gasses, liquids, highly tempered steel, and brass are examples. In comparing the elasticity of different substances, coefficients of elasticity are used. A coefficient of elasticity or restitution is defined as the stress divided by the strain.

The coefficient of elasticity most commonly determined in sports activities is that caused in the compression of balls. If one drops a ball onto a hard surface like a floor, the coefficient of restitution may be determined by

Figure 12.22   Compression of tennis ball (a) and golf ball (b) at moment of impact.
Courtesy of H. E. Edgerton.

comparing the drop height with the bounce height in the equation

$$e = \sqrt{\dfrac{\textbf{bounce height}}{\textbf{drop height}}}$$

where e = coefficient of restitution or elasticity. The closer the coefficient approaches 1.0, the more perfect the elasticity. Rules require that a basketball should be inflated to rebound to a height of 49 to 54 inches at its top when its bottom is dropped from a height of 72 inches. For the maximum bounce height, this is a coefficient of .781. In comparison, a volleyball dropped from the same height and inflated to 6 psi (pounds per square inch) rebounds to 51 inches and has a coefficient of .84. A tennis ball has a coefficient of .73, and a leather-covered softball one of .46.

The coefficient of elasticity may also be found in another way. Because the Law of Conservation of Momentum states that the total momentum in any impact between two objects must remain the same, the momentum of one object may be reduced, so long as the momentum of the other object increases proportionately. If the objects are numbered 1 and 2 and it is assumed that mass of the objects remains constant, it is possible to find the coefficient of elasticity by using the change in velocity of the two objects:

$$e = \frac{v_1 - v_2}{u_t - u_2}$$

where v_2 and v_1 are the velocities after impact and u_1 and u_2 are the velocities before impact.

Angle of Rebound

An elastic object dropped vertically onto a rebounding surface will compress uniformly on its underside and rebound vertically upward. An elastic object that strikes a rebounding surface obliquely will compress unevenly on the bottom and rebound at an oblique angle. The size of the rebound angle compared with that of the striking angle depends on the elasticity of the striking object and the friction between the two surfaces. The rebound of a perfectly elastic object is simi-

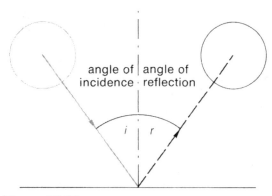

Figure 12.23   The angle of incidence and the angle of reflection in oblique rebounds.

lar to the reflection of light: **The angle of incidence (striking) is equal to the angle of reflection (rebound)** (figure 12.23). Variations from this ideal are to be expected as the coefficient of restitution varies. Low coefficients will generally produce angles of reflection greater than angles of incidence.

For example, an underinflated volleyball will not have a great coefficient of restitution. It will therefore rebound at an angle much less, or much closer to the floor, than the striking angle. The coefficient of restitution acts to affect the vertical component of rebound. In rebound at an oblique angle, friction affects the horizontal component of the rebound. An increase in friction will produce a decrease in the angle of rebound. It is possible to produce an angle of rebound equal to the angle of incidence by decreasing both the horizontal component (increased friction) and the vertical component (elasticity) proportionately. If the proportions between the two components are constant, the angle of rebound will equal the angle of incidence, but the resultant velocity of the object after impact will be decreased.

Effects of Spin on Bounce

Spin also influences rebounding angles. Balls thrown with topspin will rebound from horizontal surfaces lower and with more horizontal velocity than the surface that with which they struck. They will tend to roll farther also, an action often desirable on long golf drives. Balls hitting a horizontal surface with backspin rebound at a higher bounce and are slower. Balls with backspin also roll for shorter distances than those with topspin or no spin. Because of the compression of the ball and the friction between it and the surface, a ball with no spin hitting the surface at an angle will develop some topspin on the rebound, and a ball hitting with topspin will develop greater topspin upon rebounding. With backspin, however, the spin may be completely stopped or reversed. A ball with sidespin will rebound in the direction of the spin. A ball spinning or curving to the right will "kick" to the right upon rebounding and a left-spinning ball will do the reverse.

When spinning balls hit vertical surfaces, such as a basketball backboard or a racquetball court wall, they will respond in relation to the surface in the same manner as with horizontal surfaces. When the vertical surface is struck from below, a ball with no spin or topspin will have added spin on rebound, and the angle of reflection will be greater than the angle of incidence. With backspin the spin will stop or reverse and the angle of reflection will be less than the incidence angle. For this to be true, a backspinning ball approaching a vertical wall from above must be regarded as moving with topspin in relation to the rebounding surface. Similarly, a topspinning ball hitting the vertical surface from above is in actuality spinning backward with respect to the rebounding surface.

When a spinning ball meets a forward-moving object, as in tennis or table tennis, the ball will rebound in a direction that results from the forces acting on it at impact. For example, a ball with topspin striking a stationary vertical surface head on will rebound upward. That same ball (with topspin) striking a moving vertical surface, like a tennis racket, will also rebound upward, but not as much, because the resultant rebound has a horizontal force component from the forward-moving tennis racket. Nevertheless, the upward direction may be sufficient to send the ball out of bounds. To counteract the upward direction, the racket

face can be turned obliquely downward, thus adding a downward compensating force component as well as changing the spin of the ball.

The resultant force path of a rebounding ball is controlled by several factors. When one attempts to predict the direction of the rebound, the momentums of both the ball and the striking implement must be considered as well as the elasticity of the two objects, the spin of the ball, and the angle of impact. Awareness of these factors and the ways in which they affect play have numerous and valuable applications in sports such as handball, squash, racquetball, table tennis, paddleball, and tennis.

Fluid Forces

Water and air are both fluids and as such are subject to many of the same laws and principles. The fluid forces of buoyancy, drag, and lift apply in both mediums and have considerable effect on the movements of the human body in many circumstances. A discus sails, a baseball curves, a volleyball "wobbles," and a shuttlecock drops because of contact with air currents. Sky divers and hang gliders control their flight paths by interacting with the air currents, whereas downhill racers, swimmers, and underwater divers streamline their bodies to minimize the effect of fluid resistance.

Buoyancy

If an adult female stands in shoulder-deep water and abducts her arms as she lays her head back on the water's surface, most likely her feet will leave the bottom as her legs begin to rise. At some point between the vertical and horizontal, the swimmer will come to rest and she will be in a motionless back float. For this to occur, an upward force must counterbalance the weight (force) of her body, acting vertically downward at her center of gravity. This upward force is called *buoyancy* and, according to *Archimedes' Principle,* the magnitude of this force is equal to the weight of water displaced by the floating body. Specifically, Archimedes' principle states that

a solid body immersed in a liquid is buoyed up by a force equal to the weight of the liquid displaced. This principle explains why some objects float and others do not, why some individuals float motionless like bobbing corks, and why others struggle to keep their noses above water while attempting a back float. When a body is immersed in water, it will sink until the weight of the water it displaces equals the weight of the body. Sinking objects never do displace enough water to equal their body weight and eventually settle to the bottom. If such objects are weighed under water, they will be found to weigh less than when weighed in air. That difference in weight equals the weight of the water displaced and is the buoyant force acting on the immersed objects. Even a body that floats has some part of its volume beneath the surface and thus displaces a volume of water. The weight of the water it displaces equals the *total* weight of the floating object. Any object stops sinking when the weight of the water it displaces equals its weight.

The ratio between the weight of an object and its volume is referred to as density. The more weight per volume, the greater the density. An inflated volleyball, for example, has a slightly greater volume than a bowling ball. The bowling ball, however, weighs much more. Because the bowling ball has more weight for its volume than does the volleyball, it is said to have greater density.

The ratio between the density of any given object and that of water is called specific gravity. If an object or a body has the same density as water, or the same weight and volume ratio, it possesses a specific gravity of 1.0. Those objects with greater density will have a specific gravity greater than 1.0 and will sink. The bowling ball, being very dense, will sink very quickly. Objects with a density less than that of water will have a specific gravity less than 1.0 and will float with some part of the object or body exposed. An example is the inflated volleyball, which is composed primarily of air.

Human beings differ in specific gravity depending on individual body composition. Human bone and muscle tissue both have a specific grav-

ity greater than water and as a result tend to sink. Fat and air, on the other hand, have specific gravities much less than that of water and will float. The ease with which one floats and the floating position assumed are therefore determined by the distribution of muscle, bone, fat, and air within the body, the specific gravity of the various body parts differs accordingly.

Usually the legs have a high specific gravity and consequently are the part of the body that most often sinks during the back float. The thoracic region is the most buoyant part, having the lowest weight for its volume. A person can increase the buoyancy of this region by keeping the lungs inflated with air, thus increasing the ease of floating. Some few individuals have overall specific gravities greater than 1.0. It is impossible for these people to do a motionless float, because they are "sinkers." A practical way to determine whether a person is a floater or a sinker is to have the person assume the tucked jellyfish float position with lungs inflated. If any portion of the individual's back is on or above the surface, the individual can learn to maintain a motionless floating position that, even though it may be more nearly vertical than supine, is still called a back float.

A floater has to be concerned with two forces, the downward force of the body's weight and the upward buoyancy of the water. When these forces act on the body so that their resultant is zero, the forces will be in equilibrium and the body will be in a motionless float. The downward force acts at the center of gravity of the body, a point somewhere in the pelvis. The buoyant force acts at the center of buoyancy of the body, a point that varies with individuals but is usually closer to the head than the center of gravity. If the body were of uniform density, the center of gravity and the center of buoyancy would coincide, but because the body has less mass toward the head, the center of buoyancy is usually higher in the body than the center of gravity. The center of buoyancy is the point where the center of gravity of the volume of displaced water would be if the water were placed in a vessel the shape and size of the floater's body. Because the water is of uniform

a.   b.

Figure 12.24   A balanced float occurs when the gravity and the center of buoyancy are in the same force line. *G* = downward force of body weight. *B* = upward force (buoyancy) of water.

density, its center of gravity will be in the direction of the greater volume, that is, near the chest region. If the center of gravity and center of buoyancy are not in the same force line with each other, as shown in figure 12.24a, the body will rotate in the direction of the forces until the forces are equal and opposite in line, direction, and magnitude. At this point the floater will be in a balanced float (figure 12.24b). Individuals who float horizontally have the center of gravity and center of buoyancy in the same vertical line while in the horizontal position. These are usually individuals whose bodies contain a high percentage of fat. Those floaters whose legs tend to drop when attempting the back float will have a balanced position somewhere between the horizontal and vertical at that point where the center of gravity and center of buoyancy are in the same vertical line.

The angle of the floating position with the horizontal may be decreased by making adjustments in the position of the body segments that move the center of gravity in closer alignment with the center of buoyancy. Raising the arms over the head, bending the knees, and flexing the wrists to bring the hands out of the water all contribute to moving the center of gravity closer to the head and thus closer to the center of buoyancy (figure 12.24b).

Lift and Drag

The fluid resistance to movement through air or water consists of two forces: *drag* and *lift*. The

fluid flow that produces these two resistance forces is the result of either fluid or object velocity, which acts to produce pressure. Putting one's hand into a calm swimming pool will produce no fluid flow and no feeling of pressure because there is no velocity. Moving the hand back and forth in the pool (object velocity) or placing the hand in a fast-running stream (fluid velocity) produces definite pressure sensations because of fluid flow. Similarly, a softball thrown at 30 mph on a calm day will produce an airflow around the ball in the opposite direction of 30 mph. If the ball were thrown into a 5-mph headwind, the airflow velocity around the ball would be 35 mph. The magnitude of the fluid flow is directly proportional to the fluid and object velocities.

The resistance to forward motion experienced by objects moving through a fluid is called drag. Drag force is the result of fluid pressure on the leading edge of the object and the amount of backward pull produced by turbulence on the trailing edge. In fluid flow, the layer of fluid next to the object is called the *boundary layer*. There will usually be some amount of friction between the boundary layer and the object, which will cause resistance to forward motion. This friction is referred to as **s**urface drag. If the flow of fluid around an object is smooth and unbroken, it is referred to as *laminar flow*. Laminar flow usually occurs in fluids passing around a smooth surface at relatively slow speeds. In laminar flow, the boundary layer is slowed down slightly by sur-

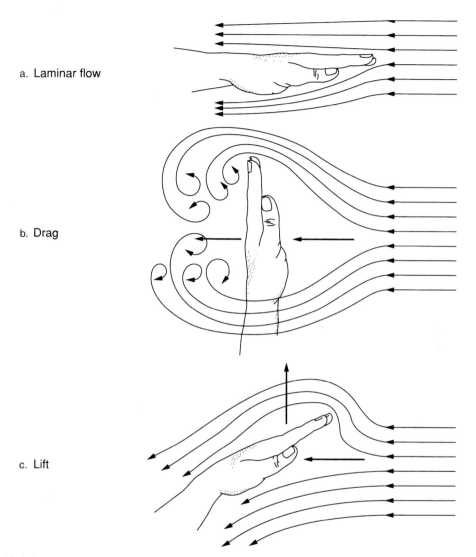

a. Laminar flow

b. Drag

c. Lift

Figure 12.25   Patterns of flow around an object vary with the shape of the frontal surface. (a) Smooth, unbroken flow is laminar flow. (b) Flow that is disrupted and creates turbulence on the trailing edge creates drag. (c) Lift is produced when flow over one side of the object is faster than flow over the other side.

face drag but continues in a smooth, unbroken flow around the object (figure 12.25a). A smooth surface will produce much less surface drag than a rough surface. New, smoother swimsuit fabrics and the practice of shaving body hair before competition are both examples of attempts to reduce surface drag in competitive swimming.

If the surface area presented by the object is great or if the flow velocity is high, there will be greater flow pressure on the leading edge of the object than on the trailing edge. In this situation, the boundary layer does not flow completely around the object. The boundary layer separates, creating a vacuum behind the trailing edge. Fluid rushes in to fill this vacuum, causing a back flow of fluid that is called *turbulence*. Turbulence produces a suction force backward, against the direction of motion. This turbulence is the result of *form drag*. In form drag the shape of the object is such that the fluid, moving at a given velocity, cannot follow the contours of the object (figure 12.25b). Drivers on interstate highways often experience turbulence caused by form drag. When approaching a large truck from behind, the driver of a small car may experience an agitated airflow that tends to make the car harder to control. The driver may also feel a pull toward the truck. Both of these are the effects of turbulence. This turbulence might also increase as the velocity of the truck increases.

Form drag often can be reduced by streamlining. Examples of streamlining are common any time one desires to move easily and quickly through air or water. The crouch position on a racing bicycle, the shape of a race car, and the sharp bow of a boat are all examples of streamlining. The shape of a discus is also meant to take advantage of the effects of streamlining. The discus is tapered at both leading and trailing edges, so the airflow does not have to make any abrupt changes in direction. This streamlining principle will work only if the discus is thrown so that air flows past the tapered edges. If the discus is thrown with the flat side leading, air must make a very abrupt change of direction. There will be increased pressure on the leading edge and turbulence on the trailing edge, creating a large form drag. For this reason, streamlining makes the angle between the long axis of the object and the direction of fluid flow very important. This angle is often referred to as the *angle of attack*.

The angle of attack is also critical in producing and utilizing the fluid force known as *lift*. Lift is the result of changes in fluid pressure as the result of differences in airflow velocities. An extremely important principle in understanding the mechanism of lift is *Bernoulli's Principle*. Simply stated, Bernoulli determined that **the pressure in a moving fluid decreases as the speed increases.** The design of an airplane wing is based on Bernoulli's principle of lift. The top side of an airplane wing has a higher curve than the bottom. To avoid creating a vacuum, airflow over the top will be at a higher velocity than the flow across the bottom. Pressure will therefore be lower on top of the wing. Lift will act upward, from the area of high pressure toward the area of low pressure, causing the wing to move upward. The swimmer uses lift in much the same way. Creating lift toward the forward surface of the hand is one force that aids in propelling the body forward. Lift, therefore, is the result of fluid on one side of an object having to travel farther in the same amount of time to avoid creating a vacuum. Lift always acts perpendicular to the fluid flow and therefore to the drag force (figure 12.25c).

Ball Spin

Bernoulli's Principle applies for moving objects passing through a stationary fluid as well as for fluids passing stationary objects and, in addition to explaining why airplanes can fly, it also explains why balls with spin follow a curved path. This latter application of Bernoulli's Principle is called the Magnus effect after the German physicist who first explained the phenomenon. A ball moving through the air will also move in the direction of least air pressure. As shown in figure 12.26a, the ball spinning in a clockwise direction drags around a boundary layer of air. At the bottom of the ball this air current is moving in the same direction as the oncoming air. At the top, the boundary air is moving in the opposite direction. The air at the bottom is moving faster, and therefore the pressure is reduced. The air at the top moves more slowly and the pressure is increased. Thus the ball will move in a downward curve in the direction of least pressure. Viewed from the side this would be the behavior of a ball with topspin imparted to it. Balls with topspin drop sooner than balls with no spin. A ball with a counterclockwise or backspin will move in an upward curve and thus stay aloft longer than a ball with no spin (figure 12.26b). Balls spinning about a vertical axis have sidespin. Right spin causes the

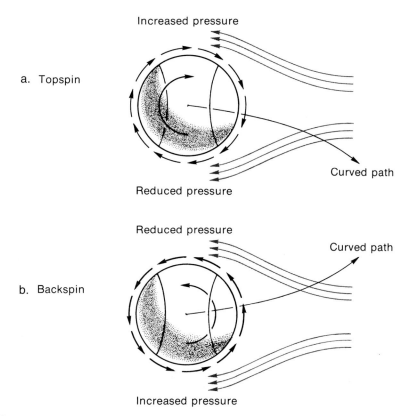

Increased pressure

a. Topspin

Curved path

Reduced pressure

Reduced pressure

Curved path

b. Backspin

Increased pressure

Figure 12.26   A spinning ball follows a curved path moving in the direction of least pressure. (The curve is exaggerated for clarity.)

ball to curve to the right and occurs when the forward edge of the ball moves to the right. Left spin is the opposite.

The amount of air a ball drags around with it when spinning depends on the surface of the ball and the speed of the spin. Rough or large surfaces, small mass, and a fast spin speed all produce a more noticeable spin and curve deflection. The small mass of a table tennis ball, the fuzz on a tennis ball, and the seams on a baseball all enhance spin, an important element in each game's strategy. The deflection will also be more pronounced if the forward velocity is slow. This may occur because of little force imparted to the ball or a strong headwind. Spin on a ball may also smooth its flight by acting as a stabilizer. Like a gyroscope, a football or discus spinning

around one axis resists spinning about another axis and therefore is less likely to tumble through the air.

FREE-BODY DIAGRAMS

In analyzing any technique, the student should consider all the external forces by methodically accounting for the effect of each one on the body. To do this it is helpful to look at the body as if it were isolated from its surroundings. The isolated body is then considered to be a separate mechanical system whose boundaries have been defined. The isolation makes it easier to identify the forces and to represent them as vectors in a diagram of the body. This type of representation is called a

TABLE 12.1	Direction and Point of Application of External Forces	
Force	**Direction of Force**	**Point of Application**
Weight (*W*)	Downward (toward center of earth)	Center of gravity of body
Normal reaction (*R*)	Perpendicular to contact surface	Point of contact
Friction (*F*)	Along contact surface (perpendicular to normal reaction)	Point of contact
Buoyancy (*B*)	Upward	Center of buoyancy of body
Drag (*D*)	Opposite the direction of oncoming fluid flow	Center of gravity of body
Lift (*L*)	Perpendicular to drag	Center of gravity of body

free-body diagram and can help settle any doubts about the application and direction of the various forces acting on the body in any given time frame. The direction of each of the external forces and the point through which each acts are summarized in table 12.1.

In figure 12.27 the magnitude of each external force acting on the body is represented by the arrow length. The direction of the force is represented by the arrowhead, and the point of application is located at the arrow tail. The body is acted on by its weight (*W*) applied through the center of gravity, the reactive force (*R*) and the friction force (*F*), both applied at the point of contact with the vault, and the horizontal force (*H*) directed through the center of gravity. In figure 12.28, the

Figure 12.27   A free-body diagram showing the application and direction of the external forces acting on the vaulter: weight (*W*), horizontal force (*H*), normal reaction (*R*), and friction (*F*).

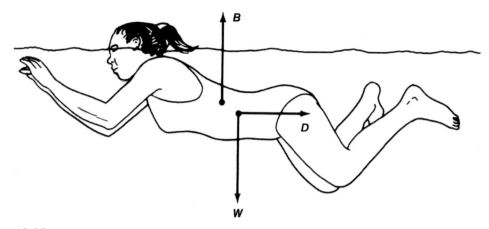

Figure 12.28   A free-body diagram showing the application and direction of external forces acting on the breaststroke swimmer: buoyancy (*B*), weight (*W*), and drag (*D*). The more streamlined the body with respect to the flow, the less will be the drag.

forces acting on the body are weight (*W*), buoyancy (*B*), and drag (*D*). The importance of visualizing all the forces acting on the body relates to the fact that the state of motion or rest of a body depends on the vector sum of all these forces. With a diagram, the forces that can be manipulated to alter the vector sum and produce the desired outcome are more readily apparent. If the swimmer in figure 12.28, for instance, wants to stress horizontal speed, attention should be paid to those factors that will maximize the propulsive force and minimize the opposing drag force, little can be done to alter the weight and buoyancy forces.

Free-body diagrams are also used to show the forces acting on an isolated body segment. In figure 12.29, the thigh has been isolated from the rest of the lower limb, and the forces acting on it are shown. The forces acting on the limb include the weight of the thigh (*W*), the resultant muscle force acting across the hip joint (M_H), the resultant muscle force acting across the knee joint (M_K), and the reactive force components acting across the hip joint (H_x and H_y) and knee joint (K_x and K_y).

WORK, POWER, AND ENERGY

Work

Simple machines such as the lever are devices designed to do work. In each instance the machine aids in the use of a force to overcome a resistance. When the resistance is overcome for a given distance, *work* is done. Mechanically speaking, **work is the product of the amount of force expended and the distance through which the force succeeds in overcoming a resistance it acts upon.** For work done in making a body move in a linear fashion, this may be expressed as

$$W = Fs$$

where *W* stands for work, *F* for force, and *s* for the distance along which the force is applied. Units for expressing work are numerous because any force unit may be combined with any distance unit to form a work unit. In the U.S. system the foot-pound is the most common work unit; the joule is the most frequently used unit in the metric system. A joule is equivalent to $10^7 \times 1$ gram of force exerted through 1 centimeter.

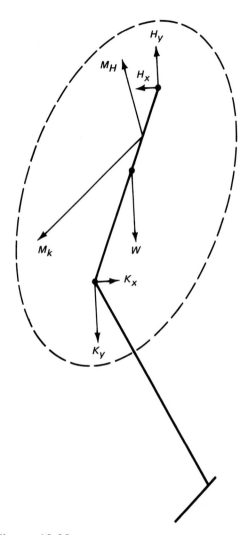

Figure 12.29   Free-body diagram of forces acting on a stationary thigh. Isolation of the limb is shown by the dotted line. Composite muscle forces are M_H and M_K. Reactive forces at the hip are H_y and H_x and at the knee are K_y and K_x. The weight force is W.

Adapted from D. I. Miller and R. C. Nelson, *Biomechanics of Sports*. Copyright © 1973 Lea & Febiger, Malvern, PA. Reprinted by permission.

In computing work, the distance *s* must always be measured in the direction in which the force acts, even though the object whose resistance is overcome may not be moving in the same direction. If one lifts a 20-N suitcase from the floor to

place it on a shelf 2 meters above the floor, the work accomplished is 40 newton-meters (Nm). If, on the other hand, that same weight is lifted an equal distance upward but along a 4-meter inclined plane, the amount of work done is still 40 Nm (figure 12.30). The work done along the incline is the same as the work done to lift the weight to the height of the incline. The horizontal distance the suitcase moves is not included.

Work done in the same direction that the body moves is called *positive* work, whereas work done in the opposite direction is called *negative* work. When an individual does a deep knee bend, the extensor muscles of the leg contract eccentrically to resist the effect of gravity on the body. The body moves in a direction opposite to the upward force of the muscles, and thus negative or resistive work is performed by the muscles. In the return to standing from the knee bend position, the body moves in the same direction as the concentrically contracting extensors, and the work of the muscles is positive. The net work accomplished during the down and up movement of the knee bend is the sum of the positive and negative work. Negative forces resisting gravity perform less work over a given distance than positive forces overcoming gravity. For example, one performs more work walking up a mountain than walking back down.

When the exertion of effort produces no motion, such as might happen during a tug of war, no work is accomplished. Static contraction of muscles may be evident and considerable physiological effort may be expended but, in the strict mechanical sense, no work is being done. The physiological measure of such efforts is determined by obtaining the energy costs, which in turn are usually measured by computing the amount of oxygen consumed during the effort and converting it to calories per minute.

Theoretically, the mechanical work performed by an individual muscle can also be determined using the equation $W = Fs$. Suppose, for instance, that there is a rectangular muscle, 10 centimeters long and 3 centimeters wide, that exerts 240 newtons of force as it turns a bony lever. Because the

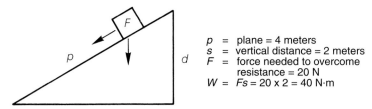

p = plane = 4 meters
s = vertical distance = 2 meters
F = force needed to overcome
resistance = 20 N
W = Fs = 20 x 2 = 40 N·m

Figure 12.30   Work is the product of force needed to overcome a resistance and the direction over which the force is applied. The force lifting the 20 N weight 2 vertical meters does 40N · m of work even though the 20 N are moved 4 meters along the plane.

average muscle fiber shortens to one-half its resting length and the fibers of a small rectangular muscle run the full length of the muscle, the force of the muscle in question is exerted over a distance of 5 cm (the amount of shortening equal to one-half the resting length). Therefore, $F = 240$ N and $s = 5$ cm, the muscle is performing 1200 newton-centimeters, or 120 newton-meters, of work. In brief: $W = F$ (240 N) $\times s$ (5/100 meters).

If the force of the muscle is not known, it is computed from the muscle's cross section. Assuming the muscle in question to be 1 cm thick and the force per square inch of cross section to be 360 N, the following steps are taken:

1. Find the muscle's cross section:
   Cross section = width × thickness.
   3 cm × 1 cm = 3 sq cm (cross section).
2. Find the amount of force exerted by the muscle:
   Average force = 360 N per sq cm.
   Cross section = 3 sq cm.
   $F = 360 \times 3 = 1080$ N.
3. Find the amount of work performed by this muscle, first in N · cm, then in N · m.
   $W = Fs$
   $W = 1080$ N $\times 5$ cm $= 5400$ N · cm.
   5400/100 = 540 N · m

For purposes of simplification, the internal structure of the hypothetical muscle used in these examples was rectangular. This means that a simple geometric cross-sectional measure could be used. For penniform and bipenniform muscles,

however, it would be essential to determine the physiological cross section. It must also be remembered that s in the work equation represents one-half the length of the average fiber in the muscle and that this may or may not coincide with the total length of the fleshy part of the muscle, depending on its internal structure. The number of pounds of force per square inch exerted by the average human muscle must be selected arbitrarily, depending on whose research the student accepts.

A single equation for computing the work performed by a muscle whose average fiber length is known and whose physiological cross section (PCS) has been determined is as follows:

$W = 360 \times$ PCS (in square centimeters) $\times$ 1/2 the length of the fibers (in centimeters)

This gives work in terms of Newton-centimeters. Because it is customary to measure work in terms of Newton-meters, the result should be divided by 100. The following equation includes this step:

$$W = \frac{360 \ (\text{PCS in square cm})(1 \ / \ 2 \ \text{the fiber length in cm})}{100}$$

Any measure of work does not account for the time involved in performing the work. When one lifts 200 N a distance of 2 meters, 400 N · m of work is done, regardless of the time it takes to do it. The *rate* at which work is done is called power and may be expressed as

$$P = \frac{Fs}{t} \quad \text{or} \quad P = \frac{W}{t}$$

where P stands for power, W for work, and t for time. Because s/t is velocity, still another form for the power equation is $P = Fv$. Any form of the equation clearly points out that the machine or person who can perform more work in a given unit of time or who takes less time to do a specified amount of work is more powerful.

In the U.S. system, power is expressed as ft · lb/sec or as horsepower (550 ft · lb/sec = 1 horsepower). The metric system unit is the watt, which is equivalent to 1 joule/second.

Energy

Energy is defined as the capacity to do work. A body is said to possess energy when it can perform work, and the energy that the body possesses is measured as the work accomplished. Energy may take numerous forms, and it is common for it to be converted from one form to another, although according to the Law of Conservation of Energy it can neither be created nor destroyed. Some forms that energy may take are heat, sound, light, electric, chemical, atomic, and mechanical. When a ball is hit with a bat, some of the mechanical energy is converted to sound and heat energy, but none of the energy is lost. **The total amount of energy possessed by a body or an isolated system remains constant.**

Potential energy and kinetic energy are two classifications of mechanical energy that have important implications in biomechanics. Potential energy is the capacity for doing work that a body has because of its position or configuration. A raised weight such as a diver standing on a platform, a bent bow, or a compressed spring all have potential energy. Measured in work units, potential energy is the product of the force an object has and the distance over which it can act. The potential energy of a 150-pound diver whose center of gravity is 20 feet above the water surface is 3000 foot-pounds. In this instance the appropriate form for the potential energy equation is

$$PE = mgh$$

where m is the mass of the body, g is the force of gravity, and h is the height between the diver's center of gravity and the water surface. The product of m and g (mg) is the same as the diver's weight.

The distance selected for h in the potential energy equation is established by choosing an arbitrary zero level. The potential energy of someone standing on a table 1 meter from the floor can be increased by boring a large hole in the floor directly in front of the table. The individual's potential for dropping farther is now greater because h is greater.

The kinetic energy of a body is the energy due to its motion. The faster a body moves, the more kinetic energy it possesses. When a body stops moving, the kinetic energy is dissipated. This is readily seen in the equation for kinetic energy

$$KE = 1/2 \ mv^2$$

where m is the mass of the object and v is its velocity. If v is zero, then KE is also zero.

Energy has been defined as the capacity to do work, and because energy can neither be created nor destroyed, the work done is equal to the kinetic energy acquired, or

$$Fs = 1/2 \ mv^2$$

This relationship is extremely helpful in explaining the value of "giving" when receiving the impetus of any moving object. In attempting to catch a fast-moving ball, one's chances of success are improved by increasing the distance used for stopping the ball's motion. The work of the kinetic energy against the hands depends on the kinetic energy the ball possesses when it hits the hand. Whether that work consists of a large F and a small s or a small F and a large s depends on the technique used by the catcher. As s increases in $Fs = 1/2 \ mv^2$, the force of the impact F must decrease. The skillful performer knows this and will decrease the possibility of injury and increase the chances of holding onto the ball with the choice of a small F and a large s. Achieving a gradual loss of kinetic energy is likewise advantageous when landing from a jump or a fall (figure 12.31).

Figure 12.31 Effecting a gradual loss of kinetic energy by bending the knees upon landing from a jump.

Energy is frequently transformed from kinetic into potential energy or conversely from potential to kinetic energy. The diver who jumps from a platform above the water begins immediately to lose potential energy in proportion to the gain in kinetic energy. At platform height all of the diver's energy is potential. At zero elevation all of the potential energy has been converted into an equivalent amount of kinetic energy. Barring no conversion of energy to other forms (heat, sound, and so forth) the potential energy at the top equals exactly the kinetic energy at the bottom.

The transformation from one energy state to another is interesting to note in a gymnast swinging on the flying rings. Like a pendulum, the swinger's energy is transformed from kinetic to potential on every swing. As the suspended body moves upward, the kinetic energy is continuously changed to potential energy, and the higher the swinger goes, the greater the potential becomes for doing work on the downswing. At the top of the swing the conversion to potential energy is complete. Once more as the gymnast begins to fall, kinetic energy again develops and becomes greatest at the bottom of the swing, when the speed is greatest and potential energy is zero. Theoretically the swinging should continue uninterrupted, but because of friction some energy is converted to heat and eventually the "pendulum" will come to rest.

THE ANALYSIS OF LINEAR MOTION

Establishing the mechanical principles that are used in the analysis of linear motion involves first identifying the nature of the forces involved in the motion of interest. As discussed in this chapter, several forces must be considered.

1. Weight—applied downward through the center of gravity.
2. Propulsive forces—forces generated by muscles, which, in turn, move segments to produce contact forces.
3. Normal reaction—applied equal and opposite to contact forces, perpendicular to contact surfaces.
4. Friction—applied perpendicular to normal reaction forces along contact surfaces opposite the direction of the propulsive force.
5. Buoyancy—acting in opposition to gravity to support the body in a fluid.
6. Drag—resistance to motion caused by fluid pressure and turbulence, acting in the direction of fluid flow.
7. Lift—acting perpendicular to the direction of fluid flow.

In the long jump example used throughout this text, weight is the resistance force that must be overcome in order for the jumper to leave the ground. The propulsive force is muscle force acting to produce forceful extension of the lower extremities and flexion of the upper extremities. The flexion of the upper extremities produces a downward reaction force. This, along with the downward-directed force produced by lower extremity extension, generates a downward-directed normal force and a backward-directed tangential force. It is the equal and opposite normal reaction force and the friction force that propel the body into the air as a projectile.

The principles that govern the mechanical aspects of a movement performance can be summarized by examining some of the basic concepts involved in the kinetics of linear motion. Some general movement principles based on these concepts might be as follows:

Inertia   An object will resist any change in motion state, based on mass or momentum (mass × velocity).

Impulse   Any change in the motion state depends on the applied force and the time over which it is applied. An impulse is required for any change in momentum.

Work   The amount of work done by the movement system is equal to the amount of force applied and the distance over which it is applied.

Kinetic energy   The amount of work done on a body or object is equal to the kinetic energy produced. Energy can be imparted to move objects or be dissipated to cause objects to stop motion.

To return to the long jump example, the inertia that must be overcome is the mass of the jumper's body. The impulse generated in the propulsion phase must be one that will give maximum linear velocity to the body for its projectile flight. When this impulse is applied, work is done on the body. The result of this work is the production of the kinetic energy necessary to carry the body forward in flight. The amount of kinetic energy generated will be directly dependent on the impulse applied.

The student must understand that the linear forces that produce motion in the human body are often the result of the rotary motion of the body segments occurring at the joints. For this reason, an analysis of linear mechanics alone cannot fully describe the mechanical attributes of performance. The following chapter will provide the student with the knowledge to analyze the rotary components of human motion.

LABORATORY EXPERIENCES

1. Define the following key terms and give an example of each that is not used in the text:
   Force
   Inertia
   Mass
   Weight
   Momentum
   Impulse

2. In the diagram of the biceps muscle in figure 12.32, find the size of the angle of pull.

3. Place a book on a table and stand a small bottle on top of it. Pull the book toward you with a quick jerk. Note the action of the bottle. Stand the bottle on the book again and pull the book across the table with a steady pull. How does the bottle move? Now pull the book and stop it suddenly. Explain the action of the bottle in all three instances.

4. Hit a softball with a bat from a tee, from a self-toss, and from a pitch. Which hit goes the farthest? Explain.

5. Lie on your back in the water with your arms over your head. Raise your legs by flexing your hips. What happens to your arms and trunk? Explain. Devise another experiment that demonstrates the same principle.

6. While both of you have on ice skates or roller skates stand facing someone whose weight is the same as yours. Push against each other. Observe

Figure 12.32   The forearm as a lever with the biceps providing the force.

and compare the distance and velocity each of you moves. Repeat the procedure with someone who weighs considerably more or less than you do. Explain the difference between the two performances.

7. Place a long wide board on some rollers (pencils, dowels, or pipes) so that there is very little friction between the board and the floor. Carefully step on the board and attempt to walk normally along it. What happens to you? To the board? Take the board off the rollers and place it on the floor. Walk along it. Explain the reason for the differences in the behavior of the board and your ability to walk along it. The use of spotters is advised for this exercise.

8. Determine the coefficient of restitution for each of the following objects dropped from a height of 2 meters onto a wooden floor:
   a. Tennis ball
   b. Racquetball
   c. Golf ball
   d. Soccer ball
   e. Baseball

Repeat the calculations for the above objects rebounding from concrete, from asphalt tile, from artificial turf, and from a tumbling mat.

9. Using a tennis racket or a paddle, impart topspin, backspin, no spin, and sidespin to a ball. Note the effect on the velocity and angle of reflection when the ball rebounds from a horizontal surface, from a vertical surface when struck from above, and from a vertical surface when struck from below.

10. Assume a back-lying position in the water with your arms at your sides. Note and explain any shift in body position. Slide your arms from your sides to a side horizontal position, keeping them close to and parallel to the surface of the water. What effect does this have on body position? Continue moving your arms until they are overhead. Next flex the wrists so the hands are out of the water. Finally, flex the legs at the knees. Explain the effect of these last three moves on your position in the water.

11. Record the body weight for each of five subjects. Using a stopwatch, record the time necessary for each subject to run up two flights of stairs. Determine the vertical distance from the bottom of the first flight to the top of the second flight. Calculate the work done by each subject and the power of each. Complete the following chart.

a. Which subjects did the most work? Why?
b. Did those who did the most work have the most power? Explain.
c. If power is an important part of an event, how should an athlete train for it?

Subject	Weight	Time	Work	Power
1.				
2.				
3.				
4.				
5.				

12. Estimate the cross section of your own biceps muscle. Approximately how much force should it be able to exert?
13. Approximately how much force should your triceps be able to exert?
14. In each of the following movement patterns identify the nature of the motion for each phase.

State the underlying mechanical objectives and describe what must occur to achieve optimum results. Consider carefully the application of linear mechanical principles.
Front crawl stroke
Bench press
High jump

REFERENCES AND SELECTED READINGS

Adrian, M. J., and J. M. Cooper. 1994. *The biomechanics of human movement.* 2nd ed. Indianapolis: Benchmark Press.

Bunn, J. W. 1972. *Scientific principles of coaching.* 2nd ed. Englewood Cliffs, NJ: Prentice Hall.

Gowitzke, B. A., and M. Milner. 1988. *Scientific bases of human movement.* 3rd ed. Baltimore: Williams & Wilkins.

Hay, J. G. 1993. *The biomechanics of sports techniques.* 4th ed. Englewood Cliffs, NJ: Prentice Hall.

Kreighbaum, E., and K. M. Barthels. 1990. *Biomechanics.* 3rd ed. New York: Macmillan.

Tözeren, A. 2000. *Human body dynamics: Classical mechanics and human movement.* New York: Springer.

Wiktorin, C. H., and M. Nordin. 1986. *Introduction to problem solving in biomechanics.* Philadelphia: Lea & Febiger.

Winter, D. A. 1990. *Biomechanics of human movement.* 2nd ed. New York: Wiley.

Zatsiorsky, V. M. 1998. *Kinematics of human motion.* Champaign. IL: Human Kinetics.

THE CONDITIONS OF ROTARY MOTION

OUTLINE

■ *Rotary Force*
   Eccentric Force
   Torque
■ *The Lever*
   External Levers
   Anatomical Levers
   Lever Arms
   Classification of Levers
   The Principle of Levers
   Relation of Speed to Range
      in Movements of Levers
   Selection of Levers
   Mechanical Advantage of Levers
   Identification and Analysis
      of Levers
■ *Newton's Laws and Rotational
   Equivalents*
   Moment of Inertia
   Acceleration of Rotating Bodies
   Action and Reaction
   Transfer of Momentum
■ *Centripetal and Centrifugal
   Forces*
■ *The Analysis of Rotary Motion*
■ *Laboratory Experiences*

OBJECTIVES

At the conclusion of this chapter the student should be able to:

1. Name, define, and use the following terms properly as they relate to rotary motion: eccentric force, torque, couple, lever, moment of inertia, and angular momentum.

2. Solve simple lever and torque problems involving the human body and the implements it uses.

3. Demonstrate an understanding of the effective selection of levers by relating speed, range of motion, and mechanical advantage to the properties of given lever systems.

4. Explain the analogous kinetic relationships that exist between linear and rotary motion.

5. State Newton's laws of motion as they apply to rotary motion.

6. Explain the cause and effect relationship between the forces responsible for rotary motion and the objects experiencing the motion.

7. Define centripetal and centrifugal force, and explain the relationships that exist between these forces and the factors influencing them.

8. Identify the concepts of rotary motion that are critical elements in the successful performance of a selected motor skill.

9. Using the concepts that govern rotary motion, perform a mechanical analysis of a selected motor skill.

ROTARY FORCE

Eccentric Force

The student already knows that the effect forces have on an object depends on the magnitude, point of application, and direction of each force. When force is applied in line with a freely moving object's center of gravity, linear motion occurs. When the direction of force is not in line, a combination of rotary and translatory motion is likely to occur. This relationship between force application and direction and the resulting motion are apparent when a book is pushed along a table. Linear motion occurs when sufficient force is applied in line with the book's center of gravity, and a combination of linear and rotary motion results from a force directed left or right of center. Similarly, an object with a fixed axis, like a door or one of the body's limbs, rotates when the force is applied "off center" but does not rotate when the force is in line with the axis of rotation. A force whose direction is not in line with the center of gravity of a freely moving object or the center of rotation of an object with a fixed axis of rotation is called an **eccentric force.** There must be an eccentric force for rotation to occur. Some examples of the application of eccentric force are shown in figure 13.1.

Torque

The turning effect of an eccentric force is called *torque,* or moment of force. The torque about any point equals the product of the force magnitude and the perpendicular distance from the line of force to the axis of rotation. The perpendicular distance between the force vector and the axis is called the *moment arm,* or torque arm. In this text, the turning effect will be referred to as torque and the perpendicular distance as moment arm. An example of torque is illustrated in figure 13.2. Neglecting the weight of the arm, the torque or turning effect caused by a 9-N weight held in the hand with the forearm flexed at the elbow to a horizontal position is the product of the weight times its perpendicular distance, or moment arm length, from the elbow. If the moment arm d is 0.3 meters, the amount of torque or downward turning force is 3 newton-meters (N·m). To keep the arm motionless in this position, the elbow flexors must exert an equal and opposite torque or upward-directed turning force of 3 N·m.

Because torque is the product of force and the length of the moment arm, it may be modified by changing either the force or the moment arm. Torque may be increased by increasing the magnitude of the force or by increasing the length of the moment arm. Decreasing either of these factors will produce a decrease in torque. In the preceding example, for instance, if the magnitude of the weight held in the hand were decreased to 6 N, the torque would also decrease, in this case to 2 N·m. Conversely, increasing the weight would increase the torque. If, however, the weight is increased but is moved closer to the axis (the elbow), the torque produced by the heavier weight would be reduced through reducing the length of the moment arm.

a. Axis of rotation

b.   Axis of rotation

c.

Figure 13.1   Examples of the application of eccentric force.

It is important to emphasize that the moment arm is the *perpendicular* distance from the direction of force to the axis of rotation. In the example just given, the moment arm length was the same as the length of the forearm because the horizontal forearm was perpendicular to the vertical direction of the force, and therefore the forearm length was equal to the perpendicular distance from the force direction to the axis. If the arm were in some position other than the horizontal, its length would no longer be equal to the moment arm distance between the force direction and axis. Suppose the forearm's position is shifted from the horizontal to one of 45 degrees of flexion with the horizontal. Now the force line of the weight is not at right angles to the forearm (figure 13.3). This means

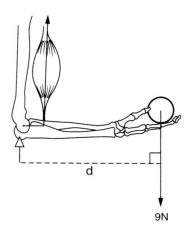

Figure 13.2   A weight applied at some distance (d) from the axis (elbow) produces torque.

Figure 13.3   The torque of the 9-N weight about the elbow joint is the product of the rotary component of the weight and the distance from the rotary component to the axis of rotation.

that the length of the moment arm is no longer the length of the forearm because, by definition, the moment arm is the perpendicular distance from the direction or line of force to the axis of motion. The moment arm now is considerably shorter. Using trigonometric relations, we find that the mo-

ment arm length is 0.2 meters. Consequently, the torque decreases from 3 N·m to 1.9 N·m, and the amount of muscular effort needed to counteract this downward force decreases proportionately.

In the human body, the mass or weight of a segment cannot be altered instantaneously. There-

a.

b.

Figure 13.4   Gravitational torque *d* decreases in going from (a) to (b) as the force line moves closer to the axis. The torque is 0 at 90 degrees.

fore, the torque of a segment that is due to gravitational force can be changed only by changing the length of the moment arm in relation to the axis. This is done by moving a body segment so that the force line of the weight is closer to or farther from the axis. The effect of doing this is quite apparent in the stages of the sit-up. Compare the gravitational torque on the trunk when the trunk is just leaving the floor with the torque when the trunk is at a 30-degree angle from the floor (figure 13.4).

Muscle forces also exert torque on rotating segments. The amount of torque depends on both the magnitude of the muscle force and the moment arm length. Unlike gravitational torque, each of these factors can be altered. The moment arm length depends on the point of insertion of the muscle and the position of the body segment at any point in a given motion. Figure 13.5 shows

how the moment arm of the biceps changes for every change of arm position during elbow flexion. The magnitude of the force of the muscle contributing to the torque changes also as its length, tension, and angle of pull change.

With changes in muscle angle of pull, the magnitude of the force effectively producing torque also changes. When muscle force vectors are resolved into their two components, it can be seen that only the rotary component—that which is perpendicular to the mechanical axis of bone— is actually a factor in torque production. The stabilizing component of the muscle force acts along the mechanical axis of the bone through the axis of rotation; thus this component is not an eccentric, or off-center, force and cannot contribute to torque. It has a moment arm length equal to zero. Once a muscle force is resolved into a rotary and a stabilizing component, the moment arm is the

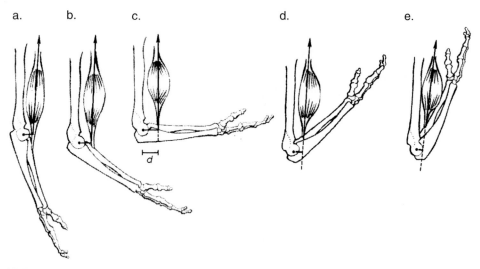

a. b. c. d. e.

Figure 13.5 The biceps at various points of elbow flexion, showing variations in the moment arm.
From B. LeVeau, *Williams and Lissner: Biomechanics of Human Motion,* 2nd ed. Copyright © 1977 W. B. Saunders, Orlando, FL. Reprinted by permission.

distance between the axis of rotation and the point of application of the rotary component of the muscle force. Because the rotary component of any known force can be calculated trigonometrically, given the angle between the line of force and the mechanical axis, torque can be calculated as the product of the rotary component of the force (F_y) times the moment arm along the lever (d) (see figure 13.9b). In the example used earlier, the angle between the line of force for the weight and the mechanical axis of the bone is 45 degrees. Using the angle and the 9-N magnitude of the force, the rotary component of the force is calculated to be 6.4 N. When multiplied by the 0.3 meter length of the moment arm, the torque is 1.9 N·m, the same value found when calculating the length of the true moment arm in figure 13.3. Either method of finding torque is satisfactory.

The important thing to remember from this discussion is that the turning effect, or torque, produced on objects free to rotate depends on two factors: the magnitude of the applied force and the perpendicular distance from the force vector to the axis. Change in turning effect occurs when either of these factors is altered. Shortening the

moment arm distance or decreasing the force magnitude will decrease the torque. Lengthening the moment arm or increasing the force magnitude will increase the turning effect and consequently the necessary effort to resist it.

Summation of Torques

The sum of two or more torques may result in no motion, linear motion, or rotary motion. When equal parallel eccentric forces are applied in the same direction on opposite sides of the center of rotation of an object, either no motion or linear motion will occur. An example of no motion is two children balanced on a seesaw. When the equal parallel forces are adequate to overcome the resistance of the object, linear motion will occur. This could be the situation with paddlers in a canoe, with one paddling on the port side and the other on the starboard side. When equal and opposite parallel forces are exerted on opposite sides of the axis of rotation, rotary motion will occur. The effect of equal parallel forces acting in opposite directions is called a *couple,* or *force couple.* An example of this type of movement is steering a car when both hands are used on oppo-

Figure 13.6   When one steers with two hands, the hands act as a force couple.

site sides of the wheel (figure 13.6). Another example is that of turning in a rowboat by simultaneously pulling on the handle of one oar while pushing on the handle of the other.

There are many examples in the human body in which two muscles rotate a bone by acting cooperatively as a force couple; for instance, trapezius II and the lower portion of serratus anterior are a force couple, rotating the scapula upward. Trapezius II and IV, acting on the two extremities of the spine of the scapula, similarly serve as a force couple to help rotate the scapula upward, as do the oblique abdominals in acting to rotate the trunk (figure 13.7).

Principle of Torques

It is common for more than one torque to act on a body at any given time. The resultant effect of these torques is expressed in the principle of the summation of torques, which states that the **resultant torques of a force system must be equal to the sum of the torques of the individual forces of the system about the same point.** Because torques are vector quantities, the summation must consider both magnitude and direction. The direction of rotation is expressed as either clockwise or counterclockwise direction. Clock-

wise torques are usually labeled as negative, and counterclockwise torques as positive. Their signs must be accounted for when they are summed.

When the sum of counterclockwise torques equals the sum of clockwise torques, no turning will occur. This idea may also be expressed by stating that rotation will be absent when the sum of the torques of all forces about any point or axis equals zero. When the sum of clockwise torques does not equal the sum of the counterclockwise torques, the resultant turning effect (torque) will be the difference between the two opposing forces and in the direction of the larger.

In figure 13.8 all the forces are applied perpendicular to the lever. Force A is 1.5 m from the axis and B is 3 m away. Both A and B are clockwise forces. Force C is a counterclockwise force that also is 3 m away from the axis. The sum of these torques produces a resultant torque of 22.5 N·m in a clockwise direction about the center of rotation.

When an eccentric force is applied at an angle to the lever other than 90 degrees, the moment arm is not along the lever line. Before the torque can be found, the length of the moment arm must be determined. This can be done using

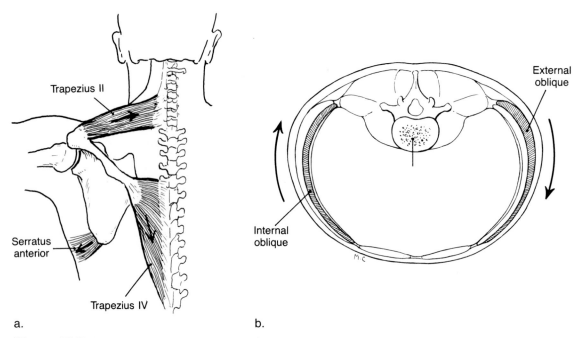

a.   b.

Figure 13.7   (a) Two force couples acting on the scapula to rotate it upward. Trapezius II and lower serratus anterior are an excellent example. Trapezius II and the lower fibers of IV also tend to act as a force couple although their pulls are not in opposite directions. (b) A cross section of the trunk in which the oblique abdominal muscles act as a force couple to rotate the trunk.

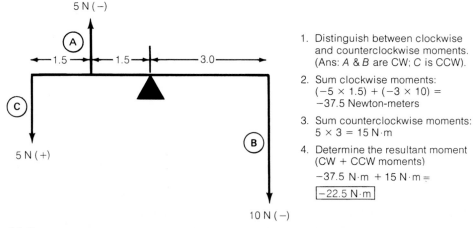

1. Distinguish between clockwise and counterclockwise moments. (Ans: *A* & *B* are CW; *C* is CCW).

2. Sum clockwise moments: $(-5 \times 1.5) + (-3 \times 10) = -37.5$ Newton-meters

3. Sum counterclockwise moments: $5 \times 3 = 15$ N·m

4. Determine the resultant moment (CW + CCW moments)

   -37.5 N·m $+ 15$ N·m $= \boxed{-22.5 \text{ N·m}}$

Figure 13.8   Summation of moments. The resultant moment about a point is equal to the sum of the moments of the individual forces about the same point. Clockwise moments are negative, and counterclockwise moments are positive. The sum of the moments about the fulcrum on this diagram is 22.5 Newton-meters in a clockwise direction.

trigonometric functions. An example of this procedure is shown in the following problem:

> What muscular force *F* pulling at an angle of 25 degrees would be required to keep the abducted arm in a position of 20 degrees with the horizontal? The muscle inserts 10 cm from the shoulder joint. The arm weighs 50 N and its center of gravity is located 30 cm from the shoulder. A 45-N weight is held in the hand 60 cm from the shoulder joint. *Note:* For the arm to be held stationary, the sum of the counterclockwise torques must equal the clockwise torques (ΣCCW = ΣCW). (See figure 13.9 for solution.)

THE LEVER

A simple machine that operates according to the principle of torques is the **lever.** A lever is a rigid bar that can rotate about a fixed point when a force is applied to overcome a resistance. When they move, levers serve two important functions. They are used either to overcome a resistance larger than the magnitude of the effort applied or to increase the speed and range of motion through which a resistance can be moved. When there is no motion, the torque produced by the effort and the torque produced by the resistance are equal and the lever system is said to be balanced.

External Levers

We use levers every day of our lives. In the kitchen the old-fashioned manual can opener, punch can opener, and bottle opener or lid pry are all examples of simple levers. Likewise, in the workshop or about the house and grounds the crowbar, pry bar, and wheelbarrow are levers. What do these implements have in common? Even though their shapes vary and their structures differ in complexity, each of these is a rigid bar. When a force is applied to one of them, it turns about a fixed point known as a **fulcrum,** and it overcomes a resistance that may, in some cases, be no more than its own weight. All the levers mentioned are designed to enable use of a relatively small force to overcome a relatively large

resistance. In levers such as these, the range of movement of the resistance is relatively slight, whereas the range of movement of the effort is large. The crowbar, for instance, lifts a rock only a few centimeters, whereas the handle moves through a much larger distance. In other words, the power to overcome a considerable resistance is gained at the expense of range of motion.

The striking implements used in sports are levers that do the opposite of this. The golf club, for instance, is used to gain range of motion at the expense of force. The length of the shaft enables the club head to travel through a large arc of motion, but it is used to overcome the relatively slight resistance of the weight of the club itself. Tennis and squash rackets, baseball bats, hockey sticks, and fencing foils are other examples of levers used to gain distance at the expense of force. These levers do not save the strength of the user, as do the household levers mentioned, but they increase the user's range and speed of movement. By striking a ball with a racket, for instance, the striker can impart more speed to it and send it a greater distance than could be done by striking it with the hand. This is because the head of the racket travels a greater distance, and therefore at a greater speed, than the hand alone is able to do.

A still different kind of lever is seen in the seesaw on the playground, the scales in the laboratory, and the mobile hanging in the art gallery. These levers gain neither force nor distance, but provide for a balancing of weights. If the loads are equal, they will balance each other when they are equidistant from the fulcrum. If they are unequal, they will balance only if the heavier load is placed closer to the fulcrum. There is an exact relationship between the magnitude of the weights and their respective distances from the fulcrum so that when the torques are summed, the resultant is zero.

This kind of lever may also be used to balance a force and a load. The skier carrying skis over one shoulder, balanced by a hand holding the other end, is an example. The amount of effort exerted by the hand depends on what portion of the ski is in contact with the shoulder. If the weight of the skis is evenly distributed on each

How much muscle force is needed to hold the arm and the 45 N weight in this position?

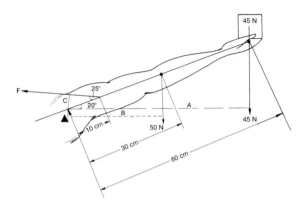

Solution Finding Rotary Components

A = 45 N force   B = 50 N force

1. Clockwise torques
    a. A_y = 45 N × cos 20
        A_y = 45 N × .940
        A_y = 42.3 N
    b. B_y = 50 N × cos 20
        B_y = 50 N × .940
        B_y = 47 N

2. CCW = CW
    a. F_y × 10 cm = (A_y × 60 cm) + (B_y × 30 cm)
    b. F_y × 10 cm = (42.3 N × 60 cm) + (47 N × 30 cm)
    c. F_y × 10 cm = 3948 N·cm
    d. F_y = 3948 N·cm/10 cm = 394.8 N
    e. F = F_y/sin 25 = 394.8 N·m/.423
    f. F = 933.3 N

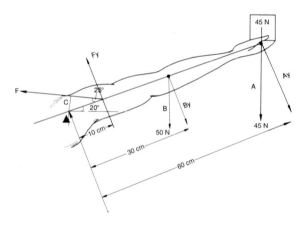

Solution Finding Moment Arm

▲ = axis
F = force of muscle
A = moment arm for 45 = N weight
B = moment arm for 50 = N weight
C = moment arm for F
To balance, clockwise torques must equal counterclockwise torques.

1. Clockwise torques
    a. 45 N × A = 45 N × (60 cm × cos 20)
        45 N × (60 cm × .940) = 2538 N·cm
    b. 50 N × B = 50 N × (30 cm × cos 20)
        50 N × (30 cm × .940) = 1410 N·cm

2. Counterclockwise torques
    a. F × C = F × (10 cm × sin 25)
        F × (10 cm × .423) = F × 4.23 cm

3. CCW = CW
    a. F × 4.23 cm = 2538 N·cm + 1410 N·cm
    b. F × 4.23 cm = 3948 N·cm
    c. F = $\dfrac{3948}{\text{N·cm}}$
    d. F = 933.3 N

Figure 13.9   Summation of torques using trigonometric functions. The amount of muscle force needed to counteract the force of gravity in this example is 933.3 N.

side of the shoulder, the hand needs to exert little or no effort.

Anatomical Levers

But where in the human body do we have anything even faintly resembling a punch can opener, hockey stick, or seesaw? When we recognize each of these levers as a rigid bar that turns about a fulcrum when force is applied to it, it is then apparent that nearly *every bone* in the skeleton can be looked upon as levers. The bone itself serves as the rigid bar, the joint as the fulcrum, and the contracting muscles as the force. A large segment of the body, such as the trunk, the upper extremity, or the lower extremity, can likewise act as a single lever if it is used as a rigid unit. When the entire arm is raised sideward, for instance, it is acting as a simple lever. The center of motion in the shoulder joint serves as the fulcrum. The effort is supplied mainly by the deltoid muscle and the resistance in this instance is the weight of the arm itself. The point at which the effort is applied to the lever is approximately the point at which the deltoid inserts into the humerus, and the point at which the resistance is applied is the center of gravity of the extended arm. If a weight is held in the hand, the resistance point is then the center of gravity of the arm plus its load and is located closer to the hand than before. If a relatively heavy weight is lifted, for practical purposes the weight of the arm may be disregarded and the resistance point may be assumed to be the center of the object's point of contact with the hand.

Anatomical levers do not necessarily resemble bars. The skull, shoulder blade, and vertebrae are notable exceptions to the definition. The resistance point, also, may be difficult to identify, especially in the seesaw type of lever. It is not always easy to tell whether the resistance is the weight of the lever itself or is the resistance afforded by antagonistic muscles and fasciae that are put on a steadily increasing stretch as the movement progresses. For instance, when the head is turned easily to the left, the resistance point may be regarded as the center of gravity of the head. We can only guess at the approximate lo-

cation of this. If the turning of the head is resisted by the pressure of someone's hand against the left side of the chin, the resistance point is the midpoint of the contact area. If the head is turned without external resistance but is forced to the limit of motion, resistance to the movement is afforded by the antagonistic rotators, and possibly by the ligaments and fasciae. The resistance *point* in such a case is the midpoint of the area over which these resisting forces act on the head. As in the first example, the location of this point can only be estimated.

Lever Arms

Lever arms are commonly defined as the portion of the lever between the fulcrum and the force points. The effort arm is the distance between the fulcrum and the effort point, and the resistance arm is the distance between the fulcrum and the resistance point. These definitions are valid, however, only when the effort and resistance are applied at right angles to the lever. When the effort and resistance are applied at some angle other than 90 degrees to the lever, these definitions are inaccurate. A better definition of a lever arm that applies regardless of the angle of force application is one synonymous to that of a moment arm. Indeed, a lever arm is a moment arm. In a lever the perpendicular distance between the fulcrum and line of force of the effort is the *effort arm (EA)*. Similarly, the perpendicular distance between the fulcrum and the line of resistance force is the *resistance arm (RA)*. In figure 13.16, *EA* is the effort arm and *RA* is the resistance arm.

Classification of Levers

Three points on the lever have been identified: the point about which it turns, the point at which effort is applied to it, and the point at which the resistance to its movement is applied or concentrated. Because there are three points, there are three possible arrangements of these points. Any one of the three may be situated between the other two. The arrangement of these three points provides the basis for the classification of levers.

Figure 13.10   Levers: (a) a lever of the first class; (b) a lever of the second class; (c) a lever of the third class.

First-Class Levers

In a first-class lever, the axis lies between the effort and the resistance (figure 13.10a). The mechanical advantage of the first-class lever is balance. The first-class lever also can be used to magnify the effects of the effort or to increase the speed and range of motion on the basis of the relative lengths of the effort moment arm (*EA*) and the resistance moment arm (*RA*). Examples of external first-class levers are the seesaw, balance scale, crowbar, scissors, and automobile jack (figure 13.11).

The head, tipping forward and backward, is a good example of a first-class lever in the body (figure 13.11). To be sure, it is a sphere rather than a bar, and the axis of motion would seem to be an imaginary one located in the frontal plane approximately between the ears. The effort is supplied by the extensors of the head, notably the splenius and upper portions of the semispinalis, and is applied to the head at the base of the skull. The resistance to the movement is furnished by the weight of the head itself, together with the tension of the antagonistic muscles and fasciae, as the limit of motion is approached. The center of concentration of the resistance is difficult to determine. If the head is acting like a seesaw, the resistance would seem to be centered in the front half of the head for hyperextension. Additional resistance is provided by the tension of opposing muscles and ligaments, the resistance point being the point at which the various resistance forces are concentrated.

Figure 13.11   The head acting as a first-class lever like the seesaw. *A* = the approximate position of the axis or fulcrum; *E* = the point where the force is applied; *R* = the approximate point where the resistance is concentrated.

Another first-class lever is seen in the foot when it is not being used for weight bearing, as when the knees are crossed in the sitting position. As the soleus pulls upward on the heel, the foot plantar flexes at the ankle joint where the

Figure 13.12 The forearm acting as a first-class lever, similar to a pair of paper shears.

fulcrum is situated. The resistance seems to be provided by the tonus of the dorsiflexor muscles. The weight of the foot apparently is not a factor here, because the foot has already relaxed into a position of partial plantar flexion. The picture would be changed, however, if the person were lying face down with the leg bent at the knee and the lower leg extended vertically upward. If the foot were then plantar flexed, the weight of the foot would be a factor in the resistance.

The forearm is another example of a first-class lever *when it is being extended by the triceps muscle against a resistance* (figure 13.12). The fulcrum is situated at the elbow joint, the effort is applied at the olecranon process, and the resistance point is located at the forearm's center of gravity when no external resistance is present, and at the hand when the latter is pushing against

an external resistance. Internal resistance does not appear to be a factor in this movement.

Second-Class Levers

In a second-class lever, the resistance lies between the axis and the effort (figure 13.10b). In this lever, the *EA* is always longer than the *RA*. This arrangement has the advantage of magnifying the effects of the effort so that it takes less force to move the resistance. Its disadvantage is that range of motion is sacrificed. Examples of external second-class levers are the wheelbarrow, door (effort applied at the knob), and nutcracker. Whether or not there are any second-class levers in the body seems to be a controversial matter among anatomists and kinesiologists. Some claim that when the foot is being plantar flexed in a weight-bearing position, as when rising on the toes, it is a second-class lever. The fulcrum is said to be at the point of contact with the ground, the effort point at the heel where the tendon of Achilles attaches and the resistance at the ankle joint where the weight of the body is transferred to the foot. Another second-class lever might be the forearm if it were being flexed by the brachioradialis alone, but this could occur only if the other flexors were paralyzed.

There are numerous second-class levers involving body segments if those actions where gravity supplies the effort for the movement and muscles control or resist the movement through eccentric contraction are included. The forearm in slow downward extension is an example. The fulcrum is at the elbow joint, and the effort may be considered to be applied at the center of gravity of the forearm and the resistance at the insertion of the elbow flexor, which for this example is considered to be the brachialis. The brachialis through eccentric contraction resists the downward-directed weight of the arm (figure 13.13). Another example is the slow lowering of the leg at the knee from an extended to a flexed position. The fulcrum is at the knee joint, the effort is the lower leg applied at its center of gravity, and the resistance is the eccentric contraction of the quadriceps at its point of insertion on the tibial tuberosity.

Figure 13.13 The forearm acting as a second-class lever, similar to pushing open a door.

Third-Class Levers

In a third-class lever, the effort lies between the axis and the resistance (see figure 13.10c). In this lever, *RA* is always the longer of the two moment arms. This means that it will take greater effort to overcome a given resistance. However, a very small motion by the effort will produce a large motion in the resistance. The advantage of the third-class lever is speed and range of motion at the expense of force.

There are not many examples of external third-class levers. One example is a screen door with a spring closing. There are, however, many examples of anatomical third-class levers, most body segments that are moved by muscular effort fall into this class. The forearm is a good example

of a third-class lever when it is being flexed by the biceps and the brachialis (figure 13.14). Another third-class lever is seen in the example cited earlier—namely, the arm as it is abducted by the deltoid muscle (figure 13.15).

The Principle of Levers

A lever of any class will balance when the product of the effort and the effort arm equals the product of the resistance and the resistance arm. This is known as the **principle of levers.** It enables us to calculate the amount of effort needed to balance a known resistance by means of a known lever or to calculate the point at which to place the fulcrum in order to balance a known re-

Figure 13.14   The forearm acting as a third-class lever, similar to a screen door.

sistance with a given effort. If any three of the four values are known, the remaining one can be calculated by using the following equation:

$$E \times EA = R \times RA$$

(effort times effort arm equals
resistance times resistance arm)

This equation restates a principle already studied under the summation of torques. When the force torques in one direction equal the force torques in the opposite direction, equilibrium exists. $E \times EA$ is a torque, as is $R \times RA$. When applied to figure 13.16, this means that it will be possible to balance the weight in the hand when the product of the weight and the perpendicular distance from its vector line of action to the ful-

crum ($R \times RA$) equals the product of the muscle effort and the perpendicular distance from its vector line of action to the fulcrum ($E \times EA$).

The lever equation also shows the importance of lever arm lengths in determining the amount of effort needed to balance a given resistance. If EA is lengthened while $R \times RA$ remains constant, the amount of effort needed to balance the lever must decrease. If, on the other hand, RA is increased, the amount of effort must increase. For this reason, second-class levers require less effort to balance or move heavier resistances, whereas third-class levers require more effort than the resistance they must balance or move (see figures 13.14 and 13.15). The first-class lever may have either a longer EA or RA, depending on the placement of the fulcrum (see figures 13.11 and 13.12).

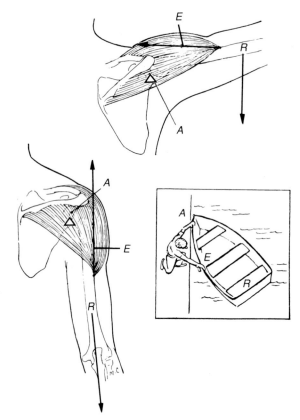

Figure 13.15   The humerus acting as a third-class lever, somewhat like a boat being pulled alongside the dock.

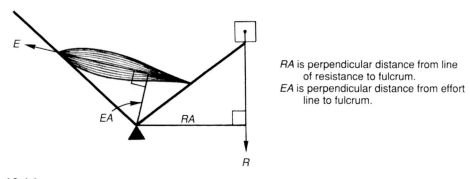

RA is perpendicular distance from line of resistance to fulcrum.
EA is perpendicular distance from effort line to fulcrum.

Figure 13.16   Lever arms, like moment arms, are the perpendicular distance between the fulcrum and the force line.

Figure 13.17   The range of motion increases as the lever arm length increases.

A lever whose effort arm is the longer of the two moment arms, whether it be a first- or second-class lever, is said to favor *force*. Less effort is required to overcome a resistance with this kind of lever than it would take to overcome the same resistance without the aid of the lever. This advantage is gained at the expense of speed and range of movement. The heavier resistance will always move through a smaller distance than the effort (figure 13.17). Conversely, a lever whose resistance arm is longer, whether it be a first- or third-class lever, is said to favor speed and distance. However, more effort is required to move it than would be the case if the relative lengths of the effort and resistance arms were reversed. Furthermore, an object of negligible weight can be moved a greater distance and more rapidly by this kind of lever than it could without the aid of the lever.

Relation of Speed to Range in Movements of Levers

The reader will have noticed that in the foregoing discussion of levers, the terms *speed* and *range* were usually linked together. There is a reason for this. In angular movements, speed and range are interdependent. For instance, if two third-class levers of different lengths each move through a 40-degree angle at the same angular velocity, the tip of the longer lever will be traveling a greater

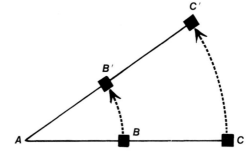

Figure 13.18   Comparison of a long and a short lever turning the same number of degrees. It takes *B* the same amount of time to reach *B'* that it takes *C* to reach *C'*.

distance or range than the tip of the shorter lever. Because it covers this distance in the same amount of time it takes the tip of the shorter lever to travel the shorter distance, the former must be moving faster than the latter. This is easily seen if the shorter lever is superimposed on the longer, as in figure 13.18. Here the shorter lever *AB* has been superimposed on the longer lever *AC*. The levers are moving from the horizontal position to the diagonal one. Because point *C* travels to its new position *C'* in the same time it takes *B* to travel to *B'*, point *C* must obviously be moving farther and faster than point *B*. This is the same relationship that was discussed in chapter 11. The linear kinematics at the end of a lever vary with the length of the radius. Thus, the greater the length of the lever, the greater the linear displacement, velocity, and acceleration that occur at the distal end point of the lever.

The effort arms in the skeletal lever systems of the human body are determined by the point of muscle attachment, usually close to the proximal end of the lever, and the muscle angle of pull. Because of these two factors, with few exceptions the effort arm in skeletal levers is shorter than the resistance arm. Thus, anatomical levers tend to favor speed and range of movement at the expense of effort. Examples of this preference are the throwing of a baseball or the kicking of a soccer ball. The hand in the one case and the foot in the other travel through a relatively long distance at considerable speed. Both movements require strong muscular action, even though the balls are relatively light in weight. This type of leverage is the reverse of the kind usually seen in mechanical implements such as the crowbar and the automobile jack, both of which are used to move heavy weights a relatively short distance. Sports implements that may serve as levers in themselves or as artificial extensions of the human arm also favor speed and range of movement. Frequently the sport implement, arm, and a large part of the rest of the body act together as a system of levers. In hitting a baseball, for instance, the trunk forms one lever, the upper arms another, the forearms another, and the hands and bat still another. This use of multiple leverage builds up speed at the tip of the bat, because the greater this speed, the greater the force that can be imparted to the ball.

Selection of Levers

Skill in motor performance depends on the effective selection and use of levers, both internal and external. Long golf clubs are selected for distance, and shorter clubs for accuracy at close range. Heavy baseball bats are chosen by those with the strength to swing them, whereas children are often taught tennis with short-handled rackets. In most instances external levers are designed for

a specific purpose and are selected accordingly. The levers of the human body, on the other hand, are not designed for one action or purpose. Body parts or segments may be held in numerous positions for any given joint action and thus provide a great variety of lever arrangements. Consequently, skill depends on the right choice of joint axis, joint action, and moment arm length. In all three instances in figure 13.19, the ball in the hand is carried forward by virtue of the counterclockwise (as seen from above) rotation of the pelvis that takes place at the left hip joint. The pelvis carries the trunk with it, but no movement occurs in any joint other than the left hip. In all three positions the resistance moment arm for the action is the perpendicular distance between the hip axis and the line of action of the resistance (the weight of the ball). However, the resistance moment arm is a different length in each situation. It is smallest in (a) and largest in (c). Consequently, when the angular velocity is the same in each instance, the linear velocity of the ball is largest in (c) and smallest in (a) (see figure 13.19). Similarly, if flexion of the shoulder is the joint action, the position of the arm that will provide the greatest linear velocity to the object in the hand at the moment of release is one in which the elbow is extended and the arm is perpendicular to the desired direction of flight (figure 13.20).

It is not always desirable to choose the longest lever, however. The positioning of body parts to form short levers enhances the angular velocity of the levers while sacrificing linear speed and range of motion at the end of the lever. And although forming the longest possible lever can increase speed and range of motion at the end of the lever, the strength needed to maintain the desired angular velocity increases as the lever lengthens. This is why the tennis player may flex the elbow in the forehand drive or the batter may "choke up" when swinging a heavy bat. As the magnitude of the resistance to be moved increases, the more the performer may want to shorten the lever. Moving very large weights produces very high levels of external torque. This

a.   b.   c.

Figure 13.19   The length of the *RA* determines the linear velocity at the end of the lever. In the positions pictured, when the pelvis rotates to the left, the linear velocity of the ball is least in (a) and most in (c). The movement occurs at the left hip and results in the lower extremity being medially rotated, relative to the pelvis.

torque can be reduced by decreasing the *RA*. One should not attempt to move heavy loads by using a long lever and high movement speeds.

Mechanical Advantage of Levers

Machines are judged good if they are efficient, poor if they are inefficient. How is the efficiency of a machine measured? Because the machines used in industry and in the workshop are usually for the purpose of magnifying force, it is customary to measure their efficiency in terms of their *mechanical advantage*—in other words, their ability to magnify force. Another way to express this ability is to state the "output" of the machine relative to its "input." In levers this is the ratio between the effort applied to the lever and the resistance overcome by the lever. It may be expressed in terms of the following equation: Mechanical advantage equals the ratio of the resistance overcome to the effort applied, or, simply,

$$MA = \frac{R}{E}$$

Because the balanced lever equation may also be expressed as

$$\frac{R}{E} = \frac{EA}{RA}$$

the mechanical advantage may be expressed in terms of the ratio of the effort arm to the resistance arm. Hence, if

$$MA = \frac{R}{E}$$

Figure 13.20   A straight arm perpendicular to the desired line of flight provides the greatest linear velocity to the ball when the joint action is shoulder flexion.

it also holds that

$$MA = \frac{EA}{RA}$$

When a muscle is said to have poor leverage, it means that it has poor mechanical advantage. In other words, the effort arm of the lever on which it is acting is short compared with the resistance arm.

Identification and Analysis of Levers

Figures 13.11 to 13.15 depict certain anatomical levers and their mechanical counterparts. These should enable the student to understand the principle of leverage as it applies in the human body and to see how the anatomical levers compare with the levers of everyday life. For each of these levers and for every lever that the student observes, these questions should be answered: (1) What are the locations of the fulcrum, effort point, and resistance point? (2) At what angle is the effort applied to the lever? (3) At what angle is the resistance applied to the lever? (4) What is the effort arm of the lever? (5) What is the resistance arm of the lever? (6) What are the relative lengths of the effort and resistance arms? (7) What kind of movement does this lever favor? (8) What is the mechanical advantage? (9) What class of lever is this?

NEWTON'S LAWS AND ROTATIONAL EQUIVALENTS

When applied to rotary motion, Newton's laws of motion may be stated as follows:

1. A body continues in a state of rest or uniform rotation about its axis unless acted upon by an external torque.
2. The acceleration of a rotating body is directly proportional to the torque causing it, is in the same direction as the torque, and is inversely proportional to the moment of inertia of the body.
3. When a torque is applied by one body to another, the second body will exert an equal and opposite torque on the first.

The laws themselves are analogous to those stated for linear motion. To comprehend their application to rotary motion, however, an understanding of the rotary equivalents of linear mass,

TABLE 13.1	Analogous Quantities in Linear and Rotary Motion	
Unit	**Linear Motion**	**Rotary Motion**
Distance	s	θ (theta)
Velocity	v	ω (omega)
Acceleration	a	α (alpha)
Mass	m	I (moment of inertia)
Force	F	T (torque)
Force equation	$F = ma$	$T = I\alpha$
Momentum	mv	$I\omega$
Impulse	Ft	Tt
Work	Fs	$T\theta$
Power	Fv	$T\omega$
Kinetic energy	$\frac{1}{2}mv^2$	$\frac{1}{2}I\omega^2$

momentum, and force is necessary. These parallel relationships between linear motion and rotary motion quantities become quite apparent when presented side by side, as in table 13.1.

Moment of Inertia

In the preceding discussion of Newton's laws, the quality of a body to resist change in its state of motion was identified as inertia. The inertia of a body with respect to linear motion was shown to be directly proportional to the mass of the object. The heavier an object is, the greater the force that is required to start it moving and to stop it. This is also true in rotary motion. Once they are set in motion, spinning bodies tend to keep spinning. As with linear motion, the amount of force needed to start or stop a spinning object is related to its mass: the heavier the object, the greater the effort that is required to start or stop its rotation. However, an additional factor needs to be considered. As an example, the hammer thrower knows that it takes more effort to start the weight moving in a circular fashion at the end of the wire than it does to start it moving in a linear fashion. It is also true that once the hammer is moving in a circular fashion, it is more difficult to slow it down than if it were moving in a straight line. Therefore, it seems that the hammer's inertia is greater when

moving in an angular pattern than when moving in a linear path. Because the mass of the hammer does not change, this increase in inertia must be due to some other element. In the same way that the torque causing rotary motion depends on the magnitude of force and the distance from the line of action of the force to the the axis, the inertia of a rotary body is affected by both the mass and the distance between the mass and the axis of rotation. A ball rotating on the end of a long string is harder to stop and start than one on a short string. As the distance between the axis and the mass increase, the inertia increases. Thus, the size of the angular inertia, called the *moment of inertia, I,* depends on both the quantity of the rotating mass and its distribution around the axis of rotation. The exact nature of this relationship is shown in the equation for the moment of inertia:

$$I = \Sigma mr^2$$

where m is the mass of a particle in the rotating body and r is the perpendicular distance between the mass particle and the axis of rotation. Thus the moment of inertia of an object is the sum of the mass of each of the particles multiplied by the square of the distance to the axis (figure 13.21). If the mass of an object is concentrated close to the axis of rotation, the object is easier to turn because the radius for each particle is less, thus

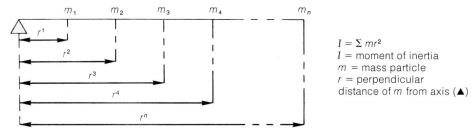

$$I = \Sigma \, mr^2$$
I = moment of inertia
m = mass particle
r = perpendicular
distance of m from axis (▲)

Figure 13.21   The moment of inertia about an axis is the sum of the mass particles multiplied by the square of the distance of each particle from the axis: $(I = \Sigma \, mr^2)$.

making I less. Conversely, if the mass is concentrated farther away from the axis, I becomes greater and the rotating body will require more force to start or stop it.

In the human body the mass distribution may be altered by changing the body position, thereby changing the moment of inertia. A runner is able to move the recovery leg forward more rapidly when it is in a flexed position than when it is extended. The mass of the leg is the same in both instances, but it is closer to the axis when the leg is flexed and the moment of inertia is less. Using data for average mass proportions of body segments and the location of the center of gravity of each segment, Dyson (1970) estimated that a person standing on a frictionless turntable with arms outstretched to the side has a moment of inertia 3 times greater than when the arms are crossed over the chest (figure 13.22). When a person lies horizontally on the table, with the arms at the sides and the vertical axis passing through the center of gravity, I becomes 14 times greater. The moment of inertia of the body is least about a vertical axis passing through the center of gravity when the arms are raised and held close to the head, and greatest when the body is in a fully extended position rotating about the hands, as in the giant swing on the high bar.

Using a method similar to finding the center of gravity of the body by the segmental method

(see chapter 14, pp. 388–393), Hay (1993) reported the moment of inertia of the human body in some common rotating positions. In the tuck position, I about the body's center of gravity was 3.5 kg·m²; in the pike position it was 6.5 kg·m² and in the layout, 15.0 kg·m². The moment of inertia about the hands of the giant swing position was 83.0 kg·m². These figures verify that inertia to rotation increases as the mass is distributed farther away from the axis.

When one is interested in the moment of inertia of a specific body segment, it is usually taken about the center of the joint serving as the axis, although other axes may be chosen. If another axis is selected, such as the center of gravity of the segment, I will change accordingly because values of r will be different in the equation $I = \Sigma mr^2$.

Acceleration of Rotating Bodies

The equation for Newton's second law of motion when applied to linear motion was shown to be $F = ma$. The rotational equivalent is $T = I\alpha$—that is, rotary force, or torque (T), is equal to the product of the moment of inertia (I) of the rotating object and the angular acceleration (α). The rotary equivalent of linear force is torque, the rotary equivalent of mass is the moment of inertia, and the rotary equivalent of linear acceleration is angular acceleration. With a little transposing of the

a.   b.

Figure 13.22   The moment of inertia about an axis decreases when the mass is concentrated close to the axis of rotation. The moment of inertia in (a) is greater than that in (b).

equation it becomes apparent how the rotary equivalent of Newton's second law of motion states that the change in rotary velocity (α) is directly proportional to the torque (T) and inversely proportional to the moment of inertia (I)—that is, $\alpha = T/I$.

Angular Momentum

Momentum is a measure of the force needed to start or stop motion. Objects undergoing angular motion have momentum in the same fashion as objects engaged in linear motion. Linear momentum is the product of mass and velocity. Angular momentum is the product of the angular equivalents of mass and velocity—that is, the moment of inertia I and angular velocity ω.

$$\text{Linear momentum} = mv$$
$$\text{Angular momentum} = I\omega$$

The momentum of a skater skating in a straight line is mv. The momentum of the skater spinning is $I\omega$.

Angular momentum can be increased or decreased by increasing or decreasing either the angular velocity or the moment of inertia. A heavy bat swung with the same velocity as a light bat has greater angular momentum. However, increasing the velocity of the lighter bat could produce an angular momentum equal to or greater than that of the heavier bat. Similarly, the angular momentum of a kicking leg can be increased by increasing its angular velocity. Conversely, it will decrease if the leg is flexed at the knee (thus decreasing this moment of inertia) while keeping the velocity constant.

Conservation of Angular Momentum

Newton's first law as applied to rotary motion can also be stated in terms related to momentum. Worded thus, it states that the total angular momentum of a rotating body will remain constant unless acted upon by external torques. This is why the law is also known as the *law of conservation of angular momentum.* Like linear momentum, angular momentum is conserved. Once a spinning body is in motion, its angular momentum will not change, provided, of course, that no outside forces are introduced. Divers, trampolinists, dancers, and any other rotating performers all make use of the conservation of angular momentum to control the speed of bodily spin. A skater starts to spin with the arms outstretched. After spinning slowly in this position, the skater brings the arms in close to the body and immediately begins to spin rapidly. The increase in angular velocity occurs with no effort on the skater's part. By bringing the arms in closer to the axis of rotation, the moment of inertia is decreased about that axis. Because the angular momentum must remain constant, a decrease in *I* produces an in-

crease in *w*. Increasing *I* by stretching the arms and perhaps a leg out to the side will again slow down the skater. A diver performing a tuck somersault can control the speed of rotation by changing the tightness of the tuck, thus changing the moment of inertia. If the diver thinks the entry into the water will be spoiled because of too rapid a rotation, the *I* can be increased and the angular velocity decreased proportionately by "opening up" or loosening the tuck (figure 13.23).

Action and Reaction

As previously explained, the force for angular motion is torque. For every torque exerted by one body on a second body, there is another torque equal in magnitude and opposite in direction exerted by the second body on the first. This is Newton's third law of motion as applied to angular movement. A force that causes a change in angular momentum must have an equal and opposite force creating an equal and opposite momentum change. In other words, angular momentum is conserved. When one jumps straight up from a trampoline bed with arms stretched upward and then swings the legs forward and up, the body will jackknife at the hips. The torque acting on

Figure 13.23   Lengthening the radius of rotation increases the moment of inertia and decreases the angular velocity. The angular momentrum of the rotating diver is conserved. (Drawn from motion picture film tracing).

the legs results in an equal and opposite torque acting on the rest of the body. A change in angular velocity is observed in both body segments, although that in the trunk segment is less because I is greater. Another jump upward followed by a sharp flexion of the wrists only will also produce an equal and opposite torque on the rest of the body. However, in this case the change in angular velocity of the arms and trunk resulting in forward-upward motion will be barely visible. I for the arms and trunk is so large compared with I for the hands that the opposite rotation will be very slight. The angular velocity of the two moving parts is inversely proportional to their moments of inertia about the axis of motion (the wrist joint in the example just given). Axes for such actions may be in any plane, but the reactions must be in the same or parallel planes. The arms swinging hori-

Figure 13.24   Angular action and reaction. As the arms swing across the body in one direction, an equal and opposite reaction occurs in the rest of the body.

zontally across in front of the trunk will produce an opposite action of the rest of the body in the transverse plane (figure 13.24). Movement of one arm downward in the frontal plane produces an equal and opposite action of the rest of the body in the frontal plane. This is the movement that may be used to regain balance on a beam or tightrope. If one falls to the left, a downward movement of the left arm produces a reaction of the rest of the body to the right and hopefully prevents a fall.

The equation describing this action–reaction relationship may be written as

$$I\,(\omega_{v1} - \omega_{u1}) = I\,(\omega_{v2} - \omega_{u2})$$

Any changes in the moments of inertia of the two bodies (I_1 and I_2) or of their respective velocities (ω_1 and ω_2) will produce equal and opposite momentum changes so that $I_1\,(\omega_{v1} - \omega_{u1})$ and $I_2\,(\omega_{v2} - \omega_{u2})$ continue to be equal and opposite.

Sometimes action and reaction in specific body parts is not desired and should be controlled. This can be done by substitution or absorption of the undesired action. In walking and running, the rotation of the pelvis and legs about a vertical axis produces an undesired reaction of the upper trunk in the opposite direction if it is not compensated in some fashion. To prevent this, the arms move in opposition to the legs to "absorb" the reaction by producing a countertwist that cancels out the reaction of the body to the leg action. The faster one moves or the more massive the legs, the more vigorous must be the arm action. The arms are used in the same fashion to prevent undesired trunk reaction to leg action in hurdling, diving, and jumping.

Transfer of Momentum

Because of the law of conservation of momentum, angular momentum may be transferred from one body or body part to another as the total angular momentum remains unaltered. In the suspended balls shown in figure 13.25, the sudden checking of motion in ball A produces a comparable action in ball E. Similarly, checking the

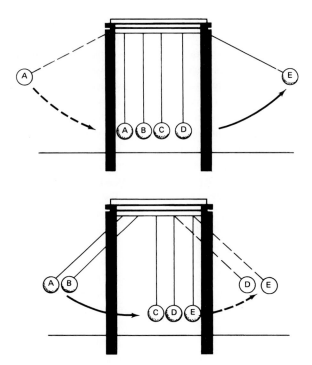

Figure 13.25   Example of conservation of angular momentum resulting in transfer of angular momentum from one body to another.

simultaneous motion in *A* and *B* produces equal momentum in *D* and *E*. Examples of transfer of angular momentum in movement patterns are numerous. As a back diver leaves the board, the arms are swung upward until the motion is checked by the limitation of range of motion in the shoulder joint. The checked momentum transfers to the body and increases its angular momentum, thus helping turn the body in the air. In the racing dive, the angular momentum of the diver's arms is also transferred to the body as the diver stops the upward movement of the arms in the forward reach, and in a jump twist the dancer transfers twisting momentum from the upper arms and trunk to the legs as the feet leave the ground. In each of these instances the body is in contact with the ground while the momentum is developing. Otherwise, an equal and opposite reaction, rather than a transfer, would occur. The

effect that the transfer of angular momentum has on unsupported bodies is discussed in chapter 21.

A very common example of the transfer of angular momentum is the series of sequential segmental rotation that occurs in throwing, kicking, and striking actions. In an efficient performer, a throwing motion involves a series of rotations of progressively smaller body segments. The initial angular momentum generated by the application of torque to the fairly massive leg and trunk segments is transferred to the much lighter upper arm. The decrease in moment of inertia between the trunk and the arm produces an increase in the angular velocity of the upper arm. By the time this angular momentum has been transferred to the hand, angular velocity will be at a maximum.

Angular momentum also can be transferred or converted into linear momentum, or the reverse can occur. The angular momentum of the hammer becomes linear momentum when it is released. Conversely, a ball that hits the ground with no spin but rebounds spinning has had some of its linear momentum converted to angular momentum. Similarly, a long jumper's linear momentum most often is partially converted to angular momentum at the takeoff. Those who advanced the somersault technique for long jumping thought that as long as the angular momentum existed, it should be used to advantage. Unfortunately there were too many disadvantages, and the style is no longer legal. The hitch kick technique that most good jumpers currently use provides the necessary "opposite" reaction to minimize the undesired forward rotation "action" of the trunk while putting the feet in an optimum landing position.

CENTRIPETAL AND CENTRIFUGAL FORCES

A weight whirling around on the end of a string is engaged in linear motion of the circular type (see p. 280), while the string itself is undergoing rotary motion about an axis. If one lets go of the string, both the string and weight fly off and experience linear motion. This is expected because, according to Newton's first law, a moving body left alone travels uniformly in a straight line. To make that body leave the straight path requires application of an additional force. In the case of the weight on the string, the force has to be applied in a manner that will cause the weight to change direction and move in a circular path about the axis. This force is called *centripetal force*. It is a constant center-seeking force that acts to move an object tangent (at right angles) to the direction in which it is moving at any instant, thus causing it to move in a circular path.

The centripetal force acting on the weight is an external force that is applied by the finger through the string to the weight. The finger, in turn, must have a force pulling on it because, according to Newton's third law, if one body exerts a force on the second body, that body will recip-

rocate with an equal and opposite force on the first body. This outward-pulling force is called *centrifugal* (center-fleeing) *force* and is felt in the tension exerted on the finger by the string attached to the circling object. Centrifugal force is equal in magnitude to centripetal force. If centripetal force ceases, there is no longer an inward pull on the object and the latter then flies off at a tangent to the direction in which it was moving at the instant the force stopped. Without centripetal force, there will be no centrifugal reaction, and the object will once more travel uniformly in a straight line.

Even though the speed of a whirling object is constant, its direction changes continually—that is, there is a constant change in velocity. This, in effect, is the same as saying that the weight is uniformly accelerating because, by definition, acceleration is the rate of change of velocity. The amount of acceleration that a whirling object possesses increases with the speed with which it is orbiting and decreases with the distance from the axis to the object. This relationship is represented in equation form as $a = v^2/r$. The substitution of this value for acceleration in the equation obtained from Newton's second law of motion, $F = ma$, results in the equation for centripetal force:

$$F_c = mv^2/r$$

The equation for centrifugal force is the same, because it is equal in magnitude and opposite in direction to centripetal force.

From the equation it can be seen that the amount of centripetal force necessary to keep an object moving in a circular path is proportional to its mass and the square of its velocity and inversely proportional to its radius. Doubling the mass doubles the centripetal force, whereas doubling the radius decreases it by half. Changes in velocity have an even greater impact and are more dramatic. Doubling the velocity along the curve increases the centripetal force fourfold, and decreasing the velocity by one-half decreases to one-fourth the force needed to keep the object in orbit.

Figure 13.26 A runner must lean in when going around a corner to balance an outward-pulling torque (F_cy). The outward-pulling torque (F_cy) will topple the runner unless it is counterbalanced by an opposite torque (Wx) so that $F_cy = Wx$.

When runners or bicyclists negotiate corners with any appreciable speed, they lean into the curve. If they did not, they would tend to topple outward. In the same manner that centripetal force was exerted by the finger on the weight at the end of the string, the ground exerts centripetal force on the body of the runner through the feet and on the body of the cyclist through the bicycle wheel.

Centrifugal force, acting equal and opposite, tends to pull the body outward, back into a linear path. This centrifugal force produces a torque on the body in an outward direction, with the foot or the bicycle wheel acting as the axis. To maintain equilibrium against this torque, the runner or the bicyclist must lean inward, using the body weight to produce an equal and opposite inward torque.

In figure 13.26a, this outward-rotating torque F_cy is shown as the product of the centripetal–centrifugal force and the distance between the center of gravity of the runner and the axis of rotation about the foot. When one leans in, an opposite re-acting torque is created, also about the feet, and is equal to the product of the weight and the perpendicular distance from the direction of weight to the axis. In figure 13.26b, the torque that is due to the lean (Wx) balances the opposite acting torque that is due to centripetal force, so $F_cy = Wx$. This relationship demonstrates that as F_c increases, the amount of lean will also have to increase. As this occurs, x increases, y decreases, and W, of course, remains the same. It also shows that the lower the center of gravity of a body negotiating a curve, the

Figure 13.27 Centripetal–centrifugal forces operating in weight event.
Photograph courtesy of Northeastern University.

smaller will be the outward-rotating force because the moment arm *y* will be less.

Where speeds are too great or radii too small for participants to negotiate curves successfully, the track may be banked. The amount of banking is determined for the particular radius and the average expected velocity so that the performer may remain perpendicular to the surface while rounding the curve. As might be expected, the greater the anticipated velocity for negotiating the curve, or the smaller the radius of the turn, the more the track must be banked.

Centripetal–centrifugal forces are evident in many instances in which the body imparts force to an external object. Overarm, sidearm, or underarm throwing patterns all involve the application of force to the object to be thrown in order to keep it moving in a circular path for all or part of the time before it is released. As soon as the object is released, its inertia causes it to move in a straight line. In the hammer throw (figure 13.27), the thrower transmits force to the head of the hammer along the flexible wire. This is centripetal force directed inward toward the axis of rotation. As the performer increases the speed of rotation, the velocity of the hammer increases, and the increased centripetal force the thrower must exert is proportional to the square of the velocity. The outward-pulling centrifugal force increases accordingly on the thrower, who must adjust by leaning back or be pulled off balance. A hammer thrower needs considerable strength to resist centrifugal force. This is also true with discus throwers who generate considerable centripetal force during the turn prior to delivery, or baseball pitchers whose elbows are subject to great forces because of the tremendous speed with which the forearm is whipped forward in the pitch. Another instance in which centripetal force is an important factor is in all swinging activities in gymnastics.

THE ANALYSIS OF ROTARY MOTION

As most motions of the human body involve rotation of a segment about a joint, any mechanical analysis of movement requires an analysis of the nature of the rotary forces, or torques, involved. In examining and evaluating performance of any movement skill, both internal and external torques must be considered. Internal torques will be generated by applied muscle forces as identified in the anatomical portion of the skill analysis. External torques now must be identified as they are produced by the external forces identified in the analysis of linear motion.

The principles that govern rotary motion are based primarily on the production of torque and the results of torque production. Some general principles of rotary motion might be stated as follows:

Torque The torque about any point equals the product of the force magnitude and its perpendicular distance from the line of action. The force rotating the body segments depends on the related joint torques, which are governed by the muscle forces and the locations of their attachments.

Summation of Torques   The resultant torque of a force system equals the sum of the individual torques. Therefore, if a maximum resultant is desired, all body segments that have the capability must contribute to their maximum. Torques may be summed either simultaneously or sequentially.

Conservation of Angular Momentum   In the absence of any outside torque, an object undergoing rotary motion will continue to rotate. Because angular momentum is conserved, alterations in the moment of inertia will produce changes in the angular velocity and vice versa. In other words, a decrease in the moment of inertia will produce an increase in angular velocity, with the opposite also being true.

Principle of Levers   Any lever will balance when the torque of the effort equals the torque produced by the resistance. The amount of effort required may be calculated using this principle if the resistance torque and the length of the effort arm are known.

Transfer of Angular Momentum   Angular momentum may be transferred from one body part to another when total angular momentum remains unchanged. In many motions, this transfer of momentum moves from more massive segments to less massive segments. When this occurs, the velocity of rotation increases with each transfer based on the conservation of angular momentum.

In the continuing example of the long jump, for instance, the force applied to generate the propulsive impulse will be the result of the joint torques generated. To be most effective, these joint torques must be summed, meaning that each body segment that has the capability must contribute to its maximum. Maximum thrust of the body in the jump depends on maximum resultant torques developed at the individual joints.

LABORATORY EXPERIENCES

1. Define the following key terms and give an example of each that is not used in the text.

   Torque
   Moment arm
   Lever
   Mechanical advantage

   Moment of inertia
   Angular momentum
   Centripetal force
   Centrifugal force

2. For each of the following anatomical levers, estimate the approximate length of the effort arm, that is, the perpendicular distance. Refer to anatomical illustrations or to a muscle mannequin to help you estimate the angle of pull of the muscles. Unless otherwise stated, assume that the segments are in their normal resting position. (*Hint:* Use the mechanical axis of the segment for the lever.)

   a. The forearm lever with the biceps providing the effort.

   b. The upper arm lever with the middle deltoid providing the effort.

   c. The upper arm lever in the side-horizontal position with the entire pectoralis major providing the effort. (*Hint:* Which view would show you the angle of pull for this movement, facing the subject or looking down from above?)

   d. Same lever as in c, with the anterior deltoid providing the effort.

3. Referring to the diagrams in figure 13.5, assume that a weight is suspended from the wrist. Find the resistance arm of the forearm lever in positions b, d, and e. Consider that the scale for these diagrams is 2 cm = 25 cm.

4. Assume that a muscle having a force of 300 N is pulling at an angle of 75 degrees. Find the components of the force (a) by the trigonometric method and (b) by the graphic method.

5. Assuming that the weight used in Laboratory Experience 3 is 8 kg, determine the rotary and nonrotary components of the weight (a) by the

trigonometric method and (b) by the graphic method.

6. Referring to figure 7.21, make a tracing of the femur and the adductor longus muscle. Draw a straight line to represent the mechanical axis of the femur and another to represent the muscle's line of pull (connecting the midpoints of the proximal and distal attachments).

   a. Using a protractor, measure the angle of pull (i.e., the angle facing the hip joint) formed by the intersection of the muscle's line of pull with the bone's mechanical axis.

   b. Measure the effort moment arm of the lever [i.e., the perpendicular distance from the fulcrum (center of hip joint) to the muscle's line of pull]. To convert this to a realistic figure use the scale 1 cm = 0.25 m.

   c. Assuming the muscle's total force to be 900 N, calculate the moment of force (i.e., the torque) of the lever.

   d. Calculate the rotary and the stabilizing components of force.

7. Place a pole across the back of a chair, hang a pail or basket containing a 3-kg weight on one end, and hold the other end of the pole. Now adjust the pole so that it becomes increasingly difficult to balance the weight of the pail with one hand. Stop when you reach the point where you are barely able to lift the pail by pushing down on the opposite end of the pole. Have an assistant measure the effort arm and the resistance arm of the lever. Without shifting the position of your hand, draw the pole toward you until you can easily lift the pail by pushing down on the opposite end of the pole with one finger. Again, have an assistant measure the effort and resistance arms of the lever. What do you conclude concerning the relative length of the two arms? In which case does the pail move through the greater distance? What do you conclude about the relationship between the effort required to move an object by leverage and the distance that the object is moved?

8. Balance a pole across the back of a chair, hanging a 3-kg weight at each end. Let one of these represent the effort and the other the resistance. The effort arm and the resistance arm should be exactly equal if the pole is symmetrical. Now add 3 more kilograms at another point on the resistance

end and adjust the pole until it balances. Measure the effort and resistance moment arms. What do you conclude about:

   a. The relationship between the resistance and the resistance arm? between the effort and the effort arm?

   b. The relationship between the resistance and the resistance arm, given a changing resistance and a constant effort?

9. Compute the amount of effort necessary to lift a resistance of 20 N with a 2-meter, first-class lever whose fulcrum is located 0.5 meters from the point at which the weight is attached and 1.5 meters from the point at which the effort is applied. Assume that both the effort and the resistance are applied at right angles to the lever.

10. Where would the fulcrum have to be located in the above-mentioned 2-meter, first-class lever if only 5 N of effort were available to balance the 20-N weight? Determine this by experiment. Check your answer by the algebraic method.

11. For each of the anatomical levers listed, identify the class of lever represented; identify the fulcrum, effort point, and resistance point; and name the kind of movement favored by this type of lever.

   a. Leg being flexed at knee by hamstrings

   b. Leg being extended at knee by quadriceps femoris

   c. Pelvis being tilted to right by left quadriceps lumborum

   d. Clavicle being elevated by trapezius I

   e. Lower extremity being abducted by gluteus medius

   f. From supine lying position, lower extremities being raised by hip flexors

   g. From supine lying position, trunk being raised by hip flexors

12. Perform the following paired movements, noting the difference in the effort needed. Diagram and explain the reasons for the difference.

   a. A push-up from the toes and a push-up from the knees

   b. A sit-up with hands on the thighs and a sit-up with a 3-kg weight held behind the head

   c. A 3-kg weight held in the hand with the arm outstretched horizontally sideward and a 3-kg weight suspended from the elbow crotch when the arm is outstretched sideward

13. Explain the difference in effort needed to hold the body levers in Laboratory Experience 12a, b, c, at

a 10-degree angle with the horizontal compared with holding them at a 30-degree angle and a 45-degree angle.

14. What muscular effort *E*, pulling at an angle of 80 degrees, would be required to keep the lower leg in a position of 10 degrees with the horizontal? The muscle inserts 8 cm from the knee joint. The lower leg and foot weigh 35 N and the center of gravity is located 18 cm from the knee joint. A 50-N weight is hung from the ankle 33 cm from the knee joint.

15. A gymnast weighing 56 kg attempts a handstand on the balance beam. Her center of gravity is 1 meter above the beam. What is the moment of force tending to pull her over if her center of gravity moves 3 cm ahead of the center of her support? 15 cm ahead?

16. Perform a vertical jump with and without the use of your arms. Have someone compare the height of the two jumps by noting the level of the top of your head. A chart with numbered horizontal lines on the wall behind you will help in scoring. The observer's eyes should be at the level of the top of your head at the peak of the jump. Repeat several times and compare your results with those of others doing the same experiment. Explain the results.

17. Stand on a frictionless turntable or sit on a swivel stool. Hold a 3-kg weight in each hand and hold the arms out to the side. Have a partner spin you around. Alternately bring your hands into your shoulders and move them out to the side. Explain the changes in your angular velocity.

18. Stand on a frictionless turntable or sit on a swivel stool. Determine how you can rotate yourself moving just your arms. Explain why your arm motions make the rotation possible.

19. Firmly tape equal-length chains of small rubber bands to a golf ball and a table tennis ball.
   a. Holding the end of the elastic, swing the golf ball around in a circle. Repeat with the lighter ball, swinging it at the same speed as the heavier ball.
   b. Swing the table tennis ball at different speeds.
   c. Swing the table tennis ball with one-half the radius length; one-fourth the radius length. What does this experiment tell about the relationship of mass, velocity, and radius to centripetal force? How can you tell whether the centripetal force is increasing or decreasing?

20. In each of the following movement patterns identify the nature of the motion for each phase. State the underlying mechanical objectives and describe what must occur to achieve optimum results. Consider carefully the application of rotary mechanical principles.

   Fencing lunge
   Bowling delivery
   Shot put
   Tennis lob

REFERENCES AND SELECTED READINGS

Adrian, M. J., and J. M. Cooper. 1994. *The biomechanics of human movement.* 2nd ed. Indianapolis: Benchmark Press.

Dyson, G. 1970. *The mechanics of athletics.* 5th ed. London: University of London Press.

Gowitzke, B. A., and M. Milner. 1988. *Scientific bases of human movement.* 3rd ed. Baltimore: Williams & Wilkins.

Hamill, J., and K. M. Knutzen. 1995. *Biomechanical basis of human movement.* Baltimore: Wiiliams & Wilkins.

Hay, J. G. 1993. *The biomechanics of sports techniques.* 4th ed. Englewood Cliffs, NJ: Prentice Hall.

Kreighbaum, E., and K. M. Barthels. 1996. *Biomechanics.* 4th ed. New York: Macmillan.

Schrier, E. W., and W. F. Allman. 1987. *Newton at the bat.* New York: Scribner's.

Tözeren, A. 2000. *Human body dynamics: Classical mechanics and human movement.* New York: Springer.

Walker, J. 1985. *Roundabout.* New York: Freeman.

Winter, D. A. 1990. *Biomechanics of human movement.* 2nd ed. New York: Wiley.

The Center of Gravity and Stability

OUTLINE

- **Center of Gravity**
  Definition of Center of Gravity
  Placement of Center of Gravity
    in Humans
- **Stability and Equilibrium**
  Factors Affecting Stability
  Principles of Stability
  Mobility
- **Finding the Center of Gravity**
  in the Human Body
  Reaction Board Method
  Segmental Method
- **Laboratory Experiences**

OBJECTIVES

At the conclusion of this chapter, the student should be able to:

1. Define the term center of gravity, and explain the basis for its location in the human body.
2. Estimate the location of the center of gravity of individuals in any position.
3. State the principles of equilibrium, and explain and demonstrate applications of each.
4. Locate the center of gravity of an individual using either the reaction board or the segmental method.

CENTER OF GRAVITY

Definition of Center of Gravity

The **center of gravity** of a body is sometimes described as its balance point or that point about which a body would balance without a tendency to rotate. For this reason, the center of gravity is often identified as the point where all the weight of the body or object is concentrated. More accurately, it is the point where the weight of the body may be said to act.

The ability to locate the center of gravity of a body is based on the knowledge of what it takes for a system to be balanced, or in equilibrium. Two conditions must be met:

1. All the linear forces acting on the body must be balanced.
2. All the rotary forces (torques) must be balanced.

Another way of expressing these necessary conditions for equilibrium is to say that the sum of all the forces acting on the body must equal zero. If there is a downward-directed linear force, there must be an equal upward force so that the vector sum of these forces equals zero. If there is a negative clockwise torque, it must be canceled out by a positive counterclockwise torque of equal magnitude (figure 14.1).

A simple experiment to locate the center of gravity, or balance point, consists of suspending an irregularly shaped object by a string and letting it hang until it ceases to move (figure 14.2). A vertical line is then drawn on the object from the point of suspension in a line that is a continuation of the string. The object is then suspended from another point, and the vertical string continuation line is drawn again. This procedure is repeated one more time. The point at which the three drawn lines intersect is the center of gravity. If the object is suspended from this point, it will hang in whatever position it is placed, because the weight of the object is equally distributed about this point and no unbalanced forces (torques) exist.

The location of the center of gravity of any object remains fixed as long as the body does not

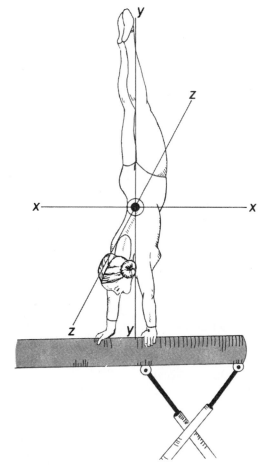

Figure 14.1 The center of gravity of a body is the point where all forces acting on the body equal zero. In this illustration it is represented as the intersection of the x, y, and z axes. It may be located by application of the principle of torques.

change shape. In rigid bodies of homogeneous mass, the center of gravity is at the geometric center. Where the density of a rigid body varies, the center of gravity is not at the geometric center but is shifted toward the more weighted section. If an object's shape or position changes, the location of the center of gravity will also change. This happens in the human body (figure 14.3). It is a

Figure 14.2   Location of the center of gravity in an irregularly shaped object.

Figure 14.3   A shift in segment configuration results in a relocation of the body's center of gravity.
(Drawn from motion picture film tracing.)

segmented structure, capable of numerous positions, and the location of its center of gravity changes accordingly. This is an important consideration in the execution of sports skills. The evolution of the technique for the high jump shows how the change of placement of the center of gravity in the body increased the height of the bar over which the jumper could project himself (figure 14.4). As one changes the relationship of the body segments to each other, the center of gravity may even be located completely outside the body itself.

Placement of Center of Gravity in Humans

The location of the center of gravity of a human being in the normal standing position varies with body build, age, and sex. It is generally accepted that in the transverse plane the center of gravity in females is located at approximately 55 percent of the standing height, whereas in males the center of gravity is at approximately 57 percent of standing height. The center of gravity will be higher in infants, whose head size is still quite large in relation

Figure 14.4   Effect of shift in center of gravity on high jump performance.

(a–j) From G. H. G. Dyson, *The Mechanics of Athletics*. Copyright © 1970 University of London Press, London. Reproduced by permission of Hodder & Stoughton, Ltd./New English Library, Ltd.

to the rest of the body. As the infant body grows and changes, the center of gravity descends to the adult position, a point level with the first sacral segment, which is approximately behind the naval and about 6 inches above the crotch.

In quiet standing, the center of gravity of the body can be considered to be held almost directly over the *center of pressure*. The center of pressure is that point at which the force vector for ground reaction force can be said to be applied. During normal standing, there will be some motion in the head region, which will in turn produce a pendulumlike motion in the center of gravity. As the center of gravity shifts slightly, the center of pressure will also shift slightly in the foot–ground interface. This slight motion is referred to as postural sway. Postural sway is normally measured in both the sagittal plane (anteroposterior or AP sway) and the frontal plane (mediolateral or ML sway). AP sway has been

found to average 5 to 7 mm, while ML sway averages 3 to 4 mm (Lundin, Feuerbach, and Grabiner 1993; Davis and Grabiner 1996).

Postural sway magnitude and velocity can be affected by a number of factors. Age, fatigue, injury, bracing, obesity, and the stability of the external environment have all been found to influence postural sway. Increased postural sway has been found to be related to falling in the elderly and in some pathological conditions. The presence of excessive postural sway should be viewed as an indication that there may be problems with stability.

STABILITY AND EQUILIBRIUM

All objects at rest are in equilibrium. All the forces acting on them are balanced; the sum of all linear forces equals zero and the sum of all

a. Stable   b. Unstable   c. Neutral

Figure 14.5   Types of equilibrium.

torques equals zero. However, all objects at rest are not equally stable. If the position of an object is slightly altered and the object tends to return to its original position, the object is in stable equilibrium. *Stable equilibrium* occurs when an object is placed in such a fashion that an effort to disturb it would require its center of gravity to be raised. Thus it would tend to fall back into place (figure 14.5a). The more its center of gravity has to be raised to upend it, the more stable it is. A brick on its side is more stable than one on end because its center of gravity needs to be raised higher to upend it. The wrestler and defensive lineman both know the value of shifting body position to increase stability by lowering the center of gravity. In fact, if for any reason the equilibrium is too precarious, assuming a crouching, kneeling, or sitting position will lower the center of gravity and increase stability.

Unstable equilibrium exists when it takes only a slight push to destroy it. This is the situation when the center of gravity of the object drops to a lower point when the object is tilted (figure 14.5b). A pencil on end or a tightrope walker displays unstable equilibrium because the center of gravity is bound to be lowered if either loses its balance. Swimmers standing on the starting block poised for the start of a race or sprint runners at the start of their race are in unstable equilibrium, as are toe dancers on point or balance beam performers. In each instance the center of gravity will be lowered if the individual is disturbed so that rotation occurs around the point of support.

The third classification of equilibrium is called *neutral equilibrium* and exists when an object's center of gravity is neither raised nor low-

ered when it is disturbed (figure 14.5c). A ball lying on a table is in neutral equilibrium. Objects in neutral equilibrium will come to rest in any position without a change in level of the center of gravity. Upon receiving a slight push, such objects fall neither backward nor forward.

Because people ordinarily hold themselves in an upright position and because the effect of gravity is always in operation on this earth, the problems of stability are ever present. Probably the only time the human body is not adjusting itself in response to gravitational force is when it is in a position of complete repose. Either consciously or unconsciously, human beings spend most of their waking hours adjusting their positions to the type of equilibrium best suited to the task.

Factors Affecting Stability

The ability to maintain one's balance under unfavorable circumstances is recognized as one of the basic motor skills. Standing on tiptoe or on one foot without losing one's balance or maintaining a headstand or a handstand for an appreciable length of time is such a skill. These particular feats are examples of static balance, and the mark of skill is to accomplish them with a minimum of motion. Familiarity with the following factors affecting the stability of a performer's equilibrium state should make analysis of the balance problem easier and may suggest means for improvement of the skill with which the technique is executed.

The three most critical factors affecting stability are the size of the base of support, the relation of the line of gravity to the base of support, and the height of the center of gravity. Other factors such as mass of the body, friction, segmental alignment, visual and psychological factors, and physiological factors may also play a role in stability.

Size and Shape of the Base of Support

The size of the base of support is a primary factor in the stability of an object. Much of the difficulty experienced in balancing on one leg on a balance beam, a tightrope, or another small surface is due to the narrow base of support. The problem is to keep the center of gravity over the base of support, a requisite for maintaining equilibrium. The wider the base, the easier this is.

The base of support includes the part of a body in contact with the supporting surface and the intervening area (figure 14.6). In a person whose weight is supported entirely by the feet, the base of support includes the two feet and the space between. If the feet are separated, the base is widened and the equilibrium improved. The person supported by crutches in figure 14.7 has a base of support that encompasses the area bounded by the feet and crutches. He will be more stable if he places the crutches forward, making a triangular base instead of a linear one. There is another factor, however, that must not be overlooked. If one takes a stride position that is wider than the breadth of the pelvis, the legs will assume a slanting position. This introduces a horizontal component of force that, if accompanied by insufficient friction between the feet and the supporting surface, as when standing on ice, obviously does not make for greater stability. In fact, the wider the stance, the less one can control the sliding of the feet. From this we see that we must observe *all* the principles that apply to a situation. Observance of only one may not bring the results expected.

In addition to the size of the base of support, the shape is also a factor in stability. To resist lateral external forces the base should be widened in the direction of the oncoming force. In figure 14.7c the position provides great stability for lateral

forces from the side but very little from the front or back. Where the forces are known to be coming from a forward-backward direction, as when catching a swift ball or spotting a performer in gymnastics, a forward-backward stance is recommended. A similar adjustment is made when one stands in a bus or a subway train. The tendency to be thrown backward when the vehicle starts up is resisted either by standing sideways with the feet in a moderately wide stance, or by facing forward and leaning forward with one foot placed forward. These automatic reactions to external forces are for one purpose only—namely, to enable one to keep the center of gravity over the base of support in spite of the disturbing lateral forces. When the direction of oncoming force cannot be predicted, a slight oblique stance is probably best.

Height of the Center of Gravity

Ordinarily, the center of gravity in an adult human being is located approximately at the level of the upper third of the sacrum, but *only* during the normal standing position. If the arms are raised or if a weight is carried above waist level, the center of gravity shifts to a higher position and it becomes more difficult to maintain one's equilibrium. Activities and stunts such as walking on stilts, canoeing, and balancing a weight on the head are difficult or dangerous because of the relatively high center of gravity. Lowering the center of gravity will increase the stability of the body because it allows greater angular displacement of the center of gravity within the bounds of the base of support (figure 14.8).

Relation of the Line of Gravity to the Base of Support

An object retains its equilibrium only so long as its line of gravity falls within its base of support. When the force that the body is resisting is the downward force of gravity, the nearer the line of gravity to the *center* of the base of support, the greater the stability (figure 14.9) and, conversely, the nearer the line of gravity to the *margin* of the

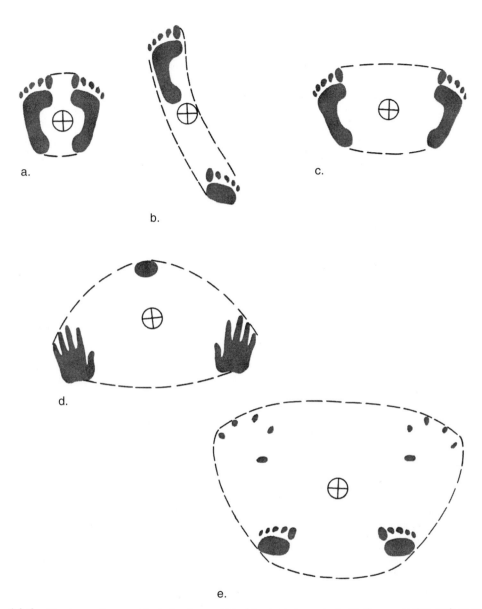

Figure 14.6   The base of support includes the part(s) of the body in contact with the supporting surface and the intervening area. What can you conclude about the stability of the base of support in these illustrations? In (a), (b), and (c) the weight is supported by the feet; in (d) it is supported by the forehead and hands during a headstand; in (e) the weight is supported by the hands and feet while the body is in a squat position. Circled crosses indicate point of intersection of line of gravity with base of support.

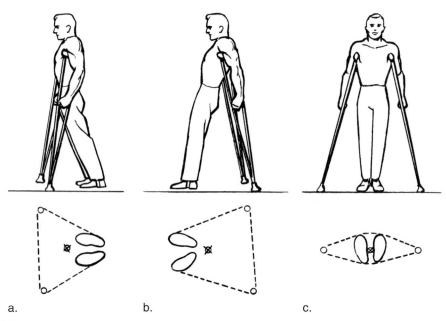

Figure 14.7   Bases of support with varying degrees of stability. Can you rank these from most stable to least stable? The subject in (a) and (b) is secure primarily in the anteroposterior direction; the position in (c) provides greater stability in the frontal plane than in the sagittal plane.

From B. LeVeau, *Williams and Lissner: Biomechanics of Human Motion,* 2nd ed. Copyright © 1977 W. B. Saunders, Orlando, FL. Reprinted by permission.

Figure 14.8   The height of the center of gravity changes with a change in body position. *X* = center of gravity. As the center of gravity moves closer to the base of support more angular displacement of the center of gravity can occur before it goes beyond the vertical line marking the edge of the base of support. The angle in (a) is greater than that in (b) and the angle in (b) is greater than that in (c). Thus, a > b> c with respect to lateral stability.

Figure 14.9 Position of the body in which the line of gravity falls approximately through the center of the base of support. This is a stable position.

Figure 14.10 Position of the body in which the line of gravity falls near the anterior margin of the base of support. This position is less stable than the one shown in figure 14.9.

base of support, the more precarious the equilibrium (figure 14.10). Once it passes beyond the margin, stability is lost and a new base must be established. This factor constitutes the major problem in some modern dance techniques, balance stunts, walking a tightrope, and building pyramids. In order to develop the neuromuscular control necessary to acquire such skills as these, there is no substitute for repeated practice. There are, however, a few devices that help keep the center of gravity centered over the base of support. One of these we do almost unconsciously. If we carry a heavy weight at one side of the body (e.g., a suitcase or a pail of water), *this constitutes a unilateral load* that, if uncompensated, would shift the center of gravity to that side, bringing it dangerously close to the margin of the base of support. By raising the opposite arm sideways, by bending or leaning to the opposite side, or by a combination of these, we counterbalance the external load and keep the line of gravity close to the center of the base

of support (figures 14.11 and 14.12). Another application of the principle of keeping the line of gravity over the center of the base of support is seen in the tightrope walker who carries a balancing pole or, to a lesser degree, in the gymnast walking on a balance beam with arms extended sideward.

When the external force acting on a body is a lateral one, stability is increased if the line of gravity is placed so that it will continue to remain over the base even when forced to move by the external force. Leaning into the wind (figure 14.13) or pushing a heavy chest are examples of when the line of gravity should be close to the edge of the base of support nearest the oncoming force. Pulling in a tug of war is an example of having the gravity line near the edge of the base of support farthest away from the external force. When one is not certain from which direction an external force may be applied, equilibrium is most stable when the line of gravity is in the center of the base of support.

Figure 14.11 Compensation for a unilateral load by inclining the entire body to the opposite side.

Figure 14.12 Compensating for a unilateral load by bending to the opposite side.

Figure 14.13 Leaning into the wind to balance the effect of its force on the body.

Mass of the Body

The mass or weight of an object is a factor in equilibrium only when motion or an external force is involved. Then, as Newton's second law states, $F = ma$. The amount of force needed to effect a change in motion (acceleration) is proportional to the mass being moved. The greater the mass, the greater the stability. It is a matter of common observation that an empty cardboard carton is more likely to blow down the street than one filled with canned goods. Likewise, a 250-pound lineman is less likely to be brushed aside than one weighing 130 pounds. In all sports involving physical contact, the heavy, solid individual stands a better chance of keeping his or her footing than does the lightweight one. When all factors are considered, however, mass is less a factor in stability than are the location of the line of gravity and the height of the center of gravity.

Friction

Friction as a factor in stability has already been suggested in relation to the size of the base of support. It has even greater influence when the body is in motion or is being acted on by an external force. Inadequate friction is what makes it difficult to keep one's equilibrium when walking on icy pavement, particularly if a frisky dog tugs unexpectedly on its leash. When the supporting surface presents insufficient friction, the footgear can make up for it. The person who must walk on icy pavement can wear "creepers" on the shoes, the golfer and the field hockey player can wear cleats, and the gymnast and basketball player can wear rubber-soled shoes.

Segmental Alignment

If, instead of being in one solid piece, an object consists of a series of segments placed one above the other, the problem of retaining its equilibrium is a multiple one. Maximum stability of a segmented body is ensured when the center of gravity of all the weight-bearing segments lie in a vertical line that is centered over the base of support. In a column of blocks, this means that each block must be centered over the block beneath. In a jointed column, as in the human body, one segment cannot slide off another, but it is quite possible for the segments to be united in a zigzag alignment. Such is all too often the case in human standing posture. In fact, the alignment of the body segments is a widely used criterion for judging standing posture. When the segments are aligned in a single vertical line, the posture is not only more pleasing in appearance to most of us, but there is less likelihood of strain to the joints and muscles. When one segment gets out of line, there is usually a compensatory misalignment of another segment in order to maintain a balanced position of the body as a whole. (In other words, for every "zig" there is a "zag.") At every point of angulation between segments there is uneven tension thrown on the ligaments and uneven tension in opposing muscle groups. This causes fatigue, if not actual strain.

The addition of an external weight to the body, as when one carries books, babies, or suitcases, may be thought of as the addition of a segment. The additional segment will add mass to the body and change its stability somewhat. More important, though, is the effect on the height of the center of gravity and the location of the line of gravity. The center of gravity will be displaced in the direction of the added weight, and the line of gravity will shift accordingly. Its new location will be governed by the nature of compensation made to accommodate the additional weight (see figures 14.11 and 14.12).

Visual and Psychological Factors

Factors that belong in this category are less easily explained than the others but are familiar to everyone. The giddiness that many experience when walking close to an unprotected edge high above the ground or when crossing a swirling river on a foot bridge is a real detriment to one's equilibrium. Even if the supporting surface is entirely adequate, the sense of balance may be disturbed. A common means of preserving the balance, both in this type of situation and when walking on a narrow rail, is to fix the eyes on a stationary spot above or beyond the "danger area." This seems to facilitate neuromuscular control by reducing the disturbing stimuli.

Physiological Factors

Besides the visual and psychological factors, there are also physiological factors related to the physical mechanism for equilibrium—namely, the semicircular canals. In addition to actual lesions of this mechanism, any disturbance of the general physical condition is likely to affect the sense of balance. Feelings of dizziness accompanying nausea or any form of debility reduce one's ability to resist other factors that threaten the equilibrium. Colds, viruses, and other problems that affect the inner ear may also interfere with balance. These physiological factors are largely beyond our control. One principle that can be derived from them, however, is that it is better to avoid situations likely to threaten the equilibrium when there is a temporary physiological disturbance.

Principles of Stability

The principles of stability are stated here as simply and concisely as possible, and several examples are suggested in each case.

Principle I

Other things being equal, the lower the center of gravity, the greater will be the body's stability.

Examples *a.* When landing from a jump one usually flexes at the knees, both to absorb force and to lower the center of gravity in order to regain one's balance.

b. In canoeing, the kneeling position represents a compromise position that combines the advantages of stability and ease of using the arms for paddling. Kneeling is preferable to sitting on the seat because the lowering of the center of gravity makes the position a more stable one. Although it is less stable than sitting on the floor of the canoe, it is a more convenient position for paddling. A position frequently recommended is kneeling and sitting against a thwart or the edge of a seat.

c. A performer on a balance beam quickly squats when he or she feels as if balance is being lost.

d. A wrestler tries to remain as stable as possible by lowering the center of gravity.

Principle II

Greater stability is obtained if the base of support is widened in the direction of the line of force.

Examples   *a.* This helps an individual keep from being thrown off balance when punching with force, pushing a heavy object, or throwing a fast ball. It also enables the puncher to "put the full body weight behind the punch" because, with a relatively wide forward-backward stance, the weight can be shifted from the rear foot to the forward foot as the force is delivered.

b. In pushing and pulling heavy furniture the whole body can be put into the act without loss of balance.

c. When catching a fast-moving object such as a baseball, or a heavy one such as a medicine ball, widening the base in line with the direction of the force enables the catcher to "give" with the catch and, in this way, to provide a greater distance in which to reduce or stop the motion of the object. It also ensures greater accuracy by reducing the likelihood of rebound.

d. The military "at ease" is more stable than the position of "attention."

e. Keeping one's balance when standing on a bus or train that is accelerating or decelerating is facilitated by widening the stance in the direction that the vehicle is moving, that is, in a forward-backward direction in relation to the vehicle.

Principle III

For maximum stability the line of gravity should intersect the base of support at a point that will allow the greatest range of movement within the area of the base in the direction of forces causing motion.

Examples   *a.* A football player knowing he will be pushed from in front should lean forward so that he can "give" in a backward direction without losing his balance.

b. A person in a tug-of-war line leans backward in preparation for absorbing a strong forward pull from the opponent.

c. A tennis player anticipating the opponent's return will keep the line of gravity centered so that the center of gravity can be shifted quickly in any direction without loss of balance.

d. Dragging a heavy box forward on a high shelf and then lifting it down is an activity in the home to which this principle applies. Assuming a forward-backward stance and leaning forward for this act gives the individual a wider distance to receive the weight of this forward-moving object. This decreases the likelihood of being thrown off balance when the box suddenly comes free of the shelf. It also enables one to take a step backward, which makes it easier to lower the box in front and to keep control of it. With a sideward stance one would be likely to be thrown off balance as the box comes free. There is also the danger of exerting so much horizontal force that, instead of lowering the box in front, the individual swings back overhead, hyperextending the spine and running the risk of straining the back.

e. Basketball and other team games involving running often require sudden reversals of direction. If the player tries to turn while the feet are close together, the momentum is likely to throw the runner off balance. This can be prevented by spreading the feet to check the forward motion and leaning back so that the line of gravity will be toward the rear. The runner can then quickly pivot to reverse direction.

Principle IV

Other things being equal, the greater the mass of a body, the greater will be its stability.

Example   In sports in which resistance to impact is a factor, heavy, solid individuals are more likely to maintain their equilibrium than lighter ones. This provides one basis for selecting linemen in football.

Principle V

Other things being equal, the most stable position of a vertical segmented body (such as a column of blocks or the erect human body) is one in which the center of gravity of each weight-bearing segment lies in a vertical line centered over the base of support or in which deviations in one direction produce torques that must be balanced by deviations producing torque in the opposite direction.

Examples   *a.* This applies to postural adjustments for achieving a pleasing, well-balanced alignment of the body segments, both with and without external loads.

   b. In balance stunts in which one person (or group of persons) supports the weight of another person or persons, the chief problem is one of either aligning or balancing the several centers of gravity over the center of the base of support.

Principle VI

Other things being equal, the greater the friction between the supporting surface and the parts of the body in contact with it, the more stable the body will be.

Example   The wearing of cleats and rubber-soled shoes for sport activities not only aids in locomotion but also serves to increase one's stability in positions held momentarily between quick or forceful movements, as in basketball, fencing, football, field hockey, lacrosse, and other sports.

Principle VII

Other things being equal, a person has better balance in locomotion under difficult circumstances when the vision is focused on stationary objects rather than on disturbing stimuli.

Example   Beginners learning to walk on a balance beam or to perform balance stunts, and others who for any reason have difficulty in keeping their balance, can minimize disturbing visual stimuli by fixing their eyes on a stationary spot in front of them, either at eye level or somewhat above eye level.

Principle VIII

There is a positive relationship between one's physical and emotional state and the ability to maintain balance under difficult circumstances.

Example   Persons should not be permitted to attempt dangerous balance stunts or activities requiring expert balance ability when their physical or emotional health is impaired.

Principle IX

Regaining equilibrium is based on the same principles as maintaining it.

Examples   *a.* After an unexpected loss of balance, such as when starting to fall or after receiving impetus when "off balance," equilibrium may be more quickly regained if a wide base of support is established and the center of gravity is lowered.

   b. Upon landing from a downward jump, stability may be more readily regained if the weight is kept evenly distributed over both feet or over the hands and feet, and if a sufficiently wide base of support is provided.

   c. Upon landing from a forward jump, the balance may be more readily regained if one lands with the weight forward and uses the hands, if necessary, to provide support in the direction of motion.

From this emphasis on stability it might seem that one should seek maximum stability in all situations. This is not true regarding certain stunts and gymnastic activities that are designed for the purpose of testing and developing body control under difficult circumstances. In many gymnastic vaults, for instance, "good form" stipulates that the performer land with the heels close, the knees separated, the arms extended sideward, and the trunk as erect as possible while the knees bend slightly to ensure a light landing. In teaching beginners it seems wiser to postpone emphasis on form from the point of view of appearance and to stress good mechanics and safety.

Mobility

There is an inverse relationship between stability and mobility. The greater the stability of a given body, the more difficult it will be to start the body moving. Conversely, the greater the mobility of the body, the less stability it possesses. A critical point in this relationship is the change from a position of stability to a state of mobility and eventually back to a position of stability. An example of this transition is seen in walking. The stationary standing position is a stable position with the line of gravity centered over the base of support. To initiate the step, a force is exerted downward and backward against the ground. The ground reaction force acts to move the center of gravity slightly up and to shift the line of gravity forward of the base of support, initiating the forward step. The swing leg then moves forward to reestablish

a base of support either to regain stability or to initiate the next step.

Often in sport and physical activity, it is necessary to alter stability intentionally to become mobile. To initiate forward motion swimmers and runners waiting for the start of a race assume a position in which they may lose balance rapidly (figure 14.14a). A football lineman in a three-point stance is also in a position to lose balance and apply forward force quickly. In many instances the ability to start, stop, or change direction quickly depends on manipulating the stability of the body.

Both the speed and the direction of the desired mobility are used to determine the nature of the change stability required to initiate the motion. To enhance the speed of a start in a given direction, the line of gravity should be as close as possible to the edge of the base of support in the direction of the desired motion. The opposite is true if a performer is attempting to stop quickly. A quick stop requires that stability be established quickly. To accomplish this, the performer must enlarge the base of support, lower the center of gravity, and

a.

b.

Figure 14.14   (a) Becoming unstable in order to move quickly. (b) Reestablishing stability to stop motion.

move the line of gravity away from the leading edge of the base of support (figure 14.14b).

FINDING THE CENTER OF GRAVITY IN THE HUMAN BODY

The location of the center of gravity in human beings is of interest to scientists in many areas. Anatomists, kinesiologists, orthopedists, physical therapists, space engineers, and equipment design engineers have all shown interest in methods of determining the location of the center of gravity. Earliest experiments located the center of gravity by balancing the body over a wedge. Various other methods have since been developed to estimate the location of the center of gravity, either at rest or in motion. Two of these procedures, easily replicated with a minimum of equipment, are described here.

Reaction Board Method

It is a fairly simple matter to find an estimate of the center of gravity of a motionless body using the *reaction board method*. Making use of the principle of moments, this procedure relies on the fact that the sum of the moments acting on a body in equilibrium is zero. Using this information, the location of the gravitational line is found for each plane. The center of gravity of the body becomes the intersection of the values for each of these three planes. Directions for locating the center of gravity in three planes follow.

Apparatus (Figure 14.15)

1. Scales: preferably either the Toledo or the spring balance type.
2. A stool or block the same height as the platform of the scales.
3. A board about 40 cm wide and 200 cm long. A knife edge should be attached to the underside of each end in such a way that when the board is placed in a horizontal position it will rest on the knife edges. In order to simplify the calculations the distance from knife edge to knife edge should measure exactly 200 cm. The front edge of

the board should be marked in centimeters. The board should be tested with a level to make certain it is horizontal.

Directions (Refer to Figure 14.15)

1. Find the subject's total weight, *W*.
2. Put one knife edge of board on the scale platform and the other edge on the box platform. Use a spirit level to make sure the board is horizontal. Note the reading on the scales. This is the partial weight of the board, *B*.
3. Have the subject lie supine on the board with the heels against the footrest at the end of the board away from the scales. The position the subject assumes should be as similar to the standing position as possible. Record the reading on the scales. This is the partial weight of the subject and board, *S*.
4. For equilibrium to exist about the pivot point *P*, the counterclockwise torques must equal the clockwise torques. If *W* is the total weight of the subject; *B*, the partial weight of the board; *S*, the partial weight of the subject and board; *L*, the length of the board; and *d*, the perpendicular distance from *P* to *W*, then

$$d \times W = (S - B)L$$

(clockwise torques = counterclockwise torques)

Rearranged,

$$d = \frac{(S - B)L}{W}$$

The distance between the subject's feet and center of gravity is *d*. This is comparable to the distance between the ground and the center of gravity when the subject is standing but must be viewed as an estimate because of shifts in body organs and tissues when lying down.

5. The percentage height of the center of gravity with respect to the subject's total height is found by dividing the value of *d* in the transverse plane (supine lying position) by the subject's total height and multiplying by 100.

$$\text{Percent} = \frac{d \text{ in transverse plane}}{\text{subject' s height}} \times 100$$

Figure 14.15   Reaction board method for locating the height of the center of gravity.

6. To locate the center of gravity in the frontal or sagittal planes the procedure must be repeated with the subject standing on the board (preferably near the middle). For the sagittal plane, the subject stands with the side to the scales (figure 14.16) and for the frontal plane location, the subject stands facing the scales. Use the same formula

$$d = \frac{(S - B)L}{W}$$

to solve for **d.** The value of **d** represents the distance from the knife edge **P** to the plane in which the subject's center of gravity is located.

7. To find the single point representing the spot where the line of gravity intersects the base of support, a piece of paper should be placed under the subject's feet for the side view measurement. The outline of the feet is traced on the paper. When the first **d** is found, the distance is measured and marked on both the left and right sides of the paper. The paper should then be removed and the points connected by a straight line. When the subject faces forward for the second measurement, the paper should be placed on the board so that the subject's feet will fit in the footprints. When the second **d** is found, the distance should be measured and marked on both edges of the paper, and the place where two lines intersect represents the approximate position of the point where the line of gravity strikes the base of support. This is a crude method of locating this point and is not strictly accurate as the subject may not be standing in exactly the same posture for both measurements. Furthermore, the element of swaying always introduces a source of error.

A modification of the reaction board method involves the use of a large triangular board supported by scales on two corners and a platform of equal height under the third corner (Waterland and Shambes 1970). Each corner makes contact with its support through a pointed bolt. Again it is important that the board be horizontal. If this triangle is equilateral, the moments are taken about lines forming two sides of the triangle, and the perpendicular distance from each line to the center of gravity is determined as follows:

Figure 14.16   Reaction board method for locating the line of gravity in the sagittal plane.

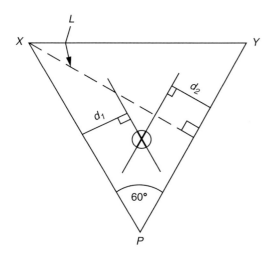

$$d_1 = \frac{(S_Y - B_Y)L}{W}$$

$$d_2 = \frac{(S_X - B_X)L}{W}$$

where

d_1 = distance between XP and center of gravity
d_2 = distance between YP and center of gravity
S_X = partial weight of subject and board on scale X
S_Y = partial weight of subject and board on scale Y
B_X = partial weight of board recorded on scale X
B_Y = partial weight of board recorded on scale Y
W = weight of subject
L = altitude of triangle (perpendicular distance from scale to line about which moment is being taken)

Figure 14.17   Immersion tanks for determination of segmental weights. Using segment landmarks as defined by Dempster, the segment is immersed in water. The displaced water is weighed and multiplied by the specific gravity of the segment to obtain the segmental weight.
From B. Gowitzke and M. Milner, *Scientific Bases of Human Movement,* 3rd ed. Copyright © 1988 Williams & Wilkins, Baltimore, MD.

Segmental Method

Experiments using the reaction board are convincing in showing how the body automatically compensates for external loads and segmental adjustments. It is revealing also to see how the body adjusts for the sideward raising of an arm, the forward bending of the trunk, a briefcase carried in one hand, or a load of books carried on the hip. Such analysis, however, is limited to the body in a stationary position. The location of the center of gravity of someone in action requires the use of another method. A highly useful procedure is one called the *segmental method.* This technique makes use of a photograph of the subject and involves finding the location of the center of gravity of each of the body segments, the position of these individual gravity points with respect to arbitrarily placed x and y axes, and knowledge of the ratio between the individual segment weights and the total body weight.

Considerable research has been done to determine values for the proportionate weights of body segments and the locations of the segmental centers of gravity. These data have been obtained through the weighing and suspension of cadaver segments, determination of the weight of segments of living subjects through the amount of water displaced by the immersed segment, and formation of mathematical models. Among the most commonly used data today are those of Dempster (1955). He weighed eight elderly male cadavers, dismembered them, weighed the segments, and determined the proportion of total weight for each segment. In addition, he located the center of gravity and specific gravity for each segment.

Using the same definitions of joint center used by Dempster, and using the segmental water volume values determined by Clauser (as cited in Plagenhoef, Evans, and Abdelnour 1983), Plagenhoef, Evans, and Abdelnour (1983) immersed the various segments of 135 subjects in water to determine segment weights as a percentage of total body weight (figure 14.17). These data are presented in figure 14.18 and table 14.1. This research team then selected a smaller sample and again used the segmental immersion technique to locate the segmental centers of gravity as a percentage of the total segment length. These data are presented in table 14.2.

With information on the proportionate mass of body segments and the location of the center of gravity of each segment, the center of gravity of the whole body in any plane may now be determined by making use of the principle of torques. The sum of the torques of the individual segments about arbitrarily placed x and y axes

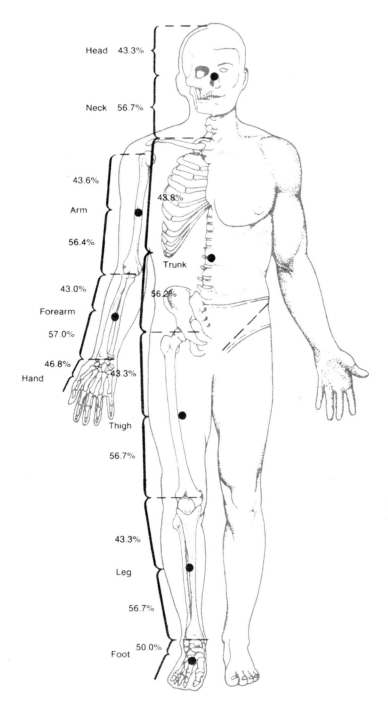

Figure 14.18   Joint centers and percentage distance of centers of gravity from joint centers in males.
Compiled from data in Plagenhoef, Evans, and Abdelnour, 1983; Hinrichs, 1990; and Dempster, 1955.

TABLE 14.1	Location of the Segment Center of Gravity as a Percentage of the Segment Length			
	Men (N = 7)		Women (N = 9)	
	Proximal	Distal	Proximal	Distal
Hand	46.8	—	46.8	—
Forearm	43.0	57.0	43.4	56.6
Upper arm	43.6	56.4	45.8	54.2
Foot	50.0	—	50.0	—
Shank	43.4	56.6	41.9	58.1
Thigh	43.3	56.7	42.8	57.2
Whole trunk[a]	63.0	37.0	56.9	43.1
Pelvis[b]	5.0	95.0	5.0	95.0
Abdomen	46.0	54.0	46.0	54.0
Thorax[c]	56.7	43.3	56.3	43.7
Head and neck[d]	55.0	45.0	55.0	45.0
Abdomen and pelvis[e]	44.5	55.5	39.0	61.0

[a]Hip joint to shoulder joint = 100%
[b]Hip joint to plane of umbilicus = 100%
[c]Pectoral line to shoulder joint (glenohumeral) = 100%
[d]Top of the head to 7th cervical = 100%
[e]Hip joint to T-11 = 100%

From S. Plagenhoef, F. Evans, and T. Abdelnour, Anatomical data for analyzing human motion, Research Quarterly 54 (2): 172, 1983. Copyright © 1983 American Alliance for Health, Physical Education. Recreation, and Dance, Reston, VA.

TABLE 14.2	Body Segment Percentages of Total Body Weight for Living Men and Woman	
Segments	Men	Women
Hands	1.3	1.0
Forearms	3.8	3.1
Upper arms	6.6	6.0
Feet	2.9	2.4
Shanks	9.0	10.5
Thighs	21.0	23.0
Trunk (including head and neck)	55.4	54.0

From data presented in Plagenhoef, Evans, and Abdelnour, 1983.

will produce the location of the center of gravity of the whole body with respect to the x and y axes. This is because the total body weight acting at the center of mass is the resultant of the combined segment weights acting at their mass centers and the resultant moment of the total body weight about the x, y axes is the sum of the individual segment torques about the same axes.

The segmental method for determining the center of gravity requires a considerable amount of measurement and calculation and therefore can be time consuming. The use of computer programs speeds up the process considerably, as

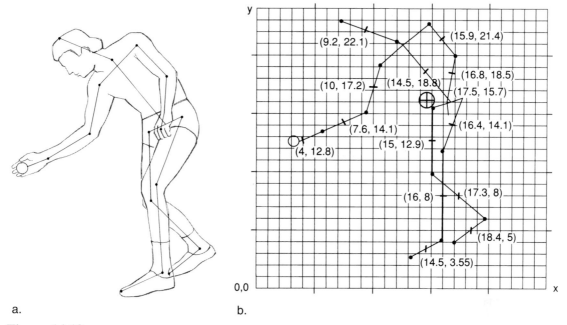

Figure 14.19   Segmental determination of the center of gravity. (a) Location of body segments. (b) The center of mass of each body segment is marked, and *x, y* coordinates are found using an arbitrarily placed *x, y* axis. With information on the proportionate mass of each body segment and the location of the center of mass of each segment, the center of gravity of the whole body may be determined using the principle of moments.

does the use of digitizers or film analyzers with built-in *x, y* coordinate systems.

Directions for locating the center of gravity using the segmental method follow.

Apparatus

1. Line drawing on graph paper taken from photographic image of subject (figure 14.19).
2. Worksheet with Plagenhoef, Evans, and Abdelnour proportions listed (figure 14.20).

Directions

1. The locations of the extremities of the individual segments must be marked according to the link boundaries shown in figure 14.18. This will result in marks at the end of the second toe, ankle, knee, hip, knuckle III of the hand, wrist, shoulders, seventh cervical vertebra, and top of the head. Where these points are obscured by other body parts, an estimate must be made. The upper trunk mark is the seventh cervical

vertebra, located slightly above the midpoint of the transverse line joining the shoulders. The lower trunk mark is the midpoint of the transverse line joining the hips.

2. The extremity limits are joined to form a stick figure consisting of 14 segments (see figure 14.19a).
3. The mass center location for each segment length is found using the data provided in table 14.1, where centers of gravity are located as a percentage of the distance between segment end points. The amount of the percentage distance from one segment end point is multiplied by the picture length of the segment. The resulting product is the distance from the selected end point to the center of gravity of the segment. The distance is measured from the end point, and the center of gravity is marked by a short slash mark intersecting the segment line.
4. *x* and *y* axes are drawn on the paper.

Body Segment	Proportion of Body Wt.	x Value	x Products	y Value	y Products
1. Trunk	.486	14.5	7.05	18.8	9.14
2. Head & Neck	.079	9.2	0.73	22.1	1.75
3. R. Thigh	.097	15.0	1.46	12.9	1.25
4. R. Lower Leg	.045	17.3	0.79	8.0	0.36
5. R. Foot	.014	18.4	0.26	5.0	0.70
6. L. Thigh	.097	16.4	1.59	14.1	1.37
7. L. Lower Leg	.045	16.0	0.72	8.0	0.36
8. L. Foot	.014	14.5	0.20	3.5	0.05
9. R. Upper Arm	.027	10.0	0.27	17.2	0.46
10. R. Lower Arm	.014	7.6	0.11	14.1	0.20
11. R. Hand	.006	4.0	0.02	12.8	0.08
12. L. Upper Arm	.027	15.9	0.43	21.4	0.58
13. L. Lower Arm	.014	16.8	0.24	18.5	0.26
14. L. Hand	.006	17.5	0.10	15.7	0.09
x - y Resultants (product total)			13.97		16.65

x Coordinate = <u>13.97</u>

y Coordinate = <u>16.65</u>

Figure 14.20   Worksheet for locating the center of gravity using the segmental method.

5. The x, y coordinates for each of the 14 segment mass centers are determined and recorded on the diagram of the figure at the respective mass centers.
6. A worksheet such as that shown in figure 14.20 is used to record the x, y coordinate values and the torques of those segments about the x and y axes. The individual torques are the products (col. 3) of the coordinate values (col. 2) and their related body segment proportions (col. 1).

7. The algebraic sum of the x products represents the x coordinate of the total body's mass center, and the algebraic sum of the y products is the y coordinate. These values are located and marked on the tracing (see figure 14.19b).

This procedure has made it possible to locate the center of gravity of the handball player at the moment of contact with the ball. It must be remembered that this location is for one brief moment during the performance of the skill, and the

● = Location of estimate of center of gravity marked at every fifth frame

Figure 14.21   The iliac crest is used as an estimate of the location of the center of gravity of a swimmer during the execution of a racing dive. The tracking of the center of gravity of a dynamic skill is done through the use of tracings of individual motion picture frames.

position of the center of gravity will shift with body segment shifts. If more information is desired about the location of the center of gravity at other critical moments during the execution of the skill, this process should be repeated using appropriate line drawings of those critical moments. Although arduous, even with the use of a computer, the process is invaluable for those individuals who need detailed analysis of dynamic skills.

Students who desire to trace the path of the center of gravity during the execution of a dynamic

skill, but who do not need the accuracy of the segmental method, may find the placement of a dot on the iliac crest to be a useful estimate for the location of the body's center of gravity (figure 14.21). This technique should be used with caution, however. It is important to remember that the center of gravity will deviate appreciably from this location in some body positions (see figures 14.1, 14.2, 14.3, and 14.4).

LABORATORY EXPERIENCES

1. Define the following key terms and give an example of each that is not used in the text:
   Center of gravity
   Stability
   Base of support

2. a. Working with a partner, determine the position of your line of gravity using the reaction board method. Locate the point where this line intersects your base of support by marking it on a tracing of your feet.
   b. Determine the position of your line of gravity, leaning as far forward as possible with the body in a straight line from the top of the head to the ankles. Repeat, leaning as far backward as possible.
   c. Locate the line of gravity in the sagittal plane while leaning as far as possible to one side.
   d. Determine the height of your center of gravity with your arms at your side and then with them stretched over your head. What percentage of your total height is your center of gravity? How does this compare with averages for your sex?
   e. Choose an original position with a small or unstable base of support. Locate the point

where the line of gravity intersects the base of support.

3. Make a tracing on graph paper of a picture of a person engaged in a motor skill. Locate the center of gravity using the segmental method.

4. Walk on a low balance beam and do the following:
   a. Look ahead at the wall.
   b. Look at a person who is in front of the balance beam doing a vigorous exercise such as a jumping jack.
   c. Walk with your eyes blindfolded.
   d. Walk along with a partner walking beside you. Without warning, the partner is to give you a slight but sudden sideward push. What measures do you take to maintain your balance? If you fail, explain why.

5. Build two columns of blocks, one with the blocks carefully centered one over the other, the second column with the blocks staggered but balanced. Grasping the lowest block of each column, slide the columns back and forth, changing the speed frequently and suddenly until the blocks tumble. Which column is the first to topple? Why?

REFERENCES AND SELECTED READINGS

Adrian, M. J., and J. M. Cooper. 1994. *The biomechanics of human movement.* 2nd ed. Indianapolis: Benchmark Press.

Chaffin, P. B., and G. Andersson. 1984. *Occupational biomechanics.* New York: Wiley.

Dainty, P. A., and R. W. Norman, eds. 1987. *Standardizing biomechanical testing in sport.* Champaign, IL: Human Kinetics.

Davis, B. L., and M. D. Grabiner. 1996. Modeling effects of muscle fatigue on unilateral postural control. *Journal of Applied Biomechanics* 12:173–84.

Dempster, W. T. 1955. *Space requirements of the seated operator.* Dayton, OH: Wright-Patterson Air Force Base (WADC TR 55-199).

Gowitzke, B. A., and M. Milner. 1988. *Scientific bases of human movement.* 3rd ed. Baltimore: Williams & Wilkins.

Hinrichs, R. N. 1990. Adjustments to the center of mass proportions of Clauser et al. (1969). *Journal of Biomechanics* 23:949–51.

Lundin, T. M., J. W. Feuerbach, and M. D. Grabiner. 1993. Effect of plantar flexor and dorsiflexor fatigue on unilateral postural control. *Journal of Applied Biomechanics* 9:191–201.

Miller, D. I., and R. C. Nelson. 1976. *Biomechanics of sport.* Philadelphia: Lea & Febiger.

Plagenhoef, S. 1971. *Patterns of human motion: A cinematographic analysis.* Englewood Cliffs, NJ: Prentice Hall, pp. 25, 27.

Plagenhoef, S., F. Evans, and T. Abdelnour. 1983. Anatomical data for analyzing human motion. *Research Quarterly* 54:169–78.

Waterland, J. D., and G. M. Shambes. 1970. Biplane center of gravity procedure. *Perceptual Motor Skills* 30:511–14.

PART

III

Motor Skills: Principles and Applications

Introduction to Part III

The most difficult aspect of the study of kinesiology is the application of anatomical and biomechanical concepts and principles so that students are able to generalize their knowledge across movement patterns and to apply it to new and unique patterns they may encounter. For students of human motion to be effective in applying their enhanced knowledge of kinesiological principles to effect improved performance, they must establish a logical framework for their analysis and engage in a systematic approach to critical observation and evaluation.

At the conclusion of Part III, students should be able to complete basic qualitative kinesiological analyses for all categories of skill classification. This means that they will have learned to observe and describe movements accurately, evaluate performance according to anatomical and mechanical principles, and prescribe corrective actions when needed. It also means that they will have developed the ability to select and evaluate the appropriateness of motor skills and exercises and related equipment.

Part III draws upon the anatomical and mechanical information presented in Parts I and II. Analyses and applications that provide the basis for the successful performance

395

of motor skills are presented on the basis of the model for kinesiological analysis developed in chapter 1.

The first eight chapters in Part III are organized according to the System for Classification of Motor Skills (p. 6–7) and are presented with the intent that the student progress from the study of relatively simple motions to more complex motions—that is, from the standing posture through exercise and locomotion, to the giving of motion to external objects and the reception of impact. Included in each chapter are a brief description of the types of motion involved, outlines of anatomical and mechanical principles for effective, efficient, and safe performance, and an in-depth qualitative analysis of at least one motor activity.

Chapter 23 concludes Part III with a description of the instrumentation and methodology currently being used for motion analysis. It is becoming more and more likely that students at all levels will have direct experience with sophisticated equipment and methodology as early as their first kinesiology course. It is, therefore, important that they understand the significance of the contributions to our growing knowledge of human motion that have occurred through the expanding use of increasingly sophisticated analysis techniques and tools.

Internet Resources

There are a number of sites on the World Wide Web which may be of interest to the student studying the applications of kinesiology. Among those that might be most helpful are the following:

http://www.per.ualberta.ca/biomechanics/
Biomechanics World Wide, a primary source for biomechanics information and links. Links to many biomechanics courses as well as biomechanists and their research. Also a good source of information about biomechanics instrumentation.

http://www.education.ed.ac.uk/cis/index.html
Biomechanics articles for coaches from the International Society for the Biomechanics of Sport (ISBS).

http://www.gcmas.org/
The official site of the Gait and Clinical Movement Analysis Society, with links to interesting gait analysis information.

http://www.sportsci.org/
Sport Sciences is an online newsletter with links to sport research and information.

http://www.mindspring.com/~jnorvill/webwalker.htm
A racewalking page for the participant, with good teaching hints for racewalking.

http://www.gssiweb.com
Gatorade Sports Science Institute website. Requires registration but it is free. Contains many articles of physical activity, some in biomechanics.

http://home.about.com/index.htm
This is a general site about many things. It lists a number of sports with a variety of articles about each one.

http://www.celos.psu.edu/kines202/index.html
Pennsylvania State University site on gait analysis, containing online research papers.

Several other sites that might be especially helpful for chapter 23 follow:

http://www.engin.umich.edu/dept/ioe/C4E/
    research—projects.html
The site belonging to the University of Michigan Center for Ergonomics. Gives a good overview of what is happening in ergonomics.

http://www.engin.umich.edu/dept/ioe/HUMOSIM/
The University of Michigan Human Motion Simulation program site with examples of this type of computer simulation.

www.biomechanics-inc.com
A commercial site with some interesting examples of real-time motion capture.

http://kwon3d.com/theories.html
This site features an online text on the 3–D analysis of motion.

http://www.peakperform.com/biomech_research_pubs_sports.htm
A commercial site with a bibliography on biomechanics using photoinstrumentation.

http://www.cc.gatech.edu/gvu/animation/
Georgia Tech site on animation with some interesting bits of human animation and explanation.

*Note: all internet sites are transient by nature and may cease to be active without warning. New sites are continually being activated.

THE STANDING POSTURE

15

OUTLINE

- **Significance of Posture**
- **Support of the Standing Posture**
  Muscular Activity in Erect
      Standing
  The Neuromuscular Mechanism
      for Maintaining Erect Posture
  Postural Stability
  Alignment of Body Segments
- **Factors Related to the Standing
  Posture**
  Energy Cost
  Evolutionary and Hereditary
      Influences
  Strength and Flexibility
  Age
  Psychological Aspects
- **Principles Applied to Posture**
- **Postural Adaptation to External
  Conditions and Special Problems**
- **Posture Screening**
- **Laboratory Experiences**

OBJECTIVES

At the conclusion of this chapter, the
student should be able to:

1. Identify and describe the
   skeletomuscular and
   neuromuscular antigravity
   mechanisms involved in the
   volitional standing position.
2. Summarize the similarities and
   differences that occur in the
   relation of the line of gravity to
   various body landmarks with
   good and poor anteroposterior
   segmental alignment.
3. Discuss the factors that affect
   the stability and energy cost of
   the erect posture.
4. Explain the effects that the
   variables of age, body build,
   strength, and flexibility have on
   the alignment of body segments
   in the standing posture.
5. Name the values, if any, of good
   posture.
6. Perform kinesiological analyses
   on the posture of individuals of
   different ages and body builds.

SIGNIFICANCE OF POSTURE

There are innumerable concepts of human posture and innumerable interpretations of its significance. Posture may well claim to be "all things to all people." To the physical anthropologist posture may be a racial characteristic, or it may be an indication of phylogenetic development; to the orthopedic surgeon it may be an indication of the soundness of the skeletal framework and muscular system; to an artist it may be an expression of the personality and the emotions; to the actor it serves as a tool for expressing mood or character; to the physician, biologist, fashion model, employer, sculptor, dancer, therapist, psychologist—to each of these—posture has a different significance. Each sees posture within the framework of his or her own profession and interest. This is no less true of kinesiologically oriented therapists and educators. To them, posture is a gauge of mechanical efficiency, kinesthetic sense, muscle balance, and neuromuscular coordination.

For all practical purposes no individual's posture can be described completely. Posture means position, and a multisegmented organism such as the human body cannot be said to have a single posture. It assumes many postures and seldom holds any of them for an appreciable time. Although characteristic patterns become apparent as we observe an individual over an extended period, it is difficult, if not impossible, to measure, or even record, these patterns. It would take a comprehensive series of pictures of an individual's varied stance and movement patterns to provide an adequate sample. Perhaps this is the reason that most posture research has been related to the volitional standing position.

Another difficulty in analyzing and evaluating human posture is the varieties of human physique represented, such as those defined many years ago by Sheldon, Stevens, and Tucker (1940). The importance of considering these in-dividual differences of build when evaluating posture was reported by Althoff, Heyden, and Robertson (1988). Each of us has had the experience of recognizing a friend from the back. It was probably, in part, that individual's habitual posture that gave the clue for visual identification.

In view of the fact that dynamic postures should be of greater concern than static postures to those who specialize in human movement, it may be well to say a word in defense of the practice of examining the posture of subjects in the erect standing position. It is admitted that the posture in such a position is of little importance in itself, unless this posture must be maintained for long periods of time. It also becomes significant when taken as the point of departure for the many postural patterns assumed by the individual, both at rest and in motion. Because there is an almost endless variety of activity postures and because these are extremely difficult to judge, a convenient custom is to accept the standing posture as the individual's basic posture from which all other postures stem. Hence, as a reflection of the individual's characteristic postural patterns, the standing posture takes on an importance it would not otherwise have. It should be kept in mind, however, that its importance is in direct proportion *to the extent to which it represents the individual's habitual carriage.*

SUPPORT OF THE STANDING POSTURE

Muscular Activity in Erect Standing

Compared with other mammals, humans have very economical antigravity mechanisms, and the muscle energy needed to maintain the erect standing position is not great. A reason for the economy of muscle effort required is the major role of the ligaments in supporting and maintaining the integrity of the joints. The muscles that are active are those that aid in keeping the weight-bearing column of bones in relative alignment and that oppose gravity's downward-directed force.

According to electromyographic studies reported by Basmajian and DeLuca (1985) and

Trepman and associates (1994), the postural muscular activity in the body segments can be expected as follows:

Foot

None of the intrinsic musculature is active during
normal standing but becomes active in the push-
off for walking or rising on the toes.

Leg

The posterior calf muscles are more active than
the anterior ones. Any swaying forward or backward produces compensatory muscle action to
bring the body back to the vertical balanced position. Rising on the toes or wearing high heels increases the activity of both the anterior and posterior muscles. The muscles of the ankle are
responsible for the control of sagtittal plane (anteroposterior) postural sway.

Thigh and Hip

Very little activity occurs in the thigh muscles
during relaxed standing. Swaying produces alternating bursts of activity in the gluteus medius and
tensor fasciae latae. This is due to the fact that the
abductors/adductors control frontal plane (mediolateral) postural sway. The iliopsoas is constantly
active, apparently to prevent hyperextension at
the hip joint.

Spine

There is very slight activity in the sacrospinalis or
abdominal muscles, depending on the relation of
the line of gravity to the spinal column. Activity
is exhibited in *one or the other* of the two sets of
muscles. Slight to moderate back muscle activity
is at least three times as likely as abdominal muscle activity (Klausen, Jeppesen, and Morgensen
1978).

Upper Extremity

The integrity of the joints in the passively hanging extremity is assisted by low-grade activity in
a number of muscles. The serratus anterior and
the fibers of the trapezius support the shoulder
girdle, and the supraspinatus resists downward
dislocation of the humerus. There appears to be
no activity in the muscles crossing the elbow or
wrist joints when the arm hangs passively.

The Neuromuscular Mechanism for Maintaining Erect Posture

The proprioceptors are responsible for most of the
reflex movements necessary for the maintenance
of the erect standing position and for the adjustments that must be made to meet changing conditions. They include the receptors of the muscles,
joints, and labyrinths and are accompanied by
two exteroceptors, one visual and the other cutaneous. The latter serves as a proprioceptor together with the pressure receptors, especially in
connection with the extensor thrust reflex. Volitional postural adjustments are made by the same
mechanism that is responsible for all volitional
movements (p. 88) and, of necessity, are governed by the structural limitations of the individual. Recently the role of the neuromuscular system in the maintenance of the upright standing
posture has been called into question. Winter and
colleagues (1998) have produced a model in
which the neuromuscular system apparently controls the initial stiffness of the lower extremity
(primarily the ankle joint). Postural sway is then
the result of the spring action produced by this
joint stiffness. It should be of interest for the student to watch the development of this theory.

There are several schools of thought regarding the method of changing habitual postural patterns. Some believe that it can be accomplished
by the frequent repetition of carefully selected exercises performed with control and with constant
attention to correct form (Lauffenburger 1987).
Others believe that the rebuilding of the necessary
neuromuscular pathways can be accomplished
only by the indirect method—that is, by influencing the individual's neuromuscular response by
means of the thought processes. In at least one
study (Fairweather and Sidaway 1993) imagery

has been found to have a more positive effect on posture than either flexibilty training or abdominal strengthening. More recently it has been hypothesized that the modification of habitual posture depends on four factors, namely (1) intent or voluntary decision toward change, (2) experience with desired posture, (3) instruction resulting in different strategies, and (4) environmental influences (Jacobs and Jacobs 2000).

Postural Stability

Hellebrandt (1940) was one of the first to demonstrate that even the erect standing posture is not literally static. "Standing," she concluded, "is, in reality, *movement upon a stationary base.*" Her experiments using scales and a reaction board revealed that the center of gravity did not remain motionless above the base of support, no matter how still the subject attempted to stand, but moved forward, backward, and sideward. This motion indicated that the subjects were constantly swaying. When the swaying was prevented by artificial means, there was a tendency to faint. Thus the involuntary swaying was seen to serve the purpose of a pump, aiding the venous return and ensuring the brain of adequate circulation for retaining consciousness.

Today, force platforms and other forms of dynamic platform posturography can automatically record postural sway magnitude, direction, and pattern. This type of data collection is making it possible to study the changes that occur in postural sway in a variety of clinical conditions, as well as in varied terrain and under varying loads.

Postural stability is currently measured on the basis of the horizontal difference in sway motion between center of gravity and center of pressure. *Center of pressure* is the single resultant of the multiple forces occurring over the entire plantar surface of the foot. In balanced standing, the line of gravity should be through the center of pressure. The greater the excursion of the center of pressure in relation to the center of gravity, the more likely that there is poor segmental align-

ment and/or poor postural stability. However close the line of gravity is to the center of pressure, this condition does not necessarily indicate good segmental alignment. One can assume an exaggerated zigzag alignment and still stand in such a way that difference in motion between the line of gravity and the center of pressure is quite small, provided the "zags" balance the "zigs," yet the posture may leave much to be desired. In this connection students may find numbers 3 and 4 of the Laboratory Experiences of particular interest.

Alignment of Body Segments

It has been assumed by many that a standing posture in which each weight-bearing segment was balanced vertically upon the segment beneath it made less demand on the muscles than a posture in which the segments formed a zigzag alignment. Good posture, it was said, takes less muscular effort to maintain than poor. The explanation given was that when a segment is not in vertical alignment, the force of gravity is not parallel with its long axis, and hence exerts a rotary component of force. Although this reasoning may seem logical, it overlooks two facts: first, that one of the most poorly aligned postures is actually a fatigue posture in which the muscles have let go and have left it to the ligaments to prevent complete collapse (figure 15.1); and second, that even in the most ideal posture some rotary force is present, owing to (1) the supporting column of the trunk (i.e., the spine) being situated closer to the posterior surface of the body than to the anterior, (2) the supporting base (the feet) being projected forward from the lower extremities instead of centered beneath them, (3) the spinal column being curved anteroposteriorly, and (4) the chest forming an anterior load upon which gravity is constantly exerting a rotary force (figure 15.2). The weight of the breasts in women constitutes an additional anterior weight and thus causes an even greater rotary component of gravitational force.

There appears to be a definite relationship between the alignment of the body segments and

Figure 15.1   Zigzag alignment of weight-bearing segments increases rotary effect of gravitational force.

Figure 15.2   Good alignment of weight-bearing segments. Rotary effect of gravitational force is minimized.

the integrity of the joint structures. It is generally accepted that prolonged postural strain is injurious to these structures. Ligaments that are repeatedly subjected to stretch become permanently stretched, and cartilages that are subjected to uneven pressures and to abnormal friction become damaged. Adequate clinical, though not experimental, evidence exists to support the contention that prolonged postural strain is a factor in the arthritic changes that take place in the weight-bearing joints.

Lack of agreement concerning the effort required for maintaining upright posture is partly due to confusion about what is meant by "upright posture." To some, it may mean merely the ability to stay on one's feet and resist the downward pull

of gravity. To others, it may mean "good" alignment as opposed to a "zigzag" alignment. Studies based on energy cost appear to indicate that, although it takes less energy to stand erect than to sit, *minimum* energy expenditure cannot be accepted as a criterion of good posture. Metabolic economy is desirable to a point, because it implies the absence of hypertonicity, but from an overall educator's point of view, well-balanced segmental alignment should not be sacrificed for it.

The energy requirement for maintaining erect posture in reasonably good alignment would seem to bear a direct relationship to the individual's habitual carriage. It is a matter of common observation that there is a wide range of body alignments seen in "upright posture." Anyone who has had the task of evaluating the posture of large groups of individuals and of giving help to those with "poor posture" is impressed with the variation in effort it takes for a student to stand in "good posture." Whereas one individual apparently has no difficulty in assuming this posture because it is the natural one, another cannot assume it even momentarily without the instructor's help and without becoming overtense. It is obvious that the second individual uses more muscular energy than the first. A single interpretation of an ideal posture is neither practical nor possible when given the large individual variations that exist among human beings. Good posture, accommodating the great variety of body types and resulting in physiological and mechanical efficiency, in both static and dynamic situations, must be broadly interpreted.

FACTORS RELATED TO THE STANDING POSTURE

Energy Cost

The increase in metabolic rate over the basal rate when standing is so small compared with the metabolic cost of moving and exercising as to be negligible. The type of posture that involves a minimum of metabolic increase over the basal rate is one in which the knees are hyperextended, the hips are pushed forward to the limit of extension, the thoracic curve is increased, the head is projected forward, and the upper trunk is inclined backward in a posterior lean (figure 15.3b). This is a typical fatigue posture requiring a minimum of energy expenditure. A common variation is a shift of the weight to one foot with accompanying asymmetrical adjustments in the spine and lower extremities.

Evolutionary and Hereditary Influences

The transformation of the human race from arboreal quadrupeds to upright bipeds is a process that is still being closely examined by anthropologists.

Lovejoy (1988) proposes that this evolutionary process is directly related to the need for the male hominid to have the hands and arms available for carrying a wider variety of foods from fairly long distances. The changes that developed in human structure, he stated, were the direct result of the shift from a vertically suspended position to a vertically supported one. This shift was responsible not only for the changes in the weight-bearing parts of the musculoskeletal structure but also for changes in the upper extremities, which were now freed for the development of a great variety of manipulative skills. Although no specific principle is derived from this explanation of the role played by the force of gravity in the evolution of human structure, an awareness of it might be of help in the analysis of individual postures.

Attention has already been called to individual variations in posture. In attempting to correct a person's posture one must be realistic and accept the limits imposed by a possible heredity factor. Improvement can doubtless be made, but one must not expect to effect a radical change in the basic shape of the spine. In addition, certain pathological conditions, such as congenitally dislocated hips, cerebral palsy, and paralysis of trunk muscles, may cause such changes in an individual's posture that the usual hereditary and environmental influences are obscured.

Strength and Flexibility

That strength and flexibility are factors in posture would seem to be a universally accepted thesis, judging by the preponderance of strength and flexibility exercises included in the majority of corrective programs and also by the strength and flexibility measurements included in posture tests. These exercises relate particularly to the strength of the abdominals, scapular adductors, and thoracic spinal extensors, and in the flexibility of the pectorals and the hamstrings. The results of research in which anteroposterior alignment was correlated with strength or flexibility have been somewhat contradictory. As is often

a.   b.   c.

Figure 15.3   (a) Individual in position of "attention." She has exaggerated lumbar curve but does not show strain. (b) Individual is overrelaxed and has zigzag alignment. (c) Individual has a nice easy posture and good alignment except for a very slight forward head and slight forward pelvic tilt.

the case, it is difficult to compare results because of significant differences in methodology, especially in the method for measuring the postural alignment and age and sex of the subjects.

Studies comparing anteroposterior alignment and strength have produced little definitive data. There have been some indications that fatigue or injury in the muscles of the lower extremity may contribute to decreasing stability in the upright posture. Strength, flexibility, and injury have, in-

stead, been found to be more closely related to the ability to perform dynamic motions from an upright postural base (Lundin, Feuerbach, and Grabiner 1993; Kuo and Zajac 1993; Li, McClure, and Pratt 1996).

Age

As the human body develops from infancy to old age, several physical and neurological factors may affect posture. The infant initially lacks either the muscular strength or the neurological development to assume an upright posture. As the trunk and upper extremities develop, the infant gains the ability to assume and maintain a sitting posture. With continued muscular and neurological development, the toddler gains the ability to stand and to take the first tentative steps. Posture, at this stage, is still more erect and less stable than in the older child or mature adult. The toddler's head is disproportionately large for the size of the body, which tends to make the toddler somewhat unstable. There is also an exaggerated lumbar curve and protruding abdomen. As the child grows and matures, the normal curvature of the spine and the growth of the body in relation to head size will produce a more upright, adult posture.

On the other end of the life span, the aging adult tends to alter posture in several ways. A common function of aging, at least in women, is the development of a stooped posture associated with osteoporosis. It is also common to see the older person lean forward more than a younger person. This forward lean has been associated with bone mineral loss, muscular weakness, and a fear of instability (Adrian, Flatten, and Lindsey 1989; Woodhull-McNeal 1992).

Psychological Aspects

The movement specialist should be prepared to deal with several psychological aspects of postural problems. For instance, not all posture problems can be explained in terms of physical causes, either musculoskeletal or environmental. Atypical postures may be symptoms of personality problems or emotional disturbances. Psychological causes for postural problems may be long term (trait), or they may be temporary (state), relating only to some short-term problem. The effect of psychological state on posture and movement is an interesting area where the study of biomechanics and the study of the psychology of physical activity are beginning to intertwine. Evidence of this resides in studies done on the correlations between mood state and performance (Huddleston et al. 2000).

PRINCIPLES APPLIED TO POSTURE

By this time the reader should understand that posture influences all we do and that it is not a static but a dynamic configuration. It should also be understood that no single ideal postural model is appropriate for all individuals. Instead, there must be an understanding of the principles that govern efficient posture. These principles must then be applied to each individual.

1. The weight-bearing segments of the body are so aligned in good standing posture that angles of inclination in the trunk and in the pelvic girdle are within "normal" limits. These limits are based on an erect posture of the pelvic girdle (lack of either posterior or anterior tilt) and the maintenance of normal spinal curves.
2. In order to be stable, the intersection of the line of gravity with the base of support will be close to the geometric center of the base. Maximum postural stability usually occurs when the line of gravity is over the center of pressure.
3. Good standing posture is a position of extension of the weight-bearing joints. This should be an easy, balanced extension and should not be accompanied by strain or tension (figures 15.3c and 15.4).
4. From the point of view of energy expenditure, good posture would seem to be a position that requires a minimum expenditure of energy *for the maintenance of good alignment.* Excess energy expenditure indicates hypertonicity or poor neuromuscular coordination, or both.
5. Good posture, in repose and in activity, permits mechanically efficient function of the

Figure 15.4   Except for a slightly forward head, the subject shows good alignment and extension without strain.

6. Good posture, both static and dynamic, requires a minimum of muscle force. This implies adequate development of the antigravity muscles to resist the pull of gravity successfully and to maintain good alignment without excessive effort or tension. It also implies a balance between antagonistic muscle groups. There is no indication, however, that "the stronger the muscles the better the posture."

7. Good posture, both static and dynamic, requires sufficient flexibility in the structures of the weight-bearing joints to permit good alignment without interference or strain. Poor flexibility may be caused by tight ligaments or fasciae, short muscles, or hypertrophied muscles. The flexibility should not be so great, however, that excessive muscular effort is needed to keep the weight-bearing joints in alignment.

8. Good posture requires good coordination. This implies good neuromuscular control and well-developed postural reflexes.

9. Adjustments in posture can be made more readily by individuals who have a good kinesthetic awareness of the postures they assume and of the degree of tension in their muscles.

10. Good posture, both static and dynamic, is favorable, or at least not detrimental, to organic function.

11. The characteristics of normal posture change with age. Young children typically have a protruding abdomen and hollow lower back. Loss of muscle strength, inactivity, and balance problems in older persons show up in a wider stance, forward head and rounded upper back, and limited flexibility in the trunk, hips, and knees.

12. In the last analysis, both the static and dynamic posture of any individual should be judged on the basis of how well it meets the demands made upon it throughout a lifetime.

joints. In other words, friction in the joints is minimized, tensions of opposing ligaments are balanced, and pressures within the joints are equalized. Hence the skeletal structure is architecturally and mechanically sound and there is a minimum of wear and tear on the joints.

POSTURAL ADAPTATIONS TO EXTERNAL CONDITIONS AND SPECIAL PROBLEMS

A number of conditions necessitate postural adjustment if one is to maintain a reasonably balanced standing position. These include standing on either an uphill or a downhill slope; standing on the level but wearing high heels; standing on a moving surface, such as bus, streetcar, subway, or train; holding a heavy bundle against the front of the body; pregnancy; and standing on one foot. In all of these the body can be relied upon to adjust automatically through the function of proprioceptors and the feedback mechanism. From the point of view of "good body mechanics," however, the nature of the adjustment may not always be desirable. For instance, one can *balance* when standing on an inclined plane by bending at the knees, hips, or spine, but it would be mechanically preferable to maintain vertical segmental alignment, as well as balance. To achieve this position one would need to stand so that the center of gravity of each weight-bearing segment was centered above the base of support. This centering can be achieved only by making the adjustment at the ankles and feet. The same is true for the person wearing high heels and for the pregnant woman, although some women lack the necessary abdominal strength for this action. It is highly desirable for them to strengthen these muscles to resist the tendency to lean back from the waist (hyperextend the spine), an adjustment that is almost sure to cause trouble in the lower back. The person carrying a heavy bundle against the front of the body may find that adjustment at the ankles is not enough, especially if the load is excessively heavy. In this case some adjustment at the knees and hips will help, but every effort should be made not to lean back at the waist (hyperextend the spine) because of the danger of lower back strain.

When standing in a moving bus, streetcar, or train, one should be prepared to make three adjustments: adjustment to acceleration, deceleration, and side-to-side sway. The same principle applies to all three—namely, establishing a comfortably wide stance in the direction of motion (forward-backward for acceleration and deceleration, and sideward for a steady speed, especially if there is a pronounced sway). During sudden acceleration, especially, the person tends to be thrown toward the back of the vehicle, in keeping with Newton's first law of motion.

The foot toward the rear, therefore, should be well braced, and more weight should be borne by the forward foot in anticipation of the jerk. The reverse is true during deceleration and stopping. In both acceleration and deceleration the body will be less likely to be thrown off balance if the knees are slightly flexed, this shortens the lever upon which the vehicle's motion acts and also lowers the center of gravity of the body.

In a crowded vehicle that makes frequent stops it may not be possible to keep adapting the stance, and one may have to rely on a hand grasp to supplement the foot adjustment. A slightly oblique stance, favoring the forward-backward direction, serves as an acceptable compromise.

The adjustment to standing on one foot is a delicate one but is usually managed automatically by the muscle, joint, and labyrinthine proprioceptors, and by the reflex response. The adjustment consists of a shift in the body weight to the single supporting limb and in the support of the pelvis on the side of the free limb. The latter adjustment requires additional effort by the quadratus lumborum and the abductors (gluteus medius and minimis, tensor fasciae latae, and oblique abdominal muscles on the support side). The iliopsoas, which is continuously active during all standing, increases its activity in steadying the lumbar spine (Basmajian and DeLuca 1985). In addition, there is probably a continuous interplay of the deep muscles of the lumbar spine and possibly of many of the lower-extremity muscles. The alternating action of the foot and ankle muscles, especially the tarsal pronators and supinators, is quite pronounced in their effort to keep the center of gravity over the narrow base of support. This problem can be helped somewhat by turning the toes slightly outward (i.e., rotating the thigh slightly outward) before the one-legged stance is assumed.

POSTURE SCREENING

Although human posture is of necessity dynamic in nature, in some instances it is beneficial to examine the static standing posture of individuals. Posture screening is one tool that may be used to evaluate the standing posture for signs of major misalignments, those that may eventually lead to problems in movement, deterioration of health, or tendency to injury.

An optimal standing posture might be described with reference to the line of gravity. Segments should be placed so that the line of gravity falls slightly anterior to the lateral malleolus and the midline of the knee joint when the knee is fully extended, slightly posterior to the hip joint axis when the hip is fully extended, and anterior to the sacroiliac joints (see figure 15.1). There is some question as to whether the line should also pass through the bodies of the lumbar and cervical vertebrae or should pass through the inflection points of the three vertebral curves. For most individuals, this alignment is controlled by the ligaments and a few appropriate muscle groups, requiring a minimal effort to maintain an erect stance.

To ascertain whether an individual has a significant postural deviation, a quick posture screening might be appropriate. The following steps need to be included:

1. The individual to be screened should wear minimal clothing (such as a bathing suit or leotard) and no shoes.
2. The individual should assume a comfortable stance. The examiner must be far enough away to view the entire body at once.
3. Observation of the relationship of the anatomical landmarks to the line of gravity is made from the side. A hanging plumb line can help in this observation.
4. Observation of the alignment of the foot, ankle, and knee is made from the front.
5. Observation for lateral deviations of the spine and unequal levels in the pelvis and shoulders are made from the rear. If scoliosis (lateral deviation) is present, one side of the back will be more prominent than the other when the individual is asked to flex the trunk.

Screening in front of a matrix expedites observation of any deviations. Marked deviations observed during static screening may be indicative of increased risk of injury. For example, when the knees, ankles, and feet are not in line, forces transmitted during running or jumping may be directed laterally, causing knee injury. Exaggerated spinal curvatures will also result in alteration of the normal transmission of forces. A serious deviation may cause significant changes in muscle strength or usage.

All misalignments create excess tensions unless the misalignment occurs as the result of "hanging from one's ligaments." However, this hanging phenomenon may eventually result in stretching of the ligaments and loss of support for segmental alignment. Greater muscle force would then be required to maintain an optimum upright posture. Faulty posture involving excess tension or requiring excess muscular involvement for motion results in fatigue and inefficient movement, which may predispose the individual to injury. Therefore, postural assessment must take into account appropriate joint alignment to minimize torque and other stresses that would require constant adjustment.

With the current data indicating postural deviations in a significant segment of the population as well as a preponderance of lower back problems in adults, it would be advisable for movement specialists to attend to a simple screening procedure and to take steps to remedy postural deviations as early as possible. Care must be taken, however, to evaluate each individual as such. Minor deviations from the suggested norm may be ignored in some cases or may require a more thorough examination to determine the root cause. It is the job of the kinesiologist to look carefully into the reasons for postural deviations and to attempt to alter only those that may be detrimental. To rework a common phrase, "If it's not broken, don't fix it."

LABORATORY EXPERIENCES

1. To demonstrate the alignment of the body segments, take from five to seven large wooden blocks, each having a vertical line painted in the center of one side. A layer of thick felt should be glued to the top and bottom of each block and a small hook screwed into each of two opposite sides.

   a. Arrange the blocks in a straight column with the painted lines in front. Connect the hooks on the sides with elastic bands. The elastic "ligaments" will be under equal tension and the felt "cartilages" under equal pressure when the column is in perfect alignment.

   b. Now insert wedges between the blocks in such a way that every other block tips to the left and the alternate blocks tip to the right. The elastic "ligaments" will now be under unequal tension and the felt "cartilages" under unequal pressure. The zigzag alignment of the painted lines illustrates graphically the poor alignment of the segments.

2. To demonstrate good and poor alignment of a single weight-bearing joint, such as the knee, two blocks arranged like those described above may be used in a similar manner.

3. Take two side-view photographs of a subject standing on a reaction board. The first photograph should represent the subject's "best" posture and the second a zigzag fatigue slump. Have another person read the scale readings at the same time the photographs are taken. Compute the distance of the line of gravity from the scale, using the method described on page 386. The length measurements (total length of board and

distance *d*) are made directly on the photograph instead of on the board itself. Draw the vertical line of gravity from the point at which the line of gravity intersects the board to a point above the head. Compare the postures and the anteroposterior positions of the line of gravity in the two photographs.

4. Take anteroposterior "line of gravity" photographs of several subjects representing various postures. Determine the location of the line of gravity for each photograph using the method described in Laboratory Experience 3. After drawing the line of gravity on each photograph, observe them carefully and note the relation of the line to the head, shoulders, upper trunk, lower trunk, pelvis, knees, and ankles.

5. Take ten anteroposterior "line of gravity" photographs of one subject within a period of one week. Compare these.

6. Take anteroposterior "line of gravity" photographs of several subjects representing different physique types. Can you make any generalizations about the relation of physique to posture?

7. Do an original posture study using a small number of subjects.

8. Perform a complete kinesiological analysis of a partner's "normal" standing posture, taking particular note of muscle participation, neuromuscular considerations, mechanical factors, and applicable principles and violations. Conclude the analysis with a prescription for improvement, including suggested methods for change and the elimination of violations of principles.

REFERENCES AND SELECTED READINGS

Adrian, M., K. Flatten, and R. Lindsey. 1989. Biomechanics and related sciences for the older adult. In *Mature stuff,* edited by D. K. Leslie. Reston, VA: AAHPERD.

Alexander, R. M. 1993. *The Human Machine.* New York: Columbia University Press.

Althoff, S. A., S. M. Heyden, and L. D. Robertson. 1988. Back to the basics: Whatever happened to posture? *Journal of Physical Education, Recreation, and Dance* 59:20–24.

Basmajian, J. V., and C. J. DeLuca. 1985. *Muscles alive.* 5th ed. Baltimore: Williams & Wilkins.

Bhatnager, V., C. G. Drury, and S. G. Schiro. 1985. Posture, postural discomfort, and performance. *Human Factors* 27:189–199.

Fairweather, M., and B. Sidaway. 1993. Idiokinetic imagery as a postural development technique. *Research Quarterly for Exercise and Sport* 64:385–92.

Fitt, S. S. 1987. Corrective exercises for two muscular imbalances. *Journal of Physical Education, Recreation, and Dance* 58:45–48.

Francis, R. S., and G. R. Bryce. 1987. Screening for musculoskeletal deviations: A challenge for the physical therapist—the Utah study. *Physical Therapy* 67:1221–25.

Franklin, M. E., and T. Conner-Kerr. 1998. An analysis of posture and back pain in the first and third trimesters of pregnancy. *Journal of Orthopaedic and Sports Physical Therapy* 28:133–38.

Hellebrandt, F. A. 1940. Physiology and the physical educator. *Research Quarterly* 11:12–29.

Huddleston, S., et al. 2000. The relationship between existing mood states and performance on a novel accuracy task. *Applied Research in Coaching and Athletics Annual* 15:85–100.

Jacobs, R., and A. B. Jacobs. 2000. Neuromuscular control strategies in postural coordination. In *Biomechanics and Neural Control of Posture and Movement,* edited by J. M. Winters and P. E. Crago. New York: Springer.

Klausen, K., K. Jeppesen, and A. Morgensen. 1978. Form and function of the erect spine in young girls. In *Biomechanics VI-B,* edited by E. Asmussen and K. Jorgensen. Baltimore: University Park Press.

Kuo, A. D., and F. E. Zajac. 1993. A biomechanical analysis of muscle strength as a limiting factor in standing posture. *Journal of Biomechanics* 26 (Suppl. 1):137–50.

Lauffenburger, S. K. 1987. Bartenieff fundamentals: Early detection of potential dance injuries. *Journal of Physical Education, Recreation, and Dance* 58:59–60.

Lehmkuhl, L. D., and L. K. Smith. 1983. *Brunnstrom's clinical kinesiology.* 4th ed. Philadelphia: F. A. Davis.

Li, Y., P. W. McClure, and N. Pratt. 1996. The effect of hamstring muscle stretching on standing posture and on lumbar and hip motions during forward bending. *Physical Therapy* 76:836–44.

Lovejoy, C. O. 1988. Evolution of human walking. *Scientific American,* November 1988, pp. 118–25.

Lundin, T. M., J. W. Feuerbach, and M. D. Grabiner. 1993. Effect of plantar flexor and dorsiflexor fatigue on unilateral postural control. *Journal of Applied Biomechanics,* 9:191–201.

Norkin, C., and P. Levangie. 1983. *Joint structure and function: A comprehensive analysis.* Philadelphia: F. A. Davis.

Pearsall, D. J., and J. G. Reid. 1992. Line of gravity relative to upright vertebral posture. *Clinical Biomechanics* 7:80–86.

Sheldon, W. H., S. S. Stevens, and W. B. Tucker. 1940. *The varieties of human physique.* New York: Harper.

Soames, R. W., and S. A. Raper. 1992. The influence of moving auditory fields on postural sway behavior in man. *European Journal of Applied Physiology* 65:241–45.

Trepman, E., R. E. Gellman, R. Solomon, K. Rameth-Murthy, L. J. Micheli, and C. J. DeLuca. 1994. Electromyographic analysis of standing posture and demiplié in ballet and modern dancers. *Medicine and Science in Sports and Exercise* 26:771–82.

Uetake, T., T. Ohtsuki, H. Tanaka, and M. Shindo. 1998. The vertebral curvature of sportsmen. *Journal of Sports Sciences* 16:621–28.

Winter, D. A., A. E. Patla, F. Prince, M. Ishac, and K. Gielo-Perczak. 1998. Stiffness control of balance in quiet standing. *Journal of Neurophysiology* 80:1211–21.

Woodhull-McNeal, A. P. 1992. Changes in posture and balance with age. *Aging: Clinical and Experimental Research* 4:219–25.

Woollacott, M. H., and A. Shumway-Cook, eds. 1989. *Development of posture and gait across the life span.* Columbia: University of South Carolina Press.

Wu, G., and W. Zhao. 1997. The role of mechanoreceptive information in the stability of human upright posture: A theoretical consideration. *Motor Control* 1:3–19.

16

KINESIOLOGY OF FITNESS AND EXERCISE

O U T L I N E

■ *Kinesiology and Exercise Programs*
Developing Flexibility
Ballistic versus Static Stretching
Active and Passive Stretching
Risk Factors in Flexibility
■ *Exercises for Muscle Strength and Endurance*
Principles Relating to Muscle
    Strength and Endurance
Risk Factors
Strength and Endurance Exercise
    Programs
■ *Modification of Common Exercises to Fit the Progressive Resistance Concept*
The Curl Sit-up
The Push-up
The Pull-up
■ *Evaluating Exercises*
■ *Laboratory Experiences*

O B J E C T I V E S

At the conclusion of this chapter, the student should be able to:

1. Define flexibility, muscular strength, and endurance, and state how each can be developed.
2. State the principles that should be followed when prescribing or engaging in exercises for flexibility.
3. Develop an appropriate exercise for improving range of motion in any joint.
4. Name and describe the five types of exercise programs used for muscle strength and development.
5. Identify the advantages and disadvantages of each type of muscle strength and endurance program.
6. Develop a graded exercise series for strengthening each of three muscle groups. Justify the selection and order of the exercises using the outline for kinesiological analysis.

KINESIOLOGY AND EXERCISE PROGRAMS

The objectives of exercise programs are to effect musculoskeletal, circulatory, and respiratory adaptations that will make possible increases in strength, flexibility, and work capacity for safer and more enjoyable motion in work, play, and activities of daily living. Indeed, the objectives are well explained by the somewhat old-fashioned term for such exercises: calisthenics. According to *Webster's Ninth New Collegiate Dictionary,* calisthenics means "the science of bodily exercise without apparatus, or with light hand apparatus, to promote strength and gracefulness."* The Greek origins of the word are indeed apropos—*kalos,* meaning beauty, and *sthenos,* meaning strength. A balance between the two is an appropriate expression of the objectives of an exercise program.

The realm of exercise is one in which the interests of the exercise physiologist and the kinesiologist overlap. Both are concerned with the energy, work, and power aspects and the musculoskeletal and neuromuscular dimensions of exercise. They diverge in their concerns with the physiologist's focus on energy sources and demands and the kinesiologist's focus on forces causing the motion and analysis of technique. Knowing what to select for an appropriate conditioning or therapeutic exercise program requires knowledge of both exercise physiology and kinesiology. As might be expected, the discussion in this chapter is limited primarily to the kinesiology of selected exercises—namely, those designed primarily to increase flexibility, develop muscular strength and endurance, and improve postural alignment. Understanding the demands of a movement will help the individual select appropriate exercises to enhance performance or rehabilitate following an injury.

DEVELOPING FLEXIBILITY

Flexibility is the ability of the tissues surrounding a joint to yield to stretching without interference or opposition and then to relax. The tissues to be stretched include not only the ligaments, fasciae, and other connective tissue related to the joints but, in many instances, the antagonistic muscles as well—that is, the muscles that oppose the movement in which the joint action is limited. For instance, the restriction in a person who is unable to bend over and touch the floor without bending the knees is even more likely to be caused by tight tendons of the hamstring muscles than by tight knee ligaments. And the person who lacks the shoulder flexibility needed for raising the arms forward-upward and past the head is hampered at least as much, if not more, by tight pectoral muscles as by tight anterior shoulder ligaments.

Joint flexibility is an important element of general health and physical fitness. Adequate flexibility is desirable for all individuals and is considered to be a possible preventer of low back pain and some of the aches and pains that accompany aging. In addition, improved performance in many sports activities, as well as prevention of injury and soreness, can result from an appropriate program of flexibility development. Using stretching exercises as part of warm-up and cooldown for other types of exercises is especially helpful in reducing injuries and soreness.

Flexibility is joint—and activity—specific. The range of motion about a joint depends on the structure of the joint and the pattern of movement to which it has been subjected. The range of motion of the shoulder is far greater than that of most other joints for all sports participants, but swimmers and baseball players require greater shoulder flexibility than do basketball players or weight lifters. Moreover, a large degree of flexibility in one joint does not mean that there will be a large degree of flexibility in another joint. For example, weight lifters often have below-average flexibility in the shoulder and above-average flexibility in the trunk, whereas swimmers often have above-average shoulder flexibility and average trunk flexibility. Individuals participating in specific activities should know the joint range of motion demands necessary for optimum performance in the activity and select appropriate flexibility exercises for each involved joint.

A general program of flexibility exercises should include those that stretch the tissues crossing the lower back, hip, shoulder, knee, and ankle. Exercises for other joints should be added as appropriate for the demands of a given activity.

Ballistic versus Static Stretching

The development of range of motion in a joint may best be accomplished using static stretching methods. In static stretching the tissues are gradually stretched up to the point of discomfort, and the resulting position is held for a minimum of thirty seconds. Ballistic stretching methods, consisting of an active bobbing or bouncing action that makes use of the momentum of the moving body part to force the involved tissues to stretch, have been shown to be equally effective in developing flexibility, but the static stretch has become the preferred method because there is less danger of tissue damage through sudden overstretching, the energy requirement is less, and there is not only less postexercise muscle soreness but this method also helps alleviate it. Another advantage is that a slow static stretch will reduce the stretch reflex contraction of the muscle being stretched. A hard ballistic stretch may trigger a phasic stretch reflex, which may then elicit a contraction of the muscle undergoing stretch. This adds to the potential for tissue damage. In spite of the potential risks, ballistic stretching programs are more likely to develop dynamic flexibility, such as that demanded in most physical activity. Ballistic stretching programs should be structured with great care. Such a program should begin with static stretches in order to establish a base flexibility. Next, slow, low-range motions should be incorporated. Gradually the program may be increased to fast, large-range motion stretches. Cau-

tion must be used to ensure that a solid base of flexibility is established before this level is reached (Alter 1996).

Active and Passive Stretching

Stretching exercises may also be classified as active or passive according to the source of the stretching force.

Active Stretching

In active stretching, the antagonists of joint actions are stretched by the concentric contraction of the contralateral muscles. In the stretch shown in figure 16.1 the muscles in the lower back and posterior leg are stretched because of the contraction of the extensors of the knee and ankle. In exercise 4.1 of appendix H the pectoral muscles and anterior shoulder structures are stretched because of the contraction of the antagonists, posterior shoulder muscles, and scapular adductors.

Active stretch patterns may be used with almost any joint or segment of the body. Other examples might be side bending stretches (with motion occurring in the spine rather than hip joints) and stretch of the anterior muscles of the thigh produced through contraction of the hip extensors while in a prone position.

Active stretching may also be assisted. In active-assisted stretching the force which produces the stretch is external. A common form of active-assisted stretching is partner stretch activity. Additionally, it is possible and popular to produce an active-assisted stretch using an external object as a point of fixation.

Passive Stretching

The passive exercise requires the help of another person or gravity unless the part of the body is one on which the subject can use another body part, such as the hands, to apply the stretch. *Except for conditions where the individual is unable to provide adequate force (as in paralysis), the assistance of another person is not a preferred method because of the danger of overstretching and injury.*

Figure 16.1   An example of active static stretching. The muscles of the lower back and posterior leg are stretched as a result of the contraction of the contralateral muscles of the legs.

Numerous exercises use the force of gravity as the stretching agent. A strong pectoral stretching exercise in which gravity does the stretching is passive hanging from a horizontal bar, or pair of rings. For a somewhat greater stretch, swinging on a trapeze or pair of flying rings is usually enjoyable as well as effective. A still different kind of pectoral stretching exercise using gravity calls for the individual to stand in an open doorway with arms extended diagonally sideward and upward with the hands braced against the door frame. Keeping them in that position, the subject leans forward from the ankles. The weight of the body in the slanting position puts the pectoral muscles and the anterior joint tissues on a stretch (see exercise 3.1 in appendix H).

Gravity also provides a stretch for the ankles in two exercises. In one, the subject stands on the bottom or next to the bottom rung of the stallbars and holds the body close to the bars by grasping a bar at about shoulder or chin level. With the feet kept parallel, the heels are lowered as far as possible in a position of dorsiflexion. This stretches the Achilles tendon as well as the posterior ligaments of the ankle (see exercise 3.3 in appendix H). In the second exercise, as the subject leans toward the wall with the feet flat on the floor, the calf muscles crossing the posterior ankle are stretched by the downward torque of the body weight applied at its center of gravity. The weight of the body also forces the heel stretch in exercise 3.2 (appendix H).

Figure 16.2   An example of passive static stretching. The anterior hip and thigh muscles are stretched by pulling up on the foot with the hand.

The quadriceps stretching exercise shown in figure 16.2 is a good example of a passive exercise in which the subject uses the hands to apply the force for the stretch. With the leg flexed at the knee, the ankle is grasped behind the body, and the anterior hip and thigh are stretched as the leg is pulled upward and posterior. Care must be taken not to apply any lateral or twisting forces, which may cause ligament, cartilage, or joint capsule damage to the knee.

A second example is used to stretch the hamstrings. While lying on the back with one knee bent to the chest the subject grasps the instep with the opposite hand. Maintaining this hold without twisting the foot, the subject pushes against the front of the knee with the other hand attempting to straighten the leg in a vertical and upward direction. A third example applied to the hip is used for stretching in the direction of abduction and outward rotation. The subject assumes the position shown in figure 3.8 in appendix H and presses down on the knees.

Proprioceptive Neuromuscular Facilitation (PNF)

In proprioceptive neuromuscular facilitation (PNF) stretching, combinations of sustained static stretch and muscular contraction are used to increase range of motion. The basic concept in PNF stretching is to avoid triggering a stretch reflex contraction in the muscle to be stretched and to make positive use of the stretch reflex, the Golgi tendon organ (GTO) response, and reciprocal innervation to further relax the stretching muscle.

Several types of PNF stretch have been identified in the literature. Among these are the repeat contraction, slow reversal, slow reversal–hold, rthymic stabilization, hold–relax, and contract–relax methods (Alter 1996). There are, in addition, several combinations of these technigues. An example of the contract–relax style of a PNF stretch would be the hamstring stretch in a long sit position. While in the long sit position the subject reaches forward slowly to grasp the ankles. In this stretch position, the subject then isometrically contracts the now-stretched hamstring muscle group to its voluntary maximum, holding the joints stationary. This static contraction should be held for ap-

proximately five seconds. Once this contraction is released, the quadriceps muscle group is contracted to produce further hip flexion while the subject uses the hands to attempt to pull the chest closer to the thighs. In this example, the sustained stretch of the hamstrings acts in the same manner discussed earlier. The contraction of the agonist hamstring muscles should produce sufficient tension in the muscle to stimulate the GTO, thereby initiating a reflex relaxation of the muscle. The following contraction of the quadriceps group further enhances this relaxation through reciprocal innervation. The PNF combination should allow for greater hip flexion than a simple static stretch.

The PNF stretch technique may be applied to any joint in the body. The key factor in PNF stretching is the active contraction of either the agonist muscle (GTO response) or the antagonist muscle (reciprocal innervation) or each in turn once the limit of range of motion has been reached. The short relaxation triggered by the two reflexes involved will allow additional stretch.

Whatever the method of stretching used, the instructor or therapist needs to be thoroughly familiar with the structure and function of the joint in question. Not only must the degree of limitation of motion be known, but it must also be known which tissues are responsible for the limitation. The effect that the various reflexes may have and the conditions under which they are likely to be active must also be considered.

Risk Factors in Flexibility

Although maintaining a level of flexibility has been found to enhance both performance and safety when applied appropriately, hypermobility, or excessive flexibility may lead to joint instability or injury. Because joint structural integrity involves soft tissues as well as bony structures, care must be taken to avoid stretches that might produce undue laxity in these supporting structures. The movement specialist should carefully examine each stretch technique to be used in order to determine the effect of the movements on the involved joint structures. The following are some examples of contraindicated stretching techniques.

Hurdler's Stretch

This technique involves sitting in a long sit position, then bringing one foot back toward the hip joint by using extreme knee flexion. This motion, utilizing knee flexion combined with hip abduction and inward rotation, stretches several of the ligamentous structures of the knee outside their normal line. This abnormal stretch places high stresses on the medial structures of the knee joint, which may lead to ligament damage and eventual instability. Similar stress in the knee may be found in the double-leg hurdle stretch, a quadriceps muscle stretch technique in which the performer sits on the heels in full knee flexion, then proceeds to lie back into full hip extension.

Standing Toe Touches

The primary concern with this exercise is the relatively high load placed on the lower back. With the small muscles of spine supporting the weight of the trunk in the stretch position, there is increased risk of low back pain or injury when returning to the upright position. One way to overcome this potentially dangerous problem is to make sure that the trunk is supported when performing back extension. One way to do this is to place the hands on the knees and use a pushing motion of the upper extremity to raise the trunk.

Deep Knee Bends (Deep Squats)

Like the hurdler's stretch, the deep knee bend places a great deal of stress on the soft tissue structures of the knee joint. Although this motion is done in the sagittal plane, which is the proper plane of motion for the knee, the torques produced in the knee can be extreme.

Alter (1996) suggests that exercises such as the bridge, torso twists, and shoulder stands may also present risks. He further indicates that inverted hanging with gravity boots, at one time popular for back pain, might also put one at risk for problems with blood pressure.

EXERCISES FOR MUSCLE STRENGTH AND ENDURANCE

The one who selects exercises for muscular strength and muscular endurance must be aware of the meaning of each of these elements of physical conditioning and understand the relationship that exists between them. *Muscle strength* is the force a muscle or muscle group can exert against a resistance in one maximum effort. *Muscle endurance* is the ability to perform repeated contractions of the muscle(s) or to sustain a contraction against a submaximal resistance for an extended period of time. These elements are related so that training with an emphasis on strength will have an effect on endurance. However, different adaptations occur within the muscle, with different training emphases. For this reason conditioning programs should be selected to be specific to the needs of a particular activity and should be patterned after the demands placed on the muscle in the activity. The most important factor in maximum strength development is the amount of resistance employed to overload the muscle. In endurance development the emphasis is placed on the number of repetitions of the movement.

Principles Relating to Muscle Strength and Endurance
Overload

This has long been recognized as the essential physiological requirement for strength development. A muscle must be exercised at or near maximal strength and endurance capacity for a specified period of time if strength and endurance are to develop. The strength of a muscle exercised against normally encountered resistances will not increase.

Specificity

Strength or endurance training activities must be specific to the demands of the particular activity for which strength or endurance is being developed. The full range of joint action, the speed, and the resistance demands of the movement pattern should be duplicated in the training activity.

Progressive Resistance

The resistance against which a muscle group is exercised must be increased periodically. Because the overload program increases strength, the original overload eventually becomes inadequate and must be supplemented with progressive increases in resistance.

Momentum

Use of momentum to initiate motion in the resistance should be minimized. Where possible, the motion should be done in a slow, controlled manner using muscle force and not momentum. One must remember, however, that speed of motion is also related to specificity. Studies have shown that high-speed resistance training with light loads can lead to improvement in performance in ballistic movements such as throwing and running (McEvoy and Newton 1998; Morrissey, Harman, and Johnson 1995).

Resistance Arm

The longer the resistance arm, the more strenuous the motion. Segments should be kept close to the body, until one is certain that individuals are capable of more strenuous effort.

Alignment and Impact

When the weight is supported by the feet, in an impact or nonimpact situation, the knees must always remain over the feet (the knee should never be twisted). When there is an alternative, low-impact work (e.g., one foot remaining on the floor) is more appropriate than high-impact work.

Frequency

A regular program of exercises should be established and followed at least three to five times per week. For muscular endurance the maximum number of repetitions used depends on the specific demands of the activity. The number of repetitions that an individual can do will depend on the actual work being performed. Because work performed will be based on repetitions, displacement, weight of the resistance, and weight of the segment, it will differ greatly from individual to individual.

Exercise Order

The order in which different muscle groups are exercised should be arranged so that each muscle group has a rest period between two exercises that stress that muscle group. The exercise order should also be planned so that the more easily fatigued muscles (the weaker ones) are exercised last.

Warm-up

All muscle strengthening and endurance workouts should be preceded by warm-up and followed by cooldown exercises. The warm-up prepares the muscles and joint tissues by increasing their temperature and permits the neuromuscular system to adjust the threshold levels, thereby making the muscles and joints less susceptible to strains and tissue tears. The cool-down helps speed recovery, removing accumulated lactic acid and, if slow static stretching is used, it also helps alleviate muscle soreness.

Maintenance

Once muscular strength and endurance are developed, they may be maintained with less frequent workout sessions. The loss of strength and endurance progresses at a slower rate than its gain. Therefore, much will be retained for an extended time. Fox, Bowers, and Foss (1988) suggest that once the difficult development phase has been accomplished, retention of strength and endurance are possible with exercise sessions once every one or two weeks, provided maximum contractions are used.

Symmetry

An appropriate balance between joint flexibility and muscle strength must be maintained for each muscle and joint as well as a balance between agonist and antagonist muscle pairs. Imbalance can lead to injury or permanent deformity.

Gravity

Maximum resistance is produced when working directly in opposition to gravity. Exercises done horizontally, or those in which the moment arm between the line of gravity of the resistance and the joint decreases, use less than maximum resistance. It is also important to remember that movements in the same direction as the line of gravity are resisted by the antagonist muscles. For example, flexion of the trunk at the hip joint while standing has a very different effect on the hip flexor muscles than the same joint action from a supine position. In the latter position the hip flexors are active, whereas in the former position they are passive.

Anthropometry

Individual differences in anthropometry must be considered in exercise. Different limb lengths produce different angular kinematics. Consequently, all individuals should not be expected to perform to the same cadence. In the same manner, all equipment is not equally well fitted to all individuals. Care must be taken in working with weight machines to see that machine lever lengths are adjusted to match each individual. Many exercise machines are not designed to fit either very large or very small bodies.

Age

As resistance training becomes more popular for young people care must be taken to prevent stress which may cause developmental problems or injury. As was discussed in chapter 2, the skeletal structure is not fully formed until the late teen years. Those who work with children are cautioned that undue, high-resistance stress on soft epiphyseal growth plates can have long-term effects such as changes in normal growth patterns. Light weights and low repetitions are recommended.

On the other end of the age spectrum, resistance training has been shown to be beneficial in elderly populations. A variety of studies have shown that balance, strength, bone density, and mobility can all be improved through resistance training. When designing a resistance training program for the elderly the movement specialist is encouraged to follow the guidelines set forth by the American College of Sports Medicine (Feigenbaum and Pollock 1999). Risk factors, discussed below, which can cause problems in healthy adults may be magnified in the elderly and caution should be used.

Risk Factors

Exercise, when properly used, is a powerful tool for positive health and well-being. It is the role of the kinesiologist to understand and to properly evaluate exercise motions and to choose those that provide a safe, enjoyable, and appropriate exercise. Because exercise is most effective when the systems of the body are required to respond to stress, potential risk is involved in exercise programs for strength and endurance. To minimize risk, some motions should be avoided. In general, in choosing exercises for strength and endurance the following guidelines should be followed:

1. **Avoid** motion to the limit of flexion and hyperextension in the cervical or lumbar regions in order to protect the vulnerable areas of the vertebral column. Therefore, when exercising, never hyperextend the trunk without stabilizing the pelvis and keeping the head in line with the neck.
2. **Avoid** combinations of motions in the vertebral column in more than one plane.

Combination motions in more than one plane executed simultaneously or in sequence increase the compressional force applied to the discs.

3. **Avoid** forcing the knee joint into extreme flexion or hyperextension. Either action may weaken ligaments and other structures in the joint.

4. **Never** hold the breath while exercising. Breathe normally through the exercise to avoid increased undue stress on the cardiovascular system through increased intrathoracic pressure.

Strength and Endurance Exercise Programs

There are five types of exercise that are used in strength and endurance programs, each using a different type of muscle action: concentric, eccentric, isometric, isotonic, and isokinetic. It is not unusual to find exercises that utilize both concentric and eccentric actions. Such exercises are referred to as isotonic exercises. Purely isotonic exercises are very difficult to produce and are not common in most exercise programs. Most common activities have elements of both concentric and eccentric exercise without being either isotonic or isokinetic.

Concentric Exercise

As generally practiced, this form of exercise involves the lifting of free weights—for example, dumbbells, disk weights, or stack weights, such as those used on the Universal Gym, through a specified range of motion. The resistance to the contracting muscles is not only the actual magnitude of the weight lifted but is the product of the weight and length of the resistance arm of the anatomical lever involved. Hence, the maximum resistance occurs only when the gravitational force is acting at right angles to the lever. The clinical value of such exercise, therefore, has been said to be "limited by its inability to impose maximum tension and work demands on a muscle

throughout its range of action." Another way of expressing this is that "resistance is constant and greatest at the extremes of the range of motion" (Rosentswieg and Hinson 1972).

During the late 1940s DeLorme and Watkins (1951) increased our awareness of the overload principle by their emphasis on *progressive resistance training,* and by the concept of the *repetition maximum* (RM). A repetition maximum is the maximum resistance a muscle group can lift a given number of times before fatiguing. Their principles for using sets of repetition maximum to develop concentric muscle strength gains are still followed in most such programs today.

Eccentric Exercise

The return movement of concentric-type exercises, when done in a slow, controlled manner, uses eccentric contraction of the antagonist muscles. Because a muscle can sustain more tension in eccentric contraction than it can develop in concentric contraction, exercise physiologists had thought that eccentric contraction exercises, or negative lifts, should be more effective in strength development than concentric exercises. The results of research to date do not support this theory. Eccentric exercises have been shown to be as effective as concentric exercises, but no more effective. Moreover, there is evidence that eccentric exercises may produce less muscle soreness than concentric exercises. On the basis of information currently available, it seems that eccentric exercise programs should not be used exclusively but that they have value if the activity to which the training is related contains eccentric contraction movement patterns.

Plyometric exercises Training programs for running, jumping, and throwing events have combined eccentric and concentric exercises into plyometric programs. These programs utilize eccentric contractions immediately followed by explosive concentric contraction. One example of a plyometric program is drop jumping. In this exercise, the individual steps or drops off a bench, allowing flexion at the knees in a normal landing. Immediately following knee flexion, one or both legs extend in a maximum explosive jump. This training works on explosiveness by taking advantage of the stretch reflex, series elastic components of muscle, and training for the synchronous firing of motor units. This combination results in a more forceful jump.

Isometric Exercise

Because an *isometric* muscle contraction is defined as involving no change in muscle length, it follows that an isometric exercise is one that involves no motion either. Isometric exercise occurs when muscles contract in a static contraction in opposition to a fixed or immovable load. Isometric exercise, although providing some strength gain, does not increase strength throughout the range of motion. Further, not all of a muscle's fibers are activated during isometric contraction. This makes isometric exercise somewhat limited in application. A primary use for isometrics currently is in the rehabilitation of muscles surrounding injured joints.

There are many drawbacks and even potential hazards when using isometric exercises. Isometric exercises increase muscle strength only and are not effective for development of other fitness components such as flexibility and cardiovascular endurance. Moreover, the strength development achieved is greatest at the specific angle of the static contraction. If the objective is the development of strength throughout the range of motion, then the isometric exercise must be done at many joint angles spread over the entire range. Finally, a static contraction activates the slow-twitch muscle fibers predominantly and therefore does not act to enhance speed of movement in any way.

Inasmuch as the extreme effort exerted in isometric exercises causes considerable internal pressure, especially if the breath is held, it is not wise for persons out of condition, such as the middle-aged or the elderly, to engage in them. The strain might be injurious to anyone with a cardiovascular impairment or with a weakness in the abdominal wall.

Isotonic Exercise

The term *isotonic* is a combination of the terms for "constant" and "tension." Hence, isotonic exercise is that in which muscular tension remains the same throughout. In fact, this state is very difficult to produce and very difficult to measure. In most exercise forms, the tension produced in muscles will vary with muscle length and with the variation in external torque. In other words, as the segment in motion moves through the range of motion, torque will vary with joint angle. A quick review of chapter 13 will refresh the student's memory of why this is true. In the 1970s fitness equipment companies started developing weight-training machines to produce isotonic exercise. The Nautilus system, as an example, employs an eccentric cam that provides a constantly changing resistance moment arm (figure 16.3). The change in the resistance arm is calculated to

Figure 16.3   One of the machines of the Nautilus system. Isokinetic exercise is possible with a different machine for each muscle group and joint action.

coincide with both the changing muscle angle of pull and changing muscle length and is intended to provide for a constant resistance torque throughout the motion. This comes close to meeting the constant tension requirements of an isotonic exercise. Equipment of this type, designed to provide this very specific type of resistance, requires a separate machine for each muscle group and joint action.

Isokinetic Exercise

Isokinetic exercise means exercise done with a constant rate of motion. An isokinetic exercise theoretically is one in which there is no acceleration and in which the velocity remains constant. To accomplish this, machines such as the Cybex (figure 16.4) have been developed. With such a machine, the angular velocity of segment motion may be preset to any selected rate within the limits of the machine. Because the machine accommodates to the force applied, it permits the individual to apply maximum force throughout the

range of motion without increasing the velocity of the motion. Maximal resistance may be applied throughout the exercise without sudden acceleration or deceleration forces. Given that optimal training requires practice of a skill at the appropriate speed (often several thousand degrees per second), use of an isokinetic device permits maximum strengthening throughout the range of motion at required speeds without endangering joints. Isokinetic devices have proved valuable in the diagnosis and rehabilitation of athletic and other joint injuries. Such devices are also widely used in research.

MODIFICATION OF COMMON EXERCISES TO FIT THE PROGRESSIVE RESISTANCE CONCEPT

Although isokinetic exercise is the superior technique for building muscular strength, it requires expensive equipment and is not feasible for class use. A practical procedure is to modify familiar exercises in such a way that the resistance to be overcome can be progressively increased. This can be done by either or both of two ways: (1) by increasing the length of the resistance arm of the involved lever and (2) by increasing the magnitude of the resistance. Among some common exercises that lend themselves well to such modifications are the sit-up, push-up, and pull-up.

The Curl Sit-up

The sit-up is a popular exercise for the development of abdominal strength and endurance. Consequently much has been written about it, and considerable research has been done on muscle and joint participation during its execution. There are many forms of the sit-up, some more rigorous than others and some more hazardous. Because of the many possible modifications, the exercise is easily adapted to form a series of safe, graded exercises once the related anatomical and mechanical factors are identified.

Figure 16.4 Isokinetic exercise for knee extensors using a Cybex machine.

Starting Position

Supine lying position with hands resting lightly on thighs, feet flat on the floor, and knee joints flexed to approximately 90 degrees.

Movement

The subject pulls in the chin and curls up to a near-sitting position. The action is then reversed and the subject curls back down to the starting position.

Essential Joint and Muscle Analysis

The format used in table 16.1 is presented as a model for the student who is just beginning to develop proficiency in motion analysis. The kinesiology student is encouraged to follow this procedure until comfortable with its use. Once the student becomes competent in this form of analysis, the level of detail may be decreased.

If the upward motion goes beyond the vertical, gravity becomes the force causing the motion, and the extensor muscles of the trunk and neck contract eccentrically to control the motion. The downward phase of the curl sit-up is the reverse motion, extension in all named joints. In this phase, gravity is the force producing the motion. The same prime movers are active but are now contracting eccentrically.

In the initial stage of the curl sit-up the rectus abdominis and external oblique muscles are acting as movers to flex the spine; the iliopsoas and other hip flexors act as stabilizers to fix the pelvis against the pull of the abdominal muscles. In the last half or two-thirds of a full sit-up, or curl-up, the hip flexors are acting as movers to flex the trunk as a whole on the thighs. If no further spinal flexion occurs, the abdominal muscles serve as stabilizers to fix the pelvis against the pull of the hip flexors. The major abdominal muscle in a straight sit-up is the rectus abdominis. If strengthening of the oblique abdominals is an objective, the sit-up action should include rotation of the spine.

Progressive Resistance Series

A set of abdominal exercises that can be performed either as a partial curl-up or a full curl-up series and that are graded from easy to more difficult according to muscular effort necessary might be as follows. All exercises are performed with the feet unsupported and the legs flexed at the knees.

1. Reverse curl. Slowly curl down from sitting position with hands on thighs. Push back up to sitting position using hands. Repeat.
2. Curl sit-up, hands under thigh to help pull-up.
3. Curl sit-up, hands resting lightly on thighs.
4. Curl sit-up, fingertips on shoulders and elbows reaching forward.

TABLE 16.1	Anatomical Analysis of the Curl Sit-up

Phase: Up Motion

Joint	Action	Segment Moved	Plane Axis	Force	Prime Movers	Contraction
Cervical spine	Flexion	Head and neck	Sagittal AP	Muscle	SCM Scalenes	Concentric
Thoracic and lumbar spine	Flexion	Trunk	Sagittal AP	Muscle	Rectus and oblique abdominals	Concentric
Hip	Flexion	Trunk	Sagittal AP	Muscle	Iliopsoas R. femoris Pectineus Sartorius	Concentric

Figure 16.5 During the course of a sit-up the length of the resistance moment arm (RA) changes, decreasing as the trunk moves toward the vertical and increasing as the trunk moves toward the horizontal.

5. Curl sit-up holding weight, increase difficulty with increased weight or move weight closer to the top of the head.
6. Curl sit-up on inclined board. (Why does the incline increase the difficulty?)

Note: The hands should never be placed behind the neck or head. Such a placement may force the neck into hyperflexion, stretching the posterior ligaments and increasing pressure on the cervical vertebrae.

Discussion

The curl sit-up provides a clear-cut example of the effect that lengthening the resistance moment arm has on the effort needed (figure 16.5). As the trunk is flexed at the hip by the hip flexors, the action is resisted by the weight of the trunk applied at the center of gravity of the trunk. The downward torque to be overcome is greatest when the trunk is nearest the horizontal because the resistance moment arm is greatest at this point. Thus, the muscular effort needed to move the trunk is also greatest at this part of the sit-up.

Muscular effort may be increased throughout the range of the action if the resistance moment arm is increased in length by moving the center of gravity of the trunk closer to the head, either by moving the arms up or by adding weights (figure 16.6). If the arms are moved and the magnitude of the weight increased, the demand made on the muscles will be increased markedly (figure 16.7).

Any sit-up motion should be done in a bent-knee position as opposed to a straight-leg position. In the straight-leg sit-up the hip flexors are on more of a stretch than in the bent-knee position, and the extended legs provide a greater force moment to resist the pull of the trunk. As might be expected, the action potentials of the hip flexors are greater in the straight-leg position than in the bent-knee position, whereas the action potentials of the rectus abdominis are greater in the bent-knee than in the straight-leg sit-up. Moreover, the results of X-ray studies suggest that there are possible dangers in the straight-leg sit-up because it causes the lordosis angle of the spine to increase, forward displacement of the fifth lumbar vertebra, and increased disc compression. For these same reasons, double leg raising and slow leg lowering from the supine position (figure 16.8) are not recommended as abdominal strengthening exercises.

There has been a good deal of controversy over whether the curl sit-up should be done with the feet anchored or unanchored. Present thinking favors the unanchored position because it is safer and requires more abdominal and less hip muscle participation than the anchored types. Anchoring the feet during the sit-up facilitates action of the hip flexors because it gives those muscles a firm anchor against which to pull. The action does result, however, in diminished electrical activity in the abdominals. Holding the feet has also been shown to produce increased lumbar curve, plac-

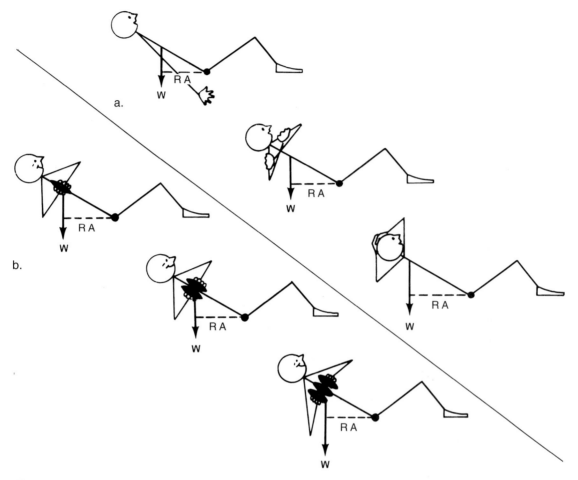

Figure 16.6   The sit-up. (a) Increasing the effort requirement by lengthening the moment arm of the trunk (RA). By moving the arms higher, the weight line W is moved higher, thus making RA longer. (b) Increasing the effort requirement by increasing the magnitude of the weight W.

ing stress on the low back (Van Leemputte, Wagemans, and Williams 1988; Mutoh et al. 1981).

The strongest action of the abdominals occurs during the first half of the traditional bent-knee sit-up motion and during the last half of the return to the ground. The curl motion, in which the head initiates movement and the trunk is flexed throughout the motion, has been found to be the most effective of the sit-up motions in strengthening the abdominals. A partial curl, often called a "crunch," involves trunk flexion to

less than 45 degrees. The crunch produces activity primarily in the abdominals, with little activity in the hip flexors. The crunch is presently accepted as the preferred abdominal exercise (figure 16.9).

A common fault in the sit-up is coming up or at least starting too quickly, using momentum rather than gradual muscle contraction. This nullifies the value of the exercise. Beginners are sometimes tempted to push off with the elbows, but this can be prevented if care is taken to see that the arms are in the correct position.

a.

b.

c.

d.

e.

Figure 16.7 Partial curl-up series for abdominal strength.

Figure 16.8 Slow leg lowering. Note the increased curve of the lumbar spine.

Figure 16.9 The partial curl-up, or "crunch." The head and shoulders are raised until the scapulae are clear of the floor.

Principles for Selecting Abdominal Exercises

1. The criterion for an abdominal exercise performed in the supine position is the performer's ability to prevent the tilting of the pelvis and the hyperextension of the lumbar spine. If the pelvic tilt and lumbar curve increase, it would seem to indicate the failure of the abdominal muscles to stabilize the pelvis and spine against the pull of the iliopsoas. Since the task is too great for these muscles, there is danger of straining them and stressing lumbar vertebrae and discs.

2. An objective in building a strong abdominal wall is to strengthen all four of the abdominal muscles: rectus abdominis, external oblique, internal oblique, and transversus abdominis. To do this successfully requires a knowledge of the exercises in which these muscles

participate and of the relative intensity of their action.

3. It seems reasonable to assume that a protruding abdomen indicates that the abdominal muscles have been stretched. It would seem to be a function of abdominal exercises, therefore, to shorten as well as to strengthen these muscles. This suggests that exercises such as back bends that put the abdominal wall in a stretched position are not desirable for strengthening.

The Push-up

The push-up is an exercise for strengthening the elbow extensors and the anterior shoulder and chest muscles. The basic exercise is described and analyzed first, and then a graded series of variations of this activity is suggested.

Starting Position

The front-leaning rest position—that is, semi-prone with the body extended, the arms extended vertically toward the floor, and the weight sup-

ported by the hands and toes. The body is in a straight line from head to heels; there is no sag at the spine or hump at the hips. The hands are approximately shoulder-width apart with the palms flat on the floor.

Movement

With the body kept straight the arms are allowed to flex at the elbow joints and the body is lowered until the chest almost touches the floor. By pushing the hands vigorously against the floor, the body is raised until it regains the starting position.

Because the hands are stabilized against the floor the segments being moved are as follows: forearm acting about the wrist joint, the upper arm acting about the elbow joint, and the trunk acting about the shoulder joints. The force causing the motion is gravity when dipping and muscle when executing the push-up.

Essential Joint and Muscle Analysis

The dip   Flexion at the elbow joint accompanied by a lowering of the body until it almost touches the floor (figure 16.10b and table 16.2).

TABLE 16.2	Anatomical Analysis of the Curl Sit-up				
Joint	**Joint Action**	**Segment Moved**	**Force for Movement**	**Muscles Active**	**Kind of Contraction**
Shoulder joints	Horizontal abduction	Trunk	Gravity	Pectoralis major Anterior deltoid Coracobrachialis	Eccentric
Shoulder girdle	Adduction	Scapula	Gravity	Pectoralis minor Serratus anterior	Eccentric
Elbows	Flexion	Upper arm	Gravity	Triceps Anconeus	Eccentric
Wrists	Reduction of hyperextension	Forearm	Gravity	Extensor carpi radialis longus and brevis Extensor carpi ulnaris	Eccentric
Maintenance of straight alignment from head to heels against the pull of gravity:					
Head and neck	None	None		Cervical extensors	Static
Lumbar spine	None	None		Rectus abdominus Obliques	Static
Hips	None	None		Flexors	Static

TABLE 16.3		**Anatomical Analysis of the Push-up**			

Joint	Joint Action	Segment Moved	Force for Movement	Muscles Active	Kind of Contraction
Shoulder joints	Horizontal adduction	Trunk	Muscle	Pectoralis major Anterior deltoid Coracobrachialis	Concentric
Shoulder girdle	Abduction	Scapula	Muscle	Pectoralis minor Serratus anterior	Concentric
Elbows	Extension	Upper arm	Muscle	Triceps Anconeus	Concentric
Wrists	Hyperextension	Forearm	Muscle	Extensor carpi radialis longus and brevis Extensor carpi ulnaris	Concentric

a.

b.

Figure 16.10   The push-up: (a) the starting and ending position; (b) the dip.

The push-up   Extension at the elbow joints until the body is again in the position shown in figure 16.10a and table 16.3.

Maintenance of straight alignment from head to heels is the same for both the dip and the push-up.

Progressive Resistance Series

In the push-up, the familiar form of the exercise represents the most difficult level in the series. Starting at what might be considered the lowest level and working up, the following push-up exercises are suggested.

1. Resting on hands and knees with legs flexed at right angles at hip and knee joints, dip and push up.
2. In semiprone position with leg extended at the hip and weight supported by hands and knees, perform a half-dip and push-up (figure 16.11a).

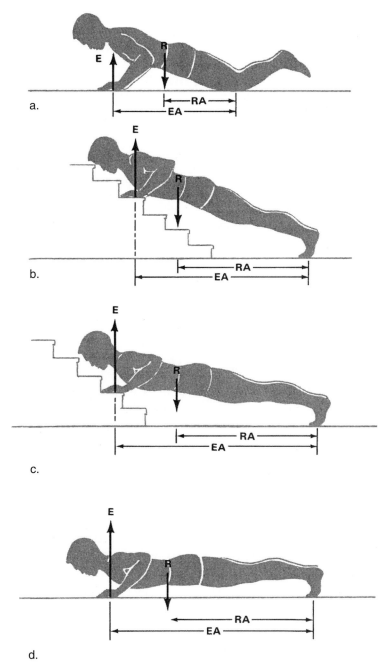

Figure 16.11   Push-up series for arm strength. As the ratio of the resistance moment arm (RA) to the effort moment arm (EA) increases in magnitude, the effort must also increase so that E × EA is greater than R × RA. Only then will the push-up occur. The order of increasing difficulty in this series is a, b, c, d.

3. Same position as for 2, but complete the full dip and push-up.
4. Front-leaning rest position, facing stairs with feet on floor and hands on fourth or fifth step, body in a straight line from head to heels, dip and push up (figure 16.11b).
5. Continue, placing hands on lower step until able to perform regulation push-up from floor (figure 16.11d).

Discussion

A student may have to work up to a full push-up in any of the positions by first performing only the negative lift phase, (letdown) or a half push-up, that is, a push-up from a half-dip position. Whatever type of push-up that is practiced, the student should be able to repeat it several times in good form before being permitted to try a more advanced type.

Two common faults must be guarded against in the push-up. They are (1) a sagging back and (2) humped up hips. The latter fault is usually caused by an "overcorrection" of the first one—namely, maintaining a flexed position at the hips to prevent the back from sagging. The correction of both of these faults lies in strengthening the abdominal muscles and training them to prevent hyperextension of the lumbar spine when the body is in the extended position. Until the subject is kinesthetically aware of this position, the use of a mirror may be helpful.

The differences in difficulty among the forms of push-up shown in figure 16.11 are primarily due to the length of the resistance moment arm in proportion to the effort moment arm. As the proportion of RA to EA increases in size, the effort in relation to the resistance also must increase ($E \cdot EA = R \cdot RA$). This can be demonstrated by placing a bathroom scale under each hand. An additional reason for the ease of the push-up from the knees (figure 16.11a) is the fact that less body weight (lower legs subtracted) is being pushed up.

The push-up from a half-dip is easier than the push-up from a full dip in any given position because the weight of the body is lifted through a shorter distance and because the joint positions permit the muscles of the elbows and shoulders to work to better advantage. The reverse dip is easier to execute than the push-up from any given level because the muscles are performing negative rather than positive work; that is, they are engaging in eccentric (lengthening) rather than concentric (shortening) contraction.

The Pull-up

The pull-up is an exercise for strengthening the elbow flexors, shoulder joint extensors, scapular adductors, and downward rotators.

Starting Position

Straight-arm hanging from a horizontal bar with the hands approximately shoulder-width apart, the palms facing the body, and the thumb in opposition to the fingers (figure 16.12c).

Movement

From a "dead hang" and with a minimum of movement of the trunk and lower extremities, the subject pulls steadily upward until the chin is level with the bar.

Return Movement

Reverse joint action of shoulder joints and girdle and elbows; same muscles but contracting eccentrically instead of concentrically; finger and thumb muscles remain in static contraction.

Graded Exercise Series
Easier pull-ups

1. Bent-arm hang, with chin above bar and with legs straight and feet off the ground (figure 16.12a).
2. Reverse pull-up—that is, slow letdown from bent-arm hanging position that can be reached by stepping onto a stool or by jumping.
3. Modified pull-up from low boom or bar with body in semisupine hanging position, arms straight, heels on floor, and body straight from heels to head.

Figure 16.12 Pull-up series for arm strength: (a) bent-arm hanging; (b) halfway position; (c) straight-arm hanging. [For pull-up, start with (c) and end with (a).)]

TABLE 16.4	Anatomical Analysis of the Pull-up				
Joint	**Joint Action**	**Segment Moved**	**Force for Movement**	**Muscles Active**	**Kind of Contraction**
Shoulder joints	Extension	Trunk	Muscle	Pectoralis major Latissimus dorsi Teres major Posterior deltoid	Concentric
Shoulder girdle	Downward rotation/ adduction	Scapula	Muscle	Rhomboids Trapezius III and IV Pectoralis minor	Concentric
Elbows	Flexion	Upper arm	Muscle	Biceps Brachialis Brachioradialis	Concentric
Wrists	Slight flexion	Forearm			Static
Fingers				Flexors	Static
Thumb	Adduction	Thumb	Muscle	Adductor pollicus	Concentric

4. Standing on bench high enough to permit subject to grasp bar (or rings) with elbows partially flexed and pull up the rest of the way.

More difficult pull-up Basic pull-up with weights attached to waist or ankles.

Discussion

The pull-up is a popular exercise for testing upper-arm and shoulder girdle strength, and some form of the exercise is commonly included in most fitness test batteries. There is no general agreement, however, about the forearm position to be taught for this exercise. Some tests specify a pronated forearm grasp and others a supinated grasp. Still others suggest the semipronated position as a compromise. Research evidence (functional tests as well as EMG studies) appears to support the supinated forearm grasp as the one most subjects find easiest. The main reason for this may be that the biceps brachii has a mechanical advantage in this position because of its straight line of pull. In the pronated position the line of pull is oblique because of the twisting of the radius to which the biceps tendon attaches.

Advocates of the supine grasp position cite its mechanical efficiency and the fact that those with low strength capabilities will have greater success with this form. Those who favor the prone position identify its use in tasks such as scaling walls or in gymnastics events on the uneven or high bars. From a kinesiological point of view it appears that the supinated grasp should be used because of its performance superiority whenever a choice is appropriate, but that both forms of pull-up should be mastered in anticipation of those situations where choice is not an option.

EVALUATING EXERCISES

If the discussions and applications of exercises that have been presented in this chapter have helped give the student a sound basis for developing an effective exercise program, the chapter will have served its purpose. Exercise instructors who have a good kinesiological background should be able to analyze and evaluate exercises, not only those with which they are already familiar, but also those that are brought to their attention by their students or are seen on television or in popular magazines. They should be able to tell whether exercises are suitable for the inexperienced performer, a performer of moderate experience and ability, or an advanced performer. They should know whether the exercises have undesirable features such as the danger of straining ligaments, encouraging posture faults, or causing excessive tension. They should also recognize the mechanical problems that may be involved, such as problems of balance, leverage, or momentum. In brief, evaluation of exercises should be based on the answers to the following questions:

1. What is the purpose of the exercise?
2. How effectively does it accomplish its purpose?
3. Does it violate any principles of good mechanics?
4. What are the chief joint and muscular actions involved in it?
5. What are its intensity and difficulty? (Is it suitable for a beginner, a moderately experienced performer, or an advanced performer?)
6. Are there any elements of danger, injury, or strain against which precautions should be taken?
7. Is it likely to call forth any undesirable or harmful responses against which the performer should be on guard?
8. If the exercise is a difficult one, what preliminary exercise would serve to prepare the performer for it?

When the exercise instructor has acquired skill in answering such questions as these and in analyzing the individual needs of students, he or she will be well on the way toward becoming a true kinesiologist. To assist in the achievement of this goal, the student should find it profitable to analyze as many exercises as possible. Table 1.1 and appendix H should prove helpful in this connection.

LABORATORY EXPERIENCES

1. Turn to appendix H. State the purpose and give the essential joint and muscle analysis for as many of the exercises as possible in Series 1 through 4.

2. Select from three to ten exercises seen in popular magazines, newspapers, videos, or on television. Using the examples in this chapter as guides, analyze and evaluate these exercises and answer the eight questions in the preceding section.

3. Observe someone doing a conditioning exercise. Analyze the exercise, using the examples in this chapter as guides.

4. Originate an exercise for stretching the hamstring muscles that will not tend to accentuate a round upper back.

5. In the straight-leg lowering exercise from supine lying, identify the resistance moment arm of the lever and also the rotary component of the resistance (see p. 424 and figure 16.8). Under what circumstances, if any, would it be appropriate for an individual to do this exercise?

6. Devise an exercise for a swimmer who wants to increase ankle flexibility, especially plantar flexion. (*Note:* Merely plantar flexing the feet volitionally is not forceful enough to increase the range of motion.)

7. Do an anatomical and mechanical analysis of a piece of "gimmick" exercise equipment. Determine to what extent the device fulfills its stated purpose. Apply each of the evaluation questions on page 432–433 to this device.

8. Devise an exercise for a person who is unable to get out of the deep end of a pool onto the deck without using the stairs. Validate its appropriateness by performing a complete kinesiological analysis following the outline presented in chapter 1.

9. Perform a complete kinesiological analysis of an exercise selected from appendix H, taking particular note of the purpose of the exercise, its classification, and the nature of the motion. Include also muscle participation, neuromuscular considerations, mechanical factors, and applicable principles and violations. Conclude the analysis with a prescription for improvement, including suggested methods for change and for the elimination of violations of principles.

REFERENCES AND SELECTED READINGS

Alter, M. J. 1996. *Science of flexibility.* Champaign, IL: Human Kinetics.

Baltzopoulos, V., and D. A. Brodie. 1989. Isokinetic dynamometer. *Sports Medicine* 8:101–16.

Bynes, W. C., P. M. Clarkson, and F. I. Katch. 1985. Muscle soreness following resistance exercise with and without eccentric contraction. *Research Quarterly* 56(3):283–85.

Corbin, C., and R. Lindsey. 1988. *Concepts of physical fitness.* Dubuque, IA: Wm. C. Brown.

DeLorme, T. L., and A. L. Watkins. 1951. *Progressive resistance exercise.* New York: Appleton-Century-Crofts.

Etnyre, B. R., and E. J. Lee. 1988. Chronic and acute flexibility of men and women using three different stretching techniques. *Research Quarterly* 59(3):222–28.

Feigenbaum, M. S., and M. L. Pollock. 1999. Prescription of resistance training for health and disease. *Medicine and Science in Sports and Exercise* 31(1):38–45.

Fox, E. L., D. W. Bowers, and M. L. Foss. 1988. *The physiological basis of physical education and athletics.* 4th ed. Philadelphia: Saunders.

Guimares, A. C. S., M. A. Vaz, M. I. De Campos, and R. Maratntes. 1991. The contribution of the rectus abdominis and rectus femoris in twelve selected abdominal exercises. *Journal of Sports Medicine and Physical Fitness* 31:222–30.

Hardy, L. 1985. Improving active range of hip flexion. *Research Quarterly* 56(2):111–14.

Hardy, L., and D. Jones. 1986. Dynamic flexibility and proprioceptive neuromuscular facilitation. *Research Quarterly* 57(2):150–53.

Kellis, E., and V. Baltzopoulos. 1995. Isokinetic eccentric exercise. *Sports Medicine* 19:202–22.

Lindsey, R., and C. Corbin. 1989. Questionable exercises: Some safer alternatives. *Journal of Physical Education, Recreation, and Dance* 60:26–32.

McEvoy, K. P., and R. U. Newton. 1998. Baseball throwing speed and base running: The effect of ballistic resistance training. *Journal of Strength and Conditioning Research* 12:216–21.

Morrissey, M. C., E. A. Harman, and M. J. Johnson. 1995. Resistance training modes: Specificity and effectiveness. *Medicine and Science in Sports and Exercise* 27:648–60.

Mutoh, Y., T. Mori, Y. Nakamura, and M. Miyashita. 1981. The relation between sit-up exercises and the occurrence of low back pain. In *International series on biomechanics: Biomechanics VIII-A,* edited by H. Matsui and K. Kobayashi. Baltimore: University Park Press.

Pollock, M. L., G. A. Gaesser, J. D. Butcher, J. P. Despres, R. K. Dishman, B. A. Franklin, and C. Ewing-Garber. 1998. American College of Sports Medicine position stand: The recommended quantity and quality exercise for developing and maintaining cardiorespiratory and muscular fitness and flexibility in healthy adults. *Medicine and Science in Sports and Exercise* 30:975–91.

Rosentswieg, J., and M. M. Hinson. 1972. Comparison of isometric, isotonic, and isokinetic exercises by electromyography. *Archives of Physical Medicine and Rehabilitation* 53:249.

Sharper, G. L., W. P. Liemohn, and L. B. Snodgrass. 1988. Exercise prescription and the low back. *Journal of Physical Education, Recreation, and Dance* 59:74–78.

Timmermans, H. M., and M. Martin. 1987. Top ten potential dangerous exercises. *Journal of Physical Education, Recreation, and Dance* 58:29–31.

Van Leemputte, M., E. Wagemans, and E. Williams. 1988. Activity and curvature of the back during different abdominal exercises. In *Proceedings of the American Society of Biomechanics,* 67–68. University of Illinois at Urbana–Champaign.

17

MOVING OBJECTS: PUSHING AND PULLING

OUTLINE

- ***Pushing and Pulling***
  Joint Action Patterns
  Nature of Force Application
- ***Principles of Pushing and Pulling Motions***
  Principles Relating to the Magnitude of Force
  Principles Relating to the Direction of Force
  Principles Relating to the Point at Which the Force Is Applied
- ***Push–Pull Applications***
  Pushing and Pulling
  Lifting, Holding, and Carrying
  Weight Lifting
  Punching
  Working with Long-Handled Implements
- ***Analysis of the Push-Pull Pattern in Ergometer Rowing***
  Anatomical Analysis
  Mechanical Analysis
- ***Laboratory Experiences***

OBJECTIVES

At the conclusion of this chapter, the student should be able to:

1. Classify activities involving push or pull patterns according to the nature of the force application.
2. Name and discuss anatomical and mechanical factors and principles that apply to representative push or pull activities.
3. Analyze the performance of someone performing a push–pull skill under each of these force application conditions: momentary contact, projection, or continuous application. Follow the kinesiological analysis outline presented in chapter 1.

PUSHING AND PULLING

A person pushes a table across the room, a boxer jabs at an opponent, a traveler lifts a suitcase onto an overhead rack, an archer shoots an arrow from a bow, and a schoolteacher lifts open a window. As widely diverse as these activities seem, they all have a common denominator: Each involves moving an external object, either directly by some part of the body or by means of an implement, in a pushing or pulling pattern.

Joint Action Patterns

In pushing and pulling patterns of motion, the basic joint actions are flexion and extension in one or more of the extremities. The joint actions in the upper extremities are characterized by flexion and extension in the elbow while the opposite movement is occurring in the shoulder. In the lower extremities, extension occurs simultaneously in the hip, knee, and ankle. This simultaneous and opposite joint action is a primary characteristic of push–pull patterns. All joint motions occur at the same time or very near the same time.

The simultaneous nature of the joint motions in push and pull patterns produces a rectilinear path of motion at the distal end point of the segments involved, as opposed to a curvilinear path. Such a rectilinear path means that all forces produced by segmental motion are applied directly to the object and that this force is applied in the direction of motion. Keeping this in mind makes it apparent that the primarily simultaneous push–pull patterns are of greatest value when it is important to apply a large force (overcome a large resistance) or to apply a force with maximum accuracy. All the forces involved are applied directly in line with the object being moved. There are no large-magnitude tangential forces.

A push, pull, or lift may be applied either directly or indirectly to an object. In the latter instance, the push or pull pattern is used to develop potential energy in an elastic device such as a bow or slingshot. When the elastic structure is released,

Figure 17.1 Push-pull patterns used in skills requiring momentary contact: (a) volleyball set; (b) heading in soccer; (c) fencing lunge.

it imparts force to the movable object, causing the arrow or shot to be projected into the air.

Nature of Force Application
Momentary Contact

Movements such as striking and hitting are characterized by momentary contact made with an object by a moving part of the body or by a held implement. The object itself may be either stationary or moving. A volleyball pass, a heading in soccer, and a fencing lunge are examples of momentary contact push and pull patterns (figure 17.1).

a.   b.   c.

Figure 17.2   Push–pull patterns used to project objects: (a) shot put; (b) chest pass; (c) free throw.

Projection

This type of force application is characterized by the development of kinetic energy in a movable object that is held in the hand or hands, followed by the release of the object at the moment of desired speed or direction. Push and pull patterns are used for projection when the projected object has considerable mass (e.g., shot put) or when great accuracy is desired (e.g., free throw in basketball, chest pass, dart throwing) (figure 17.2).

Continuous Application

Movements in this category are characterized by the continuous application of force, usually by the hand or hands, but the legs may also be included. Most activities involving moving large resistance fall into this category (e.g., weight lifting, push-

ing heavy objects), although maintaining a push or pull position while waiting for release may also be classified as continuous (e.g., archery) (figure 17.3).

PRINCIPLES OF PUSHING AND PULLING MOTIONS

However motion is given, whether by hand, foot, head, or implement, it involves the imparting of force. And force, or effort, is described in terms of its magnitude, direction, and point of application. These three aspects of force provide the basis for the principles that apply to giving motion to external objects through pushing and pulling, the objects on occasion being other human bodies. Supplementing these aspects are

Figure 17.3   Push–pull patterns used in continuous application: (a) pushing a car; (b) pulling; (c) lifting.

the factors that relate to the stability of the body at the moment of giving motion; those that relate to the interaction between the body and the surface that supports it (for unless the body is stable when it is giving impetus, much of the force is wasted); and those that relate specifically to struck objects. The underlying mechanical principles have been presented in Part II. Stated briefly in descriptive terms, they are as follows.

Principles Relating to the Magnitude of Force

1. The object will move only if the force is of sufficient magnitude to overcome the object's inertia. The force must be great enough to overcome not only the mass of the object but also all restraining forces. These include (1) friction between the object and

the supporting surface, (2) resistance of the surrounding medium (e.g., wind or water), and (3) internal resistance. Warming up helps prevent injury as well as decrease resistance. Increasing range of motion through training is also important and effective in reducing internal resistance.

2. Force exerted by the body will be transferred to an external object in proportion to the effectiveness of the counterforce of the feet (or other parts of the body) against the ground (or other supporting surface). This effectiveness depends on the counterpressure and friction presented by the supporting surface. The force applied to a ball thrown while in midair or while treading water is less than that applied to it while pushing against the ground.

3. Optimum summation of internal force is needed if maximum force is to be applied to move an object. The maximum number of segments that can safely be employed should be moved through the largest possible safe range of motion for maximum force production in a push or pull pattern.

4. For maximum accuracy, the smallest possible number of segments should be used through the smallest possible range of motion. The smaller motion limits the amount of error that is likely to be introduced into the rectilinear path.

5. For a change in momentum to occur, force must be applied over time (impulse). If maximum force is desired in projection-type activities, maximum muscle torques should be applied over as long a time as possible.

Principles Relating to the Direction of Force

6. The direction in which the object moves is determined by the direction of the force *applied* to it. If the force consists of two or more components, the object will move in the direction of the resultant of those components. After being projected or struck, the direction will be modified by gravity and air resistance.

7. If an object is free to move only along a predetermined pathway (as in the case of a window or sliding door), any component of force not in the direction of this pathway is wasted and may serve to increase friction.

8. When optimum force production is the purpose of the push or pull pattern, those segments involved should be aligned with the direction of intended force production. A misalignment of segments will produce high internal torque, thereby increasing the risk of injury.

Principles Relating to the Point at Which the Force Is Applied

9. Force applied in line with an object's center of gravity will result in linear motion of the object, provided the latter is freely movable.

10. If the force applied to a freely movable object is not in line with the latter's center of gravity, it will result in rotary motion of the object.

11. If the free motion of an object is interfered with by friction or by the presence of an obstacle, rotary motion may result, even though the force is applied in line with the object's center of gravity.

PUSH-PULL APPLICATIONS

Pushing and Pulling

The great majority of pushing, pulling, and lifting activities undoubtedly occur in everyday tasks. A number of sports, however, involve the continuous pushing or pulling of external objects. Archery is an interesting example, because it consists of pulling with one hand while pushing with the other. The same is true of using a forked-stick slingshot. Pushing is also used in football, and both pushing and pulling are used in wrestling. Weight lifting is the prime example of a sport activity involving lifting.

Rowing and paddling, although classified as forms of aquatic locomotion, may also be considered activities that involve external objects. Oars and paddles are both moved by continual pushing and pulling movements. Pole vaulting, rope climbing (previously classified as locomotor), and all suspension activities might also be included in the pushing and pulling category, provided one accepts activities that involve the moving of the body by means of pushing or pulling an external object, the object in such cases also serving as the means of body support.

The magnitude of the force used in pushing, pulling, and lifting can be increased in two ways. The immediate way is by using the lower extremities and, in some instances, the body weight to supplement the force provided by the upper extremities. In many, if not most, pushing and pulling activities the direction and point of application of force are interrelated. They both have an important bearing on the effectiveness of the force exerted, and also on the economy of effort and avoidance of strain. Economy of effort is ensured when the force is applied in line with the object's center of gravity and in the desired direction of motion. When this application of force is not feasible, the undesirable component of force should be as small as possible. For instance, if one desires to push a low trunk across the floor, it would be difficult to stoop low enough to push with the arms or even the forearms in a horizontal position. One should stoop as low as conveniently possible, however, to reduce the downward component of force that would tend to increase friction. If it were necessary to move the trunk down a long corridor, it would be more efficient to tie a rope to the handle at one end and pull it. By using a long rope, the horizontal component of force would be relatively great and the vertical or lifting component relatively small. Some lifting component would be desirable, however, as it would serve to reduce friction.

When friction is a major obstacle, as when pushing a tall object such as a filing cabinet across a carpeted floor, the horizontal push should be applied close to the cabinet's center of gravity at a point found by experimentation (figure 17.4). When this point is found, it will be possible to push the cabinet without tipping it. When it does not seem practical to slide a heavy object along the floor, one may try "walking" it on opposite corners. This involves tipping the object until it is resting on one edge of its base and then, by a series of partial rotations, alternately pivoting it first on one corner and then on the other. The arms alternate in a lever action, one hand holding the upper corner that corresponds to the lower one that is serving as the pivot, and the other hand pushing the diagonally opposite upper corner forward.

When attempting to pull an object, the same general directions apply, but with this exception. As in the case of pulling the low trunk by a rope, it may be advantageous to pull in a slightly upward direction because the lifting effect would help reduce friction. Nevertheless, unless one wishes to rotate the object, the pull should be applied in line with the object's line of gravity.

When applying a pull or a push to an object that must move on a track, such as a window or a sliding garage door or a weight on a weight machine, it is essential to apply the force in the direction that the track or runway permits. Force in any other direction is wasted and friction is increased. Trying to open a heavy window or one that sticks can be done by standing with the right side next to it, the arm close to the body, elbow fully flexed, and the heel of the hand placed beneath a crosspiece of the frame, and then pushing vertically upward. If more force is needed, the knees and hips should be flexed and the hands placed against a lower crosspiece. The extension of the lower extremities then supplements the force exerted by the arm with little increase in the length of the resistance arm. If this action is inadequate, both hands can be used by twisting the trunk to face the window. In pulling the window down, one should face it, stand as close as possi-

Figure 17.4 Using the lower extremities and body weight to supplement the upper extremities in a pushing task.

ble, and use both hands, being careful to apply the force vertically downward.

Lifting, Holding, and Carrying
Lifting

Lifting is a form of pulling; it is pulling a movable object vertically or obliquely upward. The more nearly vertical the pull and the more in line with the object's center of gravity, the more efficient is the lift. The principle involved here is that of minimizing the resistance arm of a lever to reduce the amount of effort needed to lift a given weight. For instance, to give an extreme example, less effort is needed to lift and hold a heavy package close to the body than to lift and hold it at arm's length. Likewise it takes less effort to lift a suitcase by bending the knees than by bending from the waist with the knees kept straight (figure 17.5). In bending, the resistance arm of the lever is the horizontal distance from the center of the knee joint to the body's line of gravity; in bending from the waist, the resistance arm of the lever is the horizontal distance from the center of the hip joint to the body's line of gravity. Other factors are involved here, too, but the relative length of the resistance arm is an important one. Also, because of the shorter resistance arm, it takes less effort to lift by bending with the trunk inclined slightly forward than with the trunk held in, or close to, a vertical position. That this is a mechanically more efficient method of squatting (and rising from a squat) may easily be demonstrated by the use of line-of-gravity photographs (figure 17.6).

In squatting, the thigh serves as the lever, the knee joint as the fulcrum, and the point at which the line of gravity intersects the thigh as the resistance point. The resistance moment arm is the horizontal distance from the fulcrum to the line of gravity. Figure 17.6 is based on two line-of-gravity photographs taken by Wells of one subject first (a) attempting to keep the trunk as nearly vertical as possible, and then (b) inclining the trunk slightly forward from the hips in what felt to the subject like a comfortable position. In the original photographs the moment arm of the lever in figure 17.6 a measured 17 mm and in figure 17.6 b, 14 mm. The actual (life-sized) difference in the

Figure 17.5   Picking up a suitcase: (a) efficiently; (b) inefficiently.

Figure 17.6   Squatting: (a) attempting to keep the trunk vertical; (b) inclining the body slightly forward. (*RA* = the moment arm of the thigh lever.)

two moment arms was approximately 4.5 cm. Current models are very close to these early measurements, adopting a 5-cm moment arm in industrial modeling (McGill and Norman, 1993). Although it is true that more effort is required to lift the weight of the torso itself from a full squat than from a bend at the waist, the latter method endangers the joints and muscles of the lower back (figure 17.6 b). It requires strong action of the hip and spine extensors, and the latter muscles are forced to work in a stretched condition.

If the body is used in this manner for lifting heavy objects, an additional burden is put on the muscles of the back, one that they can ill afford to take. In computer-generated models of the action of the vertebral muscles, it has been determined

Figure 17.7 Bending from the waist to reach the floor not only puts a strain on the back muscles, but also subjects the fifth lumbar vertebra to a compression force of nearly 900 N.

Figure 17.8 A safe and efficient method of lifting a heavy object.

that in a resisted flexion task against a 40-N·m applied torque, the muscle contraction force in the erector spinae reached 419 N, with an intervertebral compressive force of as high as 894 N (Ashton-Miller and Schultz 1988) (figure 17.7). The spinal extensors are not powerful muscles and are easily strained. It is unwise to expose them to the danger of strain when this can be avoided by observing the principles of good mechanics (figure 17.8).

There are several other risk factors in lifting that have been identified as causes of back pain and back injury. The first of these, high velocity or jerky lifting, has the mechanical effect of increasing the inertial load on the muscles and structures of the spine. Twisting while lifting should also be avoided at all times. This is especially true when the spine is flexed. Even small amounts of twisting during lifting have been found to greatly increase compression loads on the spine (McGill and Norman 1993).

Holding and Carrying

Although holding and carrying are not push–pull patterns, being static in nature, they are often related to the lifting motion just described. In holding, effort can be minimized by supporting the

object from underneath, with only enough force applied to counteract the downward pull of gravity. Again, as in lifting, the closer the held object is to the line of gravity, the shorter the resistance arm, thus decreasing the torque produced by the object.

An object held in a pincerlike fashion between the fingers and thumb (figure 6.30a) is an inefficient form for holding an object of any sizable mass, although it is excellent for fine control. The object held in this grip is supported by the relatively weak muscle of the thumb and hand supplying sufficient pressure to maintain the level of friction required. As these muscles fatigue, the pressure between the object and the fingers is reduced, friction decreases, and the object falls because of the downward force of gravity. Holding positions that offer support against gravity or use of the larger muscle groups of the forearm are more effective and efficient (see figure 6.30b, d, e).

The most efficient manner of carrying objects (the translation of a held object) is that which requires the least accommodation of the body's center of gravity. Objects may be carried in a variety of positions, such as on top of the head, in front of the body, to one side, or strapped on the back. In each case, the object becomes part of the moving body and therefore affects the location of the body's center of gravity. Therefore, the larger the mass of the object and the farther away from the body the object is located, the greater the change in the center of gravity of the total moving object–body system. The greater the change in the position of the center of gravity, the greater the necessity for segmental realignment of posture. As was discussed in chapter 15, any postural deviation can increase stress on the body, often creating weakness or a predisposition to injury. Objects carried on top of the head raise the center of gravity of the moving system. The objects are also precariously perched on a relatively small, rounded base of support. This carrying position, however, places the object in line with the body's line of gravity, causing no relocation of the center of gravity in either the sagittal or frontal plane and producing little or no external torque on the vertebral column. In many cultures this is the preferred method of carrying. The higher center of gravity does necessitate a more cautious approach to locomotion, as balance is somewhat precarious.

A more commonly preferred method of carrying objects is to place equal loads on either side of the body. This creates a state of equilibrium within the system. Each separate load offsets the influence of the other without necessitating a change in posture or any realignment of the segments.

Whenever objects must be carried on one hip, in back, or in front, a postural adjustment must be made to maintain stability. To minimize stress on the joints, including the vertebral column, these adjustments should be made from the ankles. Thrusting the hips out or adjusting with the back may predispose one to injury unless compensation occurs by routinely altering the location of the load.

Weight Lifting

Lifting weights, whether done for strengthening and conditioning muscles or competitive lifting contests, involves the use of the levers of the body to overcome the inertia of relatively large masses. Depending on the lift being done, either a push or a pull pattern may be used. The key to safe and successful weight lifting is in arranging the various levers involved in such a way as to minimize the torque produced by the external resistance while maximizing the available muscle torques. To produce an efficient lift, one must first establish the location of the axis of rotation for the lift. The moving weight should be kept as close to this axis of rotation as possible, reducing the resistance moment arm. In the bench press, for example, it is much safer and more efficient to lift the bar directly over the shoulders than to allow the bar any horizontal motion. To further reduce the risk of injury, the axis of rotation should be well supported. In standing lifts this means that the axis of rotation should be in line with the approximate center of the base of support. To allow the axis of rotation to move away from the base of support requires that postural torques be created for stability. These torques usually occur in the back and may lead to injury. The velocity of the lifting motion should be kept low. A high-velocity lift generates a great deal of momentum, requiring a large braking force. This braking force usually takes the form of an eccentric muscle contraction, which must act to decrease momentum.

Punching

Punches are simultaneous push-pattern motions. A punch is usually directed horizontally rather than vertically and usually terminates with contact to another body that provides the external resistance. Because the momentum of the punch is to be transferred to the opponent, it is desirable for punch velocity to be high. The purpose of the high-velocity punch can be to upset the balance of the opponent, as in boxing, or to cause injury to the opponent, as in karate and self-defense.

A boxing punch is typified by a long punch and a long follow-through. The force of the punch is transferred to the opponent over a broad area through the boxing glove. Punches to the head produce acceleration of the head and neck, which may lead to unconsciousness or may produce angular momentum, causing a loss of balance. A karate punch, on the other hand, is a shorter punch with little or no follow-through. The force of a karate blow is delivered to a very small area. Impact occurs at the peak velocity of the punch and this impact can break bone and tear tissue. For this reason, karate is practiced as a noncontact sport and judged on correctness of form and accuracy.

The simultaneous nature of many karate punches and most boxing punches allows for maximum force production with a straight-line motion intended to give the opponent little or no time for defense. In both sports, quickness of the punch is vital, both for an effective offense and to allow for a rapid return to a ready position.

Working with Long-Handled Implements

Working with implements such as a hoe, rake, mop, or vacuum cleaner involves a combination of pushing, pulling, and, in some instances, lifting. The last is usually only for short distances, but it may occur with considerable frequency. One characteristic of working with implements such as these is that the body must maintain a more or less fixed posture for relatively long periods of time, causing tension and fatigue. Hence the chief problem is that of using the body in such a way that tension will be minimized and fatigue postponed for as long as possible. If the implement is used back and forth in front of the body, the tendency of the worker is to lean forward (figure 17.9). This necessitates static contraction of the extensors of the spine in order to support the trunk against the downward pull of gravity. Because implements such as the rake and hoe are lifted at the end of each stroke and carried to position for the next stroke, the force of gravity acts on the implement as well as on the worker's body. Although the implement may not weigh much in itself, its forward position means that the lever has a long resistance arm, the effect of which must be balanced by the muscles. This gives an added burden to the back muscles and not infrequently causes a backache. A better method is to stand with the side turned toward the work site and the feet separated in a fairly wide stride, and work the implement from side to side.

Figure 17.9   Long-handled implements may force a forward-leaning posture. The wider stride is beneficial.

The reach can then be obtained by bending the knee of the leg on the same side as the implement and by inclining the body slightly to the same side. Those who are familiar with gymnastics will recognize this as a side lunge position. On the recovery, the knee and the trunk are both straightened. Thus there is an alternating contraction and relaxation of muscles and there is no necessity for any of the trunk muscles to remain in static contraction. Temporary relief can also be obtained by changing sides.

The use of a spade or snow shovel involves primarily the act of lifting. Because the load is taken on the end of a mechanical lever held in a more or less horizontal position, it is inevitable that the weight arm of the lever be relatively long. It can be shortened somewhat, however, by sliding one hand as far down the shaft as possible, using this hand as a fulcrum, and providing the force with the other hand by pushing down on the outer end of the handle. As a variation of this technique, when getting a particularly heavy load on a shovel, it is possible to bend one knee and brace the shaft against the thigh, thus using the thigh as a fulcrum. This is only for the initial lift, however; the hands must then be shifted to the position previously described in order to carry or throw the load.

Aside from taking and lifting the load on the spade, there is the factor of lowering the body to reach the load and of assuming the erect position for moving it. As in the case of stooping to lift a heavy object from the floor, the chief problems are economy of effort, maintenance of stability, and avoidance of strain. These problems are intensified by the additional factor of taking the load on a long-handled implement instead of directly in the hand. As before, separating the feet to widen the base of support, bending at the knees instead of bending from the waist to lower the body, and inclining the trunk forward only slightly will, respectively, increase stability, shorten the anatomical levers involved in the stooping, and divide the muscular work among the stronger knee, and hip, and back extensors instead of making the weaker back muscles assume too large a share of the work. Because the lower back is easily strained by heavy shoveling, it is of great importance to protect it by observing the principles of good mechanics.

ANALYSIS OF THE PUSH-PULL PATTERN IN ERGOMETER ROWING

The motion used in the rowing ergometer mimics very closely the motion used to propel a rowboat or a sculling shell through the water. The rowing motion is a combination of leg pushing action and arm pull in a continuous cycle. The row can be broken down into two primary phases—the drive phase and the recovery phase. The rower starts with the ergometer slide in the forward position. The lower extremity is fully flexed while the arms are extended horizontally forward in front of the trunk. The rowing stroke begins with the initial catch. In the water this is the point at which the oar is dropped into the water through a slight lifting of the hands. On the rowing ergometer, the catch marks the point at which the ergometer

cable is fully retracted. At this instant the performer is in the starting position, with the knees and hips fully flexed, shoulders flexed and elbows in extension.

The drive phase is initiated through extension of the lower extremity. The legs push strongly against the foot plate, pushing the body backward on the sliding seat. As the legs near full extension, the spine begins extension to maintain a smooth, continuous motion of the oar. The upper extremity now begins motion, with the upper arm pulling through shoulder horizontal abduction as the elbows flex. The stroke finishes with the knees in full extension, extension of the spine, full horizontal abduction of the shoulder and complete flexion of the elbow. The joint motion of each extremity link system (upper and lower) is done simultaneously, although the lower body initiates the stroke and the upper body finishes it. Figure 17.10 presents the sequence of the rowing stroke from starting position through leg extension to the end of the drive phase.

Anatomical Analysis (Table 17.1)

The recovery phase of the stroke varies depending on the resistance setting. In the rowing ergometer the recovery motion of lower-extremity flexion is produced by a fairly moderate concentric contraction of the flexor muscles (thus pulling the slide seat and body forward) while the forward motion of the upper extremity (shoulder horizontal adduction and elbow extension) is produced by similar contraction of the appropriate muscles, pushing the oar forward to the catch position. On the rowing ergometer, leg flexion is again produced by moderate contraction of the flexors, while arm motion may be produced primarily by the retraction of the ergometer cable (Rodriguez et al. 1990).

Mechanical Analysis

In rowing over water the primary mechanical objective of the rowing action is to produce maximum power. The rower wants to generate the

a.   b.   c.

Figure 17.10   The rowing stroke, progressing from the starting position (a), to leg extension (b), to finish with hip extension and forearm flexion (c).

TABLE 17.1	Anatomical Analysis of the Drive Phase				
Joint	Joint Action	Segment Moved	Force for Movement	Muscles Active	Kind of Contraction
Ankles	Plantar-flexion	Shank	Muscle	Gastrocnemius Soleus	Concentric
Knees	Extension	Thigh	Muscle	Quadriceps femoris	Concentric
Hips	Extension	Trunk	Muscle	Hamstrings Gluteus maximus	Concentric
Shoulder joints	Extension	Upper arm	Muscle	Pectoralis major (stern portion) Teres major Latissimus dorsi Teres minor	Concentric
Shoulder girdle	Adduction	Scapula	Muscle	Rhomboids Trapezius III	Concentric
Elbows	Flexion	Forearm	Muscle	Biceps brachii Brachioradialis	Concentric

highest possible velocity in the boat. This is accomplished through the combination of stroke length and stroke rate. The most efficient and most effective performance is one in which the force can be applied to the water through the full range of motion allowed and the fastest possible stroke rate can be maintained. Stroke rates in rowing races in the Olympic Games, for instance, are often as high as 38 to 40 strokes per minute over a distance of 2.5 kilometers (Dawson et al. 1998).

Whereas the rower in a boat does work on the water to move the boat forward, the performer on the rowing ergometer is doing work against some form of machine resistance. However, the principal objective of producing maximum power through the optimum combination of stroke length and stroke rate still applies.

Force for motion in the rowing ergometer is provided through extension of the knees and hips. It is important that this force be applied in a smooth, consistent manner. Equally important is the transfer of these forces to the hands as the hips and knees reach extension. In order to effect this transfer effiiciently the trunk must be stabilized through hip and knee extension. The rower must be careful, therefore, not to begin the flexion of the lower extremities too soon (Smith and Spinks 1995).

Ergometer rowing differs somewhat from overwater rowing. In the recovery phase of overwater rowing the oar blade must be lifted clear of the water by downward pressure on the grip, or inboard, end of the oar. The oar is then feathered, or rotated, as the hands are pushed forward so that the blade slices through the air parallel to the airflow. This requires hyperextension of the wrists, not necessary in ergometer rowing. The pull phase is then preceded by a "catch," as the hands are raised slightly, lowering the oars back into the water.

LABORATORY EXPERIENCES

1. Raise a window from the bottom:
   a. Standing at arm's length.
   b. Standing close, facing the window, and using both hands.
   c. Standing close, side to the window, and pushing it up with one hand with the elbow bent and the forearm in a vertical position.

   Which is the best method for a heavy window or a window that sticks? Explain in terms of components of force and the direct application of force.

2. Open (or close) a sliding door:
   a. Standing at arm's length.
   b. Standing close, facing the door.
   c. Standing close, facing in the direction that the door is to move, using a pushing motion with the forearm parallel with the door.

   Which is the best method? Explain in terms of direction of application of force and of components of force.

3. Push a heavy piece of furniture. Experiment to find the most efficient method.
   a. At what part of the object did you apply the force? Explain the underlying principles.
   b. What were the positions of the arms, legs, and trunk? Explain the advantage provided by these positions.

4. Observe individuals of different ages and body types:
   a. Ascending stairs.
   b. Arising from a seated position.

   Compare the performances and briefly discuss the kinesiological bases for the similarities and differences in performing pushing and pulling as applied to these activities. Note especially the position of the arms and trunk in each instance.

5. Select three or four different movements used in sports, dance, or actions of daily living. Briefly discuss how understanding the principles of push–pull motions can aid in the analysis of these skills.

6. Briefly discuss the advantages and disadvantages of pushing or pulling a vacuum cleaner or lawn mower, or assisting someone in rising from a sitting position.

7. Perform a complete kinesiological analysis of a selected push–pull skill taking particular note of the purpose of the motion, its classification, the nature of the motion, and its component parts. Include also muscle participation, neuromuscular considerations, mechanical factors, and applicable principles and violations. Conclude the analysis with a prescription for improvement, including suggested methods for change and the elimination of violations of principles.

REFERENCES AND SELECTED READINGS

Ashton-Miller, J. A., and A. B. Schultz. 1988. Biomechanics of the human spine and trunk. *Exercise and Sport Science Reviews* 16:169–204.

Brancazio, P. J. 1984. *Sport science.* New York: Simon & Schuster.

Bush, Joseph C., O. Schipplein, B. J. Anderson, and T. P. Andriacchi. 1988. Influence of dynamic factors on the lumbar spine moment in lifting. *Ergonomics* 31:211–16.

Chaffin, D. B., and G. B. J. Andersson. 1984. *Occupational biomechanics.* New York: Wiley.

Chaffin, D. B., R. O. Andres, and A. Garg. 1983. Volitional postures during maximal push/pull exertions in the sagittal plane. *Human Factors* 25:541–50.

Dawson, R. G., R. J. Lockwood, J. D. Wilson, and G. Freeman. 1998. The rowing cycle: Sources of variance and invariance in ergometer and on-the-water performance. *Journal of Motor Behavior* 30:33–43.

Dolan, P., M. Earley, and M. A. Adams. 1994. Bending and compressive stresses acting on the lumbar spine during lifting activities. *Journal of Biomechanics* 27:1237–48.

Field, R. W. 1988. Rationale for the use of free weights for periodization. *National Strength and Conditioning Association Journal* 10:38–39.

Fortin, Y. D., and D. G. E. Robertson. 1994. Lower extremity function during ergometer rowing. In *Proceedings of the Canadian Society for Biomechanics VIIIth Biennial Conference,* edited by W. Herzog et al., 248–49. Calgary, Alberta.

Garhammer, J. 1989. Weightlifting and training. In *Biomechanics of sport,* edited by C. L. Vaughan, 169–211. Boca Raton, FL: CRC Press.

Hudson, J. 1986. Coordination of segments in the vertical jump. *Medicine and Science in Sports and Exercise* 18:242–51.

Kreighbaum, E., and K. M. Barthels. 1994. *Biomechanics.* 4th ed. New York: Allyn & Bacon.

Ljunberg, A. S., A. Kilbom, and G. M. Hagg. 1989. Occupational lifting by nursing aids and warehouse workers. *Ergonomics* 32:59–78.

McGill, S. M., and R. W. Norman. 1993. Low back biomechanics in industry: The prevention of injury through safer lifting. In *Current issues in biomechanics,* edited by M. D. Grabiner, 69–115. Champaign, IL: Human Kinetics.

McLaughlin, T. N., and N. H. Madsen. 1984. Bench press techniques of elite heavyweight power lifters. *National Strength and Conditioning Association Journal* 44:62–65.

Rasch, P. J. 1989. *Kinesiology and applied anatomy.* 7th ed. Philadelphia: Lea & Febiger.

Rodriguez, R. J., R. P. Rodriguez, S. D. Cook, and P. M. Sandborn. 1990. Electromyographic analysis of rowing stroke mechanics. *The Journal of Sports Medicine and Physical Fitness* 30:103–8.

Smith, R. M., and W. L. Spinks. 1995. Discriminant analysis of biomechanical differences between novice, good, and elite rowers. *Journal of Sport Sciences* 13:377–85.

Wilson, G. J., B. C. Elliott, and G. K. Kerr. 1989. Bar path and force profile characteristics for maximal and submaximal loads in the bench press. *International Journal of Sport Biomechanics* 5(4):390–402.

Wilson, J. M. J., D. G. E. Robertson, and J. P. Stothart. 1988. Analysis of lower limb muscle function in ergometer rowing. *International Journal of Sport Biomechanics* 4:315–25.

18

MOVING OBJECTS: THROWING, STRIKING, AND KICKING

OUTLINE

- **Sequential Movements**
  Joint Action Patterns
  Nature of Force Application
- **Principles Relating to Throwing, Striking, and Kicking**
  Anatomical Principles
  Mechanical Principles
- **Examples of Throwing and Striking**
  Analysis of the Overarm Throw
  Analysis of the Forehand Drive
     in Tennis
- **Laboratory Experiences**

OBJECTIVES

At the conclusion of this chapter the student should be able to:

1. Classify activities involving sequential throwing, kicking, or striking patterns according to the nature of the force application.
2. Name and discuss anatomical and mechanical factors that apply to representative throwing, kicking, or striking activities.
3. Perform a kinesiological analysis of someone engaging in a sequential throwing, kicking, or striking skill under each of these force application conditions: momentary contact, projection, continuous application.

SEQUENTIAL MOVEMENTS

A baseball pitcher throws a baseball across the plate and the batter hits it to center field, an elderly man pitches horseshoes, a young person spikes a volleyball, student practices driving a golf ball while a college athlete practices punting a football. Once more, as is the case with pushing and pulling, a widely diverse set of activities has a common denominator. Each of these activities involves sequential movement of the body segments resulting in the production of a summated velocity at the end of the chain of segments used. The path produced by the end point of this chain of segments is curvilinear in nature.

Sequential segmental motions are most frequently used to produce high velocities in external objects. Depending on the objective of the skill, speed, accuracy, distance, or some combination, modifications in the sequential pattern may be made. Greater or fewer numbers of segments may be involved, larger or smaller ranges of motion might be used, and longer or shorter lever lengths may be chosen. Regardless of the modifications, the basic nature of the sequential throwing, striking, or kicking pattern remains the same.

Joint Action Patterns

Broer was the first to call attention to the similarity of movement patterns used in seemingly dissimilar activities such as the baseball pitch, the badminton clear, and the tennis serve (Broer and Zernicke 1979). Objective evidence of such similarities between throwing and striking activities within each of the three major upper-extremity patterns (overarm, sidearm, and underarm) was originally revealed by the Broer and Houtz EMG investigations (1967) and confirmed by Moynes and colleagues (1986). Broer and Houtz as well as Deutsch (1969) noted that representative activities from these categories across throwing patterns also showed great similarity in the muscular action of the lower extremity.

Atwater (1980) distinguished between the overarm and sidearm throwing patterns in terms of the direction in which the trunk laterally flexed. When lateral flexion occurred away from the throwing arm, an overarm pattern was used; lateral flexion toward the throwing arm indicated a sidearm pattern. The underarm pattern is distinguished by motion predominantly in a sagittal plane with the hand below the waist.

Each pattern involves a preparatory movement referred to as a backswing, or windup, followed by the establishment of a base of support prior to the initiation of the force phase and ending in a follow-through. The base of support in the direction of the force application (forward-backward) is a distinguishing feature of skill level. It has been well documented that more highly skilled individuals have longer strides. Once the base has been established, the more proximal segments begin the force application phase while the more distal segments complete the backswing. The purpose of the backswing is to place the segments in a favorable position for the force phase.

Representative joint actions for each throwing pattern are as follows.

Overarm Pattern

This kind of throw or strike is characterized by rotation at the shoulder joint. In the backswing, or preparatory, phase, the abducted arm rotates laterally, and in the forward, or force, phase the arm rotates medially. Some elbow extension, wrist flexion, and spinal rotation occur in the force phase. These movements are accompanied by rotation of the pelvis at the hip joint of the opposite limb, resulting in medial rotation of the thigh (figures 18.1 and 18.2). An immature pattern (figure 18.3) may be identified as using fewer segments, working more simultaneously rather than sequentially, and involving a more limited range of motion. This description is easily documented by referring to the developmental literature.

Figure 18.1   Overhand pattern applied in baseball pitch. The forward force phase is characterized by medial rotation of the arm, elbow extension, spinal rotation, and medial rotation of the pelvis at the contralateral hip joint.

Figure 18.2   Examples of the overarm pattern: (a) football pass; (b) javelin throw; (c) volleyball serve.

a.   b.

Figure 18.3   Overhand throw by a girl aged three years ten months who had not been given any directions regarding how to throw. Note elbow extension, pelvic rotation, step, and weight shift. (Drawn from motion picture film tracing.)

Underarm Pattern

This pattern consists of a forward movement of the extended arm in the sagittal plane, usually starting from a position of hyperextension and ending in a forward reach. The basic joint action of the arm is flexion. The actions of the wrist, spine, and pelvis are the same as those observed in the overarm pattern (figure 18.4).

Sidearm Pattern

In this pattern the basic movement is medial rotation of the pelvis on the opposite hip with the arm usually in an abducted position. The arm is moved forward in a horizontal plane because of the pelvic action and spinal rotation. The spine also laterally flexes toward the throwing arm. The range of the upper-extremity movement may also be enlarged by the addition of horizontal adduction at the shoulder. The elbow is maintained in extension or is extended from a slightly flexed position, depending on the nature of the skill in question (e.g., basketball throw for distance, tennis forehand drive, or batting). Wrist flexion may also be part of the action in some techniques (figure 18.5).

Kicking Pattern

Another form of sequential movement pattern involves use of the lower extremities and is referred to as kicking. This pattern is used, for example, when punting a football (figure 18.6) or initiating a soccer kick. Kicking is a modification of a locomotor pattern in which force is imparted to an external object during the forward swing of the non-weight-bearing limb.

To initiate the kicking motion, the left foot (of a right-footed kicker) is stabilized. The pelvis is fixed over the thigh and rotated toward the left. The right non-weight-bearing limb lags behind, resulting in thigh abduction and hyperextension at the hip joint. The right thigh then begins to flex at the hip joint followed by knee extension. This sequential segmental movement pattern results in the summation of forces and allows for maximum linear velocity of the foot at ball contact. The specific point of ball contact depends on the placement of the supporting foot and motion of the free-swinging limb during the backswing.

a.   b.   c.

Figure 18.4   Examples of the underarm pattern: (a) softball pitch; (b) badminton serve; (c) golf drive.

a.   b.

Figure 18.5   Examples of the sidearm pattern: (a) racquetball drive; (b) softball swing.

Figure 18.6   The kicking pattern as used in the football punt.

Nature of Force Application
Momentary Contact

Movements such as striking and kicking are characterized in sequential movement patterns by a momentary contact made with an object by a moving part of the body or by an implement held by or attached to a moving segment of the body. Baseball batting, golf, tennis, and soccer kicking are all examples of force imparted through momentary contact.

Projection

In sequential patterns, an object is given some velocity as the end point of a part of the body or as an implement attached to the body. At the desired point in the curvilinear path, the object is released to become a projectile. Throwing is an example of this type of projection, as are the projection of balls by implements as in lacrosse or jai alai.

Principles Relating to Throwing, Striking, and Kicking

Anatomical Principles

Regardless of which movement pattern is used, the following factors must be considered when imparting force to an object through the sequential use of body segments. To ignore the anatomical principles of sequential motion is to risk injury, because sequential motion can generate extremely high velocities, as well as impart high braking forces.

1. Muscles contract more forcefully if they are first put on a stretch, provided they are not overstretched. This principle suggests the function of the windup in pitching and of the preliminary movements in other sport skills.
2. Unnecessary movements and tensions in the performance of a motor skill mean both awkwardness and unnecessary fatigue; hence, they should be eliminated.
3. Skillful and efficient performance in a particular technique can be developed only by practice of that technique. Only in this way can the necessary adjustments in the neuromuscular mechanism be made to ensure a well-coordinated movement.
4. The most efficient type of movement in throwing and striking skills is ballistic movement. Skills that are primarily ballistic should be practiced ballistically, even in the earliest learning stages. This means that from the beginning the emphasis should be placed on form rather than on aim. Accuracy of aim will develop with practice. If the emphasis is placed on accuracy in the learning stages, the beginner tends to perform the skill as a "moving fixation" or as a slow, tense movement. Once this pattern of movement is established, it is extremely difficult to change it later to a ballistic movement.
5. When there is a choice of anatomical leverage, the lever appropriate for the task should be used—that is, a lever with a long resistance arm for movements requiring range or speed, and a lever with a long effort arm for movements requiring strength. For example, kicking is an effective way to impart force to a football because the leg provides a lever with a long resistance arm but, for the same reason, it is a poor way to move a heavy suitcase along the floor.

Mechanical Principles

Although many of the mechanical principles for throwing, striking, and kicking are similar to those cited for pushing and pulling, the applications of these principles are different. Whereas force application in push–pull patterns is maximized through using large numbers of segments simultaneously, force in throwing, kicking, and striking patterns is maximized through sequential transfer of momentum from large segments to less massive segments. To illustrate this, the mechanical principles involved in sequential movement patterns are given as they apply both to throwing and to striking.

Throwing

The efficiency of imparting force to a ball is judged in terms of the speed, distance, and direction of the ball after its release. The purpose of the throw determines which of these is given the greater emphasis. Both the speed and distance of the thrown ball are directly related to the magnitude of the force used in throwing it and to the speed of the hand at the moment of release. The speed the hand is able to achieve depends on the distance through which it moves in the preparatory part of the act and the summed angular velocities of the contributing body segments. Hence, the longer the preparatory backswing and the greater the distance that can be added by means of rotating the body, shifting the weight, and perhaps even taking a step, the greater the opportunity for accelerating. Approximately 50 percent of the ball speed is obtained from the forward step and body rotation. The remaining speed is contributed by the joint actions in the shoulder, elbow, wrist, and fingers. This is why the technique of a baseball pitcher is designed to allow maximum time and distance over which to accelerate the ball before its release. In addition, if the ground reaction force is to be maximal, the surface against which the thrower pushes must be firm and there must be no sliding between the ground surface and the foot. The more the direction of the body thrust is backward, the more important the friction becomes and the more the value of the cleated shoes is appreciated. If distance is a major objective of the throw, the angle of projection and the effects of gravitational force and air resistance must also be taken into consideration.

The accuracy with which a ball is thrown depends on accurate judgment of the distance and direction of the throw's target. The ball will leave the hand in the direction it is moving at the instant of release and continue in that direction except for modifications because of gravity and air resistance. Therefore the effect of gravity, wind, and spin must be considered, as well as the release direction. If the hand is traveling in an arc at release, the ball will follow a path tangent to the arc, and the timing of the release is highly critical.

Flattening the arc of the ball's path prior to release increases the margin of error by allowing more time over which the ball can be released in the desired direction. This may be done by taking a step and shifting the weight forward while flexing at the forward knee. The rotation of the pelvis and spine also helps.

When the object being thrown is other than a small ball, such as a javelin, discus, bowling ball, or horseshoe, the general principles are the same but must be modified according to the nature of the object and the regulations of the sport.

Principles

1. The object will move only if the force is of sufficient magnitude to overcome the object's inertia. The force must be great enough to overcome not only the mass of the object but also all restraining forces. These include (a) friction between the object and the supporting surface, (b) resistance of the surrounding medium (e.g., wind or water), and (c) internal resistance. Warming up helps prevent injury as well as decrease internal resistance. Increasing range of motion through training is also important and effective.

2. The pattern and range of joint movements depends on the purpose of the movement. If maximum force magnitude is not needed, the optimum movement pattern should be changed with respect to the range, speed, and number of joint actions until it is the most efficient for the task. Throwing a ball to a small child 10 feet away does not require the same pattern as does pitching a baseball.

3. Force exerted by the body will be transferred to an external object in proportion to the effectiveness of the counterforce of the feet (or other parts of the body) against the ground (or other supporting surface). This effectiveness depends on the counterpressure and friction presented by the supporting surface. The force applied to a ball thrown while in midair or while treading water is

less than that applied to it while pushing against the ground.

4. Linear velocity is imparted to external objects as a result of the angular velocity of the body segments. The linear velocity at the end of any segment is the product of the angular velocity and the length of the segment. Thus, for a given angular speed, the linear speed imparted to a tennis ball with a tennis racket is much greater than that of a ball hit with the hand. On the other hand, more force is needed to move the longer of the two levers.

5. Optimum summation of internal force is needed if maximum force is to be applied to move an object. For maximum velocity of each contributing body segment to occur at release of, or impact with, the external object, the slower or heavier segments must start to move first and the lightest and quickest ones last. It is preferable for the slower segments to begin their forward movements while the faster segments are still completing the backswing. This timing pattern facilitates use of the stretch reflex.

6. For a change in momentum to occur, force must be applied over time (impulse). If maximum force is desired in projection-type activities, maximum muscle torques should be applied over as long a time as possible.

7. Force applied in line with an object's center of gravity will result in linear motion of the object, provided the latter is freely movable.

8. If the force applied to a freely movable object is not in line with the latter's center of gravity, it will result in rotary motion of the object.

Striking, Hitting, and Kicking

As in the case of throwing, the effectiveness of striking, hitting, and kicking is judged by the speed, distance, and direction of the struck ball. All the factors that apply to these aspects of a thrown ball apply similarly to a struck ball. There appear to be five major factors that apply to the speed of a struck ball. These are:

1. The speed of the oncoming ball and the striking implement.
2. The mass of the ball and the striking implement.
3. The coefficient of restitution (elasticity) between the ball and the striking implement.
4. The direction the ball and the implement are moving at the time of impact.
5. The point of impact between the ball and the implement.

The speed of the approaching ball and the speed of the striking implement may be further analyzed into secondary factors. For instance, the speed of the striking implement is determined by the magnitude of the force exerted, and the magnitude of the force depends on the distance of the preparatory backswing and the speed of muscular contraction. The distance of the preparatory backswing further depends on the range of motion in the joints and the timing of the swing. Furthermore, the effectiveness of the force exerted by the body depends completely on a strong grip and a firm wrist for transmission of the force from the body to the striking implement, and a firm ground support for transmission of the normal reactive force to the body.

Objects that have been hit through their centers of gravity will have linear motion, whereas those that have been hit off center may curve because of a resultant spin. The more the striking force is eccentric in its application, the less is the linear speed imparted to the ball. Furthermore, balls that hit a striking surface at an angle to the surface will rebound at an angle approximately equal and opposite to the rebound angle.

Some examples of ball and striker velocities before and after impact are presented in table 18.1.

Principles Those mechanical principles cited as pertaining to throwing patterns are also related to striking patterns. In addition, the following fac-

TABLE 18.1	Ball and Striker Velocities before and after Impact and Time of Impact				
	Ball Velocity (ft/sec)		Striker Velocity (ft/sec)		Time of Impact (sec)
	Before	**After**	**Before**	**After**	
Baseball	Hit from tee	128	103	90	1/800
Badminton	30 ft/sec	112	97.2	95	1/800
Football punt	0	92	60	39	1/125
Football kickoff	0	85	60	47	1/125
Golf, 7 iron	0	177	155	133	1/800
Golf drive	0	225	166	114	1/1000
Handball serve	0	76	63	47	1/80
Paddleball	0	115	90	70	1/200
Soccer kick	0	85	58	42	1/125
Soccer, head	25	42	11	8.6	1/44
Squash, hard serve	0	160	145	111	1/333
Softball	Hit from tee	100	105	71	1/285
Tennis serve	0	167	123	107	1/250
Tennis forehand	0	93	71	41	1/200
Volleyball serve	0	72	65	45	1/100

From Stanley Plagenhoef, *Patterns of Human Motion: A Cinematographic Analysis.* Copyright © 1971, p. 59. Adapted by permission of Prentice Hall, Englewood Cliffs, New Jersey.

tors also must be applied when analyzing striking patterns.

1. The direction in which the object moves is determined by the direction of force applied to it. If the force consists of two or more components, the object will move in the direction of the resultant of those components. After being projected or struck, the direction will be modified by gravity and air resistance.
2. Momentum is conserved in all collisions. The momentum before impact must equal the momentum after impact, provided that none is lost through friction or other forces.
3. Any change in the momentum of colliding objects is related to the force and duration of the collision. The greater the impulse (*Ft*), the greater will be the change in momentum. This is why the follow-through is important. The longer the missile can be carried along

by the striking implement at its greatest velocity, the greater will be the change in velocity of the missile.
4. The greater the velocity of the approaching ball, the greater the velocity of the ball in the opposite direction after it is struck, other things being equal.
5. The greater the velocity of the striking implement at the moment of contact, the greater the velocity of the struck ball, other things being equal. Obviously, a full-powered swing will send the ball farther and faster than will a bunt. Both increasing the length of the lever and striking with a good follow-through help increase the velocity of the striking implement and therefore increase the force of impact.
6. The greater the mass of the ball, *up to a point,* the greater its velocity after being struck, other things being equal. A hard

baseball will travel farther and faster than a softball. Nevertheless, an iron ball would offer too much resistance for the average batter using an average bat.

7. The greater the mass of the striking implement, *up to a point,* the greater the striking force, and hence the greater the speed of the struck ball, other things being equal. A good baseball player uses a heavier bat. Too heavy a bat, however, is inadvisable because of the difficulty in swinging it with sufficient speed and control.

8. The higher the coefficient of restitution (the elasticity) of the ball and of the striking implement, the greater the speed of the struck ball, other things being equal.

9. The direction taken by the struck ball is determined by four factors: (a) the direction of the striking implement at the moment of contact; (b) the relation of the striking force to the ball's center of gravity (an off-center application of force causes spin, and spin affects direction); (c) degree of firmness of grip and wrist at moment of impact; and (d) the laws governing rebound (see pp. 321–324).

EXAMPLES OF THROWING AND STRIKING

Analysis of the Overarm Throw

To give the reader a better understanding of the coordination pattern referred to as sequential segmental actions, the force phase of the overarm pattern is analyzed as applied in a forceful throw such as in pitching. This analysis includes joint actions, muscle activity, and mechanics for the upper extremity only.

The purpose of the backswing, or preparatory, motion is to place the segments in a favorable position for the force phase. There are many ways to execute the backswing. Although some favor one method over another, any windup is appropriate that places the segments in the most advantageous position to maximize the number of

segments and the time over which force can be applied. Such a windup, allowing the joints to be placed in an optimal position to involve the greatest number of segments, includes pelvic and trunk rotation in the opposite direction from the intended throw (right for a right-hander), horizontal abduction, and lateral rotation at the shoulder joint with elbow flexion and wrist hyperextension. This sequence of arm action continues as a forward step is taken with the opposite foot. This hand–foot opposition permits the greatest range of motion in the trunk and pelvis. It also allows for a large base of support over which the force phase can be applied while preserving balance.

No pause occurs between the windup and the force phases. The windup ends with a forward stride using the opposite leg. Establishment of a base of support is followed immediately by pelvic and then trunk rotation, accompanied by lateral flexion to the left (right-handed pitcher). The trunk motion causes increased horizontal abduction with continuing lateral rotation at the shoulder joint. Elbow joint extension is followed by the initiation of rapid medial rotation at the shoulder joint, forearm pronation at the radial–ulnar joint, and then flexion and often ulnar flexion at the wrist joint. The force phase ends with the release of the ball. The angle at the elbow joint at release is approximately 105 degrees. The follow-through includes the actions from ball release until the momentum developed in the arm can be safely dissipated as the arm continues across the body in a downward direction. In addition, a forward step is also often used.

The reader should note that these actions proceed from the proximal (more massive) to the distal (lighter) segments. In characteristic sequential patterns, subsequent segments lag behind those preceding them. The subsequent segment is carried along, lagging behind until the more proximal segment attains its maximum angular velocity. The distal segment then accelerates because of a combination of the series elastic components, stretch reflex, and muscular contraction. This combination results in the reaction or slowing down of the preceding segment. Because of conservation of momentum, momentum (*mv*) is transferred from the more massive (proximal) to the less massive (distal) segments, significantly increasing their velocity. Therefore, the linear velocity at the end of the chain—that is, the ball at release—often can be over 90 miles per hour.

The legs play an important role in any successful throw. They provide the stable base over which the trunk and other segments act. In addition, the thrust they provide contributes significantly to the force of this movement. The transfer of momentum from proximal to distal, however, focuses the attention on the musculature of the upper extremity. Because this phase emphasizes the application of the force accelerating the limb, muscle contractions are mainly concentric preceded by a short eccentric phase because of the lagging of the distal behind the proximal segments.

Muscular Analysis of Upper Extermity (Table 18.2)

The lateral rotation preceding the medial rotation of the right shoulder joint is controlled by the eccentric contraction of the medial rotators of the humerus followed by the concentric contraction of the same muscles, including the subscapularis, pectoralis major, and latissimus dorsi muscles. During the acceleration phase the height of the humerus was controlled by a static contraction of the middle deltoid. The deltoid and supraspinatus muscles contract concentrically during the backswing to position the upper arm, and eccentrically during the follow-through to help decelerate the arm. The infraspinatus muscle was also very active (eccentric contraction) to assist in decelerating the arm during the follow-through.

The biceps brachii muscle activity reaches its peak as the elbow joint is flexed late into the backswing and at the beginning of the force phase. Marked activity again appears during the follow-through to protect the elbow joint in decelerating the forearm. The latissimus dorsi muscle, active during medial rotation, remains active eccentrically contracting during the follow-through to assist in controlling the arm motion across the body.

It is clear that the stretch reflex is an important facilitating mechanism in helping accelerate the lagging distal segment at the appropriate time.

TABLE 18.2	**Acceleration Phase (Initial Portion of Force Phase) of the Overarm Throw**				
Joint	**Joint Action**	**Segment Moved**	**Force for Movement**	**Muscles Active**	**Kind of Contraction**
Shoulder joints	Horizontal abduction	Upper arm	Muscle	Posterior deltoid Infraspinatus Teres minor	Concentric
	Medial rotation		Muscle	Subscapularis Latissimus dorsi Pectoralis major	Concentric
Shoulder girdle	Abduction	Scapula	Muscle	Serratus anterior Pectoralis minor	Concentric
Elbows	Extension	Forearm	Muscle	Triceps brachii	Concentric
Radioulnar	Pronation	Forearm	Muscle	Pronator teres Pronator quadratus	Concentric
Wrist	Flexion	Hand	Muscle	Flexor carpi radialis Flexor carpi ulnaris Flexor digitorum superficialis	Concentric

The more rapid the stretch (eccentric contraction), the greater will be the facilitating effect on the resulting concentric contraction of the same muscle. In this way, forces can be summated more appropriately. To gain the greatest facilitation from the stretch reflex, there should be no pause between the windup and force phases.

Because the trunk rotates under the stationary head (eyes focused on the target), the tonic neck reflex may facilitate the strong acceleration occurring during the force phase. The asymmetric tonic neck reflex facilitates the shoulder abductors and elbow extensors on the chin side. This is precisely the arm position at release.

The extensor thrust reflex may act on both the upper and lower extremities. Increasing pressure on the palmar side of the hand as the arm is being accelerated forward may facilitate the arm extensor muscles. Similarly, as the weight is transferred to the forward foot, the pacinian corpuscles are stimulated by the increased pressure, resulting in a facilitation of the lower-limb extensor muscles. When accuracy is a factor, knee flexion must be maintained to flatten the arc through which the hand is carried. This flattening permits the tangential flight path of the ball to have a broader margin for error in the timing of the release while arriving at the same target point following release.

Analysis of the Forehand Drive in Tennis
Description
The forehand drive (figure 18.7) is one of the fundamental strokes of tennis. Its objective is to send the ball over the net and deep into the opponent's court close to the baseline.

Starting position The player faces the net with the feet about shoulder-width apart and the weight on the balls of the feet. The racket is held with an eastern or shake-hands grip.

Backswing The player pivots the entire body so that the shoulder and hips of the nonracket side are toward the net. At the same time, the racket is taken back at shoulder level in either a straight or a circular manner, with the head of the racket above the wrist and its face turned slightly down. The weight of the body is over the rear foot (racket side).

Forward swing and follow-through The player flexes at the knee joints to drop the racket and racket arm below the intended contact point (still keeping the racket head above the wrist with its face turned down) and steps toward the ball with the nonracket foot. The pelvis and spine rotate so the trunk faces forward, and the weight is shifted to the forward foot as the racket is swung forward and up. The racket face is perpendicular to the court at ball impact, thus imparting topspin to the ball as it swings through and up. The follow-through continues toward the intended target, with the racket arm swinging across the body and up toward the chin.

Anatomical Factors
The action in the forehand drive is ballistic in nature and, as such, is initiated by muscular force, continued by momentum, and finally terminated by the contraction of antagonistic muscles. The chief lever participating in the movement consists of the arm, trunk, and racket together with the fulcrum located in the opposite hip joint (see figure 13.19), the point of force application at a point on the pelvis that represents the combined forces of the muscles producing the movement (mainly the gluteus medius and minimis and the adductor magnus), and the resistance point at the center of gravity of the trunk–arm–racket lever. At the moment of impact, however, the resistance point may be considered to be the point of contact of the ball with the racket face. The additional lever actions that are due to the rotation of the spine, the horizontal adduction at the shoulder, and flexion at the wrist, if present, should also be recognized.

Another important anatomical factor is the strength of the muscles responsible for keeping the arm abducted and for assisting in the forward swing as the arm is carried along by the rotating

Figure 18.7 The forehand drive.
From V. Braden and B. Bruns, *Tennis for the Future.* Copyright © 1977 Little, Brown, Boston.

spine and pelvis. Those whose muscles lack the strength to swing the outstretched arm with speed are likely to flex the arm at the elbow or adduct the arm, bringing the racket closer to the trunk and thus shortening the resistance moment arm. Among the muscles that were tested by Van Gheluwe and Hebbelinck (1986) and found active in the forward swing of the forehand drive were the anterior deltoid, pectoralis major, latissimus dorsi, biceps, brachioradialis, and triceps, the latter in two short bursts, the first at the moment of impact, and the second during follow-through (table 18.3).

Mechanical Analysis

The purpose of the forehand drive is to return the ball so that it will not only land within the oppo-

nent's court but also will land in such a place and manner that it will be difficult to return. For the player to achieve this requires both high speed and expert placement of the ball. Hence, imparting maximum speed to the ball and, at the same time, placing it with accuracy are the two major skills that the player seeks to develop.

The force of impact is determined by the speed of the racket at the moment of contact with the ball, and maximum velocity can be obtained only when maximum distance is used for accelerating. The function of the backswing is to provide this distance. There are two types of backswing, the straight and the circular. The straight backswing has the advantage of greater ease in controlling the direction of the racket and in timing the movement but the disadvantage of necessitating

TABLE 18.3	**Anatomical Analysis of the Drive Phase in the Tennis Forehand**				
Joint	**Joint Action**	**Segment Moved**	**Force for Movement**	**Muscles Active**	**Kind of Contraction**
Ankles	Plantar-flexion	Shank	Muscle	Gastrocnemius Soleus	Concentric
Knees	Extension	Thigh	Muscle	Quadriceps femoris	Concentric
Hips	Extension	Trunk	Muscle	Hamstrings Gluteus maximus	Concentric
Shoulder joints	Horizontal abduction	Upper arm	Muscle	Posterior deltoid Infraspinatus Teres minor	Concentric
Shoulder girdle	Adduction	Scapula	Muscle	Rhomboids Trapezius III	Concentric
Elbows	Flexion	Forearm	Muscle	Biceps brachii Brachioradialis	Concentric

the overcoming of inertia in order to reverse the direction from the back to the forward swing. On the other hand, the circular backswing permits the arm to move in one continuous motion over a longer path, thereby providing more than twice the distance for building up momentum. For the more skillful player who is able to control both the direction of the racket and the timing of the entire movement, it is the more efficient method.

In considering the force involved in the forehand drive, it is important to distinguish between the force applied to the lever and the force applied by the lever to the ball. Whereas the force applied to the lever is muscular force, the force applied to the ball is the force of momentum. It is determined by both the mass and velocity of the implement that makes contact with the ball. These, in turn, are related to the distance of the point of contact from the fulcrum—in other words, the length of the temporary resistance arm of the lever ("temporary" because the distance from the fulcrum to the point of contact with the ball constitutes the resistance arm of the lever only for the brief moment of impact). In addition to the rotary movement of the trunk–arm–racket lever, the linear motion produced by the forward

movement of the body (because of weight shift) adds to the force that meets the ball.

Starting with the pelvic rotation and weight shift and working out toward the racket, each movement in turn gets under way before the next one commences. If the timing is correct, the cumulative effect of these movements is to produce maximum velocity. If any of the movements is added to the preceding one either too early or too late, the potential velocity will not be realized.

Other important factors that contribute to the force applied to the ball, and therefore to the speed of the ball on its return flight, include the following:

1. The use of the arm in an almost fully extended position increases the length of the lever, thereby giving greater linear velocity to the racket head than would be the case if the upper arm were close to the body. This is only true, however, if the racket can be moved with the same angular velocity in both positions.

2. The effort needed to resist the force of the ball hitting the racket is less when the racket lever arm is shortened.

3. It takes less time to swing a shortened racket lever into the striking position than it does a fully extended one. (These first three related factors help explain why beginners and children bend the forehand elbow or choke up on the racket handle.)

4. The concentration of mass at the level of the shoulders moving forward at the moment of impact ensures maximum speed for striking.

5. A skillful player tends to use a relatively heavy racket because, other things being equal, the greater the mass of the striking implement, the greater the striking force (momentum) and hence the greater the speed of the struck ball.

6. A new ball and a well-strung racket ensure a good coefficient of restitution (elasticity), thereby increasing the speed of the struck ball.

7. The bending of the knees at the beginning of the forward swing followed by the extension of the legs and shift of weight as the racket is swung forward and up increases the ground reactive force imparted to the body and thus to the ball.

8. It has been generally accepted that a firm wrist and grip are essential for maximum impulse to be applied by the racket to the ball.

9. Placement of the ball is a matter of direction. It will be recalled that the direction taken by a struck ball is determined by four factors:
   a. The direction of the striking implement at the moment of impact.
   b. The relation of the striking force to the ball's center of gravity—in other words, the control of spin.
   c. Firmness of grip and wrist at the moment of impact.
   d. Angle of incidence.

The first of these factors is obvious. The beginner may be less aware of the importance of the other three. For successful placing of the ball, an understanding of the effect of spin and the skill of imparting the desired spin to the ball are essential. Firmness of grip depends on wrist and finger strength and is closely related to the angle at which the racket face makes contact with the ball. Because the angle of rebound equals the angle of incidence (actually slightly less than this in the case of tennis balls because of their compressibility), it will be seen that firmness of grip is therefore an important factor in the direction taken by the struck ball.

LABORATORY EXPERIENCES

1. Throw a tennis ball or baseball for distance:
   a. Standing still, facing in the direction of the throw.
   b. Standing with the left side toward the direction of the throw, with the feet apart and the weight evenly distributed, using a full arm swing and body twist with the throw.
   c. Same as in b, except with the weight on the right foot to begin with, shifting to the left as the ball is thrown.

   Compare the three methods for distance. Explain in terms of length of backswing, speed at moment of release, and total distance used in applying force to ball before releasing it.

2. If possible, observe a small child or an untrained youth and then a trained boy or girl throw a small ball as forcefully as possible at a target 20 or 30 feet away. Analyze the motions of each with reference to the pathway of the hand immediately preceding, at the moment of, and following the release. Explain the factors differentiating the good throws from the poor.

3. Observe slow-motion films of throwing, striking, and other forms of giving motion. Look for the application of the principles stated in this unit or for the lack of such application.

4. Perform a complete kinesiological analysis of a selected throwing, kicking, or striking skill, taking particular note of the purpose of the motion, its classification, the simultaneous–sequential nature of the motion, and its component parts. Include also muscle participation, neuromuscular

considerations, mechanical factors, and applicable principles and violations. Conclude the analysis with a prescription for improvement, including suggested methods for change and the elimination of violations of principles.

REFERENCES AND SELECTED READINGS

Atwater, A. E. 1980. Biomechanics of overarm throwing movements and of throwing injuries. In *Exercise and sport science reviews,* edited by R. S. Hutton and D. I. Miller, vol. 7, 43–85. Philadelphia: Franklin Institute Press.

Bollens, E. C., E. DeProft, and J. P. Clarys. 1987. The accuracy and muscle monitoring in soccer kicking. In *Biomechanics X-A,* edited by B. Jonsson, 283–88. Champaign, IL: Human Kinetics.

Broer, M. R., and S. J. Houtz. 1967. *Patterns of muscular activity in selected sport skills.* Springfield, IL: Charles C Thomas.

Broer, M. R., and R. Zernicke. 1979. *Efficiency of human movement.* 4th ed. Philadelphia: Saunders.

Clarys, J. P., and J. Cabri. 1993. Electromyography and the study of sports movements: A review. *Journal of Sports Sciences* 11:379–448.

Deutsch, H. 1969. *A comparison of women's throwing patterns.* Unpublished doctoral dissertation. Urbana: University of Illinois.

Elliot, B., J. R. Grove, and B. Gibson. 1988. Timing of the lower limb drive and throwing limb movement in baseball pitching. *International Journal of Sport Biomechanics* 4:59–67.

Elliott, B., and T. Marsh. 1989. A biomechanical comparison of topspin and backspin forehand approach shots in tennis. *Journal of Sport Sciences* 7:215–27.

Elliot, B., T. Marsh, and B. Blanksby. 1986. A three-dimensional cinematographic analysis of the tennis serve. *International Journal of Sport Biomechanics* 2:260–71.

Feltner, M., and J. Dapena. 1986. Dynamics of the shoulder and elbow joints of the throwing arm during a baseball pitch. *International Journal of Sport Biomechanics* 2:235–59.

Hamill, J., and K. M. Knutzen. 1995. *Biomechanical basis of human movement.* Philadelphia: Williams & Wilkins.

Kreighbaum, E., and K. M. Barthels. 1994. *Biomechanics: A qualitative approach for studying human movement.* 4th ed. New York: Allyn & Bacon.

MacWilliams, B. A., T. Choi, M. K. Perezous, E. Y. S. Chao, and E. G. MacFarland. 1998. Characteristic ground-reaction forces in baseball pitching. *American Journal of Sports Medicine* 26:66–71.

Moynes, D. R., J. Perry, D. J. Antonelli, and F. W. Jobe. 1986. Electromyography and motion analysis of the upper extremity in sports. *Physical Therapy* 66:1905–11.

Nelson, J. K., J. R. Thomas, K. R. Nelson, and P. C. Abraham. 1986. Gender differences in children's throwing performance: Biology and environment. *Research Quarterly* 57:280–87.

Robertson, D. G. E., and R. D. Mosher. 1985. Work and power of the leg muscles in soccer kicking. In *Biomechanics IX-B,* edited by D. A. Winter, R. W. Norman, R. P. Wells, K. C. Hayes, and A. E. Patla, 533–38. Champaign, IL: Human Kinetics.

Van Gehluwe, B., and M. Hebbelinck. 1986. Muscle actions and ground reaction forces in tennis. *International Journal of Sport Biomechanics* 2:88–99.

LOCOMOTION: SOLID SURFACE

O U T L I N E

- **Locomotion**
- **Walking**
  Description
  Anatomical Analysis
  Anatomical Principles in Walking
  Mechanical Analysis
  Mechanical Principles in Walking
  Walking Variations
- **Running**
  Description
  Anatomical Analysis
  Mechanical Analysis
  Mechanical Principles in Running
  The Sprint Start
- **Jumping, Hopping, and Leaping**
  Mechanical Principles
      in Jumping, Hopping,
      and Leaping
- **Additional Forms of Locomotion**
  Wheels, Blades, and Runners
  Rotary Locomotion
  Locomotion by Specialized Steps
      and Jumps
- **Laboratory Experiences**

O B J E C T I V E S

At the conclusion of this chapter, the student should be able to:

1. Identify and classify motor skills belonging in the categories that fall under the heading of moving one's body on the ground or on another resistant surface.
2. Describe the anatomical and mechanical nature of motor skills representative of the major types of locomotor patterns.
3. Name and state anatomical and mechanical principles that apply to the locomotor patterns of walking, running, and jumping.
4. Evaluate performance of motor skills representative of the major locomotor patterns in terms of application of the related kinesiological principles.
5. Analyze the performance of someone performing a locomotor skill. Follow the kinesiological analysis outline presented in chapter 1.

LOCOMOTION

Locomotion is the act or power of moving from place to place by means of one's own mechanisms or power. Locomotion in human beings is the result of the action of the body levers propelling the body. Ordinarily the propulsion is provided by the lower extremities, but it is occasionally provided by all four extremities, as in creeping, or by the upper extremities alone, as in walking on the hands or in suspension. It may involve the use of wheels, blades, skis, or other equipment attached to the feet, or it may involve a vehicle such as a bicycle or wheelchair, or a small craft such as a boat, canoe, or surfboard propelled by means of the arms or legs, with or without the use of a propelling implement such as oars, paddles, or poles. Locomotion may be on the ground or in the water but, at the present writing, not in the air without support. In all locomotion there must be a resistance against which the body part can push in order to generate a reaction force if motion is to occur.

All forms of locomotion performed on the ground constitute the category of motor skills of moving one's body on the ground or on other resistant surfaces.

On Foot

Walking

Running

Racewalking

Climbing (inclined plane, stairs, ladder)

Descending (inclined plane, stairs, ladder)

Jumping, leaping, hurdling

Skipping, hopping, sliding, sidestepping

Dance steps

Snowshoeing

Stilt walking

On Wheels, Blades, and Runners

Bicycling

Roller skating and skateboarding

Alpine and cross-country skiing

Ice skating

Wheelchair propulsion

On Hands and/or Knees or Hands and Feet

Walking on hands

Creeping and crawling

Crutch walking

Stunts

Rotary Locomotion

Cartwheels

Handsprings

Rolls

WALKING

To the casual observer, the movements involved in walking appear to be relatively simple, yet kinesiological analysis shows them to be exceedingly complex. The dovetailing of muscular action and the synchronization of joint movements beautifully illustrate the teamwork present in all bodily movements. Not even the most complex piece of machinery designed by the most skillful engineers exceeds the movements of the human machine in perfection of detail or in potential smoothness of function on a wide variety of terrain and in all conditions.

The work of Inman, Ralston, Steindler, Murray, and many others has served, over the course of the years, to emphasize the complexity of human walking (Rose and Gamble 1994; Murray, Kory, and Sepic 1970). In the past, researchers have been limited to studying gait and trying to compensate for those factors that often limited people in walking. Currently, a great deal of work is being done in the area of functional electrical stimulation (FES). Using computers and electrical currents, it is now possible to program the muscles of the disabled patient in such a way as to artificially stimulate the muscles of the lower extremity to reproduce the action of walking. Depending on the state of the neuromuscular system, those who once were forced to rely on wheelchairs, braces, and canes are now starting to walk with the aid of such computerized systems.

Description

Walking is accomplished by the alternating action of the two lower extremities (figure 19.1). It is an example of translatory motion of the body as a whole brought about by rotary motion of some of its parts. It is also an example of a periodic, or pendulum-like, movement in which the moving segment (in this case the lower extremity) may be said to start at zero, pass through its arc of motion, and fall to zero again at the end of each stroke. In walking, each lower extremity undergoes two phases: the swing or recovery phase and the support phase. The support phase is further divided into heel-strike, foot-flat, midstance, heel-off, and toe-off phases. The toe-off phase of one leg overlaps the heel-strike and foot-flat phases of the other leg, thus producing a period of double support when both feet are on the ground. This double support phase is characteristic of the walk and serves to differentiate it from the run.

The kinematics of the walking gait are often described in terms of strides and steps. A stride is one full lower-extremity cycle. In walking and running, a stride is defined as being from heel strike on one leg to the next heel strike with the same leg. Stride length, then, is the distance covered during a single stride. A step starts with the heel strike on one leg and ends with the heel strike of the contralateral, or opposite, leg.

Gravity and momentum are the chief sources of motion for the swing phase; hence, this phase represents a ballistic type of movement (p. 63), particularly when the individual is walking at a natural pace. The source of motion for the support phase is, for the first half, the momentum of the

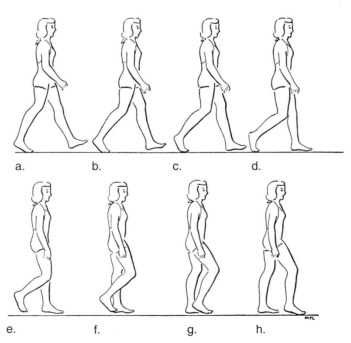

a.   b.   c.   d.

e.   f.   g.   h.

Figure 19.1   Walking is an example of linear motion of the body as a whole resulting from the angular motion of some of its parts.

forward-moving trunk (provided by the propulsive action of the other leg) and, for the second half, the contraction of the extensor muscles of the supporting leg. Whether the support phase can also be classed as ballistic movement is open to question. Even the swing phase varies in its ballistic quality according to the speed of the gait and the skill, flexibility, and build of the walker. A tense individual will tend to substitute muscular action for the pendulum swing of the lower extremity, and an individual with tight hamstrings will have to exert additional muscular force to overcome the restraining action of the short hamstrings. An individual who has knock-knees or fat thighs will also have difficulty in achieving a natural, pendulum swing because of friction and interference between the two limbs. To avoid this interference the walker would need to increase the lateral distance between the limbs and thus introduce an undesirable lateral component of motion.

Anatomical Analysis

The six major components of walking have been defined as (1) pelvic rotation, (2) pelvic tilt, (3) knee flexion, (4) hip flexion, (5) knee and ankle interaction, and (6) lateral pelvic displacement. Each of these components is essential for efficient walking, and the loss of any one will cause an increase in the energy cost.

The action taking place in the joints of the lower extremity consists essentially of flexion and extension. But, in much the same way that the shoulder girdle cooperates with the arm movements of the upper extremity, the pelvic girdle cooperates in movements of the lower extremities. The pelvis has the double task of transmitting the weight of the body alternately first over one limb, then over the other, and of putting each acetabulum in a favorable position for the action of the corresponding femur. The adaptations of the pelvic position are made in the joints of the thoracic and lumbar spine as well as in the hip joints. Thus, as first one foot and then the other is put forward, the flexion and extension move-

ments of the thigh are accompanied by slight rotary movements and abduction and adduction at the hips, and by slight lateral flexion and rotation of the spine (figures 19.2 and 19.3).

The muscular analysis presented here is a compilation of results from numerous studies on the walking gait. Wallking, both normal and pathological, is one of the most widely studied of all human movement patterns. The movement specialist would be well advised to keep abreast of the ongoing research in the area of gait analysis. Because of the relative importance and complexity of the walking gait, a complete discussion of the muscular involvement in walking is presented.

Swing Phase

The swing phase begins with toe-off and ends with heel-strike.

Spine and Pelvis

1. *Movements:* Rotation of the pelvis toward the support leg and of the spine in the opposite direction; slight lateral tilt of the pelvis toward the unsupported leg. The simultaneous opposite actions help prevent excessive motion of the trunk. Pelvic rotation also lengthens the step and decreases the lateral deviation of the center of gravity of the body, whereas pelvic tilt decreases the elevation of the center of gravity.
2. *Muscles:* Semispinalis, rotatores, multifidus, and external oblique abdominal muscles on side toward which the pelvis rotates. Erector spinae and internal oblique abdominal muscles on opposite side. (*Note:* Rotation of the pelvis to the right constitutes rotation of the spine to the left. See pp. 228–229.) The psoas and quadratus lumborum help support the pelvis on the side of the swinging limb.

Hip

1. *Movements:* Flexion; outward rotation (because of pelvic rotation); adduction at

a.   b.   c.

Figure 19.2   The muscles of the lower extremity used in walking. Key: a:1. Tensor fasciae latae; 2. sartorius; 3. pectineus; 4. biceps femoris. b:1. Rectus femoris; 2. iliopsoas; 3. vastus lateralis (medius and intermedius are not shown); 4. tibialis anterior; 5. extensor hallucis longus; 6. extensor digitorum longus; 7. peroneus tertius; 8. semitendinosus and semimembranosus; 9. soleus; 10. gastrocnemius. c:1. Gluteus medius; 2. rectus femoris; 3. soleus; 4. tibialis posterior (underneath); 5. peroneus longus; 6. peroneus brevis; 7. semimembranosus and semitendinosus; 8. vastus medialis and intermedius (lateralis not shown); 9. adductor longus; 10. gastrocnemius.

beginning and abduction at end of phase, especially if long stride is taken (also because of pelvic rotation, as well as stride length).

2. *Muscles:* The iliopsoas is the prime mover of the hip in the swing phase, with assistance from the rectus femoris, sartorius, gracilis, adductor longus, and possibly the tensor fasciae latae, pectineus, and the short head of the biceps femoris during the early part of the swing. The sartorius and the short head of the biceps are active chiefly following toe-off, while the tensor fasciae latae is also active during midswing.

In the latter part of the swing phase there is no appreciable action of the hip flexors in normal walking on level ground. This is consistent with the ballistic nature of the movement. The hamstrings contract with moderate intensity during the knee extension part of the swing and the gluteus maximus and medius contract slightly at the very end of the swing. The adductors longus and magnus, and presumably brevis, contract slightly after the swinging limb has passed the halfway mark. The function of the adductor magnus is not clear. It may help steady and guide the forward-swinging limb. In any event, its action is extremely slight, even in rapid walking.

In rapid walking there is a noticeable increase in the activity of the sartorius and the rectus femoris and also a slight increase in that of the tensor fasciae latae.

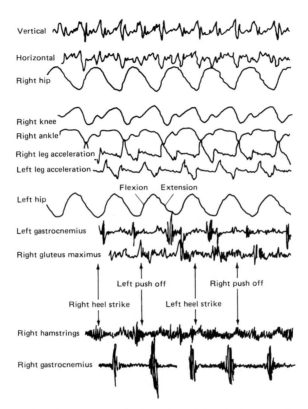

Figure 19.3   Simultaneous tracings recorded during normal walking. *From top:* vertical and horizontal accelerograms; electrogoniograms of right hip, knee, and ankle; angular accelerograms of right and left legs; electrogoniogram of left hip; electromyograms of left gastrocnemius, right gluteus maximus, right hamstrings, and right gastrocnemius.

After W. T. Liberson in *Biomechanics III (Medicine and Sport,* Vol. 8). Copyright © 1973 S. Karger AG, Basel, Switzerland. Reprinted by permission.

Knee

1. *Movements:* Flexion during the first half; extension during the second half.
2. *Muscles:* As was true in hip flexion (and for the same reason), so also in knee flexion is there remarkably little muscular action in the swing phase of normal walking. The quadriceps extensors contract slightly at the end of this phase. The action of the sartorius, a two-joint muscle, has already been mentioned in connection with the hip. The action of these muscles, as well as that of the medial hamstrings, increases in rapid walking. In an easy gait the movement

appears to be initiated by gravitational force and continued by momentum. This force is sufficient to extend the leg at the knee, except perhaps at the very end of the movement. In more vigorous walking the quadriceps femoris provides the force for leg extension.

Ankle and Foot

1. *Movements:* Dorsiflexion; prevention of plantar flexion.
2. *Muscles:* The tibialis anterior, extensor digitorum longus, extensor hallucis longus, and probably the peroneus tertius contract

with slight to moderate intensity at the beginning of the swinging phase and taper off during the middle portion of this phase. Basmajian and DeLuca (1985) found that the tibialis anterior was actually completely quiescent at midswing. They observed that the foot everted in the early phase and maintained this eversion during the middle part. This seemed to them to serve the important purpose of providing sufficient clearance between the foot and the ground. Other researchers have since found varying levels of activity in the tibialis anterior during the swing phase (Rose and Gamble 1994).

Toward the end of the swing phase this group of muscles contracts again with considerable force in preparation for the heel strike. The plantar flexors are completely relaxed throughout the entire swing phase.

Support Phase

The support phase begins with heel-strike and ends with toe-off. The portion between heel-strike of the forward foot and toe-off of the other, that is, the rear foot, constitutes a period of double support that is characteristic of walking but does not occur in running.

Spine and pelvis   Rotation of pelvis toward same side and spine to opposite side: lateral tilt away from support leg.

Hip

1. *Movements:* Extension through foot-flat to toe-off; reduction of outward rotation, followed by slight inward rotation; prevention of adduction of the thigh and dropping of pelvis to opposite side.
2. *Muscles:* During heel-strike the gluteal muscles and the hamstrings contract statically with moderate intensity. These contractions then taper off during foot-flat and disappear at midstance. A number of EMG researchers have found evidence of

gluteus maximus activity in the early part of the support phase (Basmajian and DeLuca 1985; Rose and Gamble 1994). The gluteus minimus continues to contract moderately during the middle portion. The only muscles of the hip that contract appreciably during the last part of the support phase are the adductors magnus, longus, and possibly brevis.

In rapid walking the gluteus maximus and minimus contract with appreciable intensity during the first part of the support phase, and the adductor longus during the last part. The hamstrings apparently have but a small part in the supporting phase of normal walking. Only the long head of the biceps contracts at all, and it contracts only slightly at the very beginning of this phase. In rapid walking both the long head of the biceps and the semitendinosus contract with moderate intensity during the first half of the support phase.

Knee

1. *Movements:* Slight flexion from heel-strike continuing into foot-flat, followed by extension from midstance until heel-lift when flexion for the swing phase begins. This flexion during the stance phase flattens the vertical path of the center of gravity of the body, thus increasing the efficiency of the gait.
2. *Muscles:* The quadriceps extensors contract moderately in the early part of the support phase, then gradually relax. They appear to control the slight flexion that occurs in the knee at the moment of heel-strike. The vastii continue to contract throughout the first half of this phase. As the leg reaches the vertical position, the knee apparently locks and makes contraction of the extensors unnecessary. The tension of the stretched hamstrings at the end of the swing phase, especially when a long stride has been taken, may well be the factor that initiates the slight

flexion at heel-strike. The hamstrings again show activity at the end of the support phase. In rapid walking all of these muscles contract more strongly and for a longer duration. There is an abrupt increase in their action in the second half of the support phase, which would seem to indicate that the extension of the leg at the knee is much more forceful in rapid walking than in normal walking.

Ankle and Foot

1. *Movements:* Slight plantar flexion, followed by slight dorsiflexion; prevention of further dorsiflexion, which the body weight tends to cause. Plantar flexion of ankle and hyperextension of metatarsophalangeal joints at the end of the propulsive phase, especially in vigorous walking.

2. *Muscles:* EMG studies (Basmajian and DeLuca 1985; Rose and Gamble 1994) show that there is considerable action of the tibialis anterior in the early part of the supporting phase, especially at heel-strike. This action is likely related to the controlled lowering of the foot by eccentric contraction in order to prevent the foot from slapping down too hard. Contrary to earlier opinions, the tibialis anterior does not continue to show activity during the major weight-bearing period, but it becomes active again at toe-off. The extensor digitorum longus and hallucis longus follow a similar pattern. They reach their peak of contraction almost at the moment of transition between the swing and support phases; they relax early in the support phase, commencing to contract slightly at the end of this phase.

The gastrocnemius and soleus become active from midstance to heel-off, contracting eccentrically to control ankle dorsiflexion as the center of gravity continues moving forward. Peak activity in the plantarflexors is reached from heel-off to toe-off as the foot pushes against the ground to initiate the next step.

The tibialis posterior is most active during the middle part of the support phase, one of its functions, according to Basmajian, being to prevent eversion (pronation) of the foot. He points out that the peroneus longus and tibialis posterior apparently cooperate in stabilizing the leg and foot in weight bearing. The gastrocnemius and soleus act to decelerate the lower leg and stabilize the knee at midstance (Winter and Kuryliak 1978). There is a sharp increase in gastrocnemius and soleus activity beginning after the heel lifts and continuing until the opposite heel contacts the ground initiating the period of double support. Extension of the knee in the stance phase is always accompanied by calf muscle activity. In *rapid* walking, however, their activity is much more pronounced. The peroneus longus follows a simple pattern but does not seem to contract quite so strongly as the others, except in rapid walking. The peroneus brevis does not start to contract until about the middle of the support phase, but it contracts more strongly than the longus. In rapid walking it starts earlier and contracts with intensity soon after the halfway point has been reached.

The flexor digitorum longus contracts slightly during the middle portion of the support phase and increases abruptly to moderate contraction in the last portion. In rapid walking the contraction becomes strong. The flexor hallucis longus follows the same pattern, except that it does not start to contract until the middle of the phase.

The toe muscles, flexor hallucis longus, flexor digitorum longus, and the short, intrinsic flexors of the toes contract in response to the pressure of the ground against the toes. In the propulsive phase, especially in vigorous walking, this contraction is intensified. In all parts of the support phase the contraction of the toe flexors is greater in barefoot walking than when shoes are worn. This is especially noticeable when walking on turf or sand.

Action of Upper Extremities in Walking

Unless restrained, the arms tend to swing in opposition to the legs, the left arm swinging forward as the right leg swings forward and vice versa. This reflex action is usually accomplished without obvious muscular action and serves to balance the rotation of the pelvis. When the arm swing is prevented, the upper trunk tends to rotate in the same direction as the pelvis, causing a tense, awkward gait.

Murray, Sepic, and Barnard (1967), using the technique of interrupted light photography, investigated the action of the upper extremities in walking. They noted "patterns of sagittal rotation of the shoulder and elbow," or flexion and extension of both joints. They found that, although the amplitudes of the arm swing pattern varied considerably from one subject to another, each individual had a similar pattern in all trials, even at higher speeds. Furthermore, they noted that the increased amplitude accompanying the faster speeds was due mainly to increased shoulder (hyper-) extension in the backward swing and increased elbow flexion in the forward swing. Maximum flexion of both the shoulder and elbow joints occurred at the moment of heel strike of the opposite foot and maximum extension at the moment of heel strike of the foot on the same side.

In an early investigation of the muscular action of the arms, Hogue (1969) found that although they appear to swing without muscular effort in walking at a normal pace on level ground, actually their pendular action was caused by a combination of muscular activity and gravity. The middle and posterior deltoid and the teres major were the muscles that he found to be most concerned, the latter two being active mainly during the backward swing. The posterior deltoid also contracted toward the end of the forward swing, leading one to suspect that it was serving as a brake to check the movement. The middle deltoid was found to be active during both flexion and extension of the arm at the shoulder joint. As this muscle is primarily an abductor, it seems that its function might be to keep the arms from brushing the sides of the body as they swing past it.

Neuromuscular Considerations

Walking is an action that relies heavily on reflex; little conscious control is necessary. On the contrary, if too much attention is focused on any part of the gait, tension is likely to develop and the natural rhythm and coordination are disturbed. Reflexes control not only the movements of the limbs but also the extension of both the supporting limb and the trunk in resisting the downward pull of gravity. This extension serves to give stability to the body in the support phases of locomotion, a stability that provides for effective muscular action in producing the necessary movements. Thus, in walking, as in all the motions of the body, smooth, coordinated movement requires properly functioning reflexes, normal flexibility of the joints, and optimum stability of the body as a whole in the weight-bearing phases of the act.

Two reflexes that play prominent roles are the *stretch reflex* and the *extensor thrust reflex.* The stretch reflex may be involved at the extremes in motion, particularly at the shoulder and hip joints, assisting with the change in the direction of joint motion. The extensor thrust reflex may facilitate the extensor muscles of the lower extremity as the weight rides over the foot on the support leg.

Anatomical Principles in Walking

Several key anatomical factors affect the efficiency of the walking gait. Key factors to consider in any analysis of a walking pattern are the following:

1. Alignment
   a. Good alignment of the lower extremities reduces friction in the joints and decreases the likelihood of strain and injury.
   b. The stability of the weight-bearing limb and the balance of the trunk over this limb are important factors in the smoothness of the gait. Both are improved with good alignment of the weight-bearing segments.

2. Unnecessary lateral movements decrease gait economy. Lateral movements are usually due to excessive motion in the shoulders or pelvis.
   a. Excessive trunk rotation may be caused by either exaggerated or restricted arm swing. Normally the arm swing exactly counterbalances the hip swing.
   b. The pelvis may drop on one side if the gluteus medius is not contracted for support. The result is an exaggerated hip sway.
   c. Pelvic rotation should be just enough to enable the leg to move straight forward. A straight sagittal plane action of the leg is ensured by keeping the knee and foot pointing straight forward in all phases of the gait. The feet should be placed in such a way that their inner borders fall approximately along a straight line. Deviation from this pattern of leg motion will produce a weaving, inefficient gait.
3. Normal flexibility of the joints (i.e., sufficiently long and flexible muscles, ligaments, and fasciae) reduces internal resistance and therefore reduces the amount of force required for walking.
   a. The tendons of the two-joint muscles of the lower extremity contribute to the economy of muscular action in walking.
4. Properly functioning reflexes contribute to a well-coordinated, efficient gait. Injury, disease, or substance abuse can interfere with the walking reflex.

Mechanical Analysis

Walking is characterized by the translation of the body's center of gravity forward as a result of the alternating pattern of the lower extremity joint movements during the stance and swing phases. The forces that control walking are the external forces of weight, normal reaction, friction, air resistance, and internal muscular forces. The direction and interaction of these forces determine the nature of the gait.

The inertia of the stationary body is overcome by the horizontal component of the propulsive force. Because periodic movement is characterized by an alternating increase and decrease of speed, the inertia must be overcome at every step, and the greater the weight of the body, the greater is the inertia to be overcome. As the center of gravity moves forward, it momentarily passes beyond the anterior margin of the base of support and a temporary loss of balance results. At this point the downward pull of gravity threatens a complete loss of equilibrium. A timely recovery of balance is effected, however, as the foot is placed on the ground. Thus, a new base of support is established and a new support phase is begun. The downward force of the body's weight is counteracted by the vertical reactive force through the feet. If the vertical force exceeds that needed to balance the gravitational force at the time of push-off, an exaggerated lift to the body results, causing a gait characterized by a bounce or unusual spring.

When forward motion has been imparted to the trunk by means of the ground reaction to the backward thrust of the leg and foot, it tends to continue unless restrained by another force. Once the center of gravity passes beyond the base of support, it is essential to restrain the action of the trunk until a new base of support is established. Hence, as the foot is brought to the ground in front of the body at the close of its recovery phase, a restraining phase is constituted. This diminishes as the leg approaches midstance. During the period that the foot is in front of the center of gravity, there is a forward component of force in the thrust of the foot against the ground. This results in a *backward* reactive force of the ground against the foot, which is transmitted to the leg and thence to the trunk.

The degree to which the pressure of the foot actually imparts motion to the body in the propulsive phase and restrains it in the restraining phase is in direct proportion to the counterpressure of normal reactive force of the supporting surface. If the surface lacks solidity, as in the case of mud, soft snow, and sand, it offers too little resistance

Figure 19.4   The ground reaction of force *R* is equal in action line and magnitude to the downward thrust of the foot during walking but is opposite in direction. The force is greater at heel-strike than at midstance because of the body's momentum and is greater at push-off because of the plantar flexion thrust of the calf muscles driving the body forward.
From B. LeVeau, *Williams and Lissner: Biomechanics of Human Motion,* 2nd ed. Copyright © 1977 W.B. Saunders, Orlando, FL. Reprinted by permission.

to give the needed counterpressure. The pressure of the foot results in slipping or sinking, and more pressure must be applied to achieve even a slow forward progress. Hence the efficiency of the gait depends on the right balance between the pressure of the foot and the counterpressure of the supporting surface (figure 19.4).

Like counterpressure, friction is also an essential factor in the effective application of the forces needed in walking. Because of the diagonal thrust of the leg at the beginning and end of the support phase, friction between the foot and the ground is essential in order that the counterpressure of the ground may be transmitted to the body. For efficient walking, friction must be sufficient to balance the horizontal component of force. If it is insufficient, the thrust of the foot results in a slipping of the foot itself rather than in the desired propulsion of the body. The greater the horizontal component of force (as when walking with a long stride), the greater the dependence on friction for efficient locomotion.

The forward-moving trunk meets with air resistance, which tends to push it backward. By inclining the body forward, the pull of gravity is utilized to balance the force of the air resistance. When walking against a strong wind, it is necessary to incline the body farther forward to maintain balance. If the air resistance is not balanced

by the force of gravity, it must be balanced by the contraction of the abdominal and other anterior muscles of the neck and trunk. If the body is inclined too far forward, however, the force of gravity acts too strongly on it and must be counteracted by tension of the posterior muscles. Thus, the proper degree of forward inclination is a factor in muscular economy.

Mechanical Principles in Walking

A number of mechanical principles govern the walking gait. A mechanical analysis of walking should include all of these important principles.

1. A body at rest will remain at rest unless acted on by a force. The force for walking is ground reaction force produced by extension of the lower extremity against a resistive surface. Because walking is an alternating pendular motion of the lower extremities, the inertia of the body must be overcome at every step.
2. A body in motion will remain in motion until acted on by a force. Once motion is imparted to the trunk by the backward and downward thrust of the legs, the trunk has a tendency to continue in motion, even beyond the base of support. A brief restraining action of the

forward limb serves as a brake on the momentum of the trunk.

3. Translatory movement of a lever is achieved by the repeated alternation of two rotary movements, the lever first turning about one end and then the other (Steindler 1973). In walking, the lower extremity alternates between rotating about the foot's point of contact (support phase) and the hip joint (swing phase).

4. Force applied diagonally has both horizontal and vertical components. The vertical component of the ground reaction force used in walking serves to counteract the pull of gravity. The horizontal component of this force serves to (a) check forward motion of the trunk during heel-strike and (b) produce forward motion in the trunk during heel-off and toe-off.

5. The speed of walking is increased by increasing either the stride length or the stride rate, or both.

6. The speed of the gait is directly related to the magnitude of the pushing force and to the direction of its application. This force is provided by the extensor muscles of the lower extremity, and the direction of the force application is determined by the angle of the lower extremity when the force is being applied.

7. As propulsion of the body is brought about by the backward and downward push of the foot against the supporting surface, the efficiency of locomotion partially depends on the friction and ground reaction force provided by this surface.

8. The efficiency of gait is related to its timing with reference to the length of the limbs. The most efficient gait is one that is so timed as to permit pendular motion of the lower extremities.

9. Walking has been described as an alternating loss and recovery of balance (Steindler 1973). This being so, a new base of support must be established at every step.

10. Stability of the body is directly related to the size of the base of support. In walking, the lateral distance between the feet is a minor factor in maintaining balance, because momentum (and therefore inertia) carries the body forward.

Walking Variations
Individual Variations in the Gait

Although the basic analysis of the gait is valid for all physically normal persons, individual characteristics are present to such a degree that persons are often recognized by their gaits. These variations may be either structural or functional in origin. The structural differences include unusual body proportions as well as differences in the limbs themselves, such as knock-knees and bowlegs. Extreme variations in the angle between the neck and the shaft of the femur and in the obliquity of the femoral shaft are also responsible for atypical gaits.

Variations in the forward-backward distribution of weight and in the length of stride have already been mentioned. Other variations in movement patterns that are not structural in origin are often related to characteristics of the personality. This fact was brought home forcefully to Wells when she attempted to help college students whose gaits were awkward. Almost invariably the students who walked the most awkwardly were those who were extremely shy or lacking in self-confidence. A study investigating the possible relationship between the two might be rewarding.

Age is also a factor in gait variations. As the human body ages, there is some decrease in both strength and flexibility as tissues change. Balance often becomes a significant concern. As a result of these changes, the gait of the elderly is often modified from that of a healthy young adult. Typically, the gait of a more elderly person will have the same cadence as that of a younger person, but the step length will be shorter. In addition, more time is spent in the double support phase, and propulsive force is reduced. These changes in the gait pattern, although producing a slower gait, produce greater stability (Winter et al. 1990).

Obesity has also been found to have an often negative effect on the walking gait. Obvious changes in gait would include increased impact forces in the foot-strike period, as well as a requirement for increased propulsive forces. Not as easily seen, but much more risky, are the increased medial and lateral forces that occur during walking in the obese person. These increased frontal plane forces lead to increased subtalar eversion. The combination of this eversion and the overall increase in force production may be linked to greater shear forces in the knee and increased deterioration of soft tissue structures in that region (Messier et al. 1996).

Walking Up and Down Stairs and Ramps

In walking upstairs or up a ramp, the reactive force resulting from the push of the legs should be directed through the body's center of gravity and in line with the forward-upward slope of the stairs or ramp. The most strain-free way of doing this is to incline the body forward in a straight line from the rear foot. The act of descending stairs or a ramp involves safely resisting the force of gravity on the body. The eccentric contraction of the muscles of the lower extremity enables the body to be lowered at a controlled rate, and maintaining the line of gravity toward the back of the base of support prevents forward falls (figure 19.5). In walking upstairs or up a ramp, the swing phase is characterized by an exaggerated knee lift and dorsiflexion of the ankle. According to Joseph and Watson, the hamstrings and tibialis anterior are the chief muscles involved (Basmajian and DeLuca 1985). In the support phase, when the action is chiefly extension of the knee and hip, with the ankle being either slightly plantar flexed or else maintained in the midposition on the ball of the foot, they found the chief muscular action to come from the gluteus maximus, hamstrings, quadriceps femoris, and soleus, with the gluteus medius helping maintain stability at the hip joint.

a.   b.

Figure 19.5   Going up and down stairs.

The swing phase of walking downstairs starts with a slight lifting of the rear foot to clear the step. This movement involves slight knee flexion and dorsiflexion of the ankle. It is followed by slight hip flexion, then hip and knee extension and plantar flexion of the ankle as the foot reaches for the step below the one the supporting foot is on.

The support phase starts with the ankle in plantar flexion and the knee in extension. As the foot assumes the body weight, the ankle, knee, and hip are approximately in their neutral positions with the knee very slightly flexed. As the other foot swings forward, the supporting leg engages in slight hip flexion, increasing knee flexion and dorsiflexion of the ankle. In the brief period of double support, the knee and ankle flexion reach their maximum. The main muscular action of the supporting limb, according to Joseph and Watson, consists of eccentric contraction of the hamstrings, quadriceps femoris, and soleus, with the gluteus medius contributing to hip stability as it does in ascending (Basmajian and DeLuca 1985).

Racewalking

The racewalking gait is an adaptation of walking intended to produce maximum walking speed without breaking into a run. Because the walk and

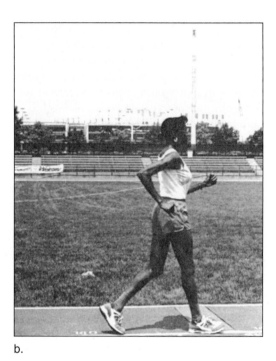

a.   b.

Figure 19.6   Racewalk gait: (a) increased lateral pelvic tilt; (b) fully extended knee during support phase.

the run are differentiated by the presence or absence of a double support phase, a racewalk must show a period of double support. A competitive racewalker attempts to minimize this double support period by increasing stride rate and decreasing stride length. In a normal walking gait, the stance phase accounts for 62 percent of the stride cycle and the swing phase makes up the other 38 percent. In the racewalk stance and swing phases, each accounts for 50 percent of the stride (Cairns et al. 1986). The peculiar straight-legged, hip swing appearance of the racewalk gait is produced by a further stipulation in competitive racewalking that requires that the knee of the support leg extend fully during the stance phase (figure 19.6).

The racewalk gait differs from the normal walking gait in several ways. In racewalking there is greater ankle dorsiflexion just prior to heel-strike and the leg is already fully extended at the knee when this contact occurs. The feet follow a line of progression closer to the midline of the body than in normal walking. There is a more exaggerated arm swing and therefore greater trunk rotation. Because of the straight support leg there is greater lateral pelvic tilt as the pelvis rises above the support leg and drops on the swing side. The combined motion of the hip, trunk, pelvis, and arms acts to compensate for the lack of knee flexion in the support leg, producing little vertical motion.

RUNNING

Description

Easy running, like walking, is a pendulum type of movement. It is doubtful, however, whether running at top speed can be so classified. The most notable factors differentiating the run from the walk are the period of double support, characteristic of the walk but not present in the run, and the

a.   b.   c.   d.

e.   f.   g.   h.

Figure 19.7   Running: (a–e) support and drive phase (right leg); (f–h) swing phase. (a) Heel-strike; (b) flat-foot; (e) toe-off and beginning of swing phase for right leg.

period of no support (a "sailing-through-the-air period"), characteristic of the run but not present in the walk. In the run the foot hits the ground in front of the body's center of gravity as in the walk, but not as far in front. As the speed of the run increases, the distance in front decreases until the foot contact is almost directly under the body's center of gravity. This position reduces the restraining part of the support phase and gives greater emphasis to the propulsive part. At maximum speed, the restraining part disappears completely. The use of the term "driving phase" for the support phase in running indicates its propulsive nature.

There are two major types of running. The first is the kind of running done for its own sake, as in competitive races or jogging. The major concerns here are time and distance in one direction. The second is the type of running that is part of games and sports. Here it is necessary also to consider matters such as change of direction or pace and stability. The technique for a run varies with

the purpose, but the basic anatomical and mechanical aspects are the same, regardless of the purpose.

Anatomical Analysis

The difference between the joint actions in walking and running is a matter of degree and coordination. The joint actions are essentially the same but the range of motion in running is generally greater. This is especially apparent in the actions of the swinging leg. The difference in coordination is evident in the period of nonsupport and the absence of the period of double support.

Swing Phase

The swing phase begins with toe-off and ends with the foot landing (figure 19.7). It is more muscular than pendular and is longer than the support phase. In fast running the initial foot contact may be the ball of the foot and, in slow running, the whole foot. The flexed leg in the swing

TABLE 19.1	Anatomical Analysis of Swing Phase in Running				
Joint	Joint Action	Segment Moved	Force for Movement	Muscles Active	Kind of Contraction
Ankles	Dorsi flexion	Foot	Muscle	Tibialis anterior Extensor digitorum longus Extensor hallicus longus	Concentric
Knees	Flexion (fast, first ⅔ of swing)	Shank	Muscle	Reflex action and momentum	
	Extension (last ⅓ of swing)	Shank	Momentum	Hamstrings	Eccentric
Hips	Flexion	Thigh	Muscle	Iliopsoas Rectus femoris	Concentric

Movements and muscular involvement in the spine and pelvis are the same as in walking but more vigorous in reaction to leg movements.

phase brings the mass of the leg close to the hip, reducing the moment of inertia and increasing the angular velocity of the forward-swinging thigh, which in turn drives the center of gravity of the body forward (table 19.1).

Support Phase

The support phase begins with the contact of the forward foot and ends at toe-off when the body is driven into the air (figure 19.7 a to e). During this time the knee and ankle "give" in flexion and then extend as the body passes over the foot and is driven into the air. The support time decreases as the speed of the run increases (table 19.2).

Mechanical Analysis

The speed of running is governed by the length of the stride and the frequency of the stride. Better runners have a greater stride length per given pace than poorer runners. The length of the stride is determined by the length of the leg, the range of motion in the hip, and the power of the leg extensors, which drive the entire body forward. Like any projectile, the distance the body will move once it is driven into the air depends on the angle of takeoff (distance that center of gravity is ahead of takeoff foot), the speed of the body's projection, and the height of the center of gravity at takeoff and landing. The stride rate of the run is affected by the speed of muscle contraction and the skill of the performer.

In running, as in walking, the forces exerted to produce and control the movement are the internal muscular forces and the external forces of gravity, normal reaction, friction, and air resistance. There is no optimal speed in running because the energy needed to run is proportional to the square of the velocity. Therefore, whether the run is an easy jog or a full-speed sprint, economy of effort is a highly desirable objective. To achieve this it is essential that the runner observe the principles that apply to efficient running.

TABLE 19.2	Anatomical Analysis of Support Phase in Running				
Joint	Joint Action	Segment Moved	Force for Movement	Muscles Active	Kind of Contraction
Ankles	Plantar flexion	Shank	Muscle	Gastrocnemius Soleus	Concentric
Knees	Flexion (initial support)	Thigh	Gravity	Quadriceps femoris	Eccentric
	Extension (at push-off)	Thigh	Muscle	Quadriceps femoris	Eccentric
Hips	Flexion	Trunk	Gravity	Gluteus maximus Hamstrings	Eccentric
	Extension	Trunk	Muscle	Quadriceps femoris	Concentric

Movements and muscular involvement in the spine and pelvis are the same as in walking but more vigorous in reaction to leg movements.

Mechanical Principles in Running

1. In accordance with the Law of Inertia, a body remains at rest unless acted on by a force. The force required to overcome inertia is greatest at takeoff and least after acceleration has ceased. The problem of overcoming inertia decreases as the speed increases.
2. In accordance with the law of acceleration, acceleration in the run is directly proportional to the force producing it. Hence, the greater the power of the leg drive, the greater the acceleration of the runner.
3. In accordance with the law of reaction, every action has an equal and opposite reaction. The force for the run is provided through the upward and forward ground reaction force in response to the downward, backward drive of the foot. The smaller the vertical component of this force, the greater the horizontal or driving component. In the most efficient run, vertical movements of the center of gravity are reduced to a minimum. There should be no bounce in running.

   In an efficient run, the foot should strike the ground as close as possible to the line of gravity. If the foot should strike ahead of the line of gravity, the reaction force to this forward and downward thrust will be a backward and upward force, acting to retard forward motion.

4. The more completely the horizontal force is directed straight backward, the greater its contribution to the forward motion of the body. Lateral motions are inefficient and detract from forward propulsion.

   The knees should be lifted directly upward and forward, with the motion of the entire lower extremity occurring within the sagittal plane. The arm swing should exactly counterbalance the twist of the pelvis and should not cause additional lateral motion.

5. Because a long lever develops greater speed at the distal end than does a short lever, the length of the leg in the driving phase should be as great as possible when speed is a consideration. Leg drive should be maximized as early as possible in the stance phase.
6. Efficiency in running, as in any movement, requires the elimination of all unnecessary forces. Internal resistance forces that are due to sarcolemma viscosity or tightness of the tendons, ligaments, and fascia can be reduced by warm-up and stretching activities.
7. Resistance forces that are due to the moment of inertia of the free leg during the swing

a.   b.   c.

Figure 19.8   The crouch start for a sprint race. The period of acceleration is characterized by a gradual decrease in the forward inclination of the trunk and a lengthening of the stride.

phase can be minimized. By flexing the free leg at the knee and carrying the heel high up under the hip, the leg is moved more rapidly as well as more economically. This high knee lift increases as speed increases.

8. The force of air resistance can be altered by shifting the center of gravity. A forward lean will work to counteract a head wind. A tailwind often enhances performance.

The Sprint Start

Because the object in sprint running is maximum horizontal velocity, sprint racers usually use the crouching start. This start enables the runner to exert maximum horizontal force at takeoff, providing maximum acceleration against inertia. In the sprint start the runner pushes against starting blocks fixed to the track surface. The blocks provide a surface against which the foot can push horizontally while utilizing maximum hip, knee, and ankle extension. Moving the rear foot farther back in the blocks can increase the push-off force but decreases the time to apply the force, which may result in a smaller impulse *(Ft)*. During the acceleration phase of the race immediately after the start, the horizontal component of the leg drive gradually diminishes until a constant level of

speed is maintained, during which period horizontal velocity remains uniform. The period of acceleration is characterized by a gradual decrease in the inclination of the trunk, a lengthening of the stride (made possible by raising the center of gravity as the trunk becomes more erect), and a decrease of the knee thrust, resulting from the gradual straightening of the knee at the moment of foot contact with the ground (figure 19.8).

JUMPING, HOPPING AND LEAPING

Jumping, hopping, and leaping are forms of locomotion familiar from earliest childhood, whether engaged in as a simple expression of joy and exuberance, as a self-testing and competitive activity, or as an integral part of a sport. In each instance the goal is to propel the body into the air with sufficient force to overcome gravity and in the direction to accomplish the desired height or horizontal distance. Like any projectile, the path of the body in the air is determined by the conditions at the instant of projection. The differences between a hop, jump, and leap relate to the landing and takeoff. In the hop, the same foot is used for the takeoff and landing. In the leap, the takeoff is from one foot and the landing on the other. A jumper takes off from one or both feet and lands on both feet. Each of these types of projection may be initiated from a stationary position (vertical jump, standing long jump) or preceded by some locomotor pattern such as running (running long jump, triple jump, high jump, hurdle).

The total horizontal distance covered by the performer of these related patterns is the sum of three distances: (1) the horizontal distance between the takeoff foot and the line of gravity of the performer, (2) the horizontal distance the center of gravity travels in the air, and (3) the horizontal distance the center of gravity is behind the body part that lands closest to the takeoff point. The total height may be considered to be divided into the distance between the ground and the line of gravity at the moment of takeoff and the maximum distance the center of gravity is projected vertically. For some activities, such as the high jump and the pole vault, the vertical distance between the center of gravity and the crossbar may be an additional important unit of distance.

All forms of these activities share the problems of adequate muscle strength to project the body against the force of gravity and the coordination needed for utilizing what might be called secondary motions for achieving maximum height or distance. The force that projects the body is provided by the forceful contraction of the extensor muscles of the hips, knees, and ankles and, to a lesser extent, by the arm flexor muscles in swinging the arms forward and upward.

Mechanical Principles in Jumping, Hopping, and Leaping

1. For movement to occur, inertia must be overcome. One of the chief problems in jumping from a stand is overcoming inertia. A preliminary motion such as swinging the arms and upper body backward and forward, taking a hop or a step, or using a preparatory run help overcome inertia in jumping.

2. Muscles can store elastic energy. When concentric contraction is preceded by a phase of active stretching, elastic energy stored in the stretch phase is available for use in the contractile phase. Work done by the muscles that are shortening immediately after stretching is greater than that done by those shortening from a static state. For this reason the strong extension required for most jumping motions is usually preceded by a flexion phase. There should be no pause between this flexion and the thrust phase of the jump. This also makes full use of the phasic response of the stretch reflex.

3. Jumpers project themselves into the air by exerting force against the ground that is larger than the force supporting their weight. It is the reaction to the force that accelerates them upward. The faster and stronger the leg movements, the more force that is produced against the ground. Some of this downward force of the legs may itself be in reaction to upward motions of the upper extremities.

4. The upward thrust of the arms seen in the high jump accelerates the support leg downward, which in turn causes a reaction thrust from the ground. Trunk motion is also stabilized, allowing an increase in torque production at the knee. Additionally, the arm swing action in jumping has the effect of raising the center of gravity immediately prior to takeoff, which may result in increased jump height or distance (Feltner, Fraschetti, and Crisp 1999).

5. The magnitude of the impulse that the jumper exerts against the ground is a product of the forces and the time over which they act. The vertical impulses in all jumps are those resulting from the swinging actions of the arms and the extension of the hip, knee, and ankle joints. The magnitude of the forces depends on the strength of the muscle, speed of joint actions, and coordination of the joint movements. The time for generating vertical impulse is greatest in jumps from a stationary

start and in those jumps that have maximum height as their goal. The time required for the generation of impulse can also vary with the jumping style. In the high jump, for instance, the Fosbury flop style generally has shorter takeoff times than the straddle. Those jump styles with shorter takeoff times have generally produced higher jumps, apparently maximizing force production to produce a greater vertical impulse in less time.

6. The path of motion of a body's center of gravity in space is determined by the angle at which it is projected, speed of projection, height of the center of gravity at takeoff, and air resistance. The angle of projection varies depending on the purpose of the jump. In the long jump, where the goal is maximum horizontal distance, the optimum angle of projection is between 20 and 26 degrees. This angle is governed by the speed of the preparatory run and the vertical velocity generated at takeoff. The majority of the takeoff velocity is horizontal. Jumping at a 45-degree angle would require equal horizontal and vertical velocities. Because run velocities in the long jump are fairly fast, it would take a very large impulse to generate an equal vertical velocity. The long jump takeoff is too quick to allow for generation of this vertical impulse. Slowing the takeoff to the point where generation of equal velocities are possible would result in such low horizontal velocities that most of the jump distance would be lost. The most commonly quoted proportion between horizontal and vertical velocities is 2:1.

   In the high jump the angle of projection is much greater. At the moment of takeoff the center of gravity should be as high as possible and the vertical velocity should be maximum. In the running high jump, some horizontal velocity is necessary at takeoff to carry the performer forward over the bar.

7. Angular momentum may be developed by the sudden checking of linear motion or by an eccentric thrust (figure 19.9).

Figure 19.9   The long jump using the hang technique. The extended body position increases the moment of inertia about the horizontal axis, thus decreasing the undesired forward rotation developed at takeoff.

ADDITIONAL FORMS OF LOCOMOTION

Wheels, Blades, and Runners

Often, human locomotion over resistive surfaces is accomplished using the mechanical aids of wheels, runners, or blades. Devices such as bicycles, various types of roller skates, skis, and ice skates are designed to allow human beings to move farther faster for less effort, or to enable them to move quickly and easily over otherwise difficult surfaces. Unlike friction in locomotion involving a body segment in contact with dry, firm ground, friction using wheels, blades, and runners must usually be *minimized* in some respect rather than maximized. In using wheels for human-powered locomotion, friction in axles and rolling friction between wheels and ground must be kept to a minimum to avoid the heat and wear caused by excessive friction. With runners and blades, reducing friction between the mechanical device and the ice or snow surface is the primary concern.

   The most common form of human-powered locomotion, the bicycle, is also one of the most

Figure 19.10   The longer force arm of the pedal crank makes the bicycle more efficient.

efficient in terms of transferring human muscle power to motion. Because the rider is constantly positioned over the center of gravity of the machine, the cycling motion has no braking or retarding phase. The continuous cyclic motion coupled with pedal and gear systems working on the principles of wheel and axles provide a mechanism in which little kinetic energy is wasted (figure 19.10).

The speed at which the bicycle travels is determined by the gear ratio at which the bike is being operated and the pedal cadence of the rider. The gear ratio of the bicycle determines the distance that can be traveled in each pedal revolution. A bicycle in first gear (smallest rear gear) need only undergo a single pedal revolution to cover the same distance as ten pedal revolutions in tenth gear, but requires much greater force because of the shortened force arm in the wheel and axle configuration.

The force that produces pedal revolutions is provided by a cyclic extension–flexion motion of the lower extremities. The magnitude of the force that must be exerted depends on the gear ratio chosen. A lower gear, with a smaller force arm, requires greater pedal force but produces a greater distance traveled for each pedal revolution than do the higher gears with larger force arms. The

pedal cycle itself has an extension, or power, phase and a flexion, or recovery, phase. Starting with the foot at the top of the pedal circle (top dead center, or TDC) and moving through the first 90 degrees of extension, the active muscles are the gluteus maximus and the rectus femoris, with the three vasti becoming active slightly later than the rectus femoris. From 90 degrees to 270 degrees the hamstring group and the gastrocnemius become active. From 270 degrees back to TDC, muscle activity is primarily in the tibialis anterior and the rectus femoris (Jorge and Hull 1985; Pons and Vaughn 1987; Clarys and Cabri 1993).

Although bicycling is an efficient form of locomotion when the system is in motion, kinetic energy is lost in stopping and starting. Each time the bicycle comes to a stop, kinetic energy is transferred to the braking system. To start the bicycle in motion, inertia must be overcome and kinetic energy reestablished. Along with inertia, rolling friction must constantly be overcome. This friction is inversely related to wheel diameter, which is why bicycles are more efficient than many other wheeled objects such as skateboards and roller skates. Rolling friction is greatest at the beginning of motion. As the wheel velocity increases, rolling friction decreases.

Increased velocity in bicycling produces increased air resistance acting against the cyclist. Drag increases as flow velocity increases. Often the cyclist will adjust the body position in an effort to reduce drag. The low handlebar position common in most racing and touring bicycles is an attempt to streamline the body, to reduce the surface area against which drag may act.

In most other forms of human-powered locomotion involving wheels, the movement involved is cyclic but not continuous, as it may be in bicycling. In roller skating and in-line skating, for example, force is produced by each leg in turn, with a period of glide occurring between strokes. During this period of glide there is a loss of velocity from friction. This means that some of the force expended on every stroke is used to regain lost velocity. Skateboards are similar but usually rely on only one leg for propulsion, the other leg maintaining constant contact with the moving board.

Both roller skates (or in-line skates) and skateboards are highly efficient during downhill motion. Velocity increases continuously because of gravity with no effort on the part of the human rider. Most will quickly remember, however, that in order to go down there must at some point have been an equivalent effort in the upward direction.

In ice skating, there is very little friction between the skate blades and the ice. This friction is reduced even further by a slight melting of the ice resulting from the pressure of the blade. Because of this extremely low coefficient of friction, it is not possible to push off in a backward direction as in running or walking. Instead the skate blade is turned perpendicular to the direction of glide. The same pressure that produces the slight melting of the ice also causes the blade to sink slightly into the ice, allowing the blade to thrust against the ice as force is applied. Thus, the slight depression in the ice provides the equal and opposite reaction necessary for forward motion (figure 19.11). Besides the lateral push-off, ice skating differs from running in that little plantar flexion occurs in the push-off. Plantar flexion at this point of the skate

stroke will probably scrape the skate toe along the ice, increasing friction.

As in other forms of human locomotion, speed in ice skating is based on stride length and stride rate. As velocity increases, the body also inclines forward to a greater degree and the feet separate. In speed skating the trunk may be inclined forward to a horizontal position to reduce drag. In figure skating, ice hockey, and recreational skating, this degree of lean is less common (figure 19.12).

Similar to ice skating but using runners instead of blades is the sport of skiing. At present there are two basic forms of skiing: nordic, or cross-country, and alpine, or downhill. In addition several other forms of sliding on snow are gaining in popularity and exposure. Ski jumping combines the speed of downhill skiing with aerodynamics and landing skills. Freestyle skiing uses the vertical velocity provided by small jumps or bumps to give the skier enough time in the air to perform a variety of gymnastic-style moves. Snowboarding replaces the familiar two skis with a single snowboard, closely related to surfing and skateboarding.

Cross-country skiing is most closely related to walking, running, and ice skating in that an alternating stride pattern is frequently used for propulsion. The most common stride pattern in cross-country skiing is the diagonal stride, in which a backward thrust with one ski produces a forward glide on the forward or gliding ski. Ski poles are used to add additional thrust (figure 19.13).

More recently, competitive skiers have been using a marathon skate stride or a V-skate stride. In both skating strides, the thrust is lateral, as in ice skating, rather than straight back. The marathon skate stride in cross-country skiing uses a single leg thrust, whereas the V-skate stride uses an alternating stride pattern. In both skate strides, the push from the rear ski is at a 30-degree angle to the glide direction (Watanabe 1987).

Alpine or downhill skiing relies primarily on gravity for a propulsive force. The skier starts at the top of a slope (usually through mechanical

Figure 19.11   The straight back push-off in figure skating.

Figure 19.12   Body lean in the speed skating stroke.

a.   b.

Figure 19.13   The cross-country ski stride: (a) diagonal stride, (b) V-skate stride.

Figure 19.14   The aerodynamic low crouch position in alpine skiing.

transportation) and glides to the bottom. The movement problems encountered by the alpine skier revolve around changing directions and maintaining balance at high speeds while undergoing a variety of horizontal and vertical disturbances. In competitive alpine skiing, speeds are such that air resistance also plays a major role. The low crouch position assumed by most alpine racers reduces the surface area and thereby reduces form drag (figure 19.14).

Rotary Locomotion

In general, the factors responsible for the successful performance of rotary locomotion are the magnitude, direction, and accurate timing of the

Figure 19.15   The body rotating around its points of contact with the supporting surface.
From William R. LaPorte and Al G. Renner, *The Tumbler's Manual.* Copyright © 1938, p. 10. Adapted by permission of Prentice Hall, Englewood Cliffs, New Jersey.

forces contributing to the desired movement of the body, including the advantageous use of the force of gravity whenever possible.

The most common activities in this category are forward, backward, and sideward rolls, cartwheels, and handsprings. Each of these is achieved by rotating about the body's successive areas of contact with the supporting surface. In forward rolls, for instance, the body rotates about the hands, shoulders, rounded back, buttocks, and feet (figure 19.15) and in cartwheels, about each hand followed by each foot with the body rotating laterally in a fully extended position. The impetus for the forward roll is given by the hands and feet, the direction of their thrust being a combination of backward and downward: backward to send the body forward, and downward to resist the downward pull of gravitational force on the head and trunk. When the hands and feet are no longer pushing, the head is tucked forward and the back is rounded with the knees bent close against the body to facilitate the roll. During the foot thrust, the hips are high, both for ensuring a stronger backward thrust with the legs and for making greater use of the force of gravity for the roll over the back.

Because a body at rest will remain at rest unless acted on by a force and a body in motion will continue in motion unless acted on by a force, it is important to keep the body moving in successive rolls and not let it come to a momentary halt following each roll. Even the briefest of interruptions necessitates the overcoming of inertia after each revolution. It takes velocity to acquire sufficient momentum to prevent these halts; therefore, each backward thrust of hands and feet against the ground should be as forceful as possible. Rotary movement is accelerated by shortening the radius. In both forward and backward rolls the radius is shortened by tucking the flexed lower extremities close to the body when the back is in contact with the floor.

Locomotion by Specialized Steps and Jumps

Other forms of ground-supported locomotion not involving the use of special equipment include two general categories. One of these consists of acrobatic stunts and athletic events, such as walking on the hands, successive jumping, and hurdling either with or without actual hurdles. The other category consists of activities used both in children's play and in forms of dance. It includes skipping, hopping, galloping, sliding, sidestepping, leaping, and standard dance steps, such as the polka and mazurka.

LABORATORY EXPERIENCES

1. Try this as a class exercise, working in pairs. A stands with heels against a wall with the feet otherwise in a comfortable, "natural" position in readiness to walk. B holds a ruler across the toes of A's feet and draws a line against the ruler. A then stands with feet parallel at right angles to the wall, and again B draws a line. Measure the distance between the two lines. This measurement is likely to vary from 0.5 cm to 2.5 cm in a sizable class. A and B now change places and repeat.

   Assume that you are to engage in a walking race of 1000 meters; also assume that if you toed straight ahead, each step would be 1 meter long. It would therefore take you 1000 steps to cover the distance. But suppose you toed out so that each step was (your measurement) _____ short. How many meters short of the finish line would you be when you had taken 1000 steps? (Answer: If the distance between the two lines had been 0.4 cm, you would be 0.4 × 1000 = 400 cm, or 4 meters, short.)

   Implication: If you are walking against an opponent who walks at the same rate as you, but who toes straight ahead, you would be 4 meters behind when you cross the finish line. Yet, presumably you took the same number of steps.

2. Observe the gait of people on the street or campus, detect individual characteristics, and analyze them using anatomical and mechanical principles.

3. Get a subject to walk in each of the following ways. Observe and note differences in the movements of the head, shoulders, hips, and so forth.
   a. Place one foot directly in front of the other.
   b. Keep a lateral distance of 20 to 25 cm between the feet.
   c. Point the toes out.
   d. Point the toes in.
   e. Point the toes straight ahead.
   f. Take a short stride.
   g. Take a long stride.

4. Select four or five individuals who differ in leg length. Get them to practice walking until each one finds the stride and speed that feels most comfortable. Compare their strides and measure the distance between footprints for each individual.

5. Observe several individuals as they run. Look for the application of the principles listed. Which are "violated" and how?

6. Using the iliac crest as an estimate of the center of gravity, trace the path of the center of gravity on a sequence drawing of some form of jump (see figure 14.21, p. 393). Determine the percentage of the distance jumped that can be attributed to each of the following:
   a. Distance center of gravity is in front of takeoff point at the moment of takeoff.
   b. Distance center of gravity travels while body is unsupported.
   c. Distance center of gravity is behind landing point.

7. Compare the segment positions at several points during the execution of a standing long jump or vertical jump as done by several "poor" jumpers and several "good" jumpers. Identify the principles of concern in these jumps. Evaluate the performance by stating the related principles. On the basis of this information, try to improve the performance of the "poor" jumpers.

8. Choose a locomotor pattern not discussed in this chapter (hurdling, for example). Perform a complete kinesiological analysis, taking particular note of the purpose of the motion, its classification, and the nature of the motion. Include also muscle participation, neuromuscular considerations, and mechanical factors. Identify those principles that will help you determine whether someone performing this pattern is doing it correctly. Conclude the analysis with a prescription for improvement, including suggested methods for change and the elimination of violations of principles.

References and Selected Readings

Basmajian, J. V., and C. J. DeLuca. 1985. *Muscles alive.* 5th ed. Baltimore: Williams & Wilkins.

Burke, E. R., and M. M. Newsom, eds. 1988. *Medical and scientific aspects of cycling.* Champaign, IL: Human Kinetics.

Cairns, M. A., R. G. Burdett, J. C. Pisciotta, and S. R. Simon. 1986. A biomechanical analysis of racewalking gait. *Medicine and Science in Sports and Exercise* 18(4):446–53.

Cavanagh, P. R., and R. Kram. 1985. Mechanical and muscular factors affecting the efficiency of human movement. *Medicine and Science in Sports and Exercise* 17(3):326–31.

Chu, D., and R. Korcemny. 1990. Sprinting stride actions: Analysis and evaluation. *National Strength Conditioning Association Journal* 11(6):6–8, 81–85.

Clarys, J. P., and J. Cabri. 1993. Electromyography and the study of sports movements: A review. *Journal of Sports Sciences* 11:379–448.

Dapena, J. 1987. Basic and applied research in the biomechanics of high jumping. In *Medicine and sport science: Current research in sports biomechanics,* edited by B. Van Gheluwe and J. Atha. Basel: Karger.

DeVita, P. 1994. The selection of a standard convention for analyzing gait data based on the analysis of relevant biomechanical factors. *Journal of Biomechanics* 27:501–8.

Enoka, R. M. 1988. *Neuromechanical basis of kinesiology.* Champaign, IL: Human Kinetics.

Feltner, M. E., D. J. Fraschetti, and R. J. Crisp. 1999. Upper extremity augmentation of lower extremity kinetics during countertmovement vertical jumps. *Journal of Sports Sciences* 17: 449–66.

Fenton, R. M. 1984. Racewalking ground reaction forces. In *Sports biomechanics,* edited by J. Terauds et al. Del Mar, CA: Academic Publishers.

Gowitzke, B. A., and M. Milner. 1988. *Scientific bases of human movement.* 3rd ed. Baltimore: Williams & Wilkins.

Hay, J. G. 1989. *The biomechanics of sports techniques.* Englewood Cliffs, NJ: Prentice Hall.

Hogue, R. E. 1969. Upper-extremity muscular activity at different cadences and inclines during normal gait. *Journal of the American Physical Therapy Association* 49:963–72.

Hubbard, M., and H. Fujikawa. 1986. Identification of skateboard rider control strategies. In *Human locomotion IV: Proceedings of the North American Congress on Biomechanics.* Montreal, Canada.

Jorge, M., and M. L. Hull. 1984. Biomechanics of bicycle pedalling. In *Sports biomechanics,* edited by J. Terauds et al. Del Mar, CA: Academic Publishers.

Jorge, M., and M. L. Hull. 1985. EMG during cycle pedalling. In *Biomechanics in sports II,* edited by J. Terauds and J. Barham. Del Mar, CA: Academic Publishers.

Krebs, D. E., D. Wong, D. Jevsevar, P. O. Riley, and W. A. Hodge. 1992. Trunk kinematics during locomotor activities. *Physical Therapy* 72:505–14.

Lovejoy, C. O. 1988. Evolution of human walking. *Scientific American,* November 1988, pp. 118–25.

Mann, R., J. Kotmel, J. Herman, B. Johnson, and C. Schultz. 1984. Kinematic trends in elite sprinters. In *Sports biomechanics,* edited by J. Terauds et al. Del Mar, CA: Academic Publishers.

Meisser, S. P., W. H. Ettinger, T. E. Doyle, T. Morgan, M. K. James, M. L. O'Toole, and R. Burns. 1996. Obesity: Effects on gait in an osteoarthritic population. *Journal of Applied Biomechanics* 12:161–72.

Mero, A., and P. V. Komi. 1987. Electromyographic activity in sprinting at speeds ranging from submaximal to supramaximal. *Medicine and Science in Sports and Exercise* 19(3):266–74.

Montgomery, W. H., M. Pink, and J. Perry. 1994. Electromyographic analysis of hip and knee musculature during running. *American Journal of Sports Medicine* 22:272–78.

Morgan, D. W., P. E. Martin, and G. S. Krahenbuhl. 1989. Factors affecting running economy. *Sports Medicine* 7:310–30.

Murray, M. P., R. C. Kory, and S. B. Sepic. 1970. Walking patterns of normal women. *Archives of Physical Medicine Rehabilitation* 51:637–50.

Murray, M. P., S. B. Sepic, and E. J. Barnard. Patterns of sagittal rotation of the upper limbs in walking.

Phys Ther. 1967 Apr;47(4):272–84. No abstract available. PMID: 6040248

Petrofsky, J. S., C. A. Phillips, and H. H. Heaton. 1984. Feedback control system for walking in man. *Computers in Biology and Medicine* 14(2):135–49.

Pons, D. J., and C. L. Vaughn. 1987. Mechanics of cycling. In *Biomechanics of sport,* edited by C. L. Vaughn. Boca Raton, FL: CRC Press.

Rose, J., and J. G. Gamble. 1994. *Human walking.* Baltimore: Williams & Wilkins.

Shiavi, R., B. McFayden, and N. Green. 1983. Electromyographic patterns in normal pediatric gait. In *Biomechanics IX-A,* edited by D. Winter et al. Champaign, IL: Human Kinetics.

Smith, G. A., and B. S. Heagy. 1994. Kinematic analysis of skating technique of Olympic skiers in the men's 50-km race. *Journal of Applied Biomechanics* 10:79–88.

Smith, G. A., J. McNitt-Gray, and R. C. Nelson. 1988. Kinematic analysis of alternate stride skating in cross-country skiing. *International Journal of Sport Biomechanics* 4:49–58.

Steindler, A. 1973. *Kinesiology of the human body.* Springfield, IL: Charles C Thomas, Lectures 37 and 38.

van Ingen Schenau, G. J., J. J. de Koning, and G. de Groot. 1994. Optimization of sprinting performance in running, cycling and speed skating. *Sports Medicine* 17:259–75.

Watanabe, K. 1987. Ski-jumping, cross-country, and nordic combination skiing. In *Biomechanics of sport,* edited by C. L. Vaughn. Boca Raton, FL: CRC Press.

Williams, K. R. 1985. Biomechanics of running. *Exercise and Sport Science Reviews* 13:389–442.

Winter, D. A., and W. Kuryliak. 1978. Dynamic stabilization in human gait: The biomechanical relationships between the triceps surae and the metatarsophalangeal joint. In *Biomechanics VI-A,* edited by E. Asmussen and K. Jorgensen. Baltimore: University Park Press.

Winter, D. A., A. E. Patia, J. S. Frank, and S. E. Walt. 1990. Biomechanical walking pattern changes in the fit and healthy elderly. *Physical Therapy* 70:340–47.

LOCOMOTION: THE AQUATIC ENVIRONMENT

OUTLINE

- **_Aquatic Locomotion: Swimming_**
  Mechanical Principles Applied
    to Swimming
  Analysis of the Sprint Crawl
- **_Aquatic Locomotion: Rowing,_**
  Canoeing, and Kayaking
  Rowing
  Canoeing
  Kayaking
- **_Laboratory Experiences_**

OBJECTIVES

At the conclusion of this chapter, the student should be able to:

1. Name those factors that contribute to the propulsion of a swimmer.
2. Name those factors that impede the progress of a swimmer.
3. Explain how the propulsive and resistive factors named affect the length or frequency of a swimming stroke.
4. Complete a kinesiological analysis of a swimming stroke by identifying the anatomical and mechanical factors important to success in the selected stroke, as well as those factors that appear to limit the particular performance

AQUATIC LOCOMOTION: SWIMMING

The problem of moving the body through water is fundamentally not so different from that of moving it on land. As in walking, it is necessary to push against something in order to move the body from one place to another. The chief differences between locomotion in the water and locomotion on land are that (1) in the water the body is concerned with buoyancy rather than with the force of gravity, (2) the substance against which it pushes affords less resistance to the push, (3) the medium through which it moves affords more resistance to the body, and (4) as a means of getting the greatest benefit from the buoyancy and of reducing the resistance afforded by the water, it is customary to maintain a horizontal, rather than a vertical, position. (Review the discussion of buoyancy on pp. 324–326.) The practical problem in swimming is not to keep from sinking, as novices are inclined to believe, but to get the mouth out of the water at rhythmic intervals in order to permit regular breathing. This is a matter of coordination, not buoyancy.

In swimming, as in all motion, the initial mechanical problem is to overcome the inertia of the body. Once the body is in motion, the problem is to overcome the forces that tend to hinder it. In terrestrial locomotion the body exerts its force against the supporting surface, the ground, to overcome inertia. The forces resisting the progress of the body are the forces of gravity and air resistance. In aquatic locomotion the water is both the supporting medium and the source of resistance. In swimming the hands and feet depend on the reaction force of the water in order that the force may be transmitted to the body. Yet, at the same time, the body must overcome the resistance afforded by the water.

The speed obtained in swimming any stroke depends on the stroke length and stroke frequency. The length of the stroke is the result of the forces that move the swimmer forward in reaction to the movements of the arms and legs, and of the resistance of the water in the opposite direction. In the front crawl the arms are the primary source of power, whereas in the breast-stroke the legs dominate. Regardless of the stroke, the actions of the arms and legs appear to result in a combination of lift and drag forces that then propel the body forward.

Four different types of water resistance act to decrease the stroke length. Form drag is the resistance that is due to the surface area of the front of the body as it meets the oncoming water. This type of resistance has the greatest effect on retarding the swimmer. Streamlining the body by changing its position in the water decreases form drag. *Surface drag* is caused by the resistance of the water next to the body. Although it has little effect on the forward progress of swimmers, they have been known to shave the hair from their bodies as a means of decreasing skin friction. A third form of drag is that which occurs at the surface as the body moves along, partially in water and partially in air. The resultant waves form an additional resistance to forward progress called wave drag. The amount of this resistance depends on both the speed and movements of the body as it progresses through the water. A fourth but minor resistance is turbulence that forms behind the body, causing it to pull some water along with it.

The *frequency* of the stroke depends on the amount of time spent per stroke cycle. This in turn is related to the nature of the stroke pattern and the muscle torques of the arms and legs. Thus, the major problem in the mechanics of swimming is the minimization of the resistance that is due to the water, which is either pushed out of the way or dragged along, and the advantageous application of the force of the arms and legs. The swimmer reduces resistance by streamlining the body position through relaxing in the recovery phase of the stroke and by eliminating useless motion and tensions. The propulsive force is increased with improvements in technique and conditioning.

Mechanical Principles Applied to Swimming

1. *Less force is needed to keep an object moving than to overcome its inertia.* Force in

Figure 20.1   Drag and lift work together to "anchor" the hand during the pull phase of the front crawl.
From James E. Counsilman, *The Science of Swimming.* Copyright © 1968, pp. 61–65. Reprinted by permission of Prentice Hall, Englewood Cliffs, New Jersey.

swimming should be applied so that the progress through the water is even rather than consisting of cycles of speeding up and slowing down. In the front crawl, the beginning of one arm pull should start before the other arm finishes its pull. In strokes such as the breaststroke and sidestroke, too long a glide will result in a reduction in momentum and the need to expend extra energy to overcome inertia in starting up again.

2. *The body will move in the opposite direction from that in which the force is applied.* For instance, a backward thrust will send the body forward, downward pressure will lift it, and pressure to the right will send it to the left. In most strokes too much force at the beginning of the arc will have too great a downward component, thereby tending to lift the body. This increases resistance and is a needless expenditure of energy. In a similar manner, a wide recovery of the arm in the front crawl or back crawl will result in an opposite lateral reaction in the legs, and thus will cause additional resistance. In the breaststroke, the two arms balance each other; hence, too great an outward force at the beginning of the stroke or inward force at the end of the stroke does not produce lateral motion but results in a waste of energy.

3. *Forward motion in swimming is produced through a combination of drag force and lift force.* In all swimming strokes the hand follows an S-shaped path through the water. The function of this curved pattern is to produce water flow laterally over the hand,

which creates lift perpendicular to the flow direction, usually forward, in the direction of motion. Drag force acts at the same time to resist motion against the direction of flow. This lift and drag combination acts to "anchor" the hand in the water, providing a somewhat stable "handle" over which the trunk is then pulled (figure 20.1).

4. *Maximum force is attained by presenting as broad a surface as possible in the propulsive movements of the limbs and by exerting a backward pressure through as great a distance as possible, provided undesirable forces are not inadvertently introduced.* The full surface of the hand should be used in arm strokes. The hand, however, should not enter the water so soon that it shortens the stroke unduly. Conversely, in the crawl stroke, care must be taken not to reach too far, which may involve lifting the shoulder and introducing lateral forces.

5. *Momentum may be transferred from one body or part to another body or part as momentum is conserved.* If the breaststroker or backstroker checks the momentum of the arms at the end of the recovery, the momentum will be transferred to the body, forcing the head and body downward and thus setting up a bobbing stroke and additional resistance.

6. *The height of the body position in the water depends on the swimmer's buoyancy and speed of moving through the water.* The buoyancy of a swimmer is primarily determined by body composition and is not

easily altered. Swimmers should not try to ride high in the water by raising the head or by pushing down, because each action will be followed by an opposite and equal reaction. However, it is possible to raise the legs somewhat by producing an efficient kick. The flutter kick contributes more to body position and stability than it does to forward propulsion.

7. *When a body is free in a fluid, movement of a part in one direction results in movement of the rest of the body in the opposite direction.* Swimming with the head out of the water, as in water polo, lifesaving, or synchronized swimming causes the feet to drop. This position produces more frontal drag than the flat horizontal position and therefore requires more energy on the swimmer's part to overcome the additional resistance.

8. *A rapidly moving body in the water leaves a low-pressure area immediately behind it.* This creates a suction effect and tends to pull the body back. Although this backward pull (drag) cannot be entirely eliminated, it can be reduced by keeping the legs close together in the crawl strokes and during the glide phase of the resting strokes. Drag of this nature can also be reduced by maintaining a streamlined body position in the water.

9. *The more streamlined the body, the less the resistance to progress through the water.* Streamlining of the body can be accomplished by carrying the head so that the water level is near the hairline in prone strokes. The body should be parallel to the surface of the water with the buttocks just below the surface. In the flutter kick and the recovery portion of the resting strokes, the feet should be kept close together.

10. *The drag on a body in any fluid increases approximately with the square of the velocity.* For this reason the recovery phase of the arm pull in breaststroke, sidestroke, or elementary backstroke and the entry of the recovery arm into the water in the crawl stroke and the butterfly stroke should not be rushed. In these instances, the arm is moving in a direction opposite that which produces forward motion in the swimmer. A rapid recovery or entry will serve to increase the drag.

11. *The sudden or quick movement of a swimmer's body, or one of its parts, at the surface of the water tends to cause whirls and eddies. These create low-pressure areas that have a retarding effect on the swimmer.* The low-pressure areas can be reduced by slicing the hand into the water and by eliminating movements that do not contribute to forward progression. In the flutter kick, movements of the feet in the air do not contribute to the propulsion of the body; hence, the feet and legs should be kept just below the surface of the water.

Analysis of the Sprint Crawl

As an example of aquatic locomotion, the sprint crawl (figure 20.2) has been chosen for analysis. The position of the head and trunk and the movement of the head in breathing are described briefly. The arm and leg strokes are described in somewhat greater detail, and their propulsive phases are analyzed anatomically.

The Head and Trunk

The head and trunk have three important functions in swimming, particularly in speed swimming. These are minimizing resistance, enabling the swimmer to breathe, and providing a stable anchorage for the arm and leg muscles to effect a maximum propulsive force. The position of the body is the key to reducing resistance. The body is as horizontal as possible, with the feet below the surface and the head breaking the water at hairline level. The flatter the body, the less drag there will be to decrease the swimmer's speed. The exact position of the body varies with the anatomical build and buoyancy of the individual, as well as with the speed of the stroke. The greater the buoyancy and speed, the higher the body will ride in the water. A common mistake is

Figure 20.2 The crawl stroke.

From James E. Counsilman, *The Science of Swimming*. Copyright © 1968, pp. 61–65. Reprinted by permission of Prentice Hall, Englewood Cliffs, New Jersey.

to lift the head too much. If the head is held too high or tipped back too far, it makes the swimmer's legs drop, causing a broader frontal surface and therefore more resistance. By static contraction of the rectus abdominis the spine is held in a position of slight flexion—or at least of incomplete extension—and the pelvis in a position of slightly decreased inclination.

Lateral movements of the trunk will also increase the resistance to forward movements and should be minimized. Any circular movement of the arms or legs causes a countermovement in the rest of the body. A wide swing of the arms on recovery produces a lateral, opposite fishtail action of the legs. Lateral flexion of the head and neck also results in a counteraction. The turning of the head for inhaling must be accomplished with the least possible interference with the rhythm of the arm and leg action and with the progress of the body through the water. It is essential not to lift the head for breathing but rather to rotate it on its longitudinal axis while tucking the chin in close to the side of the neck. In this position the face appears to be resting on the bow wave, and the mouth is just above the surface of the water. After a quick inhalation, the face is again turned forward with the eyes in the horizontal plane and the nose and chin in the midsagittal plane of the body. Although breathing with every arm cycle is preferable in distance events, sprints are better swum with fewer breathing cycles because the turning of the head, even when done properly, causes additional resistance.

To provide a firm base of attachment for the muscles of the arms and thighs the trunk must be held steady. By the alternating action of the left and right oblique abdominals and spinal extensors, the spine and pelvis are stabilized against the pull of the shoulder and hip muscles. Thus, they permit the latter to exert all their force on the limbs for the propulsive movements.

The Arm Stroke

Entry and support   Because the arm stroke provides approximately 85 percent of the total power, the entry of the arm into the water should place it in the most advantageous position for exerting force that will be effective in driving the body forward. Its position on entry is with the forearm high and the elbow pointing to the side. The hand passes in front of the shoulder in preparation for the entry and then, reaching forward, it is driven forward and downward into the water directly in front of the shoulder. The elbow is slightly flexed at the beginning of the hand entry but extends during the entry. The brief moment between entry and the beginning of the chief propulsive action is known as the support phase, and its purpose is to keep the head and shoulders high in the water. The pressure of the forearm and hand is mostly downward and then backward, thus producing an upward and forward reactive force (figure 20.2a, b).

Catch, pull, and push   The moment at which the chief propulsive action changes from downward to backward constitutes the catch. This occurs when the hand is 5 to 10 inches below the surface and involves a quick inward movement of the hand and arm that serves to bring the hand to a position in front of the axis of the body in such a way that the body weight is balanced above the arm. The upper arm is approximately vertical, a position that favors the large muscles (sternal portion of the pectoralis major and latissimus dorsi) for their task of pulling the arm downward and backward. Because the purpose of the stroke is to drive the body forward, it is essential to apply maximum force over the longest possible distance. This is best done by keeping the elbow high during the first part of the pull and by bending the elbow as the arm is pulled under the body (figure 20.2c, d). The maximum bend occurs halfway through the pull, when the hand begins to push the water backward.

This elbow action assists in producing the S-curve, which allows for the creation of propulsive lift. Flexion at the elbow also reduces the moment arm of the upper extremity, reducing resistance to motion. In the pull phase the feel is as if the hand is being pushed backward through the water. In actuality, lift and drag act to stabilize the hand in the water. The body is then pulled forward over the relatively stationary hand.

The transition from pull to push occurs as the arm passes under the shoulder. The upper arm remains nearly vertical as the forearm gradually extends until it is in front of the hip, at which time the upper arm extends and the hand gives a quick push backward (figure 20.2e, f). It would seem that the ideal direction of the swimmer's force should be directly backward for maximum forward horizontal movement. In actuality the path of the hand of most good swimmers is more like an inverted question mark. This apparent sculling motion constantly varies the angle between the surface of the hand and the direction of hand motion (angle of attack). The combination of drag forces and lift forces (see Bernouilli's principle, p. 328) that will be utilized for propulsion is extremely dependent on this angle of attack. By varying the angle of attack, the optimum lift and drag resultant for every position of the hand can

be attained. This means that as the hand velocity direction shifts with the curvilinear path of the hand, the resultant of the drag and lift forces can still be maintained in line with the body's line of motion (Toussaint and Beck 1992).

Brief anatomical analysis of propulsive phase of arm stroke Front crawl swimming is an excellent total body exercise. It has been estimated that at least 44 muscles act to produce the movements of the crawl. If all active muscles (antagonists, synergists, etc.) are considered, the estimate rises to 170 single muscles (Clarys and Cabri 1993). For this reason, only the most active prime movers will be covered in this analysis (table 20.1).

Release and recovery The elbow is now near the surface with the hand slightly lower and posterior to it and the palm facing mostly upward. The pressure of the forearm and hand now being relaxed, the elbow and shoulder are raised until the hand is out of the water. The elbow leaves the

TABLE 20.1	Anatomical Analysis of the Propulsive Phase of Arm Stroke				
Joint	Joint Action	Segment Moved	Force for Movement	Muscles Active	Kind of Contraction
Shoulder joint	Extension Oblique adduction Medial rotation	Upper arm	Muscle	Posterior deltoid Latisimuss dorsi Teres major Pectoralis major	Concentric
Shoulder girdle	Downward rotation Adduction	Scapula	Muscle	Rhomboids Pectoralis minor Trapezius	Concentric
Elbow	Flexion	Forearm	Muscle	Flexors	Concentric
Radioulnar	Pronation	Forearm	Muscle	Pronator teres Pronator quadratus	Concentric
Wrist	Held in midposition		Muscle	Flexor carpi radialis Flexor carpi ulnaris	Static
Fingers	Held in extension, adduction		Muscles	Flexors Adductors	Static

water first and swings forward and upward with the hand trailing behind it, moving from a position near the hip to a position in front of the shoulder, preparatory to a new entry (figure 20.2g, h). The movement of the arm from release to the completion of recovery is continuous. It is important that no break occur, because this would mean a loss of momentum and would necessitate an additional force for overcoming inertia, or at least for regaining the lost velocity.

As the elbow is brought forward it remains above the level of the hand throughout the recovery and entry, with the forearm virtually horizontal as the arm moves forward past the shoulder and the hand in line with the forearm. Finally, as the hand passes the head, the arm reaches forward in preparation for the entry, the shoulder girdle

remains high, the tip of the elbow is above shoulder level pointing to the side, and the forearm then points downward from the elbow with the wrist slightly flexed, the palm facing the water, and the fingers aiming forward and downward into the water. Individual differences in style in the arm recovery are likely to occur. These variations are most likely due to differences in shoulder range of motion. Unless such variations interfere with other aspects of the stroke, they are most likely insignificant (table 20.2).

The Kick

Nature of movement   The leg stroke most often used in the sprint crawl is the flutter kick. Whether or not it contributes to the propulsive force has been questioned. It is generally acknowledged that

TABLE 20.2   **Anatomical Analysis of the Recovery Phase of Arm Stroke**

Joint	Joint Action	Segment Moved	Force for Movement	Muscles Active	Kind of Contraction
Shoulder joint	Hyperextension followed by: horizontal adduction	Upper arm	Muscle	Posterior deltoid Latisimus dorsi Teres major Pectoralis major Anterior deltoid Coracobrachialis Biceps	Concentric
Shoulder girdle	Slight elevation Upward rotation Abduction	Scapula	Muscle	Trapezius Pectoralis minor Serratus anterior	Concentric
Elbow	Extension	Forearm	Muscle	Triceps Anconeus	Concentric
Radioulnar	Pronation	Forearm	Muscle	Pronator teres Pronator quadratus	Concentric
Wrist and Fingers	Relaxed until slight extension of hand at end of phase		Muscle	Extensor carpi ulnaris Extensor carpi radialis brevis Extensor digitorum indices Pollicis longus Intrinsic hand muscles	Concentric

the primary role for the kick is that of a stabilizer and neutralizer, and that therefore its timing with respect to the arm's action is critical. In this stroke the legs are relatively close together as they alternate in an up and down movement, with the feet attaining a maximum stride of about 1 to 2 feet. The width of the kick depends on such factors as the swimmer's build and strength and the speed of the stroke. In both the upstroke and downstroke, the movement, described as whiplike or lashing, starts at the hip joint and progresses through the knees to the ankle and feet. Unlike the arms, whose movements alternate between propulsion and recovery, both phases of the leg stroke are propulsive, if anything. Flexibility in the ankles is important in the kick, and those with a greater range of plantar flexion have an advantage. In the downstroke the thrust is downward and backward and, in the upstroke, upward and backward.

Downstroke The downstroke begins with a downward drive of the thigh. The thigh flexes only slightly and the knee, which was in a position of flexion at the completion of the upstroke, extends completely by the end of the downward movement. The ankle and foot remain in plantar flexion, probably being held in this position by the pressure of the water against the dorsal surface of the foot (figure 20.2a, b). It seems likely that the dorsiflexors contract statically to stabilize the foot against this pressure. Throughout the downstroke the foot remains in a slight toeing-in position. The heels should not be allowed to drift apart in an attempt to facilitate the intoeing, since this would involve rotation of the thigh and would cut down on the driving power of the limb, as well as increase the form drag (table 20.3).

TABLE 20.3	Anatomical Analysis of the Kick Downstroke				
Joint	Joint Action	Segment Moved	Force for Movement	Muscles Active	Kind of Contraction
Hip joint	Partial flexion	Thigh	Muscle	Iliopsoas Tensor fasciae latae Pectineus Sartorius Gracilis	Concentric
Knee joint	Passive flexion due to water pressure until bottom of stroke, then: forceful extension	Shank	Muscle	Quadriceps femoris	Concentric
Ankle joint	Incomplete plantar flexion probably caused by water pressure, stabilized by muscle contraction		Muscle	Tibialis anterior Peroneus tertius Extensor digitorum and hallicis longus	Static
Tarsal joints	Adduction Inversion	Foot	Muscle	Tibialis posterior Tibialis anterior Flexor digitorum and hallicis longus	Concentric

Upstroke   At the completion of the downstroke the thigh is in a position of slight flexion, the knee is completely extended, the ankle is incompletely plantar flexed. The upstroke begins with thigh extension. Slight knee flexion develops near the end of the stroke at the same time the opposite leg is finishing the downstroke. The movements of the three major segments of the lower extremity are forceful in the upstroke but are under such good control that the foot stops just below the surface of the water. To break through the surface constitutes a major error, as it causes an immediate reduction in propulsive force (figure 20.2d–f; table 20.4).

Additional Factors

Other factors of importance to the crawl stroke swimmer and to the coach are the timing and coordination of the arm and leg strokes and of the breathing, the rhythm of the stroke as a whole, the relaxation of the body, and the flexibility of the joints, particularly of the shoulders and ankles. Of these, possibly the last named is of greatest interest to the kinesiologist. The serious swimmer will want to know how to increase the range of motion in shoulder joints and ankles—that is, how to stretch the pectorals and anterior ligaments of the shoulders and how to gain greater plantar flexion of the feet. The kinesiology student should be able to originate several exercises that would accomplish this. One method that is frequently used is dry land exercise using various forms of elastic resistance.

Sample Analysis of a Common Fault in the Crawl Stroke

A *rigid flutter kick* is a common fault of beginners learning the standard crawl stroke. It is included in this text as an example of how the kine-

TABLE 20.4	Anatomical Analysis of the Kick Upstroke				
Joint	Joint Action	Segment Moved	Force for Movement	Muscles Active	Kind of Contraction
Hip joint	Strong extension	Thigh	Muscle	Hamstrings Gluteus maximus	Concentric
Knee joint	Slight flexion Shank against resistance	Shank	Muscle	Hamstrings Sartorius Gracilis Popliteus Gastrocnemius	Concentric
Ankle joint	Plantar flexion	Foot	Muscle	Gastrocnemius Soleus Peroneus longus & brevis Tibialis posterior Flexor digitorum and hallucis longus	Concentric
Tarsal joints	Plantar flexion	Foot	Muscle	Tibialis posterior Peroneus longus and brevis Flexor digitorum and hallucis longus	Concentric

siologist can analyze a common fault and use the analysis as a basis for making constructive suggestions in teaching.

Description In the rigid flutter kick the movement is one of alternate flexion and extension of the entire lower extremity, with the movement confined to the hip joint instead of being transmitted successively through the thigh to the knee joint and thence through the leg to the ankle and foot. The knee joints are fully extended throughout the kick, and the feet and ankles are held in an unchanging position of plantar flexion, the exact degree of this flexion varying with individuals. This results in a narrower kick. A rigid flutter kick is obviously less efficient than the correct kick. In brief, the rigid flutter kick deviates from the correct form in that there is an absence of knee and ankle flexion, an absence of relaxation at the end of the downkick or beginning of the upkick, and an absence of fishtail action of the sole of the foot against the water.

Anatomical analysis In the correct downkick the upward pressure of the water against the lower leg causes flexion at the knee. In the rigid kick, however, this is prevented by the tension of the quadriceps extensors. Normally, the slight flexion at the knee is followed by extension during the course of the downstroke but, when the knee is already rigidly extended, this extension cannot take place. Similarly, the reduction of the plantar flexion that should take place at the end of the downstroke fails to occur because of the continuous contraction of the plantar flexor muscles (soleus, peroneus longus and brevis, tibialis posterior, flexor digitorum longus, and flexor hallucis longus).

In the upstroke the tension of the quadriceps extensors again prevents the slight knee flexion that occurs when the kick is correctly performed (see figure 20.2). Throughout the stroke the extensors of the lower back and the abdominal muscles contract to stabilize the pelvis against the pull of the hip flexors and extensors. Normally they relax momentarily just before the legs re-

verse their direction. The tension in the muscles of the lower extremities spreads to these, however, and the excess tension of these muscles causes interference with the action of the diaphragm. This, in turn, results in less efficient breathing and is an additional factor in causing fatigue.

Mechanical analysis The propulsive component of force that drives the body forward is that which pushes the water directly backward. In the downstroke this is provided most effectively by the instep of the foot, and in the upstroke, by the sole. The amount of propulsive force developed depends on the angle at which the instep and the sole of the foot are held with respect to the surface of the water. In the upstroke the best angle for the sole of the foot is possible only when the knee is flexed. In the rigid kick the knee is straight, and the sole of the foot is therefore not in the best position for providing propulsive force.

In the correct form each limb acts as a series of levers—thigh, lower leg, and foot—but in the rigid kick each limb acts as one long lever with the force arm extending from the distal attachments of the hip flexors and extensors to the axis of the hip joint. The resistance arm consists of the entire length of the lever from the instep or from the sole of the foot to the hip joint. The force acting on this lever comes solely from the muscles of the hip joints. The muscles of the knee and ankle do not contribute to the motion of this lever, but when the limb is used as a series of levers, they provide additional force. Inertia must be overcome with each reversal of direction in the kick. Because, in the rigid flutter kick, the stroke is shorter and faster than it should be, the muscles of the hip joint, which have the double task of overcoming both the inertia of the limb and the resistance of the water, are overburdened. They must work harder and faster to meet the demands made on them by the frequent changes of direction and the increased resistance of the water due to the speed of movement. Ordinarily the upstroke has an advantage over the downstroke, because when the stroke is performed correctly, the sole of the foot is in a better position to push back against the water than is the instep on the downstroke. In the rigid kick this advantage is lost.

Teaching suggestions   The rigid crawl flutter kick is associated with undue tension of the quadriceps extensors at the knee joint, and of the plantar flexors at the ankle joint during the changes of direction in both the downkick and the upkick. There may also be unnecessary tension of the abdominal muscles and the spinal extensors. Because the kick is inefficient, it is carried on at a faster rate and through a narrower arc than would be the correct kick for the individual swimmer. Conversely, a rapid, narrow kick tends to be a rigid kick. These factors aid in its recognition. In teaching the kick, it would seem the best procedure is to insist on a slow, deep kick in the student's first attempts, and to increase the rhythm gradually to the desired rate. Motivation should not be directed toward speed in the performance of the "kick glide" in the teaching progression. Also, one should not emphasize that the legs be held straight at the knees. The emphasis should be put on the increased action at the hips and at the ankles.

AQUATIC LOCOMOTION: ROWING, CANOEING, AND KAYAKING

Boating in its various forms has become a popular recreational activity for many people. In many parts of the world rowing, canoeing, and kayaking are among the most highly regarded of the Olympic sports. Activities that engage people in movement activities are always worthy of study, even when human power is used to produce locomotion of some other object, such as a boat. On the whole, the principles that apply to swimming apply also to rowing, canoeing, and kayaking. This is particularly obvious in canoeing and kayaking, because the paddle is used in much the

same way as are the arms in swimming. The use of the oars in rowing is more limited, since they must be kept in the oarlocks at all times.

Rowing

In rowing, whether for pleasure or as part of a competitive crew, much of the propulsive force is generated by the legs. The analysis presented in chapter 17 provides an overview of the rowing motion. The rowing stroke can be broken down into two distinct phases: the pull phase and the recovery phase. The force applied to the water by the oar blade during the pull phase is a primary determinant of the distance traveled by the boat during the stroke. The pull is initiated through extension of the flexed lower extremities in a push-like motion, followed by trunk extension and then upper extremity pull.

In the recovery phase the oar blade is lifted clear of the water by downward pressure on the grip, or inboard, end of the oar. The oar is then feathered, or rotated, so that the blade slices through the air parallel to the airflow. During recovery the legs and trunk are flexed and the upper arms are horizontally adducted and elbows extended, pushing the oar into position for the next stroke (figure 20.3). In competitive rowing, the motion in the lower extremities is enhanced through the use of a sliding seat.

In rowing, the oars are held to the gunwale (top edge) of the boat by an oarlock. This oarlock provides an axis of rotation for the oar such that forward motion of the inboard end of the oar results in backward motion of the oar blade and vice versa. For this reason rowers row with their backs to the direction of forward motion.

Canoeing

The situation is somewhat different in canoeing. The paddle in canoeing is held in both hands, free of external support. The canoe paddle stroke is performed using primarily the arms, shoulders, and trunk with the lower body kept relatively

a.

b.

c.

Figure 20.3   Rowing stroke: (a) the end of recovery; (b) the catch (beginning of pull); (c) pull phase.

quiet. The paddler in a canoe faces in the direction of canoe motion. The stroke with the paddle involves reaching out in either a forward or a sideward direction and pulling the paddle blade through the water.

In paddling, as in the arm movement of the crawl stroke, too much force at the beginning of the stroke has too great a downward component, and hence too great a lifting effect. Conversely, too much force at the end of the stroke has too great an upward component, and hence a depressing effect on the canoe. To make the canoe move smoothly in a horizontal direction without unnecessary bobbing up and down, it is essential to reduce these two components to a minimum and to emphasize the backward movement of the blade.

The techniques of steering the canoe are based on this same principle (figure 20.4). One paddler paddling from the center of the canoe moves the canoe broadside to the paddling side by putting the paddle in the water, blade parallel to the keel, directly opposite the center of the canoe, and as far out as can be reached conveniently and safely. The paddler then draws the blade squarely toward the canoe at right angles to the keel of the canoe. To move broadside away from the paddling side, the paddler would slice the blade into the water opposite the center of the canoe and close to it, with the blade parallel to the keel, and then push it directly away at right angles to the keel. To turn the canoe, the paddler would have to reach either forward or backward and press the blade toward or away from the canoe at a point as far from the canoe's center of buoyancy as can be reached conveniently. A drawing stroke nearer the bow would make the canoe turn toward the paddling side; a drawing stroke nearer the stern would make the canoe turn away from the paddling side. (The direction taken by the canoe as a whole is stated in terms of the bow. As the stern of the canoe moves toward the paddling side, the bow moves away from it.) Steering a canoe is logical and

simple when one remembers the principle that movement occurs in the direction opposite to that in which the force is applied and, at the same time, remembers that a canoe tends to rotate about its center of buoyancy when force is applied at any point other than one in line with this center.

Kayaking

The kayak is similar to the canoe. The kayak rides lower in the water than either the rowboat or the canoe and has covered decks rather than an open hull. Kayaks are often used in rough water such as oceans and whitewater rivers. A key difference between kayaks and other small craft is the use of a double-bladed paddle. The blades of this paddle are set perpendicular to one another so that the wrist and arm motion involved in the propulsion phase of the stroke on one side will cause the blade on the opposite side to feather during recovery. Using this paddle, the kayaker can effectively stroke on both sides of the boat in a cyclic fashion. While one blade of the paddle is in the recovery phase the other blade is pulling. This continuous-stroke cycle eliminates the glide phase that occurs in other small craft during recovery so that little forward momentum is lost between strokes (figure 20.5).

Because the kayak is long and slender it is less stable in the water than the canoe, the rowing shell, or the rowboat. To increase stability, the kayaker sits low in the bottom of the boat with the legs extended forward, knees slightly flexed, and feet braced on a rib of the boat. The paddle stroke is produced primarily by the upper body in a continuous motion. It is important that the motion be continuous and that both sides of the body exert identical forces. Unequal forces between the two paddles cause the kayak to turn (unbalanced forces produce rotation). Varying the force applied by the two blades is how the direction of the kayak is controlled.

Figure 20.4 Movement in a canoe is in the direction opposite to that in which the force is applied. (a) Movement toward the paddling side occurs when the paddle is *drawn toward* the center of the canoe. (b) The canoe moves away from the paddling side when the paddle is *pushed away* from the canoe. (c) The sweep stroke pushes the bow away from the paddling side and draws the stern toward it, causing the canoe to move forward in a sweeping turn away from the paddling side. (Black arrows indicate the path of the paddle, and white arrows indicate the path of the canoe.)

Figure 20.5   The kayak paddle stroke.
Courtesy of the American Red Cross. All Rights Reserved
in all countries.

LABORATORY EXPERIENCES

1. Do the arm movement of the crawl stroke and deliberately press hard with the hand as soon as it enters the water, and at the end of the stroke, instead of taking the hand out of the water at the proper time, continue the movement of the arm until the hand has pressed upward against the water. What is the effect of these two errors on the body?

2. Perform a kinesiological analysis of any of the standard strokes, such as the breast, side, elementary back, back crawl. Either observe or practice the stroke before analyzing it. Use the outline for a kinesiological analysis described in chapter 1.

3. Analyze other forms of aquatic locomotion, such as paddling and rowing. Either observe or practice each before analyzing it.

4. A qualified swimmer should perform this demonstration. Try to tip a floating canoe from each of the following positions:
   a. Lying supine on the bottom with arms at the side of the body and legs together.
   b. Sitting on the bottom with legs spread, arms at side of body.
   c. Kneeling in the center of the canoes, hands on gunwales.
   d. Sitting on center thwart, hands on gunwales.

   Explain your results for each of these attempts.

5. Analyze the following common faults kinesiologically and suggest coaching points for avoiding or correcting each fault: too wide a pull with the arms in the breaststroke; a short, choppy stroke in paddling; "catching a crab" in rowing (crew style).

REFERENCES AND SELECTED READINGS

Arellano, R., P. Brown, J. Cappert, and R. C. Nelson. 1994. Analysis of 50-, 100-, and 200-m freestyle swimmers at the 1992 Olympic Games. *Journal of Applied Biomechanics* 10:189–99.

Cappaert, J. M., D. L. Pease, and J. P. Troup. 1995. Three-dimensional analysis of the men's 100-m freestyle during the 1992 Olympic Games. *Journal of Applied Biomechanics* 11:103–12.

Chatard, J. C., C. Collomp, E. Maglischo, and C. Maglischo. 1990. Swimming skill and stroking characteristics of front crawl swimmers. *International Journal of Sports Medicine* 11:156–61.

Clarys, J. P., and J. Cabri. 1993. Electromyography and the study of sports movements: A review. *Journal of Sports Sciences* 11:379–448.

Counsilman, J. E. and B. E. Counsilman. 1994. *The new science of swimming.* Boston: Allyn & Bacon.

Dal Monte, A., and A. Komor. 1987. Rowing and sculling mechanics. In *Biomechanics of sport,* edited by C. L. Vaughn. Boca Raton, FL: CRC Press.

Hay, J. G. 1989. *The biomechanics of sports techniques.* Englewood Cliffs, NJ: Prentice Hall.

Holt, L. E., and P. D. Campagna. 1985. A biomechanical and physiological comparison of Olympic flatwater canoeing. In *Biomechanics in sports II,* edited by J. Terauds and J. Barham. Del Mar, CA: Academic Publishers.

Jerome, J. 1984. *The S-stroke. Science* 84 5(6):94–95.

Keskinen, K. L., and P. V. Komi. 1993. Stroking characteristics of front crawl swimming during exercise. *Journal of Applied Biomechanics* 9:219–26.

Maglischo, E. W. 1994. *Swimming even faster: A comprhensive guide to the science of swimming.* Palo Alto, CA: Mayfield Publishing.

Maglischo, C. W., E. W. Maglischo, D. Luedtke, R. E. Schleihauf, J. Higgins, A. Thayer, and R. Hinrichs. 1987. The swimmer: A study of propulsion and drag. *Soma* 2(2):40–44.

Millward, A. 1987. A study of the forces exerted by an oarsman and the effect on boat speed. *Journal of Sport Sciences* 5:93–103.

Pelayo, P., M. Sidney, T Kherif, D. Chollet, and C. Tourny. 1996. Stroking characteristics in freestyle swimming and relationship with anthropometric characteristics. *Journal of Applied Biomechanics* 12:197–206.

Qi, Liu, J. G. Hay, and J. G. Andrews. 1993. Body roll and handpath in freestyle swimming. *Journal of Applied Biomechanics* 9:238–53.

Sanderson, B., and W. Martindale. 1986. Towards optimizing rowing technique. *Medicine and Science in Sports and Exercise* 18(4):454–68.

Shepard, R. J. 1987. Science and medicine of canoeing and kayaking. *Sports Medicine* 4:19–33.

Toussaint, H. M., and P. J. Beck. 1992. Biomechanics of competitive front crawl swimming. *Sports Medicine* 13:8–24.

21

LOCOMOTION: WHEN SUSPENDED AND FREE OF SUPPORT

OUTLINE

- **Suspension Activities**
  Principles Related to Hanging and Hand-Traveling Activities
  Principles Related to Swinging Movements
  Suspension Analysis Example
- **Nonsupport Activities**
  Principles Related to Nonsupport Activities
  Nonsupport Analysis Example
  Free Fall
  Weightlessness
- **Laboratory Experiences**

OBJECTIVES

At the conclusion of this chapter, the student should be able to:

1. Explain how each of the following influences the action of swinging bodies: weight of the body, length of the pendulum, angular momentum, potential-kinetic energy, centripetal–centrifugal force, friction.

2. Describe how to initiate pendular action, increase the height of a swing, alter the period, change grips, and dismount safely.

3. Explain how each of the following influences the flight path of unsupported bodies: angle of projection, vertical velocity, gravity, angular momentum.

4. Describe how to initiate and control rotation of unsupported bodies.

5. Analyze the performance of a suspension and a nonsupport movement, following the outline for kinesiological analysis described in chapter 1.

SUSPENSION ACTIVITIES

Climbing, hanging, swinging, and other suspension activities were more commonly engaged in by our early ancestors than by members of more recent generations. The modern version of these brachial activities is seen in the trapeze activities of the aerial artist at the circus, in gymnastics events on the high bar, parallel bars, uneven bars, and rings, and in various forms of hanging on ladders and ropes in the gymnasium and on the playground. Success in suspension activities depends on considerable strength and endurance, particularly of the hand, arm, and shoulder musculature, and the ability to adjust body positions to counteract or take advantage of the forces acting on the body (figure 21.1). Ladder, rope or rock climbing, and brachial locomotion are modifications of locomotion. Where swinging movements of a suspended body are involved, the principles of a pendulum, angular momentum, and centripetal–centrifugal forces are major considerations.

Principles Related to Hanging and Hand-Traveling Activities

1. *In hanging activities the muscles of the arm and shoulder girdle must contract to protect the joints.* The pull of the body's weight puts stress on the joints by tending to separate them.
2. *Hand traveling is a locomotor pattern governed by the principle of action and reaction.* As in walking, force applied against a supporting surface in one direction causes

Figure 21.1   Movement of the body in suspension. This maneuver on the still rings illustrates the need for good muscular development in the arms and shoulders.
Courtesy of Springfield College.

the body to move in the opposite direction. Hand traveling sideward on a bar or rail without swinging is achieved by alternately moving one hand away from the other hand, and then moving the second hand toward the first. As the first hand moves, the second hand pushes laterally against the apparatus. Both hands share the weight equally for a moment, then the second hand is released and brought toward the first hand while the first hand is pulling laterally on the apparatus.

3. *The action used in hand-climbing activities is essentially a chinning action.* In rope climbing, for instance, either with or without the use of the legs, the body is raised through a forceful pull-up action of the arms. The rock climber uses a similar motion to advance up the rock face. The gymnast using a kip motion to mount a bar or the rings uses this same pull-up action to raise the body toward the hands. This action is then often converted to a push-up type of motion, ending in a straight-arm support position.

4. *In accord with Newton's law of inertia, sequential hand support movements should be continuous. The momentum of one action contributes to the next action.* In the kip movement of the gymnast, there should be no pause between the pulling phase and the pushing phase of the hands and arms. Similarly, the rock climber tries to use the motion produced by the upward pull of one arm to contribute momentum to the next upward pull.

Principles Related to Swinging Movements

1. *The movement of a pendulum is produced by the force of gravity.* This statement presupposes a starting position in which potential energy is present. In other words, the pendulum must be moved from its resting position before the force of gravity can make it swing downward.

The initial problem of the child on the swing and of the gymnast on the rings is that of being given potential energy. Without the help of an assistant, the swinger must find a way to be put into a position with potential energy. This is usually done in one of three ways. The performer may move the apparatus to some position other than its normal position of rest before being suspended (i.e., the swing is pulled as far back and up as can be reached); the performer may initiate the swing with a push of the feet against the floor or with small running steps; or a pumping action may be used to get started. For the gymnast swinging on the rings, the last alternative involves bending the legs up in front of the body and then extending them as high as possible. The range of the arc of motion may be increased by the repetition of this procedure on the forward-upward phase of the swing. The child in the swing accomplishes the same result by inclining the trunk backward and raising the feet forward while pulling the ropes toward the body and pressing forward against the seat.

2. *As the pendulum swings downward, gravity causes its speed to increase; as it swings upward, gravity counteracts its speed, diminishing it until the zero point is reached.* Hence the pendulum's speed is greatest at the bottom of the arc and least (zero) at each end of the arc.

Caution must be exercised to maintain a firm grip on the supporting surface (rings, bar, or ropes), particularly at the bottom of the swing where the tendency to fly off is the greatest.

3. *The upward movement of a pendulum is brought about by the momentum developed in the downward movement.* The swinging body moves through an arc, first in one direction, then in the reverse direction (one-half the arc's distance is called the *amplitude*). Thus it undergoes partial rotation

about a center of motion. Because this rotation takes place in a vertical plane, the influence of gravitational pull must be taken into consideration. Whereas the force of gravity *produces* the downward swing, it *opposes* the upward swing. Nevertheless, it is indirectly responsible for the latter, inasmuch as the upward swing is caused by the momentum that was built up in the preceding downward swing.

This relationship is especially important in skills performed in gymnastics when long, swinging actions are involved. The higher the position from which the downswing is initiated, the higher will be the upswing. The range of a swing depends on the height from which the movement is initiated.

4. *The potential energy of the pendulum is greatest at the height of the swing and zero at the bottom.* Conversely, kinetic energy is greatest at the bottom and zero at the top. In a perfect mechanical system a pendulum would continue to swing with a constant amplitude with the required energy supplied by the perpetual conversion from potential to kinetic energy. Most of the potential energy is converted to kinetic energy in the downswing and reconverted on the upswing. Some is lost, however, to friction and air resistance, and a pendulum left to its own devices will gradually decrease in amplitude and stop.

To make up for the lost mechanical energy, supplemental energy in the form of properly timed muscular action of the swinger must be used. Maximum repetitions of a pendulum left to its own devices will occur if the initial height is maximum and friction is minimized.

5. *The centripetal–centrifugal force in pendular movements increases as the mass or velocity increases and decreases as the radius increases* $(C_F = \dfrac{mv^2}{r})$. The centripetal force is greatest at the bottom of the swing, where the velocity is the greatest, and decreases to

zero at the height of the swing. However, bodies develop proportionately more centripetal force and need more strength to maintain a grasp and counteract the opposing centrifugal force than do those of less weight. When centripetal force ceases to act on a swinging performer, the body will obey Newton's first law and will fly off tangent to the arc of the swing at that instant.

The grip must be the most secure at the bottom of the swing, where the tendency to fly off is the greatest. Centripetal force has been calculated to be four to five times body weight as the body swings under the bar in a giant swing. To resist the equal and opposite outward-pulling centrifugal force, strong hands and arms are essential. The bottom of the swing is the point where the beginner or the novice is most likely to lose contact with the bar.

Although actions requiring release and regrasp of a bar or ring should be done at the peak of the swing, the same is not always true of dismounts. Dismounts and cutaways should be timed to occur at a point where the tangent of the arc at the instant of release coincides with the desired line of flight.

6. *When a pendulum reaches the end of its arc, just before it reverses its direction, it reaches a zero point in velocity.* At this precise moment the force of gravity is momentarily neutralized by the upward momentum.

The performer can take advantage of this situation by using this moment to perform position changes such as changing grips, reversing direction, and performing dismounts and cutaways. The underswing half-turn on the unevens is executed best and is most easily controlled when both the twist and grip changes are completed during the height of the underswing.

7. *The height of a swing may be increased by lengthening the radius of rotation on the downswing and decreasing it on the upswing* (figure 21.2). Shortening the radius on the upswing decreases the moment of inertia and

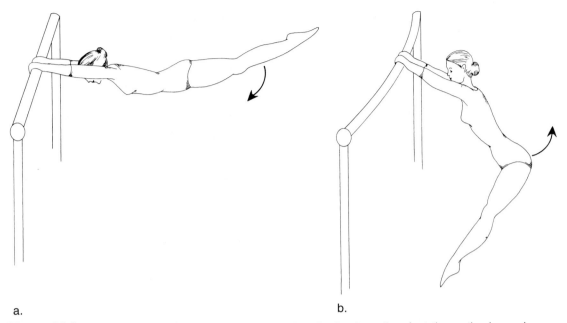

a.

b.

Figure 21.2   The height of a swing may be increased by lengthening the radius of rotation on the downswing and decreasing it on the upswing.

therefore increases the angular velocity. This occurs because the angular momentum is conserved and, because angular momentum equals $I\omega$, a decrease in I requires an increase in ω. The increased angular velocity is accompanied by an increase in kinetic energy and consequently more height results. The increased height for the start of the downswing and the lengthened radius of rotation produce a gain in angular momentum on the downswing because gravity has a longer time to act on the body before it reaches the bottom of the swing. When the shortening of the radius occurs for the next upswing, the increased momentum is conserved and, once again, there is an increase in angular velocity. The equation for angular momentum, $I\omega$, also shows that the greater the angular velocity on the downswing, the less the body has to be shortened to decrease I in order to reach its desired height on the upswing.

A swinging performer may shorten the radius of rotation by moving body parts toward the axis of rotation. This may be done by flexing at the hips, hunching the shoulders by depressing the shoulder girdle, or arching the back. A performer in the giant swing depresses the shoulder girdle and flexes at the hips on the upswing and may also arch the back slightly. In a circle from a front uprise, the head is thrown back to shorten the radius on the upswing.

8. *To increase height, the decrease in radius should be initiated at the moment the center of gravity of the body is directly under the axis of rotation.* In the movement of a pendulum, speed is greatest at the bottom of the arc. Shortening the radius at this point accelerates its angular velocity more than at any other position.

In the backward hip circle on the uneven parallel bars, for example, the movement is started with the body extended and the hips on the bar. This gives the longest possible radius of rotation on the downswing. At the moment the legs pass under the hands (the axis of rotation), the hips are flexed to shorten the radius on the upswing, thereby decreasing the moment of inertia and increasing the angular velocity.

9. *The time taken by the pendulum to make a single round-trip excursion (known as its period) is related to the length of the pendulum.* The longer the pendulum, the more slowly it swings. Specifically, the period of the pendulum is proportional to the square root of its length.

     When the hands are the axis of rotation, such as in the preparatory moves for a giant swing, the period is longer than in swings about a hip axis or a knee axis.

10. *The period of the pendulum is not influenced by its weight.* A heavy body will swing no faster than a lighter one, and vice versa. This is consistent with the behavior of freely falling bodies.

     Trapeze artists take advantage of this principle. A performer swinging from one trapeze knows that an empty trapeze of the same length, swung from an opposite platform of the same height and at the same time as the trapeze artist's, will have the same period. Consequently the performer also knows that it is safe to let go of the original bar at the height of its swing and turn around in midair, because the empty bar will be right there to be grasped, also at the height of its swing.

11. *When a body consisting of two segments reaches the vertical, with the proximal segment leading on the downswing, the distal segment will accelerate relative to the other segment and precede it into the upswing.* If, on the other hand, the distal segment reaches the vertical first, the reverse will occur. The distal segment will decelerate and the proximal segment will lead into the upswing (figure 21.3).

Action at the bottom of a swing, which forces the hips through in front of the feet, increases the acceleration on the upswing owing to hip flexion in shortening the radius. Such swings are called "beat" swings. Beat swings are used to set up release–regrasp skills on apparatus such as the uneven and even parallel bars, the high bar and the still rings.

12. *The rotation of the hands about a bar is opposed by frictional forces.* This accounts for some loss in swinging energy as it is converted into heat energy. Evidence of this is the appearance of friction blisters and skin irritations on a gymnast's hands. These friction forces tend to strengthen the gymnast's grip when the swing is in the direction the palms are facing and weakens it when the swing is in the reverse direction.

     Gymnasts reverse their grasps when the swing is reversed. This is usually done at the peak of the swing at the point of "weightlessness," when the pressure on the hands is at a minimum. Gymnasts also sand the bar before each performance to ensure its smoothness and to minimize the friction on the hands.

13. *In all mounting exercises involving swinging, the center of gravity must be brought as near as possible to the center of rotation.* This is usually done when the center of gravity is directly under the bar on the downswing.

     In the glide kip on the unevens, for instance, the performer swings the body forward and back, alternately flexing and extending to gain momentum. At the end of the glide the gymnast flexes fully at the hips so that the feet are near the bar. This sharp flexion increases the angular velocity by decreasing the moment of inertia. As the center of gravity passes under the bar on the downswing, the hips are extended vigorously. This movement raises the body and places the center of gravity close to the bar, thus further decreasing the moment of

a.

b.

Figure 21.3 (a) Double pendulum swing. If segment *a* precedes segment *b* to the vertical, segment *b* accelerates and precedes *a* in the upswing. (b) When segment *b* precedes *a* to the vertical, *a* will lead into the upswing, but the whole pendulum decelerates.

inertia and enabling the body to rotate until it is in a front support position with the center of gravity located at the fixed point of the grip.

14. *In support swings the center of gravity should be at the point of support.* Hip circles forward or backward require the center of gravity of the body to be close to the hand supports. In this position it takes less effort to keep the body against the bar while turning because the torque between the center of gravity of the body and the axis of rotation is kept at a minimum.

Suspension Analysis Example
Half-Turn Flying Hip Circle with Hecht Dismount—Uneven Parallel Bars

Gymnasts who perform on the uneven parallel bars have numerous combinations of movements from which to choose. Each routine starts with a mount and concludes with a dismount. In-between the gymnast selects from a series of movements, including those characterized as circling, swinging, or kipping movements. Grip release and regrasps must also be incorporated. Movements are classified as being of medium or superior difficulty, and each performance should contain four medium and two superior moves in its twelve to fourteen moves. The moves shown in figure 21.4 and described here are of medium difficulty. The gymnast starts in a handstand position on the high bar (a). As she begins to swing downward she performs a half-twist so that she faces in the direction of the swing (b, c). At the bottom of the swing she begins to flex at the hips in preparation for continuing in a back hip circle around the low bar (d, e). Toward the end of the hip circle she extends at the hip joint and dismounts forward over the low bar in a move called a *hecht* (f, g). She lands with her back to the bars (h).

Mechanical essentials In starting the downward swing from the handstand position, the gymnast pushes against the bar. Because of action–reaction

the bar pushes back in the opposite direction. The give of the bar adds to the reactive force and thus increases the total energy of the system. The push of the gymnast backward and the accompanying stretch increase the distance between the center of gravity and the axis of rotation and thus increase the torque on the downward swing. The time for gravity to act on the downward swinging body is also increased. The half-twist is performed at the beginning of the downswing when the forces acting on the hands are minimal and the grip change can be accomplished with ease (figure 21.4b). At the bottom of the swing the gymnast flexes at the hips, thus shortening the radius of rotation and increasing her angular velocity on the upswing. This piked position also enables her to "wrap" around the low bar as she moves into the backward hip circle (figure 21.4d). There should be no pause between one movement and the next. Any slowing down would require more energy to pick up again (Law of Inertia) and fluidity would be lost. As the gymnast's hands leave the high bar, she pushes up and forward, causing the reactive force to add to the downward trunk rotation (figure 21.4e).

The hip circle should be accomplished with the hips close to the bar so that the center of gravity is near the axis of rotation. Otherwise, centrifugal force would tend to pull the body away from the bar. Toward the completion of the hip circle the gymnast forcefully extends by lifting the upper trunk and arms forward and upward (figure 21.4f). This action causes several things to happen. In reaction, the legs also extend so that the whole body is straight. The moment of inertia about the transverse axis is increased, and the rate of rotation decreases. The body pushes down and back against the bar causing the bar to push the body forward and up. All of this results in the body rotating up and away from the bar for the dismount. Once the body has left the bar the back should be arched to again decrease the radius slightly and aid in the rotation of the body, allowing the feet to move slightly ahead of the center of gravity at the moment of landing (figure 21.4h). The success of the

a. b. c.

d. e. f.

g. h.

Figure 21.4 Half-turn flying hip circle with hecht dismount. (Drawn from motion picture film tracings.)

hecht dismount depends on sufficient angular momentum being developed in the downswing and hip circle and a forceful, properly timed extension of the body at the end of the hip circle.

Anatomical essentials   The anatomical essentials for successful performance in this movement series are strength and flexibility. Strength of shoulders, arms, and hands is especially important for swinging movements. Grip strength is essential, and until one is sure of such strength, certain swinging movements should not be attempted without the assistance of a spotter. Arm and shoulder strength can be checked by testing oneself with push-ups and pull-ups. Strong abdominal and back extensor muscles are also important. These muscle groups play a significant role in maintaining and changing the trunk position in the downward swing, the hip circle, and the hecht dismount as shown here. Range of motion is also needed for these movements, particularly in the shoulder during the swing, and in the hip and lower back during the pike of the hip circle.

NONSUPPORT ACTIVITIES

The unsupported body moves through the air along a pathway determined prior to the beginning of flight. The flight path of the body may be primarily horizontal, as in a long jump, mostly vertical, as in springboard diving or high jumping, or somewhere in between, as in vaulting and tumbling events. Principles governing the flight path of the body relate to those of the projectile. Additional principles explaining the effect of the body's lean at the moment of takeoff and the twisting movements in the air are derived from Newton's third law, the Law of Action–Reaction and the Conservation of Angular Momentum.

Principles Related to Nonsupport Activities

1. *The path of motion of the body's center of gravity in space is determined by the angle at which it is projected into space, the force of the projection, and the force of gravity.* Nothing a diver or a gymnast can do will alter the pathway of the center of gravity once the feet have left the push-off surface. The horizontal velocity of the body remains constant and the path of the center of gravity is a parabola determined by the initial force and gravity. Without the application of an external force, this path cannot be altered. For this reason the initial path must be suited to the desired result. The diver must allow for clearance of the board and sufficient air time for stunts while the gymnast must either produce a vertical path to land on a trampoline, balance beam, or vaulting horse or must produce sufficient air time for stunts on the floor.

2. *The time a body remains unsupported depends on the height of its projection, which is governed by the vertical velocity of the projection* (figure 21.5). The more complicated or lengthy the stunt a diver or gymnast wishes to perform, the higher the peak of projection must be. A diver must emphasize vertical rather than horizontal distance.

3. *Most rotary movements are initiated before the performer leaves the supporting surface.* To possess angular momentum during a nonsupport activity, an eccentric force must be used for takeoff. In a front somersault, for example, the center of gravity must be in front of the feet at the moment of takeoff in order for torque to exist. In a somersault with a twist (figure 21.6), the push must be sideways as well as diagonally backward as the upper body leads the twist in the opposite direction. In keeping with Newton's third law, the direction of the twist is opposite to the direction in which the feet push against the supporting surface.

4. *The angular momentum ($I\omega$) of an unsupported body is conserved. It cannot be increased or decreased.* A performer executing a somersault may increase the

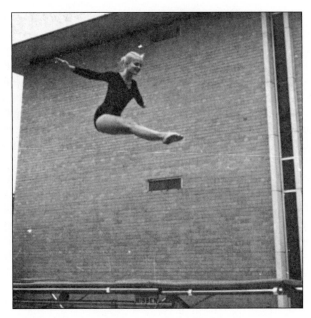

Figure 21.5   Movement of the body in the air, free of support. The height of projection depends on its vertical velocity.

Figure 21.6   Back one-and-one-half somersault, one-and-one-half twist, free.
From D. A. Armbruster et al. *Swimming and Diving,* 5th ed. Copyright © 1968 C. V. Mosby, St. Louis. Reprinted by permission.

angular velocity by decreasing the moment of inertia. This is done by decreasing the radius of rotation, that is, by increasing the amount of tuck. A tuck somersault has a smaller moment of inertia than a pike somersault, and a pike somersault has less than a layout. To stop rotation in anticipation of landing or entry into the water, the moment of inertia is increased, thereby decreasing the angular velocity.

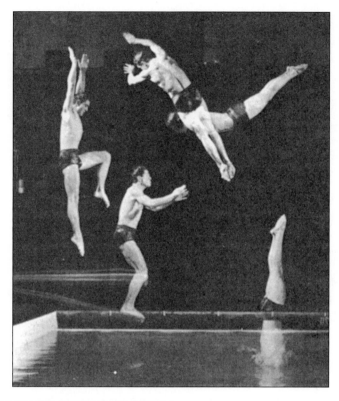

Figure 21.7   The reverse dive layout with one-half twist.
From G. Batterman, *The Techniques of Springboard Diving,* copyright © 1968 MIT Press, Cambridge, MA.

If a somersault starts with a twist from the push-off surface, the twist can be increased by decreasing the arch or the pike of the spin and by moving the arms closer to the body. Each of these moves decreases the moment of inertia and increases the angular velocity of the twist.

5. *When a body is free in space, movement of a part in one direction results in movement of the rest of the body in the opposite direction.* In a back dive in the pike position, the diver should wait until the legs have rotated past the vertical before the pike is opened. As the trunk and arms move back, the legs will react in the opposite direction and therefore move back to the vertical position.

A reverse dive layout with a one-half twist (figure 21.7) may be performed by initiating the twist in the air rather than from the board. The diver will cause the body to twist to the opposite direction by moving one arm across the chest after the body is in a layout position in the air. The arm must then be moved overhead, keeping it close to the body so that another equal and opposite reaction does not occur. This method for initiating a twist is slow and is not usually used for more than a half-twist.

6. *A performer who is rotating about a horizontal axis in the air may initiate a twist about a vertical axis by tilting the body to one side.* In any twisting somersault, a diver can tilt to the side by moving one arm from the side horizontal to a position over the head and the other arm sideward downward across the body. This happens because of

Figure 21.8 Double-twisting back somersault.

action–reaction. As the arms move in one direction in the frontal plane, the body moves in the other direction. The twist will occur in the direction of the raised arm and be directly proportional to the spin. That is, the faster the performer is rotating forward or backward, the faster will be the twist (figure 21.8).

Nonsupport Analysis Example
The Reverse Dive Layout with One-Half Twist

A twisting dive is one in which the body makes at least one-half turn about the vertical axis. Twisting dives may be combined with somersaults in the tuck, pike, or layout positions. Divers may face forward and leave the board with a forward-spinning action or a backward-spinning action (reverse spinning dives). They may also initiate dives from a backward stance and spin backward or forward (inward spinning dives). In the reverse dive layout with a one-half twist pictured in figure 21.7, the diver starts the dive facing the end of the board. He performs a reverse spinning

somersault about a transverse axis in a layout position completing a one-half revolution. At the same time, he twists one-half a revolution about the vertical axis.

Mechanical essentials In starting a reverse dive the diver must end the forward approach by pushing backward toward the back end of the board with the feet. The rebounding board will push back with an equal and opposite reaction, causing the legs to move forward. This action of the board causes the reverse spin to develop in the body as the feet and legs move forward and the head and upper trunk rotate backward. It also causes the entire body to move forward away from the board. Because the feet push back against the board in reverse dives and force the body forward, less lean is needed on takeoff than with forward dives, where the feet push forward toward the tip of the board. The amount of rotation (spin) about the transverse axis must be determined in large measure at takeoff of this dive because usual methods of controlling the rate of spin by decreasing the moment of inertia through tucking or piking are not permitted. The angular momentum of the dive is determined and conserved at takeoff and cannot be altered, although some control may be exercised by varying the arch in the back in the initial layout. An increase in the arch will increase the rate of rotation.

The twist in this dive is accomplished through the use of two methods of initiating twists. As the diver leaves the board, he not only pushes back to create the reversed spin, but he also pushes slightly to the right to initiate a twist to the left. Once the diver is in the air the principle of action–reaction is used to complete the twist. As the diver twists to the left the left arm is brought across the chest, causing his body to move in the opposite direction (left) in reaction. He continues to aid the twist by circling the arm down next to the body, close to the axis of rotation. Keeping the head in line with the body and the right arm overhead during the twist decreases the moment of inertia of the rotating body and increases the speed of the twist. Turning the head left toward the water helps in the turn and the diver's orientation. The diver's twist is completed so that he enters the water with the back to the board and at the point where the center of gravity was predetermined to land the instant the feet left the board. In spite of the spin of the body about both a vertical and a horizontal axis, the body's center of gravity follows a perfect parabolic curve controlled only by the velocity and angle of projection and the downward acceleration of gravity.

The entry of the dive must consider that the forward rotation of the dive will continue because of the Law of Conservation of Momentum. The stretched position of the body with the arms overhead creates the greatest moment of inertia possible and therefore the slowest rotation, but there is still some rotation. For this reason the diver should continue to turn underwater in the same direction. The angle of entry of the dive should be a natural continuation of the parabolic path of the center of gravity of the body. For reverse dives the entry would be almost vertical.

Anatomical essentials As with all dives from a diving board, this dive requires good strength, flexibility, and control, particularly in the trunk and legs. Good range of motion in the ankle joint is essential because the feet contact the end of the board, dorsiflex as the board is depressed, and then ride it upward and extend until the toes leave the board. Strength in the extensors of the hip and knee is also important in lifting the body from the board and maintaining the extended position in the air. Strength of the abdominals and back extensors is of prime importance to divers. Vertical alignment in the air relies on control by these muscles, as does the entry position. The abdominals also are important in the initiation and control of rotations and in the prevention of overarching the back. Contrary to popular belief, extreme extension mobility of the back is not desirable in dives and should be avoided. In the dive described here, overarching would decrease the height of the dive and slow the twist, as it causes an increase in the moment of inertia about the vertical axis. Flexibility of the back and hips for full flexion in tuck and pike positions is desirable, however.

Free Fall

Although all unsupported bodies follow the law of falling bodies, most return to earth in a very short time, having performed the desired stunts on the way. Yet there are times when the human body is in a state of free fall for much longer periods of time. Skydiving and parachuting are examples of human bodies in free fall. The human body will reach terminal velocity between 100 and 200 mph, depending on the surface area presented to the airflow (Brancazio 1984). In a nose dive, or head down, position it takes about 20 seconds to reach terminal velocity, close to 200 mph. Increasing the surface area presented to the airflow by assuming a "spread-eagle" position reduces the terminal velocity to 100 mph, reached in about 15 seconds. By manipulating the shape of the body in this way, the rate of descent can be partially controlled. Direction can also be modified by flexing

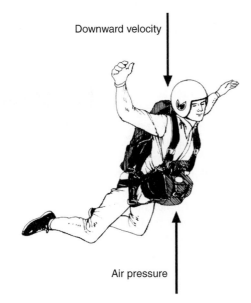

Downward velocity

Air pressure

Figure 21.9 The spread-eagle position used to increase air pressure in skydiving.

and extending the extremities on one side of the body. Arm and leg flexion will decrease drag on that side of the body, producing a sideslipping or sideways motion. Reducing drag at one point of the body will produce rotation (figure 21.9).

Weightlessness

Once human beings ventured into space, dealing with a gravity-free environment became a matter for serious study. With the planning and construction of orbiting space stations, more and more people will be confronted with the necessity of living and working in weightless conditions.

One critical fact must always be remembered in dealing with human motion in weightless conditions: *The laws of motion still apply.* Objects still possess inertia based on mass or momentum, acceleration is still directly related to force and mass, and every action has an equal and opposite reaction. The only difference is that the force of gravity no longer provides a constant downward accelera-

tion. In a weightless environment the terms "down" and "up" are relatively meaningless.

The implications of a gravity-free environment deserve some attention in any study of human motion. In such an environment a force equal to or greater than the mass of an object or body is still required to start that object in motion. A force equal to the product of mass and acceleration is also required to stop a body in motion. A ball thrown in space requires the same throwing force and will strike the catcher's hand with the same force as on earth. However, because of a lack of gravity pulling downward, it will travel in a straight line, not a parabolic path.

Of great concern in manned spaceflight is the loss of bone mineral that occurs with prolonged weightlessness. In an environment with gravity such as that experienced on earth, humans must constantly resist the effects of gravity. In a weightless environment, this stress is removed. Because bone reacts to the stresses placed on it, a reduction of stress produces a reabsorption of bone material. For this reason, researchers and other space scientists are working to devise exercise programs that will continue to stress the musculoskeletal system in a weightless environment. A major obstacle to providing adequate exercise programs is the lack of adequate resistance. In space, if the astronaut pushes against something, such as a treadmill in running, there is still an equal and opposite reaction. Because the astronaut is not subject to the pull of gravity, rather than push off into a running step, the astronaut will push completely off the treadmill. Likewise, lifting weights is as likely to move the astronaut down as to move the weight up.

Because of the lack of gravity, the concept of up and down has little meaning in space, since once a position is assumed through concentric muscle contraction the segment or body remains in the new position unless moved by another force, such as further muscle contraction, or through contact with an external force. Reflexes are greatly affected by weightlessness. The extensor thrust reflex is less important because no deep pressure is experienced by the pacinian corpuscles. Also, in the absence of gravity, information from the proprioceptors is confusing, resulting in disorganization within the system. Until the individual adjusts, this disorganization often results in nausea, a serious problem in space travel.

LABORATORY EXPERIENCES

1. Hang motionless from a rope or a pair of rings. Now start swinging without the help of anyone else. How was the swing accomplished? Explain.

2. Swing on a pair of rings without attempting to get much height. Perform the following movements. Explain the results by stating the underlying principles. Be sure to have mats placed under the swinging area.
   a. Reverse the grasp of one hand. At which point in the swing is this accomplished most easily?
   b. Dismount at various positions along the arc of the swing. Note the effect on the body.

3. Perform the following movements in the water and explain the actions by stating underlying principles. (Except for the factor of increased resistance, the actions simulate those of an unsupported body.)
   a. Lie on the side and swing both legs forward vigorously, keeping the knees straight. Note the effect on the trunk.
   b. Lie on the back with the arms in a side horizontal position. Keeping the elbows straight, swing both arms in a clockwise direction across the surface of the water in a 90-degree arc as you roll to the right into a prone float. Note the direction in which the feet now point compared with the starting position.

4. Perform a complete kinesiological analysis of a selected swinging or airborne activity, taking particular note of the purpose of the motion, its classification, and the nature of the motion. Include also muscle participation, neuromuscular considerations, mechanical factors, and applicable principles and violations. Conclude the analysis with a prescription for improvement, including suggested methods for change and the elimination of violations of principles.

REFERENCES AND SELECTED READINGS

Adrian, M. A., and J. M. Cooper. 1994. *The biomechanics of human movement.* 2nd ed. Indianapolis: Benchmark Press.

Brancazio, P. J. 1984. *Sport science.* New York: Simon & Schuster.

Carr, G. 1997. *Mechanics of sport.* Champaign, IL: Human Kinetics.

Cooke, P. 1984. Acrobatics: Physics with a twist. *Science 84* 5(5):86–87.

Enoka, R. M. 1988. *Neuromechanical basis of kinesiology.* Champaign, IL: Human Kinetics.

Gowitzke, B. A., and M. Milner. 1988. *Scientific bases of human movement.* 3rd ed. Baltimore: Williams & Wilkins.

Hamill, J., D. M. Golden, and M. A. Williams. 1985. Dynamics of selected tower dive take-offs. In *Biomechanics in sports II,* edited by J. Terauds and J. Barham. Del Mar, CA: Academic Publishers.

Hamill, J., M. D. Ricard, and D. M. Golden. 1986. Angular momentum in multiple rotation nontwisting platform dives. *International Journal of Sport Biomechanics* 2:78–87.

Hay, J. G. 1989. *The biomechanics of sports techniques.* Englewood Cliffs, NJ: Prentice Hall.

Kreighbaum, E., and K. M. Barthels. 1990. *Biomechanics.* New York: Macmillan.

Yeadon, M. R. 1993. The biomechanics of twisting somersaults. Part III: Aerial twist. *Journal of Sports Sciences* 11:209–18.

Yeadon, M. 1997. Twisting double somersault high bar dismounts. *Journal of Applied Biomechanics* 13:76–87.

22

IMPACT

OUTLINE

■ *Meaning of Impact and Its Reception*
  Problems and Concepts
  Falls and Landings
  Catching
■ *Principles in Receiving Impact*
  Related to Avoiding Injury
  Related to Maintaining and
     Regaining Equilibrium
  Related to Accuracy and Control
■ *Laboratory Experiences*

OBJECTIVES

At the conclusion of this chapter, the student should be able to:

1. Name the common problems associated with the diverse forms of receiving impact.
2. Explain how the work–energy, impulse–momentum, and pressure-area relationships apply to receiving the impact either of one's own body or of external objects.
3. State the principles related to avoiding injury while receiving impact and furnish an application for each.
4. State the principles related to maintaining and regaining equilibrium while receiving impact and furnish an application for each.
5. State the principles related to accuracy and control while receiving impact and furnish an application for each.

MEANING OF IMPACT AND ITS RECEPTION

The word *impact* is derived from the Latin word *impingere,* "to press together." Impact is further defined as force of contact, violent collision, striking together. Receiving impact is opposing or resisting in some manner the force with which a moving body tends to maintain its speed and direction. Impact may be from one's own body, as in landing from a jump or fall, or imparted by external objects, as in catching or spotting.

Impact of one's own body is experienced following any fall through space. Such falling motion, which occurs subsequent to a jump, a dive, or an accidental fall, has a rapidly increasing velocity because of the uniform acceleration effect of gravitational force. When the body lands on a supporting surface, impact has been said to occur. The impact is felt as the force of contact. Likewise, impact is experienced in a horizontally moving body when the motion is stopped as a result of contact with a resisting surface, such as a wall or another obstacle.

Examples of receiving impact from external objects are commonly seen in sports. Baseballs are caught or fielded with the hands, hockey balls and pucks are received with a stick, soccer balls are trapped with the feet, and blows from an opponent's fist are received by various parts of the body. Examples of receiving impact are also seen in industry and in daily life. Cartons and tools are tossed from one person to another, red-hot rivets are caught in tongs, and victims from a fire are caught in nets or air bags.

Problems and Concepts

What are the particular problems involved in these diverse forms of receiving impact, and what are the principles that enable us to solve these problems satisfactorily? In the reception of the body's own impact, the chief problems seem to be those of *avoiding injury* and *regaining equilib-*

rium promptly. Three problems appear to be involved in receiving the impact of external objects: (1) *avoiding injury,* (2) *maintaining equilibrium,* and (3) *receiving the object with accuracy and control.*

Whether the moving object is one's own body or an external object, the basic concepts enabling us to understand and solve these problems are the same. The first concept is the *kinetic energy–work relationship: When a body or object is "received" it has work done on it equal in amount to the change in kinetic energy of the moving body* (see p. 334). If, for example, velocity of an object is reduced to zero, all of its kinetic energy would be used to do work on the receiver. Because work equals the product of force and distance, the work done in "receiving" may consist of any combination of force and distance as long as the product of the two is equivalent to the kinetic energy lost by the moving object.

The second applicable concept is the *momentum–impulse relationship* (see pp. 313–315): *Any change in momentum requires a force applied over a period of time (impulse) and is equal to the product of that force and the time.* Again, the reduction in momentum of any object can be accomplished by any equivalent product combination of force and time. Both impulse and kinetic energy are proportional to the mass and velocity (momentum) of any object and will change if the momentum does.

The third concept involves *pressure* and is especially important with respect to avoiding injury: *The pressure that any part of the body must absorb is inversely proportional to the area over which the force is applied.*

Falls and Landings

The abrupt loss of motion resulting from collision with an unyielding surface is likely to cause an injury in landing after falls and landings. To avoid injury it is necessary to find some means of losing the body's kinetic energy more gradually. This is achieved by increasing the distance and time over which the kinetic energy and momentum are lost. Landing on "giving" surfaces, such as mats or sawdust, controlled flexion at the joints of the landing extremities through eccentric contraction of the antagonist muscles, and rolling are important contributors to the gradual decrease in momentum without injury. Landings are often catagorized as "soft" or "stiff" based on joint involvement. The knee is a major contributor to force dissipation in most landings. In soft landings, the involvement of both the ankle and the hip increase. In stiff landings, the contribution of the ankle is greater while the contribution of the hip decreases. A similar pattern occurs with landings from different heights. As the height of landing increases, the involvement of both the hip and the ankle increase (McNitt-Gray 1993; Zhang, Bates, and Dufek 2000)

Another factor in injury that should not be overlooked is the relationship of the force of impact to the size of the area that bears the brunt of the impact. A force of 450 N concentrated on 1 square centimeter of body surface, for instance, is likely to cause more serious injury than the same amount of force spread over an area of 50 square centimeters. Hence the problem is to increase the size of the area that receives the force of the impact. This is especially important when there is limited opportunity for increasing the distance over which the kinetic energy is lost.

Athletes in activities involving landing from substantial heights adopt a variety of landing strategies based on the requirements of the sport. Jumpers such as high jumpers and pole-vaulters decrease the trauma to the body by landing on very deep crash pads. Gymnasts, on the other hand, land a mats of varying thickness, based on the event. As mat thickness decreases, the gymnast uses an increased angle of hip and knee flexion on landing in order to increase the time over which kinetic energy is lost (McNitt-Gray, Yokoi, and Millward 1993).

The problem of regaining equilibrium in falling and landing is largely a problem in controlling the placement of the limbs in preparation for landing, because equilibrium is regained when an adequate base of support is established. This requires sufficient control to place the feet, or perhaps both the hands and the feet, in a position that will provide a favorable base of support. The problem of regaining equilibrium is closely related to that of avoiding injury, since establishing an adequate base depends on the integrity of the bones and joints that receive the force of impact.

Various methods of falling are taught in classes in tumbling, martial arts, and modern dance. Perhaps one of the most effective measures for the prevention of injury in accidental falls is this kind of instruction, followed by the practice of a variety of falls until the techniques have been mastered. Practice helps establish the right patterns, patterns that will be followed automatically when accidental falls occur.

Catching

As in the case of receiving the impact of one's own body, avoidance of injury in catching or receiving external forces is achieved by increasing the distance over which the object's kinetic energy is lost. When catching a fast-moving baseball, the experienced player will not hold the hands rigidly in front of the body but will give with the ball. By moving the hands toward the body through a distance of 10 to 20 inches as the ball is received, the catcher is making it possible for the ball's kinetic energy to be lost gradually. This same principle is likewise true for the player who is reaching for a high ball with one hand. The extended arm acts as a lever, the force being applied by the impact of the ball on the palm. The torque is therefore the product of the force of impact and the perpendicular distance from the shoulder joint to the ball's line of flight at the instant it is caught. If the line of flight is perpendicular to the outstretched arm, the torque is the product of the force of impact and the length of the arm. Catching a fast ball with the arm extended can put a tremendous strain on the shoulder joint, as well as endanger the bones of the hands. To avoid injury the player should give by reaching somewhat forward for the ball and drawing the arm back at the moment of impact and by rotating the body and stepping back if the force is sufficiently great. If the elbow flexes slightly, the lever of the arm will be shortened and the torque reduced.

Another factor in avoiding injury when catching fast balls is the position of the hands. Beginners often reach with outstretched arms and point their fingers toward the approaching ball. This leads to many a "baseball finger." The fingers should be pointed either down or up, according to whether the ball is below or above waist level. Balls approaching at approximately waist level can be caught above the waist if the player bends the knees.

The second problem in receiving the impact of external objects, that of maintaining equilibrium, is often neglected. The receiver should prepare for it in advance, because a fast ball or a sudden blow can easily cause anyone caught off balance to lose equilibrium. The stance is of great importance here. The base of support needs to be widened in the direction of the ball's flight, thus making it possible for the catcher to shift the weight of the body from the forward to the rear foot at the moment of impact. This action not only increases the chances of maintaining equilibrium but also contributes to the gradual reduction of the ball's motion. Widening the stance in a direction at right angles to the flight of the approaching ball does little to increase the catcher's stability.

The third problem—that of receiving the ball or another object with accuracy and control—is perhaps the one given the most emphasis in game situations. As in the attempt to avoid injury, one of the key factors is the gradual loss of the object's kinetic energy. This reduces the danger of the ball's bouncing off the hands. Accurate vision, judgment, and positioning of the body are of vital importance. "Keeping the eye on the ball" is essential to judging its speed and direction, and hence to adjusting the position of the body. Thus accurate judgment depends on accurate vision, and accurate adjustment of the body depends on both of these, as well as on agility and smoothness of neuromuscular response. Together, these factors make up what is known as "hand–eye" and "foot–eye" coordination." To a certain extent this is innate, but it is also developed and improved by practice.

Intercepting a ball or a puck is another illustration of receiving impact. Ice hockey, field hockey, soccer, basketball, and football are all games in which a player tries to intercept a pass. The same principles that apply to catching apply to intercepting, but with this difference: Whereas in catching there is usually time to place oneself in a favorable position and to use one's arms, hands, or feet advantageously, in intercepting, one must take advantage of the opportunity when it comes. There is no time for preparation. The important principle to observe is to give with the hands, feet, or stick the moment that contact is made with the ball or puck in order to keep control of it; otherwise it is likely to bounce off.

In receiving both the impact of one's body and that of external objects, an important factor to be considered is the subsequent movement one expects to make. It may be the determining factor in deciding what stance to assume. For instance, if a run is anticipated, a forward–backward stance will be more favorable than a lateral one. Furthermore, it will be desirable to have the weight over the forward foot. If a catch is to be followed immediately by a throw, the movements used for giving may be blended into the preparatory movements of the throw. These are fine points that have much to do with the degree of one's skill in an activity.

A summary of the principles to observe in receiving impact, both that of one's own body and that of external objects, is presented in the next section, together with some representative applications of these principles.

PRINCIPLES IN RECEIVING IMPACT

Related to Avoiding Injury

1. *The more gradual the loss of momentum (or kinetic energy) of the moving body or object, the less the force exerted on the body.* In other words, increasing either the time or the distance used in stopping the motion will decrease the forces imparted in the deceleration. When landing from a jump, for instance, the performer should use eccentrically controlled flexion in the ankles, knees, and hips to increase both the time and the distance for losing momentum (figure 22.1). High jumpers and pole-vaulters often increase the time and distance even more through the use of thickly padded landing pits. Any amount of padding,

whether by fatty or muscle tissue such as in the buttocks, or artificial padding such as in shoe insoles, uniform padding, or on playing surfaces, helps reduce the forces of impact. If the hands and arms must be used in the landing, care must be taken to allow the joints to give into flexion to avoid injury.

Often in falling there is horizontal as well as vertical momentum to be absorbed. Using a roll or a series of rolls is an effective way to increase the time and distance over which this momentum is lost (figure 22.2). Rolls are commonly taught in the martial arts as falling techniques. If a roll is not possible, a few running or hopping steps may serve the same purpose.

When catching a ball or receiving a blow, giving with the impact will increase time and distance over which momentum is transferred to the body. In catching a ball, the performer gives by pulling the arms back toward the body at the moment of impact and, if necessary, shifting the weight backward or taking a backward step or two. The speed of the joint motion due to the momentum of the incoming object will be controlled by eccentric contraction of the antagonist muscles. If the ball is caught with only one hand, the arm should be allowed to

Figure 22.1   Landing from the running long jump. The momentum of the moving body is decreased through the controlled flexion at the ankles, knees, and hips and the "give" of the landing surface.
Courtesy of Northeastern University.

Figure 22.2   To avoid injury when landing from a jump or fall, the horizontal motion should be decreased gradually. An effective technique is the shoulder roll. The action is controlled by landing and rolling on the more heavily padded parts of the body.

move horizontally backward and the body should rotate. This catching motion may be adapted to serve as the preparatory phase in a subsequent throw. A similar giving action is used when absorbing blows to the head or body. Moving the body or body part in the same direction as the motion of the blow will decrease the force of the blow.

As in landing and falling, any padding that can be added to the catching or striking surface will aid in the gradual decrease in momentum, as well as increasing the area over which stress is absorbed. The gloves worn by softball and baseball players, boxers, and some karetekas (martial arts performers) all help to reduce impact forces (figure 22.3).

2. *The larger the area receiving the impact, the less will be the force per unit of surface area.* Falls in the martial arts often include slapping motions with the arms. The arm slap increases the surface area over which the fall is broken, thus reducing the force on any

given area. Turning during a fall in order to land on a broad area such as the back (with the head tucked), the thighs, and buttocks, or rocking onto the chest are all methods of increasing the surface area for impact.

3. Repeated impacts, such as in running, gymnastics, aerobic exercise classes, and other activities may lead to overuse injuries. Repeated impact landings should be "soft" whenever possible. Attention should also be given to the nature of the landing surface. Energy absorbing surfaces are preferable for repeated impacts.

Related to Maintaining and Regaining Equilibrium

4. *Other things being equal, the larger the base of support in the direction of the impetus, the greater will be the body's equilibrium.* In any jump or fall, the body's equilibrium is temporarily lost. To gain prompt control of the body upon landing, a favorable base of support can be established by adjusting the position of the feet prior to landing in such a way that they will provide an adequate base when the landing is made. This foot position should be such that it will facilitate equal distribution of the body weight over the two feet. If the force of the landing makes it difficult to establish an adequate base of support with the feet alone, one or both hands may be used to temporarily broaden this base long enough for equilibrium to be established. In any case, the larger dimension of the base of support should be parallel with the horizontal direction of movement. This is exemplified by the forward lengthening of the stride, which occurs almost automatically when one trips while running or walking.

When preparing to receive an external impetus, the base of support should be widened in the direction of the expected force. This can be applied to catching a heavy object, maintaining standing balance

Figure 22.3 Catching a baseball with the aid of a glove. The shock of impact is reduced because of the broad area of the glove and its thick padding.
Courtesy of Northeastern University.

Figure 22.4   Catching a medicine ball. The principles of stopping a heavy object are demonstrated. The feet are separated in the direction of the oncoming ball; the line of gravity is forward in preparation for catching the heavy ball; there is a gradual "give" in the joints of the arms and legs and a backward weight shift so that the momentum of the ball may be reduced gradually; the stability of the receiver is improved by lowering the center of gravity.

on a moving vehicle such as a train or bus, or receiving a push, pull, or blow (figure 22.4).

5. *At the moment of impact, the line of gravity should be centered above the base.* This position will provide maximum distance in any direction should it be necessary to adjust for any horizontal forces upon contact. To provide maximum distance for the establishment of balance after landing from a forceful horizontal movement, the line of gravity should be located close to the near edge of the base of support at the moment of landing. In the same way, the line of gravity

should be near the front edge of the base of support and the knees should be bent in preparation for receiving an object with large horizontal momentum. In this way, the horizontal distance over which the center of gravity can move and still stay over the base of support is maximal (figure 22.5).

Related to Accuracy and Control

6. *The more gradually the velocity of an external object is reduced, the less likely is the object to rebound when its impact is received.* All the methods suggested for avoiding injury and maintaining equilibrium when receiving the impact of external objects also apply to preventing rebound.

7. "*Keep the eye on the ball.*" Whether the object whose impact is about to be received is a ball, carton, or fist, keeping the eyes on it will enable one to judge its speed and direction and to respond accordingly. The tendency of some novices to shut the eyes should be corrected at the outset.

8. *Catching an external object with accuracy and control depends largely on the position of the catcher relative to the direction of the approaching object.* Putting oneself in the most favorable position possible is an essential objective for accurate catching. This precaution applies also to such everyday tasks as lifting a heavy suitcase or carton down from a high shelf, as well as to catching objects that are approaching more or less horizontally (figure 22.6). This is basic to the prevention of injury and the maintenance of equilibrium.

Figure 22.5   Stability in landing is increased by lowering the center of gravity and moving the line of gravity toward the front edge of the base of support.

a.   b.

Figure 22.6   Lifting a suitcase down from a high shelf: (a) inefficiently; (b) efficiently. In (b) the woman is prepared to take a step backward if necessary and to bring the suitcase down close in the front of her body. The base of support is widened in the direction of the force being received, and the center of gravity is located over the front edge of the base of support.

LABORATORY EXPERIENCES

In each of the following Laboratory Experiences (1–5), select the preferable method of executing the movement. Justify your selection by citing the anatomical and mechanical principles demonstrated, as well as those that are violated.

1. Jump from a low bench to the floor, landing on both feet.
   a. Landing with minimum give (stiff landing)—that is, with as little flexion at the ankles, knees, and hips as possible.
   b. Landing with maximum give (soft landing)—that is, allowing the ankles, knees, and hips to flex to a full squat position. The head should be kept erect.
   c. Landing as in b but looking down at the feet. Which method is preferable? Why?

2. Trip on the edge of a mat and fall forward, landing first on the knees, then on the hands.
   a. Keeping the arms rigid, elbows straight.
   b. Letting the elbows flex, arching the back, rocking down onto the abdomen and chest, with the head turned sideways.

3. Jump down from a table or gymnasium box, using the parachute landing technique—that is, landing on the toes with the feet together, bending the knees slightly and turning sideward, rolling onto the side of the leg, thigh, and hip, then onto the back of the shoulder, keeping the arms close in front of the chest and the head flexed forward.

4. Catch a medicine ball thrown straight toward your chest.
   a. With your arms rigidly outstretched.
   b. With your hands held close in front of your chest.
   c. With your arms outstretched at first but brought in toward your chest at the moment of impact.
   Which method is preferable? Why?

5. Receive a hard drive in field hockey, (a) with and (b) without giving with the stick. Compare the results of both as to control of the ball and sensation in the hands.

REFERENCES AND SELECTED READINGS

Dufek, J. S., and B. T. Bates. 1991. Biomechanical factors associated with injury during landing in jump sports. *Sports Medicine* 12:326–37.

Hay, J. G. 1989. *The biomechanics of sports techniques.* Englewood Cliffs, NJ: Prentice Hall.

Kirby, R., and J. A. Roberts. 1985. *Introductory biomechanics.* Ithaca, NY: Mouvement Publications.

Kreighbaum, E., and K. M. Barthels. 1995. *Biomechanics.* 4th ed. New York: Allyn & Bacon.

Kovacs, I., J. Thianyi, P. DeVita, L. Rácz, J. Barrier, and T. Hortobágyi. 1999. Foot placement modifies kinematics and kinetics during drop jumping. *Medicine and Science in Sports and Exercise* 31:708–16.

McGinnis, P. M. 1999. *Biomechanics of Sport and Exercise.* Champaign, IL: Human Kinetics.

McNitt-Gray, J. L. 1993. Kinetics of the lower extermities during drop landings from three heights. *Journal of Biomechanics* 26:1037–46.

McNitt-Gray, J. L., T. Yokoi, and C. Millward. 1993. Landing strategy adjustments made by female gymnasts in response to drop height and mat composition. *Journal of Applied Biomechanics* 9:173–90.

Schrier, E. W., and W. F. Allman, eds. 1987. *Newton at the bat.* New York: Scribner's.

Zhang, S. N., B. T. Bates, and J. S. Dufek. 2000. Contributions of lower extremity joints to energy dissipation during landings. *Medicine and Science in Sports and Exercise* 32:812–19.

INSTRUMENTATION FOR MOTION ANALYSIS

OUTLINE

- ***Instrumentation for Kinematic Analysis***
  Basic Photoinstrumentation
    Procedures
  Other Kinematic Instrumentation
- ***Instrumentation for Kinetic Analysis***
- ***Electromyography***
- ***Computer Models and Simulation***
- ***Using Quantitative Analysis***
  Optimization of Performance
  Injury Prevention
  Rehabilitation
- ***Summary***

OBJECTIVES

At the conclusion of this chapter, the student should be able to:

1. Identify and discuss instrumentation for the collection and analysis of kinematic data in human movement.
2. Identify and discuss instrumentation for the collection and analysis of kinetic data in human movement.
3. Discuss the limitations of biomechanical instrumentation.
4. Critically examine the research literature in the field of human movement with an understanding of the methodologies used.

The scholarly study of people in motion has interested scientists for centuries, and their contributions have established the foundation for the advances made in kinesiology and biomechanics research in the twentieth century. Methodology has progressed from exclusive dependence on observations by the naked eye to the use of sophisticated photographic and electronic equipment for analyzing and quantifying the anatomical and mechanical nature of human performance. Although the student in the undergraduate course in kinesiology is not expected to have much experience with using some of the more highly sophisticated equipment and methodology, much of the technology used in movement analysis is readily available. Because of this increased availability of analysis technology and the increased interest in undergraduate research, the student should be aware of the available instrumentation and more advanced approaches to movement analysis.

INSTRUMENTATION FOR KINEMATIC ANALYSIS

Kinematic data, or data that describe a motion, are collected with a variety of instruments ranging from still cameras through high-speed film and video to sophisticated motion-tracking systems. The primary purpose of all such instrumentation is to enable people to analyze motion beyond the capabilities of their own physical senses. The human eye, for instance, can take in information at a rate of only ten to twelve items per second. When you are looking at motions that take less than 1 second to complete, a great deal of the visual information is lost. By "freezing" sequential pieces of the movement artificially, it becomes possible to analyze any given movement pattern in detail, including those bits of information that may be lost to the human eye or quickly forgotten by the brain.

One of the simplest and least expensive forms of kinematic instrumentation is the still camera. Still cameras are useful in motion analysis when used with special adaptations. For example, if the camera shutter is left open during the filming, and the exposure is controlled by a flashing strobe light, multiple images on a single picture are the result (see figure 18.7). Another technique is to attach tiny light bulbs to the joints and extremities. When photographed in a dark room with an open shutter, the motion appears as a light streak and the nature of the movement pattern is revealed.

Similar results may also be obtained by attaching a motor drive to a camera, allowing for rapid film advancement and exposure. Simple forms of motor-driven cameras are available, whereas other cameras may require the addition of an external motor drive unit. Although simple still camera techniques are not commonly used in research today, they are still an inexpensive and effective tool for undergraduate study (figure 23.1).

For many years the most frequently used kinematic research instrument was the high-speed motion picture camera coupled with a stop-motion film analyzer. Cameras with speeds up to 500 frames per second and variable shutters provide an ample number of clear data points for analyzing the fastest of human motions. Cameras with speeds up to 20,000 frames per second are often used to study projectiles and impacts. Such a camera can freeze a bullet in flight or at impact and can photograph the lighting of a match as several dozen individual pictures.

The quantitative analysis of movement techniques recorded on high-speed processed film requires the use of some type of projector that permits single-frame projection so that measurements may be made of the image. The most efficient method of measurement is to digitize the data and feed them into a computer. The term digitize simply means that specific data points from each frame are input into the computer as pairs of x and y coordinates. The computer program then uses these coordinates to perform trigonometric functions similar to those presented in chapter 10, in order to arrive at measures of displacement, velocity, and acceleration.

a.   b.

c.   d.

Figure 23.1   Movement pictures using a motor-driven still camera.

Since the late 1980s most kinematic motion analyses have been done using video. Video analysis can be as simple and rough as tracing from a video monitor onto acetate film or as complex and sophisticated as automatic computerized digitizing. Videotape has the advantage of being much lower in cost than movie film and offering instant playback rather than waiting for film processing. It is now routine to interface the video playback unit directly with a computer. With this interface in place, the image may then be digitized from the monitor by a human operator or digitized directly by the computer if the subject has been marked with reflective or light-emitting markers. Video motion analysis instrumentation may be configured to produce either two-dimensional or three-dimensional analysis. Three-dimensional analysis techniques are more complex, requiring some form of synchronization between two or more cameras. Newer technology also makes use of the magnetic field imaging techniques used in virtual reality to produce a real-time (though not instantaneous) three-dimensional model of motion (figure 23.2).

Motion analysis systems are available in a range of prices, depending on the level of automation and the complexity of the system. For the movement specialist without access to the

Figure 23.2　Representation of a three-dimensional human form in motion as seen by a computer.

more costly automated computer systems, videotape can still be a valuable tool. When played with a high-quality playback system with single-frame advance capabilities, it is possible to see the motion being analyzed in much greater detail than the human eye can follow at normal speed (figure 23.3). It is also possible to do tracings on acetate film applied to the monitor, or to use a computer digitizing tablet. Advances in software have also made it possible to input a video image directly into a computer, either as a movie or by "grabbing" a single frame at a time. This capability makes motion analysis available to a much broader segment of the population of movement analysis professionals.

Basic Photoinstrumentation Procedures

In any consideration of kinematic motion analysis, some fundamental procedures must be followed regardless of the instrumentation that is to be used. Because the basic measurements in kinematics are time and displacement (both angular and linear), care must be taken to ensure maximum accuracy in these two measurements.

The measurement of time in most photographic instrumentation is based on the frame rate, or the rate at which images are photographed. In still photography this rate is controlled by the rate at which the light source is emitted (stroboscopic) or at which the motor drive operates. In cinematography and videography, frame rate is the rate at which the film moves through the camera. The typical home movie camera has a frame rate of 24 frames per second, home video a frame rate of 30 frames per second. High-speed movie cameras and video cameras can have frame rates as high as 20,000 frames per second. For the appropriate frame rate to be chosen, something must be known about the motion to be investigated. Walking at a normal pace can be adequately filmed at frame rates (often referred to as Hz) as low as 24 frames per second (24 Hz) without losing much data. The faster the motion, the faster the frame rate needs to be. Most human motion can be filmed at 60 to 100 Hz. If the analysis is to include an impact of some sort or the release of an object, frame rates need to be higher—from 300 to 500 Hz. Once frame rate has been established, the time elapsed between frames or the time over which displacement occurs is equal to the frame rate divided into 1 second. At a frame rate of 60 Hz, therefore, the frame time would be 1/60 of a second, or .017 seconds.

The second basic kinematic measure is displacement. To accurately measure displacement, there are two primary concerns. First, when working in two dimensions, care must be taken to place the camera in a position exactly perpendicular to the plane of the motion. If the camera is placed at an angle to the motion, parallax errors will occur.

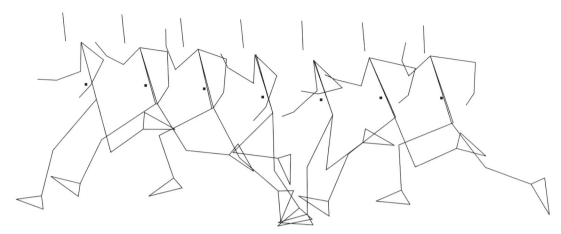

Figure 23.3   Computer-generated stick figure of running.

To see what a parallax error looks like, hold a pencil in front of you so that you are able to see its full length. Now rotate the point of the pencil slowly away from you. Note how the pencil seems to grow shorter. This foreshortening is due to parallax. Filming anywhere other than perpendicular to the plane of motion can produce similar effects that cause large errors in measures of displacement.

The second consideration in measuring displacement is to have some scale reference in the picture. It is necessary to have some way of relating the image size on film to real-life distances. A simple way to do this is to place a meter stick in the field of view of the camera in such a way that it is in the same plane as the motion and the same distance from the camera. This may be done by photographing the meter stick first, before the performance or at the end of the film. This scale reference could also be taped on a floor, a wall, a goal post, or some other surface. Any known length can be used (figure 23.4).

Once the scale reference has been photographed, it should be measured again on the image. This measurement is then divided into the real length of the scale reference to produce a conversion factor. For example, if the scale reference is actually 1 meter long but measures only 11 cm on the video or film image, the conversion factor would be 1/11 or .091. The conversion factor is a constant and has no units. This means that all linear measures (done in centimeters) taken from the film in this example need to be multiplied by .091 to give real-life displacements in meters. Scale references and conversion factors are not necessary for angular measurements. The angles viewed in any given frame remain constant regardless of image size.

When taking photos, movie film, or videotape for motion analysis, the camera must be absolutely level and still. A tripod and a carpenter's level are strongly recommended. It is also important to set the shutter speed of the camera as high as possible. The higher the shutter speed, the less time the shutter is open for each frame and the image recorded on the film is less likely to be blurred. There is a trade-off between shutter speed and light, however: The higher the shutter speed, the more light that is required.

To ensure that measures of displacement are made consistently from frame to frame, it is also advisable to mark the joints or parts of the body to be analyzed. A simple method for doing this is to use a felt tip marker or place adhesive tape crosses on the significant bony landmarks or joint centers. These markings need to be clearly visible on the film image throughout the motion.

Figure 23.4   A meter stick used as a scale reference.

Figure 18.6 shows several frames of film with the subject marked appropriately at the joints of interest. Usually, markers are placed to indicate proximal and distal end points of segments, or are placed as close to joint centers as is possible by palpation. Correct placement of markers helps ensure accuracy of measurement.

Optoelectronic systems

In many motion analysis systems, the cameras used do not record pictures but instead record the position of light sources. These optoelectronic devices require that the subject of the motion analysis be carefully marked with light-emitting diodes (LEDs) or some form of reflective marker (figure 23.5). The cameras are sensitive to these light sources and transmit their locations in space to a computer as a series of *x, y* coordinates. Kinematic calculations are done on the basis of changes in these coordinate locations. In this type of system the pictorial output usually takes the form of a stick figure or computer-generated model rather than an actual video picture. Most optoelectronic systems are used in laboratory settings rather than in field-based studies, because lighting must be very carefully controlled.

Three-Dimensional (3-D) Systems

Both photoinstrumentation systems and optoelectronic systems are commonly configured to collect data in three planes, or three-dimensional data. In order to conduct a three-dimensional analysis of motion it is necessary to have more than one camera. The simplest configuration for this analysis method is to position two cameras such that the two camera axes are close to perpendicular. Because kinematic calculations are based on both position and time, it is important that the two cameras' frame rates be carefully synchronized. This is usually done through a genlock mechanism connecting the two cameras. This "black box" locks the two cameras' operating systems together. In addition, the system must be calibrated in three dimensions. The simple meter stick calibration that was described above is not sufficient in this case. In most three-dimensional systems calibration is done using a cube or a multiarmed device. Reflective markers are placed on the calibration device at carefully measured points. These makers are then recorded by the system and their locations are input to the computer. The computer can then use these known locations to perform kinematic calculations.

Figure 23.5   Reflective markers are used with a number of optoelectronic data collection systems.

Each camera used in a three-dimensional analysis records marker positions in two dimensions only. Conversion of these data from two-dimensional data into three-dimensional data is done by combining data from all cameras mathematically. The process used for this conversion is usually one referred to as direct linear transformation (DLT). It is an advanced process that involves construction of a series of matrix equations which are then usually programmed into the computer of the motion analysis system.

Real-Time Systems

Motion tracking systems that operate in real time are becoming commonplace in biomechanics analysis. Although the primary use of these systems seems to be in the production of virtual reality simulations and video animation, biome-chanists also use motion tracking for complex three-dimensional analysis of motion. Real-time motion tracking systems are currently either light based or electromagnetic in nature. Light-based systems depend on a series of pulsed light markers attached to the subject. The light from these markers is detected by a sensor system. Each marker has a characteristic rapid pulse pattern that allows the sensing system to continuously identify each individual marker. Two-dimensional motion is tracked through marker displacement vertically and horizontally, whereas the third dimension of motion (distance from the sensors) is calculated instantaneously on the basis of the time required for the light signal to travel to the sensor.

Electromagnetic tracking devices, such as those used in virtual reality, usually consist of a set of electromagnetic transmitter/sensor pairs with one pair component attached to the body, the other to a computer. Signals from the moving body are transmitted to the computer for processing. Current systems can handle several dozen receiver points at once (although the larger the number of receivers being tracked, the slower the rate of data collection). The advantage of such systems is that the signal to the computer is not blocked by the motion of the extremities as often happens in film or videotape. These virtual reality systems show a great deal of promise for rapid and accurate collection of three-dimensional data.

Regardless of the nature of the transmitter/ sensor devices in real-time motion tracking, these systems are all capable of analyzing motion with six degrees of freedom. The term *degrees of freedom* refers to the number of unique directions in which a system can move. In human motion, six degrees of freedom account for motion in each of the three planes and around each of the three axes.

Many real-time, six degree of freedom systems are primarily used in laboratory settings, with subjects connected to computer and sensor system by cables. Some newer systems are using small, individual transmitters attached to the body, freeing subjects from cable systems. As technology in this area progresses, this system will become more accessible and more adaptable.

Figure 23.6   Elbow and wrist elgons on right arm; index finger and forearm elgons on left arm.
From M. J. Adrian, An Introduction to Electrogoniometry, *Kinesiology Review 1968*, copyright © 1968 American Association for Health, Physical Education and Recreation, Washington, DC.

The student of kinesiology in the next several years is quite likely to encounter one of these real-time motion tracking systems.

Excellent examples of kinematic data collection systems are easily found on the Internet. The student who wishes to view these systems, see examples of the analysis that can be done, or, in some instances, interact with sample data from such systems is advised to spend some time on-line perusing the large number of sites available. Refer to the introduction to Part III for a list of Internet sites to start the search.

Other Kinematic Instrumentation

Two other instruments sometimes used in kinematic measurement are the electrogoniometer, or elgon, and the accelerometer. The elgon is a double-arm goniometer (see p. 33) with a potentiometer for an axis (figure 23.6). A potentiometer, acting like a light dimmer switch, converts changes in angular displacement to changes in electrical current. These changes in electrical current may be recorded on an oscilloscope, a chart recorder, or a computer. An elgon recording provides no information concerning movement other than joint angle changes over time. Elgons can be constructed to measure movement in one or all three planes.

The accelerometer is an instrument that, when used singly, measures linear acceleration. These measurements are based on variations in electrical current in response to pressure changes, caused by the inertia of the accelerometer. The output from an accelerometer, like the elgon, may be recorded on an oscilloscope or a chart recorder or input into a computer. Accelerometers are most frequently used to study impact, where objects or limbs undergo rapid, high levels of acceleration.

Both accelerometers and elgons involve rigid, bulky items that must be attached to the body. Each also may involve wires leading to the output device or to a radio transmitter also worn on the body. Because of these necessary attachments, both forms of instrumentation may interfere with the performance of the movement skill. For this reason, accelerometers and elgons are most often used in laboratory situations for experimental research.

INSTRUMENTATION FOR KINETIC ANALYSIS

Kinetic data are usually collected through the use of dynamometers or force transducers. Dynamometers are primarily spring-and-cable tension instruments that measure static muscle strength, or strength in a single position. Examples of dynamometers are the grip-strength dynamometer and the leg-strength dynamometer.

Recently force transducers have been used more and more often in kinetic analysis. One example of a force transducer frequently used in kinetic studies is the strain gauge. In the strain gauge, altered resistance due to strain on the mechanism, which may be made of wire or a semiconductor substance, produces a change in

Figure 23.7   Force-sensing resistors (FSRs) and piezoelectric film used to collect force and pressure data.

is best to look at these data as being relative to some known measure, such as body weight.

Perhaps the most common use of force transducer technology in kinetic motion analysis is the force plate. This force, or pressure-sensing, instrument is placed in the floor, ground, or wall so that ground reaction forces may be recorded in all six possible modes (vertical, two horizontal, and about each of the three axes) while walking, running, jumping, landing, or making any of a vast number of movements. As the foot or any other body part lands on the platform, linear forces and torques acting at the point of impact are identified through output, usually to a computer system (figure 23.8). From data generated in this manner, especially when combined with kinematic data, a mathematical process referred to as inverse dynamics may often be used to calculate the joint torques that are acting throughout the motion.

ELECTROMYOGRAPHY

Most studies that have been done to determine muscle action during any given movement have been done using electromyography. In electromyography (EMG), the electrical activity generated by the differences in action potential between two sites on the same muscle is measured through the use of electrodes, which are sensitive to changes in electrical current. These electrodes may be small metallic plates attached to the skin, or they may be indwelling needle or fine wire electrodes (see figure 3.13). The action potentials from the muscles are sensed by these electrodes, and the signal that is generated is amplified and transmitted to some form of processing and recording device such as an oscilloscope, a paper recorder, or a computer. An analysis of the recorded EMG signal can then provide information on the intensity of muscle contraction and the temporal and sequential order of muscle activation. Such information can provide great insight into the muscular demands of specific activities. Figure 23.9 is a sample of the EMG data recorded by a paper trace recorder.

output voltage, which may then be recorded by an output device. Strain gauges can be manufactured to fit almost any analysis situation. Strain gauge systems have been fabricated to measure forces on uneven parallel bars, impact on a tennis racket, the strain in a hammer throw chain, and many other applications. Strain gauges or piezoelectric force transducers (which respond to pressure) have been used extensively in gait analysis. The small transducers are placed at strategic points on the sole of the foot, and the force present during gait is measured.

Two types of adaptable pressure-sensing materials that are used in kinetic analysis are piezoelectric film and force-sensing resistors (FSRs). Both sensors come in a variety of sizes and configurations and can easily be adapted to a variety of movement problems (figure 23.7). Each is also easily connected to a computer containing an analog-to-digital converter. This type of technology is highly affordable and easy to work with. For this reason the student is cautioned to carefully examine data produced by these devices. Both piezoelectric film and FSRs are difficult to calibrate. It

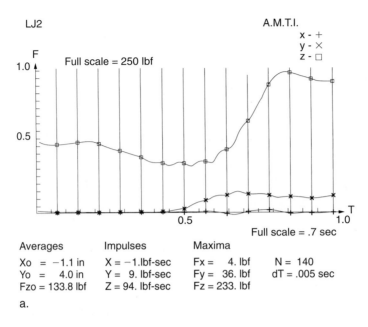

LJ2

A.M.T.I.

x - +
y - ×
z - □

F
1.0

Full scale = 250 lbf

0.5

T

0.5   1.0

Full scale = .7 sec

Averages	Impulses	Maxima	
Xo = −1.1 in	X = −1.lbf-sec	Fx = 4. lbf	N = 140
Yo = 4.0 in	Y = 9. lbf-sec	Fy = 36. lbf	dT = .005 sec
Fzo = 133.8 lbf	Z = 94. lbf-sec	Fz = 233. lbf	

a.

Full scale = 250 lbf

b.

Figure 23.8   Force-time data collected by a force plate and computer: (a) force-time history of the takeoff in a standing long jump; (b) force vector diagram of the same jump.

Although EMG is an excellent tool for determining the existence of muscle activity at any given point in time, the recorded data are simply indicative of action potential. EMG data provide no information concerning the type of muscular contraction (static, concentric, or eccentric) or the force produced by the muscle contraction. The primary purpose of EMG for the movement spe-

cialist is to identify and verify the presence or absence of muscle activity in a given muscle at a given point in time.

Some quantitative analysis of EMG signals is done by "normalizing" the EMG output. This technique involves the transformation of the EMG signal during activity to a percentage of the signal recorded for a maximum voluntary con-

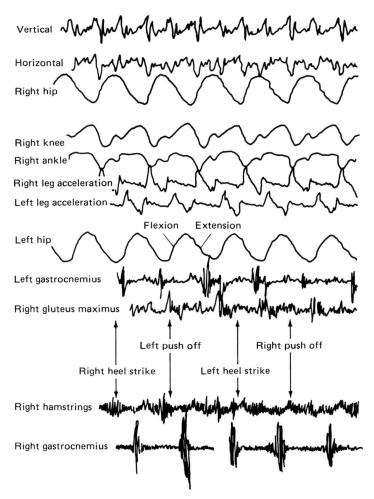

Figure 23.9   EMG trace of muscles of the legs during walking.

traction of the muscle being investigated. This normalizing technique is often used to compare the changes that occur in muscle activity with changes in activity conditions such as load, muscle angle of pull, joint angle, movement speed, and fatigue. The student is cautioned, however, to remember that many factors can affect EMG output, and conclusions based on EMG results should be carefully examined.

COMPUTER MODELS AND SIMULATION

Kinematic, kinetic, and electromyographic data about human motion are often compiled and synthesized into sets of equations that describe the motion mathematically. These sets of equations are referred to as mathematical models or, more frequently, as computer models. A computer

Figure 23.10 Computer model of the human body represented as a series of segmental levers.

model is a mathematical description of the body in motion compiled into a computer program. Often these equations are used to produce a graphic representation of motion. Figures 23.3 and 23.10 are examples of the graphic representations of computer models.

When a computer model is manipulated experimentally by changing the value of the variables, the result is a computer simulation. Computer simulations allow for the exploration of the limitations and capacities of human movement systems without endangering human subjects. The values for the variables one wishes to test are entered into the computer program, and the computer simulates the desired motion using the given values. As an example, several angles of takeoff may be simulated for the long jump without the necessity of using an actual jumper. These simulations may be done quickly and optimal performance predicted once an accurate computer

model has been designed. Computer simulations have been used to predict limits to human performance that are even now being challenged by athletes. Figure 23.11 illustrates a simple computer simulation.

One of the more forbidding challenges in the work of computer modeling and simulation of human movement is to represent accurately the complexity of the human body in the model. When one considers the makeup of the human system, with all the possible combinations of joint and muscle, the task seems overwhelming. Most computer models, therefore, use greatly simplified representations of the various biological components of any given motion. An example of this is the way in which muscle action is frequently simulated. When analyzing closely the action of a given muscle, one must consider not only the contractile element of the muscle but also the elastic components. A simplified model of muscle might be somewhat like that depicted in figure 23.12, consisting of a contractile element, a series elastic component, and a parallel elastic component. Each of these components must then be assigned a value based on the researcher's knowledge of the body. This simple muscle model then gains rapidly in complexity if it is applied to each of the muscles that might be active in a given motion. For this reason, computer simulations often vary greatly from what one might expect from actual human performance. Still, they provide the movement specialist with increased knowledge about the movement potential of the human body.

In the very near future, it is likely that software for simulating various human movements will become readily available. However, one must remember that the computer simulation, although useful, cannot yet completely model human neurology, physiology, or psychology. Regardless of the complexity of the model used to produce a computer simulation, such simulations are still simplifications of actual motion.

Figure 23.11   Computer simulation of unweighting skis through fast flexion and extension.

PE = parallel elastic component
SE = series elastic component
CE = contractile element

Figure 23.12   A simplified model of the contractile properties of muscles, as represented in a computer-generated model of human movement.

USING QUANTITATIVE ANALYSIS

As the task of collecting data on human movement becomes easier and more automated, there is a risk of producing such data for their own sake, with no thought toward application. When one sets out to collect movement data, there should be some clear purpose in mind. It is the purpose of the analysis that will determine the type of data that need to be collected and the methodology and instrumentation to be used. A sound plan is to base the collection of biomechanical data on a carefully designed analysis plan, using a model such as that introduced and used throughout this text. The analysis that one undertakes should be aimed toward some end result.

In the various fields that deal with human movement there are several purposes to which the collection of movement analysis data might be directed. Examples of the purposes for performing a movement analysis include such things as the optimization of performance, the prevention of injuries, and rehabilitation.

Optimization of Performance

Often, when considering the efficiency and effectiveness of performance, the maximum is not the most desirable. For instance, in shooting free throws, the basketball player who applies maximum force is more than likely to overshoot the target, resulting in a missed shot. The long jumper who generates maximum horizontal velocity may have trouble converting to a vertical velocity. The computer operator who types at the fastest possible speed may find many errors. In instances such as these and countless others, what is needed is an *optimum* performance. Optimal performance implies that all the factors which make up the motion are combined in such a way as to produce the most effective result. The optimization of human performance has been the goal of much of the quantitative biomechanical analysis that has been done.

Quantitative biomechanical data are useful in the process of optimizing performance in that they provide a mathematical description of the relationships between various factors that comprise the performance. As an example, it is well known that running speed depends on the combination of stride length and stride frequency. At first glance it would seem that producing the longest stride length of which an individual is capable and taking these strides as fast as possible would generate the fastest running speed. In actuality, there is a point where increased stride length simply adds to the braking force of the stride by producing too much horizontal force in the wrong direction. It is possible, through kinematic motion analysis and force plate studies, to determine the stride length at which the individual produces the greatest pos-

sible impulse in the desired direction. This, then, becomes the optimum stride length. Once this stride length is mastered, further increments in running speed will be due to increases in stride frequency. Stride frequency might be enhanced by examining the quantitative data on the angular velocities that are generated as the swing leg is brought forward on each step. As will be remembered from earlier chapters, the velocity of the swing leg can often be improved by decreasing the moment of inertia of the lower extremity through greater hip and knee flexion. Thus, the running stride has been optimized to produce the best possible performance for that individual runner.

Injury Prevention

Injuries are often the result of forces applied to the body in excessive or inappropriate ways. Torques that are too great in magnitude or that are applied in the wrong direction, high acceleration forces, impact, and sudden forceful stretch can all produce injuries. Quantitative data collection can provide valuable information about the risk of injury in any movement. Most people are now familiar with the impact studies that have been done by the automobile industry. By using heavily instrumented "crash test dummies" to quantify the force acting on the human body during an automobile accident, newer and more effective safety devices have been developed. The same sort of studies have been done on football and bicycle helmets, playing surfaces, mats and landing pads, and a variety of other impact surfaces. Data have been collected on the forces transmitted to the body in a variety of movement activities, including walking, running, and jumping. It has been found, for instance, that walking down stairs produces 2.5 times the load on the body that level walking does. Running and jumping can impose loads as high as seven or eight times body weight (Loy and Voloshin 1991).

One area that has long been of concern in injury prevention is the study and modification of load-lifting techniques. Researchers in ergonomics (the study of work) have gathered data not only on the forces generated by lifting various loads but also on the limitations of the structures doing the lifting. A number of studies have been done to establish the loads at which the various structures of the vertebral column begin to fail. These data have been used to build general models of safe load limits and safe lifting practices.

Rehabilitation

A large amount of the work that has been done in quantitative gait analysis, electromyography, and load handling has been done by researchers in the rehabilitation field. Immediately following World War II, many hospitals and clinics began studying gait in depth, hoping to produce a model of the "normal" gait in order to aid in efforts to rehabilitate wounded soldiers. From the early work by researchers such as Murray and coworkers (1964, 1970), Inman, and Ralston (Rose and Gamble 1994) came the bases for clinical rehabilitation work that is done today. In most therapeutic and rehabilitation settings, quantitative data are collected on patients on a regular basis. These data are then compared with the models of normal patterns, and from these comparisons, programs of rehabilitation and remediation are designed. The extent to which quantitative biomechanics has

been used in physical therapy and rehabilitation fills volumes in most university and clinic libraries. The reading of current rehabilitation research should become a habit for any student of human movement.

SUMMARY

This closing chapter has included a brief overview of some of the technology that is being used by those who work with human movement. As technology becomes more available, the use of once complex systems will become commonplace. Therefore, it is imperative that the student of human movement be comfortable with computer technology. As this book is being written, technology is spreading to larger and larger segments of the population. Physical therapists regularly use video-based gait analysis systems, computer-driven rehabilitation devices, and computer-based treatment plans. Teachers are using computer technology to work with physical education students throughout the school years. Middle school students are using videotape to examine their own performances. With sophisticated technology available to a large segment of the population, movement professionals are obligated to examine and search constantly for ways to use technology to further the work they do.

REFERENCES AND SELECTED READINGS

Adrian, M., and J. M. Cooper. 1994. *Biomechanics of human movement.* 2nd ed. Dubuque, IA: Wm. C. Brown Communications.

Bauer, W. L. 1987. Physical models in sports biomechanics. In *Medicine and sport science: Current research in sports biomechanics,* edited by B. Van Gheluwe and J. Atha. Basel: Karger.

Dainty, D. A., and R. W. Norman. 1987. *Standardizing biomechanical testing in sport.* Champaign, IL: Human Kinetics.

Delp, D., and S. Delp. 1989. Understanding human movement with computer graphics. *Soma* 3(3):17–25.

De Luca, C. J. 1997. The use of surface electromyography in biomechanics. *Journal of Applied Biomechanics.* 13:135–63.

Erdman, A. G., E. D. Rekow, M. Hartfel, and M. Chin. 1986. The tools of biokinematics. *Soma* 1(1):30–38.

Frederick, E. C. 1986. In search of the asymptote: Projecting the limits of human performance. *International Journal of Sport Biomechanics* 2:1–5.

Gowitzke, B. A. 1984. Muscles alive in sport. In *Biomechanics: The 1984 Olympic Scientific Congress Proceedings,* edited by M. Adrian and H. Deutsch. Eugene, OR: Microform Publications.

Loy, D. J., and A. S. Voloshin. 1991. Biomechanics of stair walking and jumping. *Journal of Sports Sciences* 9:137–49.

Murray, M. P., A. B. Drought, and R. C. Kory. 1964. Walking patterns of normal men. *Journal of Bone and Joint Surgery* 46A:335–60.

Murray, M. P., R. C. Kory, and S. B. Sepic. 1970. Walking patterns of normal women. *Archive of Physical Medicine Rehabilitation* 51:637–50.

Rose, J., and J. G. Gamble. 1994. *Human walking.* Baltimore: Williams & Wilkins.

Vaughn, C. L. 1984. Computer simulation of human motion in sports biomechanics. *Exercise and Sport Sciences Reviews* 12:373–416.

Yeadon, M. R., and J. H. Challis. 1994. The future of performance-related sports biomechanics research. *Journal of Sports Sciences* 12:3–32.

Zatsiorsky, V. M., and V. L. Fortney. 1993. Sport biomechanics 2000. *Journal of Sports Sciences* 11:279–83.

Glossary

A

abduction   Movement of a segment in the frontal plane away from the midline of the body

acceleration   The rate at which velocity changes

adduction   Movement of a segment in the frontal plane toward the midline of the body

afferent neuron   Neuron that carries impulse toward the central nervous system; sensory neuron

agonist   Muscle primarily responsible for motion; prime mover

angle of attack   The angle between the long axis of a projected object and the direction of airflow

angle of incidence   The angle at which an object strikes a hard surface

angle of projection   The angle between the horizontal and the initial velocity vector of a projectile

angle of pull   The angle between the mechanical axis of bone and the line of pull of a muscle

angle of reflection   The angle at which an object will leave a hard surface after striking it

angular acceleration   The rate at which angular velocity changes

angular displacement   Any change in angle

angular impulse   A torque applied over some period of time

angular momentum   The quantity of angular motion a level possesses, equal to the product of the moment of inertia and the angular velocity

angular velocity   The rate at which angular displacement takes place

anteroposterior (AP) axis   The axis which passes horizontally from front to back, perpendicular to the frontal plane

Archimedes' principle   Law governing buoyancy, which states that a body immersed in water is buoyed up by a force equal to the weight of the fluid displaced by the body

B

backward tilt   Pelvic motion in which the posterior surface moves somewhat backward and downward

base of support   Any part of the body in contact with the supporting surface and the intervening area

Bernoulli's principle   Law governing fluid forces, which states that when flow velocity is high, fluid pressure is low, and when flow velocity is low, fluid pressure is high

bilateral axis   The axis which passes horizontally from side to side, perpendicular to the sagittal plane

biomechanics   The study of the mechanics of biological systems

boundary layer   A layer of fluid that is immediately adjacent to the surface of an object

buoyancy   An upward force that acts to support a body immersed in water

C

cardinal plane A primary plane, one that passes through the center of gravity

center of buoyancy That point in the body at which the upward force of buoyancy acts

center of gravity The "balance point" of the body; the center of mass; the intersection of the three cardinal planes

centrifugal force The "center-fleeing" force acting on an object undergoing circular motion; a reaction force to centripetal force

centripetal force The "center-seeking" force constraining an object to a circular path

coefficient of elasticity A number that represents the ability of a material to resist deformation and to return to its original state

coefficient of friction A number that represents the resistance to rolling or sliding motion that exists between any two surfaces

coefficient of restitution See **coefficient of elasticity**

compression Force that acts to press or compact

concentric muscle contraction Contraction in which the muscle fibers shorten

concurrent forces Forces acting at the same time and point of application but at different angles

conservation of angular momentum In the absence of any angular impulse, momentum remains constant

conservation of momentum In the absence of an impulse, momentum remains constant

curvilinear motion Motion that follows a curved path

D

deceleration The rate at which velocity decreases

density The amount of mass per unit of volume

diagonal planes Infinite number of planes of motion lying on the diagonal between the cardinal planes

displacement A vector quantity that reflects any change in position

distance A scalar quantity that reflects the amount of space moved

drag A fluid force that acts to resist motion

dynamics The study of objects or systems subject to acceleration

E

eccentric contraction A lengthening muscle contraction

eccentric force An "off-center" force, one that is not in line with the center of gravity or the axis and therefore tends to cause rotation

efferent neurons Neurons that carry impulses away from the central nervous system; motor neurons

effort arm (EA) The perpendicular distance between the applied effort force and the axis of a lever

elasticity The ability to resist deformation and to return to the original shape

energy The ability to do work, based on either position or motion

equilibrium A state of balance

extension The return from flexion

F

first-class lever One in which the effort and the resistance are on opposite sides of the axis

flexion A reduction in joint angle

force A push or a pull

force couple Parallel forces on either side of the axis acting in opposite directions

form drag Fluid resistance to forward motion based on the cross-sectional area of a body

free-body diagram A schematic representation of all the forces and levers that make up a defined system

friction A resistance to rolling or sliding, based on the nature of the two interacting surfaces

frontal plane Vertical plane passing through the body from side to side, dividing it into anterior and posterior halves

fulcrum An axis; the point about which rotation occurs

G

gravity An acceleration toward the center of the earth

ground reaction force Equal and opposite reaction produced by the supporting surface

H

horizontal abduction   Movement of a segment in the transverse plane away from the midline of the body

horizontal adduction   Movement of a segment in the transverse plane toward the midline of the body

I

impulse   The product of a force and the amount of time over which it is applied

inertia   A resistance to motion based on the mass of an object

K

kinematics   The "measurement of motion"; those variables that describe motion with respect to time

kinetic energy   Energy based on motion; a product of mass and velocity

kinetics   The study of the forces that act to produce motion

L

laminar flow   Smooth, unbroken fluid flow

law of reaction   The law of motion that states that for every action there will be an equal and opposite reaction

lever   A rigid bar that is fixed at a single point, about which it may be made to rotate

lift   A fluid force that acts in response to the pressure differential produced by differing flow velocities around an aerodynamic shape; acts perpendicular to fluid flow

line of gravity   A line that extends from the center of gravity of an object toward the center of the earth

linear forces   Forces applied in the same direction and along the same line of action

linear motion   Motion in a line, in which all parts of the object move in the same direction and at the same speed

M

Magnus effect   An explanation of the lift forces that cause a spinning object to curve in the direction of the spin

mass   The quantity of matter an object contains

mechanical advantage   The ratio of effort arm to resistance arm, or the ratio of resistance to effort in a lever

mechanical axis of bone   A line drawn from the proximal joint center to distal joint center

moment arm   The perpendicular distance from any force to an axis in a lever system

moment of inertia   The quantity of a rotating mass and its distribution around the axis of rotation

momentum   The amount of motion an object possesses; the product of mass and velocity

motor unit   A single motor neuron and all the muscle fibers it innervates

P

parallel forces   Forces that act parallel to each other; polar coordinates

potential energy   Energy based on the position of an object, usually its height from the surface

power   The rate at which work is done

principle of levers   For a lever to be in equilibrium, the clockwise torques must equal the counterclockwise torques; $E \times EA = R \times RA$

projectile   An object that is given some initial velocity and then is released

R

radian   A unit of angular measure, 57.3°

reciprocating motion   Repetitive motion

relative motion   Motion with respect to some reference object

resistance arm (RA)   Perpendicular distance between the resistance force vector and the axis of a lever

resultant   The combined effect of two or more vector quantities

rotary component   That vector component of force which acts perpendicular to a lever

S

sagittal plane   Vertical plane passing through the body from front to back, dividing it into right and left halves

scalar   A single quantity, measuring only amount

second-class lever   One in which the resistance is closer to the axis than is the effort

specific gravity   Ratio between the density of an object and that of water

speed   Scalar quantity quantifying the rate of motion

stability   The ability to remain in or return to a state of equilibrium

stabilizing component   That vector component of force which acts parallel to a lever

statics   The study of the mechanics of systems or objects in equilibrium

strain   The amount of deformation experienced by an object when stressed

stress   The force applied per unit of area

surface drag   Resistance to forward motion produced by the interaction of a fluid with a surface

T

tension   A form of stress that involves pulling forces

third-class lever   One in which the effort is closer to the axis than is the resistance

transverse plane   Horizontal plane that passes through the body, dividing it into upper and lower halves

torque   The tendency for rotation; turning effect

torsion   A form of stress that involves twisting

turbulence   Chaotic fluid motion at the trailing edge of a moving object

V

vector   A double quantity; one that specifies both magnitude and direction

velocity   A vector quantity describing the rate of displacement

vertical axis   The axis which is perpendicular to the ground

W

weight   The product of the mass of an object and the acceleration that is due to gravity

work   The product of a force and the distance over which that force produces motion

Classification of Joints and Their Movements

APPENDIX B

Type	Articulation	Movement
	Diarthrodial: Nonaxial	
	Shoulder girdle	
	Sternoclavicular	Limited motion of outer end of clavicle in all three planes
		Elevation–depression
		Forward-backward
		Rotation: forward-downward; backward-upward
	Acromioclavicular	Movements of scapula (including motion in both joints)
Irregular;		Elevation–depression
Arthrodial;		Rotation: upward-downward
Plane		Abduction–adduction
		Upward tilt—reduction of same
	Intercarpal	Slight gliding movements in cooperation with movements of wrist and metacarpals
	Intertarsal	Slight gliding movements in cooperation with movements of talonavicular and ankle joints
	Diarthrodial: Uniaxial	
	Elbow	
	Humeroulnar	Flexion–extension–hyperextension (slight)
	Knee	
	Tibiofemoral	Flexion–extension–hyperextension (slight)
Hinge;	Ankle	
Ginglymus	Talotibial and talofibular	Dorsiflexion—plantar flexion (extension)
	Fingers and thumb	Flexion–extension
	Interphalangeal	
	Toes	
	Interphalangeal	Flexion–extension

Type	Articulation	Movement
Pivot; Screw; Trochoid	Forearm Proximal and distal radioulnar Neck Atlantoaxial (first and second cervical)	Supination–pronation Rotation: right-left
Diarthrodial: Biaxial		
Condyloid; Ovoid; Ellipsoidal	Wrist Radiocarpal Fingers Metacarpophalangeal Toes Metatarsophalangeal Head Occipitoatlantal	Flexion–extension–hyperextension Abduction–adduction Flexion–extension Abduction–adduction Flexion–extension–hyperextension Abduction–adduction (limited) Flexion–extension–hyperextension Lateral flexion: right-left
Saddle; Seller; Reciprocal reception	Thumb Carpometacarpal	Flexion–extension–hyperextension Abduction–adduction Opposition (combination of abduction, hyperflexion, and possibly slight inward rotation)*
Diarthrodial: Triaxial		
Ball-and-socket; Enarthrodial	Shoulder Glenohumeral Hip Femoroacetabular	Flexion–extension–hyperextension Abduction–adduction Rotation: outward-inward Horizontal adduction (from abduction) Horizontal abduction (from flexion) Flexion-extension-hyperextension Abduction-adduction Rotation: outward-inward Horizontal adduction (from abduction) Horizontal abduction (from flexion)
Shallow ball-and-socket	Foot Talonavicular	Dorsiflexion—plantar flexion (very slight) Abduction–adduction (slight) Inversion–eversion (very slight)

Type	Articulation	Movement
Combination Diarthrodial Nonaxial and Fibrocartilaginous Synarthrodial		
Triaxial simulated ball-and-socket	Vertebral bodies Intervertebral cartilages	Flexion Extension Hyperextension
Nonaxial irregular	Vertebral arches	Lateral flexion: right-left Rotation: right-left

*Opinions differ with respect to inward rotation.

APPENDIX C

Figure C.1   Range of elbow joint motion: flexion–extension and hyperextension.

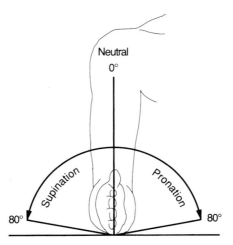

Figure C.2   Range of forearm motion: pronation and supination.

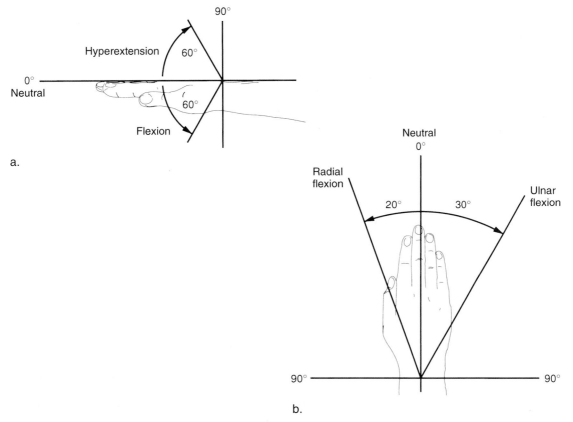

Figure C.3   Range of wrist joint movement: (a) flexion–extension and hyperextension; (b) radial and ulnar flexion.

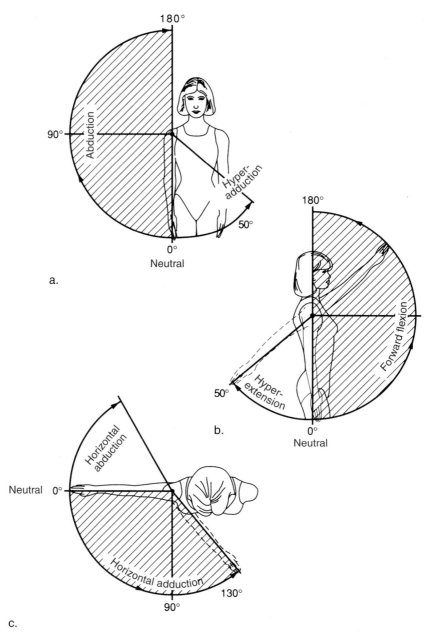

Figure C.4   Range of arm movement on trunk (involving both shoulder joint and shoulder girdle): (a) abduction and adduction; (b) flexion and hyperextension; (c) horizontal adduction and abduction.

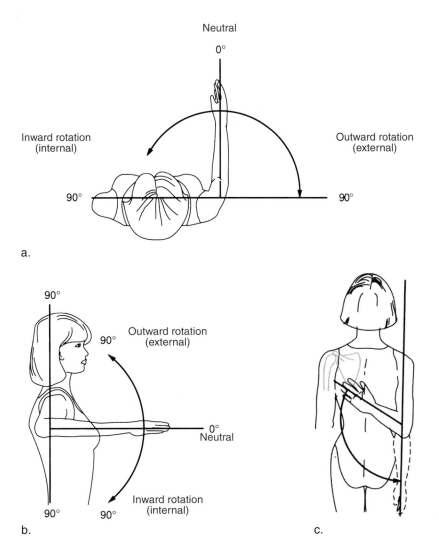

Figure C.5   Range of arm movement on trunk (involving both shoulder joint and shoulder girdle): (a) rotation with arm at side; (b) rotation with arm in abduction; (c) internal rotation posteriorly.

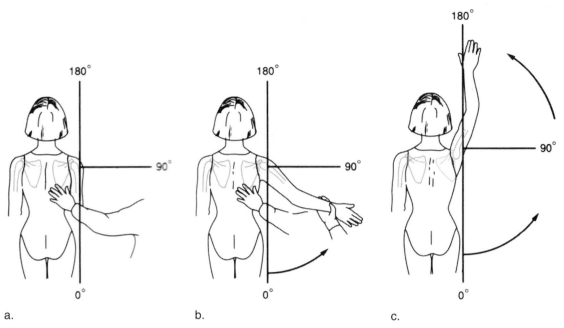

a.   b.   c.

Figure C.6   Range of shoulder joint (glenohumeral) motion: (a) starting position; (b) abduction; (c) sideward-upward elevation of arm (combining abduction of arm and upward rotation of scapula).

110°

0° Neutral

a.

120°

0° Neutral

b.

Figure C.7   Range of hip joint flexion: (a) starting position; (b) maximal flexion without rotating pelvis.

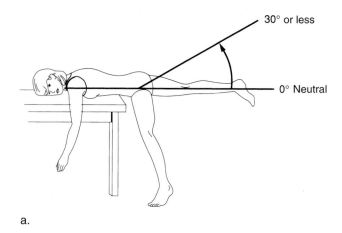

30° or less

0° Neutral

a.

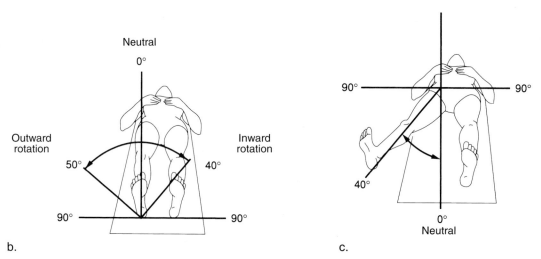

Neutral

0°

Outward
rotation

Inward
rotation

50°   40°

90°   90°

90° ———————— 90°

40°

0°
Neutral

b.   c.

Figure C.8   Range of hip joint movement: (a) hyperextension; (b) inward and outward rotation; (c) abduction.

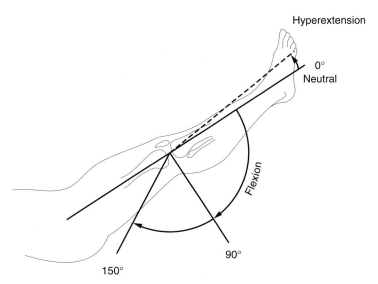

Figure C.9   Range of knee joint motion: flexion–extension and hyperextension.

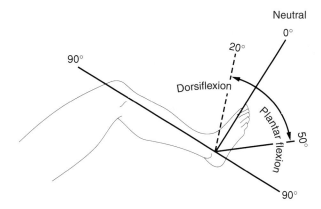

Figure C.10   Range of ankle joint dorsiflexion and plantar flexion with knee in flexed position.

a.

b.

Figure C.11   Range of motion in the thoracic and lumbar spine: (a) hyperextension; (b) lateral flexion.

APPENDIX D

The Upper Extremity*

Muscle	Proximal Attachments	Distal Attachments	Nerve Supply
		Shoulder Joint	
Coracobrachialis	Coracoid process of scapula	Inner surface of humerus opposite deltoid attachment	Musculocutaneous nerve
Deltoid	Anterior: anterior border of outer third of clavicle Middle: acromion process and outer end of clavicle Posterior: lower margin of spine of scapula	Lateral aspect of humerus, near midpoint	Axillary (circumflex) nerve
Infraspinatus and teres minor	Axillary border and posterior surface of scapula below scapular spine	Posterior aspect of greater tuberosity of humerus	Suprascapular and axillary nerves
Latissimus dorsi	Spinous processes of lower six thoracic and all lumbar vertebrae; posterior surface of sacrum; crest of ilium; lower three ribs	Anterior surface of humerus below head by flat tendon just anterior to, and parallel with, tendon of pectoralis major	Thoracodorsal (middle subscapular) nerve
Pectoralis major	Medial two thirds of clavicle; anterior surface of sternum; cartilages of first six ribs; slip from aponeurosis of external oblique abdominal muscle	Lateral surface of humerus just below head by flat tendon 2 to 3 inches wide	Medial and lateral anterior thoracic nerves
Subscapularis	Entire anterior surface of scapula	Lesser tuberosity of humerus	Subscapular nerve
Supraspinatus	Medial two-thirds of supraspinatus fossa above scapular spine	Top of greater tuberosity of humerus	Suprascapular nerve
Teres major	Posterior surface of inferior angle of scapula	Anterior surface of humerus below head, just medial to latissimus dorsi tendon	Lower subscapular nerve

*See chapters 5 and 6.

Shoulder Girdle

Muscle	Attachment	Nerve Supply
Coracobrachialis	Coracoid process of scapula	Inner surface of humerus opposite deltoid attachment	Musculocutaneous nerve
Levator scapulae	Transverse processes of first four cervical vertebrae	Vertebral border of scapula between medial angle and scapular spine	Dorsal scapular and branches from third and fourth cervical nerves
Pectoralis minor	Anterior surface of third, fourth, and fifth ribs near cartilages	Tip of coracoid processes of scapula	Medial anterior thoracic nerve
Rhomboids: major and minor	Spinous processes of seventh cervical and first five thoracic vertebrae	Vertebral border of scapula from spine to inferior angle	Dorsal scapular nerve
Serratus anterior	Outer surface of upper nine ribs at side of chest	Anterior surface of vertebral border and inferior angle of scapula	Long thoracic nerve
Trapezius	Occipital bone; ligamentum nuchae; spinous processes of seventh cervical and all thoracic vertebrae	Part I: posterior border of lateral third of clavicle; Part II: top of acromium process; Part III: upper border of scapular spine; Part IV: root of scapular spine	Spinal accessory and branches from third and fourth cervical nerves

Elbow and Forearm

Muscle	Attachment	Nerve Supply
Anconeus	Posterior surface of lateral epicondyle of humerus	Lateral side of olecranon process and posterior surface of upper part of ulna	Branch from radial nerve
Biceps brachii	Long head: upper margin of glenoid fossa; Short head: apex of coracoid process of scapula	Bicipital tuberosity of radius	Musculocutaneous nerve
Brachialis humerus	Anterior surface of lower half of	Anterior surface of coronoid process of ulna	Musculocutaneous and branch from radial nerves
Brachioradialis	Upper two-thirds of lateral supracondylar ridge of humerus	Lateral side of base of styloid process of radius	Radial nerve
Pronator teres	Medial epicondyle of humerus and medial side of coronoid process of ulna	Lateral surface of radius near middle	Medial nerve

The Upper Extremity (continued)

Muscle	Proximal Attachments	Distal Attachments	Nerve Supply
Pronator quadratus	Anterior surface of lower one-fourth of ulna	Anterior surface of lower one-fourth of radius	Branch from median nerve
Supinator	Lateral condyle of humerus; adjacent portion of ulna; radial collateral and annular ligaments	Lateral surface of upper third of radius	Branch from deep radial nerve
Triceps brachii	Long head: infraglenoid tuberosity Lateral head: posterior surface of upper half of humerus Medial head: posterior surface of lower two-thirds of humerus	Olecranon process of ulna	Radial nerve
Wrist			
Extensor carpi radialis brevis	Lateral condyle of humerus	Posterior surface of base of third metacarpal	Radial nerve
Extensor carpi radialis longus	Lateral epicondyle of humerus and supracondylar ridge above	Posterior surface of base of second metacarpal	Radial nerve
Extensor carpi ulnaris	By two heads from lateral epicondyle of humerus and middle third of posterior ridge of ulna	Posterior surface of base of fifth metacarpal	Deep radial nerve
Flexor carpi radialis	Medial epicondyle of humerus	Anterior surface of base of second metacarpal	Median nerve
Flexor carpi ulnaris	By two heads from medial condyle of humerus and medial border of olecranon process of ulna	Palmar surface of pisiform and hamate carpal bones, and base of fifth metacarpal	Ulnar nerve
Palmaris longus	Medial epicondyle of humerus	Transverse carpal ligament and palmar aponeurosis	Median nerve
Thumb and Fingers			
Abductor pollicis longus	Dorsolateral surface of ulna below anconeus, dorsal surface of radius near center, and intervening interosseous membrane	Lateral surface of base of first metacarpal	Deep radial nerve
Extensor digiti minimi	Proximal tendon of extensor digitorum	Fifth finger's extensor digitorum tendon	Deep radial nerve

Muscle	Attachment	Nerve Supply
Extensor digitorum	Lateral epicondyle of humerus	By four tendons, one to each finger, each tendon dividing into three slips, the middle one attaching to dorsal surface of second phalanx and the other two uniting to attach to dorsal surface of base of distal phalanx	Deep radial nerve
Extensor indicis	Dorsal surface of lower half of ulna	Index finger's extensor digitorum tendon	Deep radial nerve
Extensor pollicis brevis	Dorsal surface of radius below abductor pollicis longus	Dorsal surface of base of first phalanx	Deep radial nerve
Extensor pollicis longus	Dorsal surface of middle third of ulna	Dorsal surface of base of distal phalanx	Deep radial nerve
Flexor digitorum profundus	Upper two-thirds of anterior and medial surfaces of ulna	By four tendons (one to each finger) to base of distal phalanx, after passing through tendon of flexor digitorum superficialis	Interosseous branch of median nerve
Flexor digitorum superficialis	Humeroulnar head: medial epicondyle of humerus, ulnar collateral ligament, medial margin of coronoid process; Radial head: oblique line on anterior surface of radial shaft	By four tendons to the four fingers, each tendon splitting to attach to either side of base of middle phalanx	Median nerve
Flexor pollicis longus	Anterior surface of middle half of radius	Anterior surface of base of distal phalanx of thumb	Volar interosseous branch of median nerve
Abductor digiti minimi	Pisiform bone and tendon of flexor carpi ulnaris	Ulnar side of base of first phalanx of fifth finger and ulnar border of aponeurosis of extensor digiti minimi	Ulnar nerve
Abductor pollicis brevis	Anterior surface of transverse carpal ligament, greater multangular and navicular bones	Radial side of base of first phalanx of thumb	Median nerve
Adductor pollicis	Carpal (oblique) head: deep carpal ligaments, capitate bone, and bases of second and third metacarpals; Metacarpal (transverse) head: lower two-thirds of anterior surface of third metacarpal	Ulnar side of base of proximal phalanx of thumb	Deep palmar branch of ulnar nerve

The Upper Extremity (continued)

Muscle	Proximal Attachments	Distal Attachments	Nerve Supply
Flexor digiti minimi brevis	Hook of hamate bone and adjacent parts of transverse carpal ligament	Ulnar side of base of first phalanx of fifth finger	Palmar division of ulnar nerve
Flexor pollicis brevis	Superficial head: greater multangular bone and adjacent part of transverse carpal ligament	Superficial head: radial side of base of first phalanx of thumb	Median nerve
	Deep head: ulnar side of first metacarpal	Deep head: ulnar side of base of first phalanx of thumb	
Interossei dorsales	By two heads from adjacent sides of metacarpals in each interspace	Base of proximal phalanx and aponeurosis of extensor muscles on each side of middle finger, on thumb side of index finger, and on ulnar side of fourth finger	Palmar branch of ulnar nerve
Interossei palmares	First: ulnar side of second metacarpal	First: ulnar side of base of first phalanx of index finger and expansion of extensor digitorum tendon	Ulnar nerve
	Second: radial side of fourth metacarpal	Second: radial side of base of first phalanx of fourth finger and expansion of extensor digitorum tendon	
	Third: radial side of fifth metacarpal	Third: radial side of base of first phalanx of fifth finger and expansion of extensor digitorum tendon	
Lumbricales	Tendons of flexor digitorum profundus in center of palm	Extensor aponeuroses on radial side of proximal phalanges	First and second: median nerve; third and fourth: ulnar nerve
Opponens digiti minimi	Hook of hamate bone and adjacent parts of transverse carpal ligament	Entire length of ulnar border of fifth metacarpal	Deep palmar branch of ulnar nerve
Opponens pollicis	Anterior surface of greater multangular bone and transverse carpal ligament	Entire radial border of anterior surface of first metacarpal	Median nerve

The Lower Extremity*

Muscle	Proximal Attachments	Distal Attachments	Nerve Supply
		Hip Joint	
Adductor brevis	Outer surface of body and inferior ramus of pubis	Line from lesser trochanter to linea aspera and upper fourth of linea aspera	Obturator and accessory obdurator nerves
Adductor longus	Anterior surface of pubis	Medial lip of middle half of linea aspera	Obturator nerve
Adductor magnus	Inferior rami of pubis and ischium and lateral border of inferior surface of ischial tuberosity	Linea aspera, medial supracondylar line, and adductor tubercle on medial condyle of femur	Obturator nerve
Biceps femoris, long head	Lower and medial impression on tuberosity of ischium	Lateral side of head of fibula and lateral condyle of tibia	Sciatic nerve
Gluteus maximus	Posterior gluteal line of ilium and adjacent portion of crest; posterior surface of lower part of sacrum and side of coccyx	Posterior surface of femur on ridge below greater trochanter; iliotibial tract of fascia lata	Inferior gluteal nerve
Gluteus medius	Posterior surface of ilium between crest, posterior gluteal line, and anterior gluteal line	Oblique ridge on lateral surface of greater trochanter	Superior gluteal nerve
Gluteus minimus	Posterior surface of ilium between anterior and inferior gluteal lines	Anterior border to greater trochanter	Superior gluteal nerve
Gracilis	Anterior aspect of lower half of symphysis pubis and upper half of pubic arch	Medial surface of tibia just below condyle	Obturator
Iliopsoas	Psoas major: sides of bodies and intervertebral cartilages of last thoracic and all lumbar vertebrae; front and lower borders of transverse processes of lumbar vertebrae Iliacus: anterior surface of ilium and base of sacrum	Both: lesser trochanter of femur and for a short distance below along medial border of shaft	Femoral nerve

*See chapters 7 and 8.

The Lower Extremity (*continued*)

Muscle	Proximal Attachments	Distal Attachments	Nerve Supply
Pectineus	Pectineal line between iliopectineal eminence and tubercle of pubis	Pectineal line of femur, between lesser trochanter and linea aspera	Femoral nerve
Rectus femoris	Anterior inferior iliac spine and groove above brim of acetabulum	Base of patella, as part of quadriceps femoris tendon; by means of patellar ligament it attaches to the tibial tuberosity	Femoral nerve
Sartorius	Anterior superior iliac spine and upper half of notch below it	Anterior and medial surface of tibia just below condyle	Femoral nerve
Semimembranosus	Upper and lateral impression on tuberosity of ischium	Horizontal groove on posterior surface of medial condyle of tibia	Sciatic nerve
Semitendinosus	Lower and medial impression on tuberosity of ischium with biceps femoris	Upper part of medial surface of shaft of tibia	Sciatic nerve
Six deep outward rotators	Outer and inner surfaces of sacrum and of pelvis in region of obturator foramen	Posterior and medial aspects of greater trochanter	Third, fourth, and fifth lumbar and first and second sacral nerves
Tensor fasciae latae	Anterior part of outer lip of iliac crest and outer surface of anterior superior iliac spine	Iliotibial tract of fascia lata on lateroanterior aspect of thigh, about one-third of the way down	Superior gluteal nerve
Knee Joint			
Biceps femoris	Long head: lower and medial impression on tuberosity of ischium Short head: lateral lip of linea aspera	Lateral side of head of fibula and lateral condyle of tibia	Sciatic nerve
Gracilis	See hip joint		
Popliteus	Lateral surface of lateral condyle of femur	Posterior surface of tibia, above popliteal line	Tibial nerve
Rectus femoris, sartorius, semimembranosus, semitendinosus	See hip joint		

Muscle	Origin	Insertion	Nerve Supply
The three vasti	V. lateralis: upper part of intertrochanteric line; anterior and lower borders of greater trochanter; lateral lip of gluteal tuberosity; upper half of linea aspera V. intermedius: anterior and lateral surface of upper two-thirds of shaft of femur V. medialis: lower half of intertrochanteric line; medial lip of linea aspera; upper part of medial supracondylar line	The tendons of the three vasti muscles unite with that of rectus femoris to form the quadriceps femoris tendon; this attaches to the base of the patella and, indirectly, by means of the patellar ligament, to the tuberosity of the tibia	Femoral nerve
Ankle Joint, Foot, and Toes			
Extensor digitorum longus	Lateral condyle of tibia and upper three-fourths of anterior surface of fibula	Dorsal surface of second and third phalanges of four lesser toes	Deep peroneal nerve
Extensor hallucis longus	Middle half of anterior surface of fibula	Dorsal surface of base of distal phalanx of hallux (great toe)	Deep peroneal nerve
Flexor digitorum longus	Posterior surface of middle three-fifths of tibia	Plantar surface of base of distal phalanx of each of the four lesser toes	Tibial nerve
Flexor hallucis longus	Posterior surface of lower two-thirds of fibula	Plantar surface of base of distal phalanx of hallux (great toe)	Tibial nerve
Gastrocnemius	Posterior surface of each femoral condyle and adjacent parts by two separate heads	Posterior surface by calcaneus by means of calcaneal tendon (tendon of Achilles)	Tibial nerve
Peroneus brevis	Lateral surface of lateral two-thirds of fibula	Tuberosity on lateral side of base of fifth metatarsal	Superficial peroneal nerve
Peroneus longus	Lateral condyle of tibia; lateral surface of head and upper two-thirds of fibula	Lateral margin of plantar surface of first cuneiform and base of first metatarsal	Superficial peroneal nerve

The Lower Extremity (continued)

Muscle	Proximal Attachments	Distal Attachments	Nerve Supply
Peroneus tertius	Anterior surface of lower third of fibula	Dorsal surface of base of fifth metatarsal	Deep peroneal nerve
Soleus	Posterior surface of head of fibula and upper two-thirds of shaft; popliteal line and medial border of middle third of tibia	Posterior surface of calcaneus by means of calcaneal tendon (tendon of Achilles)	Tibial nerve
Tibialis anterior	Lateral condyle and upper two-thirds of lateral surface of tibia	Plantar surface of base of first metatarsal and medial surface of first cuneiform	Deep peroneal nerve
Tibialis posterior	Posterior surface of upper two-thirds of tibia beginning at popliteal line; medial surface of upper two-thirds of fibula	Tuberosity of navicular bone with branches to sustentaculum tali of calcaneus, to three cuneiforms, to cuboid, and to bases of three middle metatarsal bones	Tibial nerve

The Spinal Column*

Muscle	Proximal Attachments	Distal Attachments	Nerve Supply
Deep posterior spinal muscles	Posterior surface of sacrum and posterior processes of all the vertebrae	Spinous and transverse processes and laminae of vertebrae slightly higher than lower attachments	Branches of spinal nerves for all but levatores costarum, which is innervated by intercostal and eighth cervical nerves
Erector spinae	Thoracolumbar fascia; posterior portions of lumbar, thoracic and lower cervical vertebrae; angles of ribs	Angles of ribs; posterior portions of cervical and thoracic vertebrae; mastoid process of temporal bone	Posterior branches of spinal nerves
Hyoid muscles	Suprahyoid: hyoid bone Infrahyoid: sternum, clavicle, and scapula	Temporal bone and mandible Hyoid bone	Facial, inferior alveolar, hypoglossi, and ansa hyperglossi
Levator scapula	See shoulder girdle		
Obliquus externus abdominis	Anterior half of crest of ilium; aponeurosis from ribs to crest of pubis	Lower border of lower eight ribs by tendinous slips that interdigitate with those of serratus anterior	Lower seven intercostal nerves and iliohypogastric nerves

*See chapter 9.

Muscle			Nerve Supply
Obliquus internus abdominis	Inguinal ligament; crest of ilium; thoracolumbar fascia	Anterior and middle fibers into crest of pubis, linea alba, and aponeurosis on front of body; posterior fibers, by three separate slips, into cartilages of lower three ribs	Lower three intercostal nerves, the iliohypogastric and the ilioinguinal nerves
Prevertebral muscles	Anterior surfaces of various parts of cervical vertebrae and of upper three thoracic vertebrae	Anterior portions of occipital bone and of cervical vertebrae	Cervical nerves
Psoas	See hip joint		
Quadratus lumborum	Crest of ilium and iliolumbar ligament	Lower border of twelfth rib and tips of transverse processes of upper four lumbar vertebrae	Branches from the upper three or four lumbar nerves
Rectus abdominis	Crest of pubis	Cartilages of fifth, sixth, and seventh ribs	Anterior branches of lower six intercostal nerves
Scalenes (three)	First two ribs	Transverse processes of cervical vertebrae	Branches from second to seventh cervical nerves inclusive
Semispinalis thoracis, cervicis, and capitis	Transverse processes of all thoracic and seventh cervical vertebrae; articular processes of lower four cervical vertebrae	Spinous process of upper four thoracic and lower five cervical vertebrae; occipital bone	Posterior branches of cervical and upper six thoracic nerves
Splenius capitis and cervicis	Lower half of ligamentum nuchae; spinous processes of seventh cervical and upper six thoracic vertebrae	Mastoid process of temporal bone and adjacent part of occipital bone; transverse processes of upper three cervical vertebrae	Branches from second, third, and fourth cervical nerves
Sternocleidomastoid	By two heads from top of sternum and medial third of clavicle	Mastoid process of temporal bone and adjacent portion of occipital bone	Accessory and branches from the second and third cervical nerves
Suboccipitals	Posterior portions of atlas and axis	Occipital bone and transverse process of atlas	Branches from the first two cervical nerves

Major Respiratory Muscles*

Muscle	Peripheral Attachment	Central Attachment	Nerve Supply
Diaphragm	Circumference of thoracic outlet	Central tendon, a cloverleaf-shaped aponeurosis	Phrenic nerve
	Upper Attachments	**Lower Attachments**	
Intercostales externi	Lower border of each rib but last	Upper border of rib immediately below	Branches from corresponding intercostal nerves
Intercostales interni	Inner surface and costal cartilage of each rib but last	Upper border of rib immediately below	Branches from corresponding intercostal nerves
Levatores costarum	Transverse processes of seventh cervical and upper eleven thoracic vertebrae	Upper eight: each to rib immediately below, between tubercle and angle. Lower four: by two bands each, one to rib immediately below and other to second rib below	Branches from corresponding intercostal nerves
Serratus posterior inferior	Lower borders of lower four ribs	Spinous processes and ligaments of lower two thoracic and upper two or three lumbar vertebrae	Branches from ninth, tenth, and eleventh intercostal nerves
Serratus posterior superior	Upper borders of second, third, fourth, and fifth ribs	Spinous processes and ligaments of lower two or three cervical and upper two thoracic vertebrae	Branches from the first four intercostal nerves
Transversus abdominis	Linea alba and crest of pubis	Inguinal ligament, crest of ilium, thoracolumbar fascia, and cartilages of lower six ribs	Branches of lower six intercostal nerves, iliohypogastric, and ilioinguinal nerves
Transversus thoracis	Lower half of inner surface of sternum and adjoining costal cartilages	Lower borders and inner surfaces of costal cartilages of second, third, fourth, fifth, and sixth ribs	Branches from upper six thoracic intercostal nerves

Additional Muscles That Participate in Respiration

Muscles of shoulder joint or shoulder girdle
Pectoralis major
Pectoralis minor
Trapezius I and II

Muscles of the spinal column
Quadratus lumborum
Scalenes: anterior, posterior, medialis
Sternocleidomastoid

Mathematics Review

1. **Order of Arithmetic Operations**

   Certain arithmetic operations take precedence over others. In completing problems with a series of operations the following guidelines apply:

   a. Addition or subtraction may occur in any order.

   Example: $4 + 8 - 7 + 3 = 8$ or
   $8 + 3 + 4 - 7 = 8$

   b. Multiplication or division must be completed before addition or subtraction.

   Example: $48 \div 6 + 2 = 10$

   Example: $4 + (2/3)(1/2) = 4\ 1/3$

   c. Any quantity above a division line, under a division line or a radical sign ($\sqrt{}$), or within parentheses or brackets must be treated as one number.

   Example: $\sqrt{36 - 25} = \sqrt{11}$

   Example: $2(5 + 3 - 4) = 8$

   Example: $\dfrac{9 + 2}{3} = \dfrac{11}{3}$

2. **Fractions, Decimals, and Percents**

   a. To add (or subtract) fractions, the denominator in each term must be the same. (Choose the lowest common denominator for each term. Multiply each term by the common denominator and then add [or subtract].)

   Example: $\dfrac{3}{4} + \dfrac{5}{3} = \dfrac{29}{12} = 2\dfrac{5}{12}$

   (lowest common denominator = 12)

   Solution:

   $$\frac{\left(\dfrac{3}{4} \times 12\right)}{12} + \frac{\left(\dfrac{5}{3} \times 12\right)}{12} = \frac{9}{12} + \frac{20}{12} = \frac{29}{12} = 2\frac{5}{12}$$

   Example: $\dfrac{cd}{x} + \dfrac{x}{c} = \dfrac{c^2 d + x^2}{xc}$

   (lowest common denominator = xc)

   Solution:

   $$\frac{\left(\dfrac{cd}{x} \cdot xc\right)}{xc} + \frac{\left(\dfrac{x}{c} \cdot xc\right)}{xc} = \frac{c^2 d}{xc} + \frac{x^2}{xc} = \frac{c^2 d + x^2}{xc}$$

   b. To multiply fractions, multiply the numerators by each other and the denominators by each other.

   Example: $\dfrac{3}{8} \cdot \dfrac{2}{3} = \dfrac{6}{24} = \dfrac{1}{4}$

   Example: $pq\left(\dfrac{p}{q}\right) = \dfrac{p^2}{q} = p^2$

c. To divide fractions, invert the divisor and multiply.

Example: $\dfrac{3}{8} \div \dfrac{9}{2} = \dfrac{3}{8} \times \dfrac{2}{9} = \dfrac{6}{72} = \dfrac{1}{12}$

Example: $\dfrac{n}{r} \div \dfrac{s}{t} = \dfrac{n}{r} \times \dfrac{t}{s} = \dfrac{nt}{rs}$

Example: $\left(\dfrac{1}{a} + \dfrac{1}{b}\right) \div \left(\dfrac{1}{a} - \dfrac{1}{b}\right)$

$\qquad = \dfrac{b+a}{\cancel{ab}} \cdot \dfrac{\cancel{ab}}{b-a} = \dfrac{b+a}{b-a}$

d. To convert a fraction to a percentage divide the numerator by the denominator and multiply by 100.

Example: $\dfrac{3}{8} = .375 \times 100 = 37.5\%$

Note: To convert a percentage to a decimal move the decimal point two places to the left.

e. When *dividing* by a decimal divide by the integer and add sufficient zeros to move the decimal point the appropriate number of digits to the *right*.

Example: $36 \div .04 = 900$ or

$\qquad 36 \div 4 = 9$ plus $00 = 900$

(appropriate number of digits to right = 2)
When *multiplying* by a decimal multiply the integer and add enough zeros to move the decimal point the appropriate number of digits to the *left*.

Example: $6 \times .012 = .072$ or

$\qquad 6 \times 12 = 72$ plus 0 to left .072

(appropriate number of digits to left = 3)

f. Decimals may be expressed as positive or negative powers of 10:

$$10^0 = 1$$
$$10^1 = 10$$
$$10^2 = 100$$
$$10^3 = 1000$$

Example: $5624 = 56.24 \times 10^2$
$\qquad\qquad = 5.624 \times 10^3$
$\qquad\qquad = .5624 \times 10^4$

$$10^{-1} = 0.1$$
$$10^{-2} = 0.01$$
$$10^{-3} = 0.001$$
$$10^{-4} = 0.0001$$

Example: $.0379 = 3.79 \times 10^{-2}$
$\qquad\qquad = 37.9 \times 10^{-3}$
$\qquad\qquad = 379 \times 10^{-4}$

3. **Proportions, Formulas, and Equations**
The location of values in proportions, equations, or formulas may be shifted provided that whatever addition, subtraction, multiplication, or division is performed on one side of the equation is also performed on the other side.

Example: $\dfrac{a}{b} = \dfrac{c}{d}$

Solve for d: $d \cdot \dfrac{a}{b} = \dfrac{c}{\cancel{d}} \cdot \cancel{d}$

$\qquad d \cdot \dfrac{\cancel{a}}{\cancel{b}} \cdot \dfrac{\cancel{b}}{\cancel{a}} = c \cdot \dfrac{b}{a}$

$\qquad\qquad d = c \cdot \dfrac{b}{a}$

Example: $v^2 = u^2 + 2as$

Solve for s: $2as = v^2 - u^2$

$\qquad\qquad s = \dfrac{v^2 - u^2}{2a}$

4. **Right Triangles and Trigonometric Equations**

a. In a right triangle one angle always equals 90°. The other two angles will always be acute angles and the sum of these two angles will be 90° since the sum of the angles in any triangle is 180°.

b. In a right triangle the *sides* are related to each other so that the square of the longest side or *hypotenuse* (c) is equal to the sum of the squares of the two sides: $c^2 = a^2 + b^2$. This is the Pythagorean theorem.

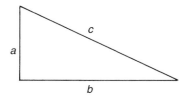

c. In triangle *ABC,* side *a* is called the side opposite angle *A,* side *b* is opposite angle *B,* and the hypotenuse, *c,* is opposite the right angle. Side *b* is named the side *adjacent* to angle *A* and side *a* is the side adjacent to angle *B.*

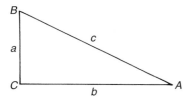

d. *Trigonometric functions* are ratios between the sides of a right triangle and are determined by the value of one of the acute angles. There are six trigonometric functions—the sine, cosine, tangent, cotangent, secant, and cosecant—but it will be necessary to consider only the first four here.

In △ *ABC* the ratio between the side opposite one of the acute angles and the hypotenuse is called the *sine* of the angle. For angle *A* it would be written as

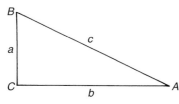

the sine $\angle A = \dfrac{a}{c}$, or $\sin A = \dfrac{a}{b}$;

the sine $\angle B = \dfrac{b}{c}$, or $\sin B = \dfrac{b}{c}$.

The *cosine* expresses the ratio between the side adjacent and the hypotenuse. For angle

A, $\cos A = \dfrac{b}{c}$; for angle B, $\cos B = \dfrac{a}{c}$.

The *tangent* and *cotangent* represent ratios between the two sides of the

triangle. For A, $\tan A = \dfrac{a}{b}$ and $\cot A$

$= \dfrac{b}{a}$; for angle B, $\tan B = \dfrac{b}{a}$ and $\cot B$

$= \dfrac{b}{a}$. A glance at these values shows

that $\sin A = \cos B$, and that $\tan A = \cot B$.

As can be seen from studying these ratios, two functions may have the same ratio. For instance, the $\sin A = \cos B$ and the $\tan A = \cot B$.

In general terms these trigonometric functions are expressed as follows:

$\sin \theta* = \dfrac{\text{side opposite}}{\text{hypotenuse}}$ or $\sin \theta = \dfrac{\text{opp}}{\text{hyp}}$

$\cos \theta = \dfrac{\text{side adjacent}}{\text{hypotenuse}}$ or $\cos \theta = \dfrac{\text{adj}}{\text{hyp}}$

$\tan \theta = \dfrac{\text{side opposite}}{\text{side adjacent}}$ or $\tan \theta = \dfrac{\text{opp}}{\text{adj}}$

$\cot \theta = \dfrac{\text{side adjacent}}{\text{side opposite}}$ or $\cot \theta = \dfrac{\text{adj}}{\text{opp}}$

e. Values of trigonometric functions may be obtained from tables of trigonometric functions (see appendix F) or from handheld calculators with trigonometric function capability.
   Example: $\sin 60° = .8660$
   $\cos 30° = .8660$
   $\tan 22° = .4040$
   $\cot 68° = .4040$

*θ (Greek letter, *theta*) is the symbol for angle.

Tables of trigonometric functions usually go up to 90°. Angles greater than 90° may be handled as follows:

(1) Functions of angles greater than 90° but less than 180° are the same as functions of an angle equal to 180° minus the angle in question. All functions of angles in this range are negative except the sine.
Example: sin 120° = sin 60°
tan 150° = – tan 30°

(2) Functions of angles greater than 180° but less than 270° are the same as functions of an angle equal to 270° minus the angle in question. Functions of angles in this range are negative except for the tan and cot.
Example: cos 220° = – cos 50°
tan 195° = tan 75°

(3) Functions of angles greater than 270° but less than 360° are the same as functions of an angle equal to 360° minus the angle in question. All functions of angles in this range are negative except the cosine.
Example: cot 300° = – cot 60°
sin 330° = – sin 30°

f. Through the use of trigonometric functions, it is possible to determine the values of all components of a triangle when the values of *one side and one angle* or the values of *two sides* are known.
Example 1: In triangle *ABC*, angle $A = 25°$ and the length of the hypotenuse is 15 m. Find the length of the other two sides.

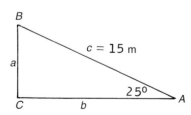

Solution:

(1) $\sin 25° = \dfrac{a}{c} = \dfrac{a}{15}$

$a = 15 \sin 25°$

$a = (15)(.4226)$

$\boxed{a = 6.34 \text{ m}}$

(2) $\cos 25° = \dfrac{b}{c} = \dfrac{b}{15}$

$b = 15 \cos 25°$

$b = (15)(.9063)$

$\boxed{b = 13.59 \text{ m}}$

Example 2: In triangle *ABC* the lengths of the sides are 3 cm and 5 cm. What is the length of the hypotenuse and the size of both acute angles?

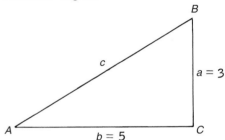

Solution:

(1) $\tan A = \dfrac{a}{b} = \dfrac{3}{5}$

$A = \arctan .600$

(i.e., *A* = angle whose tan is .600)

$\boxed{A = 31°}$

(2) $B = 90 - A;\ \boxed{B = 59°}$

(3) $\sin A = \dfrac{a}{c} = \dfrac{3}{c}$

$C = \dfrac{3}{\sin A} = \dfrac{3}{\sin 31°}$

$C = \dfrac{3}{.5150} = \boxed{5.83 \text{ cm}}$

Note: C may also be found using the Pythagorean theorem: $C^2 = a^2 + b^2$

5. Geometry of Circles

a. The circumference of a circle is calculated using the formula $C = 2\pi r$, where C is the circumference, r is the radius, and π (pi) is a constant value of 3.1416. Pi is the ratio that exists between the diameter of a circle and its circumference.

b. In making one complete turn about a circle the radius goes through one revolution, 360° or 2π radians. A radian is the angle subtended by an arc of a circle equal in length to the radius. One radian equals $\dfrac{360°}{2\pi}$ or 57.3°. Some equivalents for these angular units of measure are as follows:

Revolutions	Radians			Degrees
1	2π	or	6.28	360°
0.5	1π	or	3.14	180°
0.25	0.5π	or	1.57	90°
2	4π	or	12.56	720°

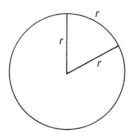

(1) To convert degrees to revolutions divide by 360.
  Example: 1260° = 3.50 rev
(2) To convert radians to revolutions divide by 6.28.
  Example: 15.75 radians = 2.51 rev
(3) To convert degrees to radians divide by 57.3.
  Example: 360° = 6.28 radians
(4) To convert revolutions to radians multiply by 6.28.
  Example: 2.3 rev = 14.44 radians
(5) To convert revolutions to degrees multiply by 360.
  Example: 2.3 rev = 828°
(6) To convert radians to degrees multiply by 57.3.
  Example: 7.6 radians = 435.5°

APPENDIX F

Degrees	Sines	Cosines	Tangents	Cotangents	
0	.0000	1.0000	.0000		90
1	.0175	.9998	.0175	57.290	89
2	.0349	.9994	.0349	28.636	88
3	.0523	.9986	.0524	19.081	87
4	.0698	.9976	.0699	14.301	86
5	.0872	.9962	.0875	11.430	85
6	.1045	.9945	.1051	9.5144	84
7	.1219	.9925	.1228	8.1443	83
8	.1392	.9903	.1405	7.1154	82
9	.1564	.9877	.1584	6.3138	81
10	.1736	.9848	.1763	5.6713	80
11	.1908	.9816	.1944	5.1446	79
12	.2079	.9781	.2126	4.7046	78
13	.2250	.9744	.2309	4.3315	77
14	.2419	.9703	.2493	4.0108	76
15	.2588	.9659	.2679	3.7321	75
16	.2756	.9613	.2867	3.4874	74
17	.2924	.9563	.3057	3.2709	73
18	.3090	.9511	.3249	3.0777	72
19	.3256	.9455	.3443	2.9042	71
20	.3420	.9397	.3640	2.7475	70
21	.3584	.9336	.3839	2.6051	69
22	.3746	.9272	.4040	2.4751	68
23	.3907	.9205	.4245	2.3559	67
24	.4067	.9135	.4452	2.2460	66
25	.4226	.9063	.4663	2.1445	65
26	.4384	.8988	.4877	2.0503	64
27	.4540	.8910	.5095	1.9626	63
28	.4695	.8829	.5317	1.8807	62
29	.4848	.8746	.5543	1.8040	61
30	.5000	.8660	.5774	1.7321	60
31	.5150	.8572	.6009	1.6643	59
32	.5299	.8480	.6249	1.6003	58
33	.5446	.8387	.6494	1.5399	57
34	.5592	.8290	.6745	1.4826	56
35	.5736	.8192	.7002	1.4281	55
36	.5878	.8090	.7265	1.3765	54
37	.6018	.7986	.7536	1.3270	53
38	.6157	.7880	.7813	1.2799	52
39	.6293	.7771	.8098	1.2349	51
40	.6428	.7660	.8391	1.1918	50
41	.6561	.7547	.8693	1.1504	49
42	.6691	.7431	.9004	1.1106	48
43	.6820	.7314	.9325	1.0724	47
44	.6947	.7193	.9657	1.0355	46
45	.7071	.7071	1.0000	1.0000	45

Note: With angles above 45° be sure to use the headings that appear at the bottom of the columns.

APPENDIX G

To Convert from	To	Multiply by
Inches	Centimeters	2.54
Centimeters	Inches	0.39
Feet	Meters	0.305
Meters	Feet	3.28
Yards	Meters	0.91
Meters	Yards	1.09
Miles	Kilometers	1.61
Kilometers	Miles	0.62
Pounds	Kilograms	0.45
Kilograms	Pounds	2.21
Pounds	Newtons	4.45
Newtons	Pounds	0.225
Slugs	Kilograms	14.59
Kilograms	Slugs	0.068
Ft · lb	Joules	1.36
Joules	Ft · lb	0.735
Ft · lb/sec (power)	Watts	1.36
Watts	Ft · lb/sec	0.735

Exercises for Kinesiological Analysis

APPENDIX H

These exercises and techniques, intended as laboratory material for the student, are presented for analysis (major joint and muscle action) of movements. Many are commonly used to develop strength, increase flexibility, and improve posture. In most instances they are organized according to the major body segments (the upper and lower extremities and the trunk–head–neck). Many of the exercises are illustrated by three views: (1) the starting position, (2) the movement, and (3) the return to the starting position. The various exercises were selected on the basis of their use in (1) physical fitness and posture programs, (2) conditioning programs for improving athletic performance, and (3) tests for assessing strength and muscular endurance. The sports and gymnastics techniques are representative of movements involving the imparting of motion to one's own body and to external objects. The exercises are organized in the following series:

> Series 1 Weight-Training Exercises (barbells and weights)
> Series 2 Isometric Tension Exercises (singly and with partners)
> Series 3 Flexibility Exercises
> Series 4 Posture Exercises
> Series 5 Selected Sports and Gymnastics Techniques

The exercises within each series are numbered consecutively in the following manner: The first exercise in Series 1 is numbered 1.1, the second, 1.2. The first exercise in Series 2 is numbered 2.1, followed by 2.2, and so on in similar fashion.

Series 1. Weight-Training Exercises
The Upper Extremity

Starting Position	**Movement**	**Return to Starting Position**

Exercise 1.1

Exercise 1.2

Exercise 1.3

Series 1. Weight-Training Exercises
The Upper Extremity

Starting Position	**Movement**	**Return to Starting Position**

Exercise 1.4

Exercise 1.5

Exercise 1.6

Series 1. Weight-Training Exercises
The Upper Extremity

Starting Position   **Movement**   **Return to Starting Position**

Exercise 1.7

Exercise 1.8

Exercise 1.9

Series 1. Weight-Training Exercises
The Upper Extremity

Starting Position	**Movement**	**Return to Starting Position**

Exercise 1.10

Exercise 1.11

Exercise 1.12

Exercise 1.13

Series 1. Weight-Training Exercises
The Lower Extremity

| **Starting Position** | **Movement** | **Return to Starting Position** |

Exercise 1.14

Exercise 1.15

Exercise 1.16

Series 2. Isometric Tension Exercises
The Upper Extremity

Exercise 2.1 Pull down.

Exercise 2.2 Pull up.

Exercise 2.3 Push out.

Push   Push
up   down

Exercise 2.4

Push   Push
down   up

Exercise 2.5

Pull   Pull
down   up

Exercise 2.6

Series 2. Isometric Tension Exercises
The Lower Extremity and Trunk

Push up

Exercise 2.7

Pull leg down

Exercise 2.8

Press lumbar
spine back

Exercise 2.9

Exercise 2.10   Push down, pull up.

Exercise 2.11   Pull up, push down.

Exercise 2.12   Pull neck backward.

Series 3. Flexibility Exercises for Major Joints

Exercise 3.1   Exercise 3.2   Exercise 3.3   Exercise 3.4

Exercise 3.5   Exercise 3.6   Exercise 3.7

Exercise 3.8   Exercise 3.9   Exercise 3.10

Series 4. Posture Exercises

Exercise 4.1

Exercise 4.2

Exercise 4.3

Exercise 4.4

Series 4. Posture Exercises

Exercise 4.5

Exercise 4.6

Series 5. Sports and Gymnastics Techniques

a.

b.

c.

d.

e.

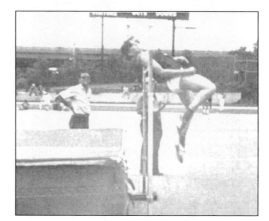

f.

Exercise 5.1   High jump. (Time between each frame is .094 sec.)

Series 5. Sports and Gymnastics Techniques

g.

h.

i.

j.

k.

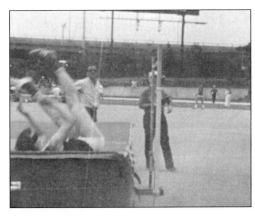

l.

Exercise 5.1   (continued).

Series 5. Sports and Gymnastics Techniques

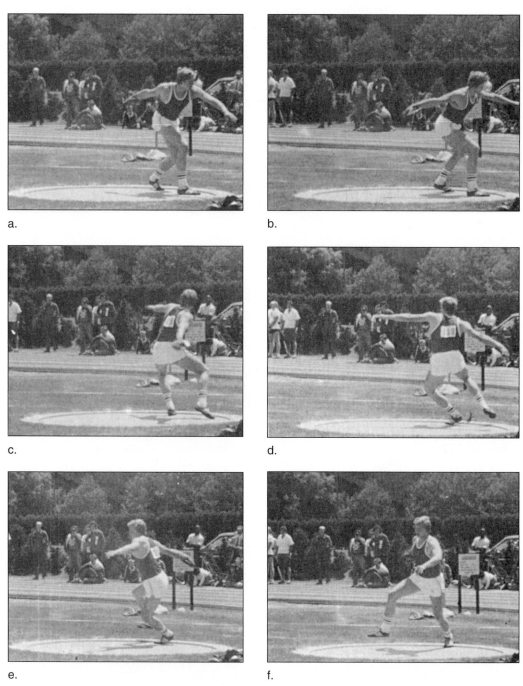

a.

b.

c.

d.

e.

f.

Exercise 5.2 Discus throw. (Time between each frame is .125 sec.)

Series 5. Sports and Gymnastics Techniques

g.

h.

i.

j.

k.

l.

Exercise 5.2   (continued).

Series 5. Sports and Gymnastics Techniques

a.   b.   c.   d.

Exercise 5.3   Volleyball serve.

a.   b.   c.

Exercise 5.4   Soccer throw-in.

Series 5. Sports and Gymnastics Techniques

a.   b.   c.   d.   e.

Exercise 5.5   Baseball swing.

a.   b.   c.   d.   e.   f.

Exercise 5.6   Backward somersault.

Series 5. Sports and Gymnastics Techniques

a.   b.   c.

d.   e.   f.

Exercise 5.7 Back walkover.

Series 5. Sports and Gymnastics Techniques

a.   b.

Exercise 5.8   Vertical jump: (a) good technique; (b) poorer technique. (Time between each frame is .094 sec.)

CHAPTER 10

2. a. 111.25 N
   b. 73 kg
   c. 27.94 cm
   d. 6.1 m/s
   e. 2.84 liters

3. a. 5 cm
   b. 2.24 cm
   c. 5.4 cm
   d. 7.2 cm

4. a. $x = 40.78$ m/sec; $y = 19.02$ m/sec
   b. $x = -60.1$ lb; $y = 60.1$ lb
   c. $x = 75.85$ kg; $y = -90.39$ kg
   d. $x = -21.65$ m/s^2; $y = -12.5$ m/s^2

5. $s = 28$ meters; $d = 12$ meters
6. $x = 627.8$ N; $y = 168.2$ N
7. $V = 28.65$ m/s; $v = 93.98$ ft/s;
   $\theta = 29.25$ degrees or .51 radians
8. Horizontal $(x) = 103.4$ N; vertical $(y) = 37.6$ N
9. c. 1992 m at 106°
   e. Rectangular $= -535$ m, 1919 m
      Polar $= 1992$ m, -74 degrees or 106 degrees
      from start
10. $x = 112.5$ lb; $y = 51$ lb; $R = 123.5$ lb; $\omega = 24°$
11. b. x (stabilizing) ≈ 834.5 N; y (rotary) ≈ 337 N
12. 1359 N; $\omega = 20$ degrees

CHAPTER 11

3.   1500 m = 12.19 m/s
     5000 m = 11.27 m/s
     10,000 m = 11.09 m/s

5. $t = .177$ sec
7. $t = 3.9$ sec up; total = 7.8 s
   $y = 38.2$ m/s

11. $t = 3.46$ sec; $s = 58.7$ meters
    $t = 2.4$ sec; $s = 49.88$ meters
12. Start of force: $\omega = 1089.7$ deg/sec (19 rad/sec)
    Contact: $\omega = 1153.8$ deg/sec (20 rad/sec)
    $v = 7$ m/s

CHAPTER 13

4. x (stabilizing) = 77.6 N; y (rotary) = 289.8 N
9. $E = 6.7$ N
10. $EA = 1.6$ meters; $RA = 0.4$ meters

14. $E = 285$ N
15. 3 cm: $T = 1.7$ kg $\cdot$ m
    15 cm: $T = 8.3$ kg $\cdot$ m

INDEX

A

abdominal muscles, 228–33
  in respiration, 246, 250
abdominal wall, 232–33
abduction, 40
abductor pollicis brevis muscle, 143, 147, 148
abductor pollicis longus muscle, 143, 146, 148
acceleration
  angular kinematics, 293–96
  defined for kinematics, 284
  of free-falling bodies, 287–88, 289
  linear kinematics, 286–93
  of rotating bodies, 360–62
  uniformly accelerated motion, 287–88, 289
Acceleration, Law of, 313–15, 358
accelerometer, 544
acetabular labrum, 165, 166
acetabular ligament, 165, 166
acetabulum, 165, 166
Achilles tendon, 203
acrobatic stunts, locomotion by, 491
acromioclavicular joint, 95–96
acromioclavicular ligament, 96
acromioclavicular sprain, 120–21
acromion process, 95, 96
actin filament, 47, 48
active movement, 63
active stretching, 414, 415
adduction, 40
adduction, diagonal, 118, 120
adductor brevis muscle, 174–75, 176, 177, 178
adductor gracilis muscle, 176
adductor longus muscle, 177, 178
adductor magnus muscle, 175, 176, 178
adductor minimus muscle, 175
adductor pollicis muscle, 143, 147
afferent neuron, 70–71, 72
age
  gait variations, 478–79
  in muscle strength and endurance, 419
  standing posture and, 405–6
agonist muscles, 57, 60

air resistance, 283–84
alignment
  joints and, 41
  in muscle strength and endurance, 418
all-or-none principle of muscular
    contraction, 74
alpha fibers, 78
alpine skiing, locomotion by, 488, 490
American Society of Biomechanics (ASB), 258
analysis, kinesiological. *See* kinesiological
    analysis
anatomical analysis, of motor skills, 11, 12
anatomical levers, 349
anatomical pulleys, 306–7
anconeus, 133–34, 136
angle of attachment, 52
angle of attack, 328
angle of incidence, 323
angle of projection, 292–93
angle of pull, 304–6
angle of rebound, 322–23
angle of reflection, 323
angular kinematics, 284, 293–98
angular momentum, 361–62
  conservation of, 368
  transfer of, 363–65, 368
angular motion. *See* rotary motion
ankle, 193–209
  injuries, 212–13
  ligaments, 194–95
  movements, 35, 199–200, 208
  muscles, 200–208
  range of motion, 35
  in running, 481–83
  strains, 212
  structure, 194, 195
  in walking, 472–73, 474
annular ligament, 129, 130
annulospiral (AS) ending, 78
antagonistic muscles, 58–60
anterior cruciate ligament, 185
anterior intercondyloid fossa, 184
anterior lateral malleolar, 194, 195
anterior ligament (elbow), 129

anterior longitudinal ligament, 218, 219
anterior sacroiliac ligament, 160, 161
anterior scalene muscle, 237, 246, 251
anterior talofibular ligament, 195
anterior talotibial ligament, 194, 195
anteroposterior (AP) ais, 37
anthropometry, in muscle strength and
    endurance, 419
antigravity reflex, 84
aponeurosis, 48–49
aquatic locomotion, 496–508
  canoeing, 506, 508
  kayaking, 508–10
  rowing, 506–7
  swimming (*see* swimming)
arches, maintenance of foot, 208–9
Archimedes' principle, 324–25
area, units of measurement, 264
arm movements, 113–19, 562–63
arthritis, 32–33
articular disc, 96, 97
assessment
  in kinesiological analysis, 4
  of range of motion, 33, 34
atlantoaxial joint, 27, 222, 223, 226
atlanto-occipital joint, 219–22, 226, 239
atlas, 221, 222
atmospheric pressure, in joint stability, 32
autonomic nervous system, 70
axes
  anteroposterior (AP) ais, 37
  bilateral, 37
  mechanical axis of a bone, 23, 25
  vertical, 37
axon, 71

B

back
  injuries, 252–53
  low back pain, 253
back walkover, technique, 606

609

backward somersault, technique, 605
balance, 408
ball and socket joint, 27, 29
ballistic movement, 63
ballistic stretching, 414
ball spin, 328–29
basal ganglia, volitional movement, 88, 89
baseball swing, technique, 605
base of support, 376, 377–79, 533–34
Basmajian, J. V., 66
Bernoulli's Principle, 328
biarticular muscles, 61–62
biceps brachii muscle, 52, 104, 105
    characteristics and functions, 107, 109,
        131, 132, 133
biceps femoris muscle, 171–73, 177, 187,
        190–91, 192
bicycle, locomotion by, 486–88
biomechanics, 258
    defined, 262–63
    quantities in, 263–65
bipenniform skeletal muscles, 50
blades, locomotion by, 486–90
bodily movements, types of, 62–63
bones
    diagram, 24
    as levers, 349
    mechanical axis, 23, 25, 303
    number of skeletal, 23, 24
    skeletal changes, 23, 25
    types, 23
bounce, effects of spin on, 323–24
boundary layer, 326
brachialis, 131, 133
brachioradialis, 131–32, 133, 134
brain. *See also specific areas*
    volitional movement, 88–90
brainstem, 88, 89, 90
Brunnstrom's Clinical Kinesiology, 238
buoyancy, 324–26, 330, 335
    in swimming, 496

C

calcaneocuboid joint, 198
calcaneofibular ligament, 195
calcaneotibial ligament, 194, 195
calcaneus, 194, 195–96, 197
calisthenics, 413
cameras, used for kinematic analysis, 538, 540
canoeing, as locomotion, 506, 508
capitulum, 128
cardinal plane, 37
carpal joints, 27, 136
carpal tunnel syndrome, 153
carpi radialis brevis muscle, 143, 145
carpi radialis longus muscle, 143, 145
carpi radialis longus tendon, 145
carpi ulnaris muscle, 143, 145
carpometacarpal joints, 136, 138, 139–41
carrying and holding, 443–44
carrying angle, 129–30
cartilaginous joints, 29–30
catching, avoiding injury with, 530–31
center of gravity, 34, 36, 372–74
    defined, 372–73
    in humans, 373–74
    in stability, 376

center of gravity, locating the, 385–93
    reaction board method, 385–87
    segmental method, 388–93
center of pressure, 374, 402
central nervous system (CNS), 70
    pyramidal and extrapyramidal tracts, 90
    in volitional movement, 88–90
centrifugal force, 365–67
centripetal force, 365–67
cerebellum, volitional movement, 88, 89–90
cerebral cortex, volitional movement, 88–89
cervical vertebrae, 216, 217, 220, 221
cervicis muscles, 227, 234
chondromalacia, 212
Chopart's joint, 198
circular motion, 280
circumduction, 40–41
clavicle, 95, 96, 97
    fracture of the, 121
climbing. *See also* suspension activities
    stairs, 479
coactivation, 91
coccyx, 216, 217
cochlea, 80, 81
cocontraction, 60–61
coefficient of elasticity, 322–23
computers
    modeling and simulation, 547–49
    used for kinematic analysis, 540
concentric contraction, 52–53, 56
concentric exercise, 420
concurrent forces, 309–10
concurrent movements, 61, 62
condyloid joint, 27, 29
connector neurons, 72
conservation of angular momentum, 368
Conservation of Angular Momentum, Law
        of, 362
Conservation of Momentum, Law of, 316–17,
        358, 362
contact forces, 319–21
contractility, 45–46
contraction, skeletal muscle, 52–54
contusions, 178
    knee, 210
    leg, 209–10
    spinal, 252
coordination of muscular system. *See*
        muscular system coordination
coracoacromial ligament, 104, 105
coracobrachialis
    angle of pull, 306
    characteristics and functions, 107,
        108, 109
coracoclavicular ligament, 96
coracohumeral ligament, 104, 105
coracoid process, 96
coronal plane, 36
coronoid process, 128, 129
costochondral joints, 242
costoclavicular ligament, 96, 97
countercurrent movements, 61–62
couple, force, 344–45, 346
cross-country skiing, locomotion by,
        488, 490
crossed extensor reflex, 83
cruciate ligaments, 185–86
cuboid, 195
cuneiforms, 196, 197
Cureton, Thomas, 258

curl sit-up (modified for progressive
        resistance training), 422–27
curvilinear motion, 279–80
cutaneous receptors, 80

D

dance, locomotion and, 491
deceleration, 286
deep knee bending, 211–12, 417
deep posterior spinal muscles, 227, 235, 236
deep squats, 417
degrees of freedom, 543
deltoid ligament, 194, 195
deltoid muscle, 105, 107, 108, 109–10, 111
dendrites, 71, 72
density, and buoyancy, 325–26
description, in kinesiological analysis,
        4, 5–10
diagonal adduction, 118, 120–21
diagonal planes of motion, 37
diaphragm, in respiration, 246–47
diarthrodial joint, 28–29
direction, of force, 302–4
discus throw, technique, 602–3
dislocations, shoulder, 121–22
displacement, 284
    angular kinematics, 293–94
    in kinematics, 284, 540–42
    in linear kinematics, 284
dissection, muscle, 63
distal radioulnar joint
    movements, 130–31
    structure, 130
distance, 284
    in linear kinematics, 284
diving
    nonsupport activities (*see* nonsupport
        activities)
    reverse dive layout with one-half twist,
        analysis of, 524–25
dorsal basal ligament, 140
dorsal carpometacarpal ligament, 139, 140
dorsal interossei muscle, 202, 206
dorsal radiocarpal ligament, 137
dorsal radioulnar ligaments, 130
drag
    in fluid resistance, 326–28, 330, 335
    swimming and, 496
Duchenne, G. B., 64
dynamics, defined, 263
dynamometers, kinetic analysis with, 544

E

ear, reflexes, 87–88
ears, labyrinthine proprioceptors, 80–81
eccentric contraction, 53, 56
eccentric exercise, 420–21
eccentric force, 340, 341
effectiveness, kinesiology and, 2, 3
efficiency, kinesiology and, 2, 3
effort arm (EA), 349
elasticity, 321–22
    coefficient of elasticity, 322–23
    strain, 321
    stress, 321

elbow joint
　dislocation, 153
　epicondylitis, 153
　fracture, 153
　gradations of contraction, 74
　movements, 130
　range of motion, 35, 560
　structure, 127–30
　in swimming, 500–502
elbow muscles, 131–35
　anconeus, 133–34, 136
　antagonist muscles and, 58
　biceps brachii, 131, 132, 133
　brachialis, 131, 133
　brachioradialis, 131–32, 133
　location, 131
　pronator quadratus, 132, 134
　pronator teres, 132, 134
　supinator, 133, 134, 135
　triceps brachii, 133, 135, 136
electrogoniometer, kinematic analysis
　　with, 544
electromyography (EMG), 65–66, 85,
　　545–47
elgon, kinematic analysis with, 544
Emerson's law, 31
endomysium, 46, 48
energy
　defined, 334
　potential and kinetic, 334–35, 336
　work and, 334–35
epicondylitis, 153
epimysium, 46, 48
epiphysis, 23, 25, 26
equilibrium, 81, 374–75. *See also* stability
　classification of, 375
　maintaining and regaining during impact,
　　533–34
　neutral, 375
　stable, 375
　unstable, 375
erector spinae muscle, 227, 234, 246, 250
ergometer, analysis of push-pull pattern with
　　rowing, 446–48
evaluation
　of exercises, 432
　in kinesiological analysis, 4
　of range of motion, 33, 34
exercise programs, objectives, 413
exercises
　evaluating, 432
　exercise order, in muscle strength and
　　endurance, 418
expiration, 246, 251–52
extensibility, 45–46
extension, 39
extensor carpi radialis brevis muscle, 143, 145
extensor carpi radialis longus muscle, 143,
　　145, 146
extensor carpi ulnaris muscle, 143, 145
extensor digitorum brevis muscle, 206
extensor digitorum muscle, 143, 146, 147,
　　148, 201, 202
extensor hallucis longus muscle, 201, 202
extensor pollicis longus muscle, 143, 147, 148
extensor thrust reflex, 82, 83, 475
external force, 302, 307–9
external levers, 347–49
external resistance, 283–84
exteroceptive reflexes, 82–83

exteroceptors, 75–76
extrafusal fibers, 77, 78
extrapyramidal tracts, 90
extrinsic muscles, 143

F

falls, impacts and, 529–30
fan-shaped skeletal muscles, 50
fascia, in joint stability, 32
fascia lata, 184
fasciculus, 48
fast-twitch muscle fibers, 48
femur, 165–66, 182–83
　movement of femur at hip joint, 166–69
fibrous joint, 30
fibula, 194
fibular collateral ligament, 184, 185
fingers
　avulsion fracture, 153
　carpometacarpal joints, 141
　cooperative actions of wrist and digits,
　　150–52
　grasping, 151–52
　interphalangeal joints, 143
　metacarpophalangeal joints, 141–43
　movements, 141–42, 143, 148
　muscles, 143, 146–48
　structure, 136, 139–40, 141–42
　in swimming, 500–502
first-class levers, 350–51
fixator muscles, 57–58, 60
flat bones, 23
flexibility, 41
　defined, 413
　developing, 413–17
　exercises, 597
　risk factors in, 416–17
flexor carpi radialis muscle, 143, 144, 146
flexor carpi ulnaris muscle, 143, 144, 146
flexor digitorum longus muscle, 201,
　　206, 207
flexor digitorum superficialis muscle, 143,
　　145, 146, 147
flexor digitorum superficialis tendon, 145
flexor hallucis longus muscle, 201, 206
flexor pollicis longus muscle, 143, 146,
　　147, 148
flexor reflex, 82
flower-spray (FS) endings, 78
fluid forces, 324–29
foot, 193–209
　arches, maintenance of, 208–9
　calcaneocuboid joint, 198
　Chopart's joint, 198
　intermetatarsal joints, 198, 199
　interphalangeal joints, 199, 200
　intrinsic muscles, 206–7
　joints, 196–99
　metatarsophalangeal joints, 198,
　　199–200
　midtarsal joint, 198, 199
　movements, 199–200, 208
　muscles, 200–208
　standing posture, 401
　structure, 193–94, 195–96
　subtalar joint, 196, 198
　talonavicular joint, 198

tarsometarsal joints, 198, 199
transverse tarsal joint, 198, 199
　in walking, 472–73, 474
force, 262
　anatomical pulleys, 306–7
　ball spin, 328–29
　buoyancy, 324–26, 330, 335
　as cause of motion, 278
　composite effects of two or more forces,
　　309–11
　concurrent forces, 309–10
　contact forces, 319–21
　defined, 302
　direction of force, 302–4, 439
　drag, 326–28, 330, 335
　eccentric, 340, 341
　elasticity (*see* elasticity)
　external force, 302
　external force, resolution of, 307–9
　fluid forces, 324–29
　free-body diagrams, use of, 329–31, 332
　friction, 320–21, 330, 335
　internal force, 302
　lift, 326–28, 330, 335
　linear forces, 309
　magnitude of force, 302–3, 438–39
　momentary contact in striking or
　　kicking, 456
　nature of, 302–11
　normal reactive, 319, 330, 335
　parallel forces, 310–11, 312
　point of application, 302–3, 439
　pushing and pulling, application of,
　　436–37
　rebound (*see* rebound)
　resolution of, 304–9
　rotary force, 340–48
　spin, effects of, 323–24
　strain, 321
　stress, 321
　summation of forces, 317–18
　torque (*see* torque)
　units of measurement, 264–65
　weight, 318, 330, 335
force couple, 344–45, 346
force transducers, kinetic analysis with,
　　544–45, 546
force-velocity relationship in skeletal muscle
　　function, 55, 56
forearm
　fractures, 152
　movements, 135–36
　muscles, 135–36
　range of motion, 35, 561
form drag, 328
fovea capitis, 165
fractures
　ankle, 213
　avulsion, 153
　elbow, 153
　forearm, 152
　leg, 210
　rib, 252–53
　transverse process of lumbar
　　vertebra, 252
free-body diagrams, 329–31, 332
free fall, 525–26
free nerve endings, 80
frequency, in muscle strength and
　　endurance, 418

friction
  in contact forces, 318–21, 330, 335
  motion and, 283–84
  in stability, 380–81
frontal plane, 36
fulcrum, 282, 348
functional electrical stimulation (FES),
        64–65, 468–69
fundamental standing position, 37, 38
fusiform skeletal muscles, 50
fusimotor fibers, 77, 78

G

Galileo (Galileo Galilei), 288
gamma fiber system, 78
gastrocnemius muscle, 61, 187, 192–93, 201,
        203–4
gemellus inferior muscle, 173, 174
gemellus superior muscle, 173, 174
general motion, 281
glenohumeral joint. *See* shoulder joint
glenoid fossa, 95, 103, 105
glenoid labrum, 103, 104
gluteus maximus muscle, 173–74, 175,
        177, 178
gluteus medius muscle, 176–77, 178
gluteus minimus muscle, 177, 178
Golgi tendon organ (GTO), 76, 79–80
  tendon reflex, 86–87
goniometer, 33
gracilis muscle, 175–76, 177, 178, 187,
        189, 192
gradations of contraction, 74
grasping, 151–52
Gravitation, Law of, 318
gravity
  center of gravity (*see* center of gravity)
  line of, 36, 376, 379
  movement of body caused by, 281, 283
  muscle function and, 54–55
  in muscle strength and endurance, 419
  projectiles and, 289–93
  stretching and, 415–16
  in uniformly accelerated motion,
        288–89
  weightlessness, 526–27
greenstick fractures, 121, 152
gymnastics
  back walkover, technique, 606
  backward somersault, technique, 605
  half-turn flying hip circle with hecht
        dismount, analysis of, 519–21
  nonsupport activities (*see* nonsupport
        activities)
  rotary locomotion, 490–91
  suspension activities (*see* suspension
        activities)

H

hamstring muscles, 61–62, 171–73, 177, 187,
        190–91
  strains, 178
hand. *See also* wrist
  avulsion fracture, 153
  carpal tunnel syndrome, 153

carpometacarpal and intermetacarpal
        joints, 139–41
  cooperative actions of wrist and digits,
        150–52
  grasping, 151–52
  intermetacarpal joints, 141
  interphalangeal joints, 143
  ligaments, 139–40
  metacarpophalangeal joints, 136, 141–43
  movements, 140–41, 142–43, 148–50
  muscles, 143–49
  structure, 139–40, 141–42
  thumb (*see* thumb)
hanging. *See* suspension activities
head
  movements, 239–40, 242
  in swimming, 498, 500
hecht, 519
height of release, 291–92, 293
herniated disc, 252
high jump, technique, 600–601
hinge joint, 27, 28
hip joint, 165–78
  injuries, 178
  ligaments, 165–66
  movement of femur at the, 166–69
  range of motion, 35, 565–66
  structure, 165, 166
hip joint muscles
  abductor muscles, 162
  adductor brevis, 174–75, 176
  adductor gracilis, 176
  adductor longus, 175, 176
  adductor magnus, 175, 176
  adductor minimus, 175, 176
  adductor muscles, 162
  biceps femoris, 171–73
  characteristics and functions, 169–78
  extensor muscles, 162
  flexor muscles, 162
  gemellus inferior, 173, 174
  gemellus superior, 173, 174
  gluteus maximus, 173–74, 175
  gluteus medius, 176–77
  gluteus minimus, 177
  gracilis, 175–76
  hamstrings, 171–73
  iliacus, 169–70
  iliopsoas, 169–70
  inward rotator muscles, 163
  location, 169
  obturator externus, 173, 174
  obturator internus, 173, 174
  pectineus, 170
  piriformis, 173, 174
  psoas major, 169–70
  psoas minor, 169–70
  quadratus femoris, 173, 174
  rectus femoris, 170, 171
  sartorius, 170, 171
  semimembranosus, 171–73
  semitendinosus, 171–73
  six deep outward rotators, 173, 174
  tensor fasciae latae, 170–71, 174
hip pointer, 178
hips
  in running, 481–83
  standing posture and hip
        musculature, 401
  in walking, 470–71

hitting, mechanical principles, 456, 458–60
holding and carrying, 443–44
hopping, 484–86
horizontal plane, 36, 37
humeroradial joint, 130
humeroulnar joint, 127–28, 130
humerus, 58, 60, 95, 96, 127–29
hunching, 119–20
hurdler's stretch, 417
hyoid muscles, 227, 228, 229
hyperabduction, 40
hyperadduction, 40
hyperextension, 39
hyperflexion, 39

I

ice skates, locomotion by, 488, 489
iliacus muscle, 169–70
iliocostalis muscles, 227, 234
iliofemoral ligament, 166, 167
iliolumbar ligament, 160, 161
iliopsoas muscle, 169–70, 177, 178
iliotibial tract, 184, 186
ilium, 159, 160, 165
impact, 529–35
  accuracy and control, 534–35
  avoiding injury, 530–31, 532–33
  catching, 530–31
  concepts, 529
  defined, 529
  falls and landings, 529–30
  maintaining and regaining equilibrium
        during, 533–34
  in muscle strength and endurance, 418
  problems, 529
  receiving impact, principles in, 532–35
impulse, in Newton's Law of Acceleration,
        313–14, 336
incidence, angle of, 323
inertia
  defined, 311, 313, 336
  moment of inertia, 359–60
Inertia, Law of, 311, 313, 358, 359–60
infrahyoid muscles, 227, 228, 229
infrapatellar bursae, 184
infraspinatus, 105, 107, 111, 112
injury prevention
  in kinematic analysis, 550–51
  in kinetic analysis, 550–51
  in quantitative analysis, 550–51
in-line skates, locomotion by, 488
insertion, muscular attachments and, 48–49
inspection, of muscles, 63–64
inspiration, 245–46, 251
intercarpal joint, 138–39
interchondral joints, 242
interclavicular ligament, 96, 97
intercondyloid eminence, 182, 183
intercondyloid fossa, 182, 183
intercondyloid tubercles, 182
intercostales externi muscle, 246, 247–48
intercostales interni muscle, 246, 247–48
intermetacarpal joints, 139–41
intermetatarsal joints, 198, 199
internal force, 302
internal resistance, 284
International Society of Biomechanics, 258

Internet resources, 19, 396–97
internuncial neurons, 72
interoceptors, 75–76
interossei, 194
interosseous basal ligament, 140
interosseous carpometacarpal ligament, 139
interosseous sacroiliac ligament, 160, 161
interphalangeal joints, 143, 199, 200
interspinales muscles, 235, 236
intersternal joints, 242
intertransversarii muscles, 235, 236
intervertebral discs, 217–18
intrafusal fibers, 77, 78
intrinsic muscles, 143
irregular bones, 23
irregular joints, 28
ischiofemoral ligament, 166, 167
ischium, 159, 160, 165
isokinetic contraction, 54
isokinetic exercises, 422
isometric contraction, 53–54, 56
isometric exercise, 421, 595–96
isotonic exercise, 53–54, 421–22

J

joint flexibility, 413–14
joint proprioceptors, 80
joints
  alignment, 41
  articulations, 25–26, 27
  atlantoaxial, 27
  atmospheric pressure, 32
  ball and socket, 27, 29
  carpal, 27
  cartilaginous, 29–30
  classification of, 557–59
  condyloid, 27, 29
  fascia and skin, 32
  fibrous, 30
  flexibility, 41
  hinge, 27, 28
  ligamentous, 29, 30, 31
  motions, analyzing, 41
  muscular arrangement, 31–32
  naming joint action in complex
    movements, 41
  pivot, 27, 29
  range of motion (*see* range of motion
    (ROM))
  saddle, 27, 29
  shape of bony structure, 31
  stability, 30–32
  structural classification, 26–30
  structure, 26–30
  synarthrodial joints, 29–30
  thorax, 242–44
jumping, 484–86

K

kayaking, as locomotion, 508–10
kicking
  kicking pattern, 453, 455
  mechanical principles, 456, 458–60
  momentary contact, 456
  principles relating to, 456–60

projection, 456
  swimming, 502, 503, 504, 505
kinematic analysis, 538–44
  accelerometer, 544
  basic photoinstrumentation procedures,
    540–44
  computer models and simulation, 547–49
  displacement in, 540–42
  electrogoniometer, 544
  electromyography, 545–47
  elgon, 544
  injury prevention, 550–51
  instrumentation for, 538–44
  optimization of performance, 550
  optoelectronic systems, 542
  potentiometer, 544
  quantitative analysis, 549–51
  real-time systems, 543–44
  rehabilitation, 551
  three-dimensional systems, 542–43
  time in, 540
kinematics, 284–98
  angular acceleration, 295–96
  angular displacement, 293–94
  angular velocity, 294–95
  defined, 263, 284
  linear acceleration, 286–87
  linear displacement, 284
  linear distance, 284
  linear kinematics, 284–93
  linear velocity, 284–86
  projectiles (*see* projectiles)
  speed, 284–86
  uniformly accelerated motion, 287–88, 289
kinesiological analysis, 4–14
  anatomical analysis, 4, 11, 12
  components of, 4–14
  description in, 4, 5–10
  evaluation in, 4, 10–14
  exercises for, 589–607
  mechanical analysis, 4, 11–14
kinesiology
  analysis, kinesiological (*see* kinesiological
    analysis)
  defined, 2, 262
  function of, 2–3
  methods of study, 3
  nature of, 2–3
  study, reasons for, 2–3
kinesthesis, 90–91
kinetic analysis, 544–45
  computer models and simulation, 547–49
  injury prevention, 550–51
  optimization of performance, 550
  quantitative analysis, 549–51
  rehabilitation, 551
kinetic energy, 334–35
kinetics, defined, 263
knee cap, 183–84
knee joint, 182–87
  chondromalacia, 212
  collateral ligament sprain, 210–11
  contusions, 210
  deep knee bending, 211–12
  injuries, 210–12
  ligaments, 184, 185–86
  menisci, 182, 184–85
  movements, 186–87
  movements of the leg at the, 193
  Osgood-Schlatter disease, 212

range of motion, 35, 567
  in running, 481–83
  structure, 182–84
  vulnerability of, 210
  in walking, 472, 474–75
knee joint muscles, 187–93
  biceps femoris, 187, 190–91, 192
  gastrocnemius, 187, 192–93, 204
  gracilis, 187, 189, 192
  hamstring group, 187, 190–91
  location, 187
  popliteus, 187, 192
  quadriceps femoris group, 187–91
  rectus femoris, 187–91
  sartorius, 187, 188, 191
  semimembranosus, 187, 190–91, 192
  semitendinosus, 187, 190–91, 192
  vastus intermedius, 187–91
  vastus lateralis, 187–91
  vastus medialis, 187–91
kyphosis, 216

L

laboratory study, of kinesiology, 3
labyrinth, reflexes, 87–88
labyrinthine proprioceptors, 80–81
laminar flow, 326, 327
landings, impacts and, 529–30
lateral collateral ligament, 185, 194
lateral flexion, 40
lateral lumbosacral flexor muscles, 162
lateral meniscus, 184, 185
latissimus dorsi muscle, 107
leaping, 484–86
leg
  contusions, 209–10
  fracture, 210
  injuries, 209–10
  movements of the, at knee joint, 193
  shin splints, 210
length
  length-tension relationship, 55, 56
  units of measurement, 264
lengthening contraction, 53
lengthening reaction, 87
levatores costarum muscles, 235, 236, 246,
    248–49
levator scapulae muscle, 228, 233, 237–38
  characteristics and functions, 99, 101
levers, 347–59
  anatomical, 22, 349
  classification of, 349–52, 353, 354, 355
  defined, 347
  external, 347, 349
  first-class levers, 350–51
  fulcrum, 347
  identification and analysis of, 358
  lever arms, 349, 354, 355
  mechanical advantage of, 357–58
  principle of, 352–55, 368
  second-class levers, 350, 351–52
  selection of, 356–57
  speed to range, relationship of, 355–56
  third-class levers, 350, 352, 353, 354
lift, in fluid resistance, 326–28, 330, 335
lifting, 441–43
ligamentous arrangements, 31

ligamentous joints, 29, 30
ligamentous reinforcements, 104, 105
ligaments. *See also specific ligaments*
   elbow, 128–29
   foot, 196–99
   hand, 139–40
   hip joint, 165–66
   and joint stability, 31
   knee joint, 184, 185–86
   shoulder joint, 104–5
   spinal column, 218, 219, 220–22, 227
   wrist, 137–40
linear forces, 309
linear kinematics, 284–93, 294, 296–98
linear motion
   acceleration, 286–87
   analysis of, 335–36
   defined, 279
   displacement, 284
   distance, 284
   linear kinematics, 284–93
   projectiles (*see* projectiles)
   relationships between angular and, 294,
      296–98, 359
   types, 279–80
   uniformly accelerated motion, 287–88, 289
   velocity, 284–86
line of gravity, 36, 376, 379
line of pull, 51–52
locomotion
   aquatic (*see* aquatic locomotion;
      swimming)
   defined, 468
   jumping, hopping and leaping, 484–86
   nonsupport activities (*see* nonsupport
      activities)
   propulsion, 468
   resistance, 468
   rotary locomotion, 490–91
   running (*see* running)
   by specialized steps, 491
   suspension activities (*see* suspension
      activities)
   walking (*see* walking)
   wheels, blades, and runners, 486–90
locomotor mechanisms, 88
long bones, 23
long-handled instruments, working with,
     445–46
longissimus capitis muscle, 234
longissimus cervicis muscle, 234
longissimus thoracis muscle, 234
longitudinal arch, 195–96
longitudinal skeletal muscles, 49
long jump, phases of, 8, 9
long plantar ligaments, 198
longus capitis muscle, 228
longus colli muscle, 228
lordosis, 217
low back pain, 253
lower extremity
   ankle (*see* ankle)
   foot (*see* foot)
   knee (*see* knee joint; knee joint muscles)
   relationship of trunk, pelvis, and lower
      extremities, 163–64
lumbar spine, movement, 239–42, 568
lumborum muscle, 234
lumbosacral rotator muscles, 163

lumbosacral spinal extensor muscles, 162
lumbosacral spinal flexor muscles, 162
lumbricales muscle, 206
lunate bone, 137

M

magnitude
   of force, 302–3
   of the resistance, 278
Magnus effect, 328–29
maintenance, in muscle strength and
     endurance, 418–19
major rhomboid muscle, 101–2
malleoli, of tibia and fibula, 194, 195
mass, units of measurement, 264–65
mathematical modeling, 547–49
mathematics review, 581–85
maximum accuracy, 289–90
maximum horizontal displacement, 289
McCloy, C. H., 257
measurement, units of, 263–65
mechanical advantage, 357–58
mechanical analysis, of motor skills, 11–14
mechanical axis of a bone, 23, 25, 303
mechanics, defined, 262
medial collateral ligament, 184, 185
medial malleolus, 194
median plane, 36
medius scalene muscle, 246, 251
Meissner corpuscles, 80
men, center of gravity in, 389, 390
menisci, 182, 184–85
metacarpal bones, 136, 137, 138
metacarpophalangeal joints, 136, 141–43
metatarsal arch, 196
metatarsals, 195–96, 197
metatarsophalangeal joints, 198, 199–200
metric system, 264–65
metric-U.S. equivalents, 588
midcarpal joint, 138–39
midtarsal joint, 194, 198, 199
minor rhomboid muscle, 101–2
mobility
   relationship between stability and, 384–85
   of spinal column, 226–27
modeling, study of human movement
     through, 548–49
models, in analyzing skeletal muscles, 64
moment arm, 340–43
moment of inertia, 359–60
momentum
   angular, 361–65
   Conservation of Momentum, Law of,
     316–17
   in Law of Acceleration, 314–15
   in muscle strength and edurance, 418
monoarticular muscles, 61
motion, 262, 278–84
   angular motion (*see* rotary motion)
   causes of, 278
   circular motion, 279, 280
   classification of, 278–81
   curvilinear motion, 279–80
   defined, 278, 284
   experienced by the body, 281
   factors modifying, 283–84

   general motion, 281
   kind of motion, factors determining, 281–83
   modifying motion, factors, 283–84
   Newton's laws of (*See* Newtonian Laws)
   planes of (*see* planes of motion)
   reciprocating, 280–81
   rectilinear motion, 279, 281
   relative motion, 278
   rotary motion (*see* rotary motion)
   study of (*see* kinematics)
   translatory motion (*see* linear motion)
motor neuron, 70–71
motor skills
   anatomical analysis, 4, 11, 12
   classification of, 5–8
   description of, 4, 5–10
   evaluation and, 4, 10–14
   mechanical analysis, 4, 11–14
   mechanical principles, 13–14
   movement phases, 5, 7
   nature of forces causing impeding
     motion, 13
   prescription for improvement, 4, 14
   primary purpose of a motor skill, 5, 6
   simultaneous-sequential nature of the, 8, 10
   system for classification of, 6–8
   underlying mechanics objective, 13
motor unit, 74–75
movement
   abduction, 40
   active, 63
   adduction, 40
   ballistic, 63
   circumduction, 40–41
   classification, 5–8
   extension, 39
   in frontal plane about an anteroposterior
     axis, 40
   hyperabduction, 40
   hyperadduction, 40
   hyperextension, 39–40
   hyperflexion, 39
   lateral flexion, 40
   motor skills (*see* motor skills)
   naming joint action in complex
     movements, 41
   nonaxial, 41
   outward and inward rotation, 40
   passive, 62
   pronation, 40
   reflex (*see* reflex movement)
   rotation left and right, 40
   in sagittal plane about a bilateral axis, 38–40
   supination, 40
   in transverse plane about a vertical axis, 40
   volitional movement (*see* volitional
     movement)
movement phases, of motor skills, 5, 7
mover muscles, 57, 60
multifidi muscles, 235, 236
multipenniform skeletal muscles, 50
muscle
   contractions, 74–75
   contusions, 178
   stimulation, 64–65
muscle endurance
   defined, 417
   exercises for (*see* muscle strength and
     endurance, exercises for)

muscle fiber, 46–48
  slow and fast-twitch fibers, 48
muscles
  coordination of (*see* muscular system coordination)
  and joint stability, 31–32
  muscular attachments and nerve supply, 570–80
  myositis ossificans, 178
  skeletal muscles (*see* skeletal muscle analysis; skeletal muscle function; skeletal muscle structure; *individual muscles*)
Muscles Alive, 238
muscle spindles, 76–79
muscle strength, defined, 417
muscle strength and endurance, exercises for, 417–22
  age, 419
  alignment and impact, 418
  anthropometry, 419
  concentric exercise, 420
  eccentric exercise, 420–21
  evaluating exercises, 432
  exercise order, 418
  frequency, 418
  gravity, 419
  isokinetic exercises, 422
  isometric exercises, 421
  isotonic exercises, 421–22
  maintenance, 418–19
  momentum, 418
  overload, 417
  plyometric exercises, 420–21
  progressive resistance, 418
  resistance arm, 418
  risk factors, 419–20
  specificity, 418
  symmetry, 419
  warm-up, 418
muscular attachments, 48–49
muscular system coordination, 57–63
  antagonists, 58–60
  biarticular muscles, action of, 61–62
  bodily movements, types of, 62–63
  cocontraction, 60–61
  different roles of muscles in total movement, 60
  movers or agonists, 57, 60
  muscles, roles of, 57–60
  neutralizers, 58, 60
  stabilizing, fixator and supporting muscles, 57–58, 60
  synergists, 57, 60
musculoskeletal framework, 22
musculotendinous junction, 86–87
myofibrils, 46, 47
myosin filament, 47, 48
myositis ossificans, 178

N

navicular bone, 194, 195–96, 197
neck
  injuries, 252
  proprioceptors, 80–81
  reflexes, 87–88

negative work, 332
nerves, 72
  muscular attachments and nerve supply, 570–80
nervous system
  basic structures, 70–74
  motor unit, 74–75
  nerves, 72
  neuromuscular analysis, 91
  neurons, 70–72
  sensory receptors (*see* sensory receptors)
  synapse, 72–74
  volitional movement (*see* volitional movement)
neurons, 70–72
neutral equilibrium, 375
neutralizer muscles, 58, 60
Newton, Sir Isaac, 311
  Laws (*see* Newtonian Laws)
Newtonian Laws, 311–18
  Acceleration, Law of, 313–15, 358
  applied to rotary motion, 358–65
  Conservation of Angular Momentum, Law of, 362
  Conservation of Momentum, Law of, 316–17, 358, 362
  Inertia, Law of, 311, 313, 358, 360–61
  Reaction, Law of, 315–18, 362–63
nonsupport activities, 521–27
  free fall, 525–26
  nonsupport activities, principles related to, 521–24
  reverse dive layout with one-half twist, analysis of, 524–25
  weightlessness, 526–27
normal reactive force, 318, 319, 320, 330, 335

O

obesity, gait variations, 479
oblique popliteal ligament, 184, 185
obliquity of femoral shaft, 182–83
obliquus capitis inferior muscle, 227, 233
obliquus capitis superior muscle, 227, 233
obliquus externus abdominis muscle, 227, 228, 229, 231
obliquus internus abdominis muscle, 227, 228–29, 230, 231
obturator externus muscle, 173, 174
obturator internus muscle, 173, 174
olecranon process, 128, 129
opponens pollicis muscle, 143, 147, 148
optoelectronic systems for kinematic analysis, 542
orientation of body, 33–34, 36–38
  anatomical standing position, 37, 38
  axes of motion, 37
  center of gravity, 34, 36
  fundamental standing position, 37, 38
  line of gravity, 36
  orientation planes, 36–37
  standard standing positions, 37–38
origin, muscular attachments and, 48–49
oscillation, 281
Osgood-Schlatter disease, 212
osteoporosis, 25
otoliths, 80

overarm throw
  analysis of, 460–62
  pattern, 451–53
overload, in muscle strength and endurance, 417

P

pacinian corpuscles, 80
palmaris longus muscle, 143, 144, 145
palmaris longus tendon, 145
palpation, of muscles, 63–64
parachuting (free fall), 525–26
parallel forces, 310–11, 312
passive movement, 62
passive stretching, 414–16
patella, 183–84
patellar ligament, 184, 185
pectineus muscle, 170, 177, 178
pectoralis major muscle, 105, 246, 251
  characteristics and functions, 107–8
  line of pull, 51, 52
pectoralis minor muscle, 99–100, 246, 251
pelvic girdle
  contusions, 178
  injuries, 178
  movements, 160–61, 163–64
  muscles, 161–63
  myositis ossificans, 178
  primary movement of, 164
  relationship to trunk and lower extremities, 163–64
  secondary movement of, 164
  structure, 159–61
pelvis, in walking, 470, 473
pennate type of muscles, 50
performance, optimization of, 550
perimysium, 46, 48
peripheral fiber, 71–72
peripheral nervous system, 70, 72, 73
peroneus brevis muscle, 201, 202, 203
peroneus longus muscle, 201–2, 203
peroneus tertius muscle, 201, 203
phases, movement, 5, 7
phasic, stretch reflex, 84, 86
phasic muscle spindle stimulation, 79
Physiologie des Mouvements, 64
piriformis muscle, 173, 174
pivot joint, 27, 29
planes
  movement in frontal plane about an anteroposterior axis, 40
  movement in sagittal plane about a bilateral axis, 38–40
  movement in transverse plane about a vertical axis, 40
planes of motion, diagonal, 37
planes of the body
  axes of motion, 37
  cardinal plane, 37
  combination of planes, movements in, 40–41
  frontal plane, 36, 40
  orientation planes, 36–37
  sagittal plane, 36, 40
  transverse plane, 36, 37, 40

plantar calcaneonavicular ligament, 194, 195, 197, 198
plantar fascia muscle, 201, 207–8
plantaris muscle, 200
plyometric exercises, 420–21
point of application, 302–3
polar coordinate system, 268, 269
pons-medulla. *See* brainstem
popliteus muscle, 187, 192
positive work, 332
posterior cruciate ligament, 185, 186
posterior dislocation of the shoulder, 121
posterior lateral malleolar, 194, 195
posterior ligament (elbow), 129
posterior longitudinal ligament, 218, 219
posterior sacroiliac ligament, 160, 161
posterior scalene muscle, 246, 251
posterior talofibular ligament, 195
posterior talotibial ligament, 194, 195
posture, 400–409
    adaptations to external conditions and special problems, 408
    alignments of body segments, 402–4
    defined, 400
    exercises, 598–99
    mechanisms, 88
    neuromusculature mechanism for maintaining erect, 401–2
    postural stability, 402
    principles applied to, 406–7
    screening, 409
    standing posture (*see* standing posture)
    support of the standing posture, 400–401
potential energy, 334–35
potentiometer, kinematic analysis with, 544
power, 333–34
precision handling, 152
pre-expiration, 246
prehension, 151–52
preinspiration, 246
prepatellar bursae, 184
prescription, in kinesiological analysis, 4
prevertebral muscles, 227, 228
primary ending, 78
primary movement of pelvis, 164
principle of levers, 352–54
progressive resistance, in muscle strength and edurance, 418
progressive resistance training, 420
    curl sit-up, modified as, 422–27
    modification of exercises to fit, 422–32
    pull up, modified as, 430, 431–32
    push up, modified as, 427–29
projectiles, 288–93
    forces acting on, 290–93
    path, 290
    projecting in sport, reasons for, 289–90
    range, factors controlling, 290–93
projection, 456
pronation, 40
pronator quadratus, 132, 134
pronator teres, 132, 134
proprioceptive neuromuscular facillitation (PNF), 416
proprioceptive reflexes, 82, 83–88
proprioceptors, 76–81
    erect posture and, 401
    Golgi tendon organ, 76, 79–80
    joint and skin, 80

labyrinthine and neck, 80–81
    muscle proprioceptors, 76–80
    muscle spindles, 76–79
proximal radioulnar joint, 130–31
psoas major muscle, 169–70
psoas minor muscle, 169–70
psoas muscle, 228, 238–39
pubis bone, 159, 165
pubofemoral ligament, 166, 167
pulleys, anatomical, 306–7
pulling, pushing and. *See* pushing and pulling
pull up, modified for progressive resistance training, 430, 431–32
punching, pushing and pulling during, 444
pushing and pulling, 436–48
    activities, 439–41
    applications, 439–46
    continuous application, 437, 438
    direction of force, principles related to, 439
    ergonomic rowing, analysis of push-pull pattern in, 446–48
    force application, 436–37
    holding and carrying, 443–44
    joint action patterns, 436
    lifting, 441–43
    long-handled instruments, working with, 445–46
    magnitude of force, principles related to, 438–39
    momentary contact, 436
    point at which force is applied, principles related to, 439
    principles of, motions, 437–39
    projection, 437
    punching, 444–45
    weight lifting, 444
push up, modified for progressive resistance training, 427–28, 429
pyramidal tracts, 90

Q

quadrate skeletal muscles, 49, 50
quadratus femoris muscle, 173, 174
quadratus lumborum muscle, 228, 238–39, 246, 251
quadratus plantae muscle, 206
quadricep muscle, contusions, 178
quadriceps femoris group, 187–90
quadriceps tendon, 184
quadrilateral skeletal muscles, 49
quantitative analysis, 549–51

R

racewalking, 479–80
radial collateral ligament, 129, 137
radial extensor muscles, 145
radial fossae, 129
radial notch, 128, 130
radiocarpal joint, 136–38
radioulnar joints, 129, 130, 137
    movements, 130–31
    muscles, 131–36
    structure, 130
    in swimming, 500–502

radius, 128–29
range, in movements of levers, 354–56
range of motion (ROM), 32–33, 34, 35
    assessment of, 33, 34
    average ranges, 33, 35
    factors affecting, 32–33
    joints and, 41
rapid movements, 63
Reaction, Law of, 315–18, 362–63
reaction board method for locating center of gravity, 385–87
real-time systems for kinematic analysis, 543–44
rebound, 322–24
    angle of rebound, 323
    strain, 321
    stress, 321
receptors, sensory. *See* sensory receptors
reciprocal activation, 91
reciprocal inhibition, 91
rectangular coordinate system, 268, 269
rectilinear motion, 279, 281
rectus abdominis muscle, 227, 230–31
rectus capitis anterior muscle, 228
rectus capitis lateralis muscle, 228
rectus capitis posterior major muscle, 227, 233
rectus capitis posterior minor muscle, 227, 233
rectus femoris muscle, 61, 62, 170, 171, 177, 178, 187–91
reflection, angle of, 323
reflex arc, 81–82
reflex movement, 81–88
    antigravity reflex, 84
    crossed extensor reflex, 83
    defined, 81
    extensor thrust reflex, 82, 83, 475
    exteroceptive reflexes, 82–83
    flexor reflex, 82
    labyrinth and neck reflexes, 87–88
    neuromuscular analysis, 91
    posture and locomotor mechanisms, 88
    proprioceptive reflexes, 82, 83–88
    stretch reflex, 84–86, 475
    tendon reflex, 86–87
    withdrawal, 82
regular muscle fibers, 77
rehabilitation, in quantitative analysis, 551
relative motion, 278
repetition maximum (RM), 420
repetitive stress injuries (RSIs), 153
resistance
    air resistance, motion and, 283–84
    locomotion, 468
    swimming, 496
resistance arm (RA), 349, 418
respiration
    expiration, 246, 251–52
    inspiration, 245–46, 251
    movement of thorax during, 245–46
    phases, 245
respiration, muscles of, 246–52
    abdominals, 246, 250
    diaphragm, 246–47
    erector spinae, 234, 246, 250
    extensors of cervical and thoracic spine, 236–37, 246, 250
    intercostales externi, 246, 247–48
    intercostales interni, 246, 247–48
    levatores costarum, 246, 248–49

pectoralis major, 246, 251
pectoralis minor, 246, 251
quadratus lumborum, 246, 251
scalenes, 246, 251
serratus posterior inferior, 246, 249
serratus posterior superior, 246, 249
sternocleidomastoid, 238, 246, 251
transversus thoracis, 246, 249–50
trapezius I and II, 246, 251
resultant vector, 266–67
reverse muscle action, 49
rhomboids muscles, 59, 99, 101–2
ribs. *See also* thorax
    fractures, 252–53
    movement of, in respiration, 245–46
    structure, 241–44
righting reflexes, 87
rigid flutter kick, 503–6
roller skates, locomotion by, 488
rotary force, 340–48
rotary locomotion, 490–91
rotary motion, 279, 280
    acceleration, 295–96
    analysis of, 367–68
    angular kinematics, 284, 293–98
    centrifugal force, 365–67
    centripetal force, 365–67
    displacement, 293–94
    levers (*see* levers)
    moment of inertia, 359–60
    Newtonian laws applied to (*see* Newtonian laws)
    relationships between linear and, 294, 296–98
    velocity, 294–95
rotation, 40
rotator cuff, 108, 111
    strains, 122
rotatores muscles, 235, 236
rowing
    ergometer, analysis of push-pull pattern, 446–48
    as locomotion, 506–7
Ruffini endings, 80
running, 480–84
    anatomical analysis, 481–82
    description of, 480–81
    locomotion by, 486–90
    mechanical analysis, 482–83
    mechanical principles in, 483–84
    sprint start, 484
    stride, 482
    support phase, 482–83
    swing phase, 481–82
    types, 481

S

saccule, 80, 81
sacroiliac articulation, 159, 160, 161
sacrospinous ligament, 160, 161
sacrotuberous ligament, 160, 161
sacrum, 159, 160, 216, 217
saddle joint, 27, 29
safety, kinesiology and, 2
sagittal plane, 36
sarcomeres, 47–48

sartorius muscle, 170, 171, 177, 178, 187, 188, 191
    as biarticular muscle, 61
scalar quantities, defined, 265
scalenus anterior muscle, 228, 237
scalenus medius muscle, 228, 237
scalenus posterior muscle, 228, 237
scaphoid bone, 137
scapula, 59, 95, 96
    stabilization of, 58
scapulohumeral rhythm, 95
scoliosis, 217
secondary movement of pelvis, 164
second-class levers, 350, 351–52
segmental alignment, 381
segmental method for locating center of gravity, 387–93
semicircular canals, 80–81
semilunar cartilage, 182
semilunar notch, 128
semimembranosus muscle, 171–73, 178, 187, 190–91, 192
semispinalis capitis muscle, 227, 235–36, 237
semispinalis cervicis muscle, 227, 235–36, 237
semispinalis thoracis muscle, 227, 235–36, 237
semitendinosus muscle, 171–73, 178, 187, 190–91, 192
sensory neuron, 70–71, 72
sensory receptors, 75–81
    classification, 75–76
    defined, 75
    exteroceptors, 75–76
    Golgi tendon organ, 76, 79–80
    interoceptors, 75–76
    joint and skin proprioceptors, 80
    labyrinthine and neck proprioceptors, 80–81
    muscle proprioceptors, 76–80
    muscle spindles, 76–79
    proprioceptors, 76–81
    reflexes (*see* reflex movement)
sequential movements, 451–56
    joint action patterns, 451–55
    kicking pattern, 453, 455
    overarm throwing pattern, 451–53
    underarm pattern, 453, 454
sequential use of body segments, 8, 10
serratus anterior muscle, 99, 100
serratus posterior inferior muscle, 246, 249
serratus posterior superior muscle, 246, 249
Sherrington, Sir Charles, 70
shin splints, 210
short bones, 23
shortening contraction, 52–53
short plantar ligaments, 198
shoulder
    lifting, 119–20
    protraction, 120
    retraction, 120
shoulder girdle, 95–96
    acromioclavicular articulation, 96
    movements, 97–99, 119–20
    sternoclavicular articulation, 96–97
    in swimming, 500–502
shoulder girdle muscles, 99–103
    and arm movements, 113–19
    levator scapulae, 99, 101
    location, 99
    pectoralis minor, 99–100

rhomboids, 99, 101–2
    serratus anterior, 99, 100
    subclavius, 99, 100–101
    trapezius, 99, 102–3
shoulder injuries, 120–22
    acromioclavicular sprain, 120–21
    chronic dislocations, 122
    clavicle, fracture of the, 121
    dislocations, 121–22
    rotator cuff strains, 122
shoulder joint, 95
    ligamentous reinforcements, 104–5
    movements, 105–7, 120
    muscular reinforcements, 104–5
    range of motion, 35, 564
    structure, 103–4
    in swimming, 500–502
shoulder joint muscles, 107–13
    and arm movements, 113–19
    biceps brachii, 107, 109
    coracobrachialis, 107, 108, 109
    deltoid, 107, 108, 109–10, 111
    infraspinatus, 107, 111, 112
    latissimus dorsi, 107, 111–12
    location, 107
    pectoralis major, 107–8
    subscapularis, 107, 108–9
    supraspinatus, 107, 110–11, 112
    teres major, 107, 112
    teres minor, 107, 111, 112
    triceps brachii, 107, 112–13
side arm throwing pattern, 453, 454
simulation, study of human movement with, 548–49
simultaneous use of body segments, 8, 10
skating, locomotion by, 488, 489
skeletal muscle analysis, 63–66
    conjecture and reasoning, 63
    dissection, 63
    electromyography, 65–66
    inspection and palpation, 63–64
    models, 64
    muscle stimulation, 64–65
skeletal muscle function, 51–56
    angle of attachment, 52
    concentric contraction, 52–53, 56
    contraction, types of, 53–54
    eccentric contraction, 53, 56
    force-velocity relationship, 55, 56
    gravity, influence of, 54–55
    isokinetic contraction, 54
    isometric contraction, 53, 56
    isotonic contraction, 53–54
    in joint stability, 31–32
    lengthening contraction, 53
    length-tension relationship, 55, 56
    line of pull, 51–52
    in range of motion, 32
    shortening contraction, 52–53
    static contraction, 53
    stored elastic capabilities, 55–56
skeletal muscle structure, 45–51
    bipenniform skeletal muscles, 50
    contractility, 45–46
    elasticity, 45–46
    extensibility, 45–46
    fan-shaped skeletal muscles, 50
    fiber arrangement, classification based on, 49–50

force and range of motion, 50
fusiform skeletal muscles, 50
longitudinal skeletal muscles, 49
multipenniform skeletal muscles, 50
muscle fiber, 46–48
muscular attachments, 48–49
properties of muscular tissue, 45–46
quadrate skeletal muscles, 49, 50
reverse muscle action, 49
spindle-shaped skeletal muscles, 50
triangular skeletal muscles, 50
unipenniform skeletal muscles, 50
skeletomotor fibers, 77
skeleton
    bones (*see* bones)
    changes, skeletal, 23, 25, 26
    diagram, 24
skiing, locomotion by, 488, 490
skin
    in joint stability, 32
    proprioceptors, 80
skydiving (free fall), 525–26
slow-twitch muscle fibers, 48
soccer throw-in
    movement phases of, 7
    technique, 604
soft landings, 530
soleus muscle, 201, 204–5
specificity, in muscle strength and
            endurance, 418
speed, 284–86
    defined, 284
    in linear kinematics, 284–86
    range in movements of levers, relationship
            of speed to, 355–56
speed of release, 293
spin
    ball spin, 328–29
    effects of, on bounce, 323–24
spinal column, 216–27
    atlantoaxial joint, 222, 226
    atlanto-occipital joint, 219–22, 226, 239
    contusions, 252
    fractures of transverse process of lumbar
            vertebra, 252
    herniated disc, 252
    injuries, 252
    joints, 217–22
    ligaments, 218–22, 227
    low back pain, 253
    movements, 222–26, 239–42
    range of motion, 35
    stability and mobility, 226–27
    standing posture and spine musculature, 401
    structure, 216–17
    in walking, 470, 473
    whiplash, 253
spinal column muscles, 227–42
    abdominal muscles, 228–33
    abdominal wall, 232–33
    deep posterior spinal muscles, 227,
            235, 236
    erector spinae, 227, 234
    hyoid muscles, 227, 228, 229
    levator scapulae, 228, 233, 237–38
    location, 227–28
    obliquus capitis inferior, 227, 233
    obliquus capitis superior, 227, 233

obliquus externus abdominis, 227, 228,
        229, 231
obliquus internus abdominis, 227, 228–29,
        230, 231
prevertebral muscles, 227, 228
psoas, 238–39
quadratus lumborum, 228, 238–39
rectus abdominis, 227, 230–31
rectus capitis posterior major, 227, 233
rectus capitis posterior minor, 227, 233
scalenes, 228, 237
semispinalis capitis, 227, 235–36, 237
semispinalis cervicis, 227, 235–36, 237
semispinalis thoracis, 227, 235–36, 237
splenius capitis, 227, 233
splenius cervicis, 227, 233
sternocleidomastoid, 228, 237, 238
suboccipital group, 227, 233
thoracolumbar fascia, 232, 236–37
transverse abdominis, 227, 231, 232
transversospinalis muscles, 236, 237
spinal cord, 70, 71–72
    volitional movement, 90
spinalis muscles, 235
spindle-shaped skeletal muscles, 50
splenius capitis muscle, 227, 233
splenius cervicis muscle, 227, 233
sprains
    ankle, 212–13
    back, 252
    collateral ligament sprain in knee joint,
            210–11
    wrist, 153
spring ligament, 194, 198
sprint start, 484
stability. *See also* equilibrium
    base of support in, 376, 377–79
    factors affecting, 375–81
    friction, 380–81
    joint, 30–32
    mass of the body, 380
    mobility, relationship between stability
            and, 384–85
    physiological factors, 381
    postural stability, 402
    principles of, 381–84
    relation of the line of gravity to the base of
            support, 376, 378–79
    segmental alignment, 381
    of spinal column, 226–27
    visual and psychological factors, 381
stabilizing muscles, 57–58, 60
stable equilibrium, 375
standing long jump, phases of, 8, 9
standing positions, body orientation and, 37–38
standing posture. *See also* posture
    age and, 405–6
    alignments of body segments, 402–4
    factors related to, 404–6
    neuromusculature mechanism for
            maintaining erect, 401–2
    psychological aspects, 406
    screening, 409
    support of the standing posture, 400–401
standing toe touches, 417
statics, defined, 263
static stretching, 414
sternoclavicular joint, 95–97

sternoclavicular ligament, 96, 97
sternocleidomastoid muscle, 64, 228, 237,
        238, 246, 251
sternocostal joints, 242, 244
sternum, 95, 96, 97, 242
stiff landings, 530
stored elastic capabilities in skeletal muscle
        function, 55–56
strains, 321
    back, 252
    strain gauge, kinetic analysis with,
            544–45
strap muscles, 227, 228
stress, 321
stretching. *See also* flexibility
    active versus passive, 414–16
    ballistic versus static, 414
    deep knee bends, 417
    hurdler's stretch, 417
    proprioceptive neuromuscular
            facilitation, 416
    standing toe touches, 417
stretch reflex, 84–86, 475
striking
    anatomical principles, 456
    forehand drive in tennis, analysis of,
            462–65
    mechanical principles, 456, 458–60
    momentary contact, 456
    principles relating to, 456–60
    projection, 456
subclavius muscles
    angle of pull, 306
    characteristics and functions, 99, 100–101
subcoracoid dislocation of the shoulder, 121
subcostal angle, 242
subglenoid dislocation of the shoulder, 121
suboccipital muscle group, 227, 233
subscapularis muscle, 105, 107, 108–9
subtalar joint, 194
supination, 40
supinator muscle, 133, 134
supporting muscles, 57–58, 60
suprahyoid muscles, 227, 228, 229
suprapatellar bursae, 184
supraspinatus muscle, 104, 107, 110–11, 112
surface drag, 326, 496
suspension activities, 513–21
    half-turn flying hip circle with hecht
            dismount, analysis of, 519–21
    hanging and hand-traveling activities,
            principles related to, 513–14
    swinging movements, principles related to,
            514–19
sustentaculum tali ligament, 194
swimming, 496–506
    arm stroke, analysis of, 500–502
    faults in crawl stroke, analysis of, 504–6
    head and trunk, analysis of, 498, 500
    kick, analysis of, 502, 503, 504
    mechanical principles applied to, 496–98
    resistance, 496
    rigid flutter kick, 504–6
    sprint crawl, analysis of the, 498–506
swinging. *See* suspension activities
symmetry, in muscle strength and
            endurance, 419
synapse, 72–74

synarthrodial joints, 29–30
synergist muscles, 57, 60
synovial fluid, 284
synovial membrane of knee joint, 184

T

talocalcaneal joint, 196, 198
talocalcaneal ligaments, 196, 198
talonavicular joint, 198
talus bone, 194, 195, 196, 197
tarsal bones, 194, 196
tarsal joints, movement, 199–200, 208
tarsometatarsal joints, 198, 199
tendon reflex, 86–87
tendons, 48–49
    and joint stability, 31–32
    in range of motion, 32
tennis, analysis of the forehand drive, 462–65
tensor fasciae latae muscle, 170–71, 174, 177, 178
teres femoris, 165, 166
teres major muscle, 58, 105, 107, 112
teres minor muscle, 105, 107, 111, 112
terminal velocity, 288
thigh, 177–78
    contusions, 178
    injuries, 178
    muscles, 177–78
    myositis ossificans, 178
    standing posture and thigh musculature, 401
third-class levers, 350, 352, 353, 354
thoracic muscles, 227, 234
thoracic vertebrae, 216, 217
thoracolumbar fascia, 232, 236–37
thorax
    injuries, 252–53
    joints, 242–44
    movements, 239–42, 245–46
    respiration and (see respiration; respiration, muscles of)
    rib fractures, 252–53
    structure, 241–44
three-dimensional systems, for kinematic analysis, 542–43
threshold level, 73–74
throwing
    anatomical principles, 456
    forehand drive in tennis, analysis of, 462–65
    joint action patterns, 451–54
    mechanical principles, 456–58
    movement phases of, 5, 7
    overarm pattern, 451–53
    overarm throw, analysis of, 460–62
    principles relating to, 456–60
    side arm pattern, 453, 454
    underarm pattern, 453, 454
thumb. See also hand
    cooperative actions of wrist and digits, 150–52
    grasping, 151–52
    movements, 140–41, 143, 148–50
    muscles, 143, 146–48
    structure, 136, 139–40, 143
tibia, 182, 183, 194

tibial collateral ligament, 184, 185
tibialis anterior muscle, 200, 201, 202
tibialis posterior muscle, 201, 205–6
tibionavicular ligament, 194, 195
time
    in kinematic analysis, 540
    units of measurement, 264, 265
time of flight, 289, 292–93
toes, 196
    movements, 199–200, 208
tonic muscle spindle stimulation, 79
tonic reflexes
    labyrinth, 87–88
    neck, 87–88
    stretch, 84, 86
torque, 340–48, 367–68
    defined, 340
    modifying, 340–44
    principle of torques, 345–48
    summation of, 344–45, 346
translatory motion. See linear motion
transverse abdominis muscle, 227, 231, 232
transverse acetabular ligament, 165, 166
transverse arch, 195, 196
transverse ligament, 185, 186
transverse metacarpal ligament, 140
transverse plane, 36, 37
transverse tarsal joint, 198, 199
transverse tibiofibular ligament, 194
transversospinalis muscles, 236, 237
transversus thoracis muscle, 246, 249–50
trapeziometacarpal joint, 139
trapezius muscle, 59
    characteristics and functions, 99, 102–3
    trapezius I muscle, 246, 251
    trapezius II muscle, 246, 251
trapezoid ligament, 96
triangular skeletal muscles, 50
triceps brachii, 105, 133, 135, 136
    characteristics and functions, 107, 112–13
trigonometric functions, table of, 586–87
triquetral bone, 137
trochlea, 128
trunk, in swimming, 498, 500
turbulence, 328

U

ulna, 128–29
ulnar collateral ligament, 129, 137
unbalance, 263
underarm throwing pattern, 453, 454
uneven parallel bars, analysis of half-turn flying hip circle, 519–21
unilateral load, 379, 380
unipenniform skeletal muscles, 50
units of measurement, 263–65
unstable equilibrium, 375
upper extremity
    elbow (see elbow joint; elbow muscles)
    forearm (see forearm)
    hand (see hand)
    overarm throw, muscular analysis of, 461–62
    radioulnar joints (see radioulnar joints)

standing posture and upper extremity musculature, 401
    thumb (see hand; thumb)
    in walking, 475
    wrist (see wrist)
U.S.-metric equivalents, 588
utricle, 80, 81

V

vastus intermedius muscle, 187–91
vastus lateralis muscle, 187–91
vastus medialis muscle, 187–91
vector analysis, 265–74
    combination of vectors, 266–67
    graphic resolution, combination of vectors using, 268–71
    locations of vectors in space, 268
    resolution of vectors, 267–68
    trigonometric resolution, combination of vectors using, 271–74
    value of, 274
    vector representation, 265–66
vector quantities, defined, 265
velocity
    angular kinematics, 294–95
    computation, 284–86
    defined, 284
    in kinematics, 284–86, 294–95
    in linear kinematics, 284–86
    projectiles and, 289–93
    terminal velocity, 288
vertebral spine. See spinal column
vertical axis, 37
vertical jump, technique, 607
video, used for kinematic analysis, 539–40
visceroceptors, 76
volar basal ligament, 140
volar carpometacarpal ligament, 139, 140
volar radiocarpal ligament, 137, 139
volar radioulnar ligaments, 130
volitional movement, 88–91
    kinesthesis, 90–91
    pyramidal and extrapyramidal tracts, 90
    reciprocal inhibition and coactivation, 91
volleyball serve, technique, 604
volume, units of measurement, 264

W

walking, 468–80
    anatomical analysis, 470–75
    anatomical principles in, 475–76
    description of, 469–70
    gait, individual variations in, 478–79
    mechanical analysis, 476–77
    mechanical principles in, 477–78
    neuromuscular considerations, 475
    racewalking, 479–80
    stairs, climbing and descending, 479
    upper extremities in, 475
    variations, 478–80
warm-up, in muscle strength and endurance, 418
water resistance, motion and, 283–84

weight
    as force, 318, 330, 335
    mass of the body, in stability, 380
    units of measurement, 264–65
weightlessness, 526–27
weight lifting, pushing and pulling
      during, 444
weight training, exercises, 589–94
wheels, locomotion by, 486–90
whiplash, 253
wind resistance, 283–84
withdrawal reflexes, 82
women, center of gravity in, 390

work, 331–34
    computation, 332–34
    defined, 331
    and energy, 334–35
    positive and negative, 332
wrist. *See also* hand
    bones, 137
    carpal tunnel syndrome, 153
    cooperative actions of wrist and digits,
      150–52
    joint, 136–38
    ligaments, 137–40
    midcarpal and intercarpal joints, 138–39
    movements, 147

    movements of hand at wrist joint,
      137–38, 139
    muscles, 143–46
    range of motion, 35, 561
    sprained or strained, 153
    structure, 136–37, 138
    in swimming, 500–502

Y

Y ligament, 166